Gerontological Nursing

DATE DUE

BRODART   Cat. No. 23-221

Gerontological Nursing

SIXTH EDITION

Charlotte Eliopoulos, RNC, MPH, PhD

Specialist in Holistic Gerontological Care
President, Health Education Network
Glen Arm, Maryland

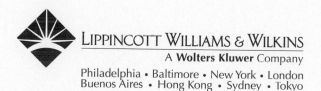

LIPPINCOTT WILLIAMS & WILKINS
A Wolters Kluwer Company
Philadelphia • Baltimore • New York • London
Buenos Aires • Hong Kong • Sydney • Tokyo

Senior Acquisitions Editor: Quincy McDonald
Managing Editor: Helen Kogut
Editorial Assistant: Marie Rim
Senior Production Editor: Sandra Cherrey Scheinin
Director of Nursing Production: Helen Ewan
Managing Editor/Production: Erika Kors
Art Director: Carolyn O'Brien
Design Coordinator: Brett MacNaughton
Senior Manufacturing Manager: William Alberti
Indexer: Ellen Brennan
Compositor: Peirce Graphic Services
Printer: R.R. Donnelley—Crawfordsville

6th Edition

9 8 7 6 5 4 3 2 1

Library of Congress Cataloging-in-Publication Data

Eliopoulos, Charlotte.
    Gerontological nursing / Charlotte Eliopoulos.— 6th ed.
        p. ; cm.
Includes bibliographical references and index.
    ISBN 0-7817-4428-8 (alk. paper)
    1. Geriatric nursing. I. Title.
    [DNLM: 1. Geriatric Nursing. WY 152 E42g 2005]
RC954.E44 2005
618.97'0231—dc22

                                    2003026731

Care has been taken to confirm the accuracy of the information presented and to describe generally accepted practices. However, the authors, editors, and publisher are not responsible for errors or omissions or for any consequences from application of the information in this book and make no warranty, express or implied, with respect to the content of the publication.

The authors, editors, and publisher have exerted every effort to ensure that drug selection and dosage set forth in this text are in accordance with the current recommendations and practice at the time of publication. However, in view of ongoing research, changes in government regulations, and the constant flow of information relating to drug therapy and drug reactions, the reader is urged to check the package insert for each drug for any change in indications and dosage and for added warnings and precautions. This is particularly important when the recommended agent is a new or infrequently employed drug.

Some drugs and medical devices presented in this publication have Food and Drug Administration (FDA) clearance for limited use in restricted research settings. It is the responsibility of the health care provider to ascertain the FDA status of each drug or device planned for use in his or her clinical practice.

LWW.com

This book is dedicated to my husband, George Considine, for his continuing encouragement, support, and love

Reviewers

Glenda Avery, BSN, MSN, PhD
Professor
Auburn University
Auburn, Alabama

Victoria Brown, RN, PhD, HNC
Professor
Georgia College & State University
Milledgeville, Georgia

Christine Castagne
Instructor
College of the North Atlantic
Gander, New Foundland, Canada

Helene Clark, RN, PhD
Assistant Professor
The Catholic University of America
Washington D.C.

Patricia Garrett Clark, RN, MSN
Associate Professor
Abraham Baldwin College
Tifton, Georgia

Anne Denney, RN, MSN
Assistant Professor
Thomas More College
Crestview Hills, Kentucky

Susan Ford, RN, MN, CS, OCN
Nursing Program Chair
Tacoma Community College
Tacoma, Washington

Betty Henderson, RN, MN
Assistant Professor
Texas Woman's University College of Nursing
Houston, Texas

Karol Burkhart Lindow, RN, C, CNS, MSN
Associate Professor of Nursing
Kent State University
New Philadelphia, Ohio

Joyce Maynor, RN, MSN, BC
Assistant Professor
Southeastern Louisiana University
Baton Rouge, Louisiana

Valarie Petersen, MN, CS, APRN, BC
Nursing Faculty
Bob Jones University
Greenville, South Carolina

Mary Quintus, RN, MSN
Nursing Instructor
Miles Community College
Miles City, Montana

Alice Ray, RN, MSN
Assistant Professor of Nursing
Abraham Baldwin Agricultural College
Tifton, Georgia

Violetta Ribeiro, DNSc, MS, BNSc
Associate Professor
Memorial University of Newfoundland School of
 Nursing
Newfoundland, Canada

Kathy Rovere, RN, BSN
Instructor
Malaspina University–College
Nanaimo, British Columbia, Canada

Tracy Szirony, RNC, CHPN, PhD
Associate Professor
Medical College of Ohio
Toledo, Ohio

Jeanine Tweedie, RN, MSN
Assistant Professor
Hawaii Pacific University
Kaneohe, Hawaii

Kathleen Wankel, RN, MN
Nursing Program Director
Miles Community College
Miles City, Montana

L. Diane Weed, MSN, CRNP
Clinical Assistant Professor
University of Alabama
Huntsville, Alabama

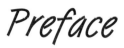

Preface

It is difficult to believe that a quarter century has passed since the first edition of *Gerontological Nursing* was published. In 1979, the specialty of gerontological nursing was in its adolescence: youthful as a result of recently being born into the ranks of nursing specialties, exuberant at the potential to discover and develop, yet quite immature with a limited knowledge base. Often with excitement and sometimes with trepidation, those with the label of "gerontological nurse" ventured down uncharted paths and laid the groundwork for those who would later advance the specialty. The challenge at that time was to bring core knowledge concerning basic care of the elderly to nurses who cared for this population. The specialty has advanced considerably since then as a result of impressive research and experience.

Sixth Edition

While the first edition of *Gerontological Nursing* attempted to provide basic knowledge to form a foundation for specialty practice, this **sixth edition** takes the specialty down a few new paths through its **integration of holistic concepts and practices**. Greater emphasis is placed on the **emotional and spiritual aspects of aging and gerontological care**. In addition, heightened attention is given to the **self-care and nurturing of the gerontological nurse** with the recognition that this work must be done in order for nurses to truly be healers. **Integrative care approaches** are offered with discussions of the **responsible and effective use of complementary and alternative therapies**.

Text Organization

This edition consists of 42 chapters, divided into six units.

Unit I, Understanding the Aging Experience
Provides basic facts about the aging population and the aging process.

Unit II, Foundations of Gerontological Nursing
Includes
- the growth of the specialty
- a new holistic model for gerontological care
- legal aspects
- ethical issues
- diverse roles of gerontological nurses in diverse practice settings.
- *new chapter* on self-care for the gerontological nurse that honors nurses' role as healers and discusses self-care practices that enable nurses to maximize their healing presence

Unit III, Fostering Connection and Gratification
Provides *new material* on strategies to help elders connect with self, others, and their spirituality

Unit IV, Facilitating Physiological Balance
Includes updated content on basic physical needs

Unit V, Selected Health Conditions
Reviews the unique presentation and treatment of illnesses in older adults, accompanied by integrative approaches that foster holistic care

Unit VI, Gerontological Care Issues
Includes
- practical guidance for safe medication use

- living with chronic conditions
- rehabilitation
- acute care
- nursing in long-term care facilities
- family caregiving
- end-of-life care

Features

The book is intended to be practical and user-friendly, with plentiful tables, figures, full color photographs, and displays.

POPULAR FEATURES

Chapter Outlines and *Learning Objectives* introduce each chapter.

Nursing Diagnosis Highlights and *Care Plans* demonstrate practical application of content.

Key Concepts underscore crucial information contained within the text.

Points to Ponder challenge readers to reflect on their own views, experiences, and behaviors.

Critical Thinking Exercises challenge readers to apply the chapter content to help them grow in their depth and breadth as healers.

NEW FEATURES

Nursing Diagnosis Tables alert the reader to potential nursing diagnoses.

Visit the Connection web site, a companion web site that alerts the reader of important information found on   to further enhance learning.

Web Connect highlights useful web sites that can be the gateway for additional information on the chapter topic.

Student and Instructor Resources

RESOURCES FOR STUDENTS

Connection web site. This offers additional background information on specific topics to enhance learning and the latest updates on what's new in Gerontological Nursing.

RESOURCES FOR INSTRUCTORS

Instructor's Resource CD-ROM to Accompany Gerontological Nursing, 6e. This CD-ROM contains the following:

- *Instructor's manual* with syllabi to aid in adapting this book to a gerontology course or to integrate throughout the curriculum, lecture outlines, and answers to case studies and care plans
- *Test bank* containing multiple-choice questions
- *PowerPoint slides* based on lecture outlines

I maintain that if done properly, gerontological nursing is among the most complex, dynamic specialties nurses could select. To do it justice, nurses need to have a sound knowledge base in gerontology and geriatric care, an appreciation for the richness of unique life experiences, and the wisdom to understand that true healing comes from sources that exceed medications and procedures. May this book serve as a tool to help nurses provide competent, holistic care to older adults in a variety of clinical settings and to discover new facets to this maturing gem of a specialty.

Peace and Blessings,
Charlotte Eliopoulos

Acknowledgments

From the time a Lippincott editor by the name of Bill Burgower encouraged me to write the first edition of *Gerontological Nursing* to the present, numerous people have played important roles in the growth and refinement of this book. Some were experienced editors who guided me through the hurdles of manuscript preparation; others were clinical nurses who offered feedback on their experiences of putting the book into practice. Friends and colleagues who possessed integrity and cared enough about me to offer honest criticism also played a role.

I am deeply indebted to the team at Lippincott Williams & Wilkins: Quincy McDonald, Claudia Vaughn, and especially, Helen Kogut. They shared and committed to visions for expanding features to enhance the usefulness of the book; more importantly, their professionalism, patience, and guidance made the process of writing this revision a smooth and painless one. For the many people who assisted behind the scenes—reviewers who gave helpful suggestions, the Art Department who added visual appeal, the Sales Department who provided feedback from the field, the technological gurus who developed the CD-ROMs and website for this text—special thanks is offered.

I continue to be significantly grateful to the many elders who have touched my life and taught me the wisdom and beauty of age, and for God who makes all things possible.

Charlotte Eliopoulos

Contents

UNIT III
*Fostering Connection
and Gratification*

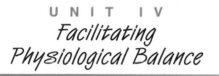

U N I T   I V
Facilitating Physiological Balance

U N I T   V
Selected Health Conditions

U N I T   V I
*Gerontological
Care Issues*

Connection Web Site

The following tables and displays from the text will be available on the Connection web site.

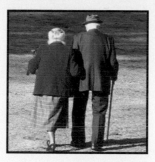

Understanding the Aging Experience

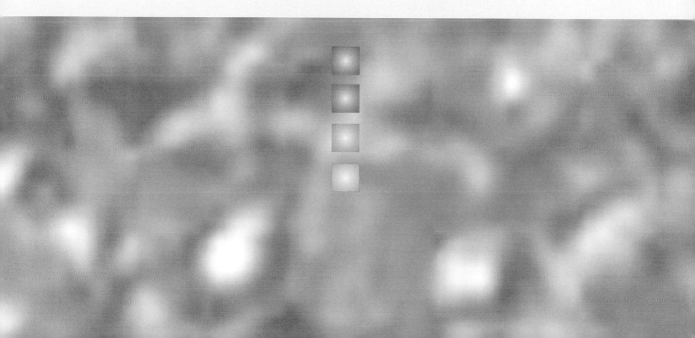

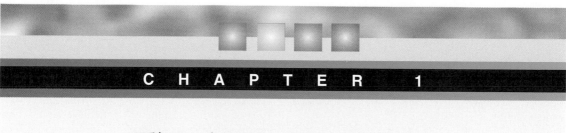

The Aging Population

■ Chapter Outline

The aged through history
Ancient Chinese respect for aged
Early Egyptian interest in maintaining youth
Biblical emphasis on respect for elders
Legislative efforts to improve quality of life
and services

Growth of the older population
Increasing life expectancy
Growing number of old-old
Unique subsets of elderly
Geographic distribution

Race and gender differences
White people outlive black people
Women outlive men

Income and employment
Declining percentage of elderly people at
poverty level

Education
Increase in educational attainment with
each generation

Health status
Elderly people experience fewer acute but
more chronic illnesses

Use of resources
High government payment of older
persons' health care
Challenges for nurses
Balancing quality care with cost-
containment efforts

Impact of the baby boomers

■ Learning Objectives

After reading this chapter, you should be able to:

- explain the different ways in which the elderly have been viewed throughout history
- describe characteristics of today's elderly population in regard to:
  - life expectancy
  - gender and race differences
  - marital status
  - living arrangements
  - education
  - acute and chronic illness
  - causes of death
  - health insurance coverage
- discuss projected changes in future generations of elderly people

"Families forget their older relatives . . . most people become senile in old age . . . Social Security provides every elderly person with a decent retirement income . . . a majority of the elderly reside in nursing homes . . . Medicare covers all health care-related costs for older people. . . ." These and other myths continue to be perpetuated about older people. Misinformation about the elderly is an injustice not only to this age group but also to persons of all ages who need accurate information to prepare realistically for their own senior years. Gerontological nurses must know the facts about the older population to effectively deliver services and educate the general public.

The Aged Through History

Today's elders have offered the sacrifice, strength, and spirit that made this country great. They were the proud GIs in world wars, the brave immigrants who ventured into an unknown land, the bold entrepreneurs who took risks that created wealth and opportunities for work, and the unselfish parents who struggled to give their children a better life. They have witnessed and participated in profound informational, technological, and social growth and change. They have earned respect, admiration, and dignity. Today the elderly are viewed with positivism rather than prejudice, intelligence rather than myth, and concern rather than neglect. A brief reflection of the view of the old in past societies demonstrates that this positive view was not always the norm, however.

Historically, societies have reacted to their aged members in a variety of ways. In the time of Confucius, there was a direct correlation between a person's age and the degree of respect to which he or she was entitled. Taoism viewed old age as the epitome of life, and the ancient Chinese believed that attaining old age was a wonderful accomplishment that deserved great honor. On the other hand, the early Egyptians dreaded growing old and experimented with a variety of potions and schemes to maintain their youth. Opinions were divided among the early Greeks; myths portray many struggles between old and young. Plato promoted the aged as society's best leaders, whereas Aristotle denied the elderly any role in governmental matters. Ancient Romans had limited respect for their elders; in the nations that Rome conquered, the sick and aged were customarily the first to be killed.

Woven throughout the Bible is God's concern for the well-being of the family and desire for people to respect elders (*Honor your father and your mother* . . . Exodus 20:12). Many key biblical figures, such as Moses and Abraham, made significant contributions in their advanced years. Yet, the honor bestowed upon the aged was not sustained. The Dark Ages were especially bleak for older persons; the Middle Ages did not bring considerable improvement. Strong feelings regarding the superiority of youth occurred during medieval times; these feelings were expressed in uprisings of sons against fathers. The art of this period, depicting figures such as Father Time, also portrayed an uncomplimentary image of older adults. The elderly were among the first to be affected by famine and poverty and the last to benefit from better times. In the early 17th century, England developed Poor Laws that provided care for the destitute and enabled older persons without family resources to have some modest safety net. Many gains in the treatment of the elderly that were made during the 18th and 19th centuries were lost because of the cruelties of the Industrial Revolution. Although child labor laws were developed to guard minors, the aged were left unprotected. Those unable to meet industrial demands were placed at the mercy of their offspring or forced to beg on the streets for sustenance.

Although Dr. I. L. Nascher, known as the father of geriatrics, wrote the first geriatric textbook in 1914, American literature during the first half of the 20th century reflects little improvement in the status of older adults. The first significant step in improving the lives of older Americans was the passage of the Federal Old Age Insurance Law under the Social Security Act in 1935, which provided some financial security for elderly persons. The profound graying of the population started to be realized in the 1960s, and the United States responded with the formation of the Administration on Aging, enactment of the Older Americans Act, and the introduction of Medicaid and Medicare, all in 1965. Since that time, society has demonstrated a growing concern for its older members (Table 1-1).

The past few decades have brought a profound awakening of interest in older persons as their numbers in society have grown. A more humanistic attitude toward all members of society also has affected the aged, and improvements in health care and general living conditions ensure that more people have the opportunity to attain old age and live longer, more fruitful years in this segment of life than previous generations (Fig. 1-1).

TABLE 1-1 ● *Publicly Supported Programs of Benefit to Older Americans*

1900	Pension laws passed in some states
1935	Social Security Act
1961	First White House Conference on Aging
1965	Older Americans Act: nutrition, senior employment, and transportation programs
	Administration on Aging
	Medicare (Title 18 of Social Security Act)
	Medicaid (Title 19 of Social Security Act) for poor and disabled of any age
1972	Supplemental Security Income (SSI) enacted
1991	Omnibus Budget Reconciliation Act (nursing home reform law) implemented

Growth of the Older Population

Persons older than 65 years of age represent more than 12% of the population in the United States. Advancements in disease control and health technology, the greater number of people able to survive the previously hazardous period of infancy and other dangers throughout the life span, improved sanitation, and better living conditions have increased life ex-

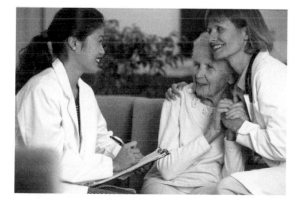

FIGURE 1-1

It is important for gerontological nurses to be as concerned with adding quality to the elders' lives, as they are with increasing the quantity of years.

pectancy for most Americans. More people are surviving to their senior years than ever before. In 1930, slightly more than 6 million persons were aged 65 years or older, and the average life expectancy was 59.7 years. The life expectancy in 1965 was 70.2 years, and the number of elderly exceeded 20 million. Life expectancy has now reached 77.1 years, with over 34 million persons exceeding age 65 years (Table 1-2). Not only are more people reaching old age, but they are living longer once they do; the number of people in their seventies and eighties has been steadily increasing and is expected to continue to increase (Table 1-3). The population over age 85 represents approximately 40% of the elderly population, and the number of centenarians is steadily growing. It is predicted that growing numbers of persons will reach their senior years, with an anticipated 20% of the population being older than 65 years of age by the year 2020.

KEY CONCEPT
More people are achieving and spending longer periods of time in old age than ever before in history.

UNIQUE SUBSETS OF ELDERLY

At one time all persons over age 65 years were grouped together under the category of *old*. Now it is recognized that much diversity exists among different age groups in late life, and persons age 65 years and over can be categorized as follows:

- young-old: 65 to 75 years
- old: 75 to 85 years
- old old: 85 to 100 years
- elite old: over 100 years

The profile, interests, and health care challenges of each of these subsets can be vastly different. For example, a 66 year-old may desire cosmetic surgery to stay competitive in the executive job market; a 72 year-old may have recently remarried and want to do something about her dry vaginal canal; an 82 year-old may be concerned that his arthritic knees are limiting his ability to play a round of golf; and a 95 year-old may be desparate to find a way to correct her impaired vision so that she can enjoy television. Any stereotypes

TABLE 1-2 ● *Life Expectancy at Birth From 1920-2000 With Projections to 2010*

	US Population		White Population			Black Population		
Year	Total		Total	Men	Women	Total	Men	Women
1920	54.1		54.9	54.4	55.6	45.3	45.5	45.2
1930	59.7		61.4	59.7	63.5	48.1	47.3	49.2
1940	62.9		64.2	62.1	66.6	53.1	51.5	54.9
1950	68.2		69.1	66.5	72.2	60.8	59.1	62.9
1955	69.6		70.5	67.4	73.7	63.7	61.4	66.1
1960	69.7		70.6	67.4	74.1	63.6	61.1	66.3
1965	70.2		71.0	67.6	74.7	64.1	61.1	67.4
1970	70.9		71.7	68.0	75.6	65.3	61.3	69.4
1975	72.6		73.4	69.5	77.3	68.0	63.7	72.4
1980	73.7		74.4	70.7	78.1	69.5	65.3	73.6
1985	74.7		75.3	71.8	78.7	69.3	65.0	73.4
1990	75.4		76.1	72.7	79.4	69.1	64.5	73.6
1995	75.8		76.5	73.4	79.6	69.6	65.2	73.9
2000	77.1		77.7	74.8	80.4	72.4	68.9	75.6
2010 (projected)	78.5		79.0	76.1	81.8	74.5	70.9	77.8

(From U.S. Department of Commerce. [2001]. *Statistical abstract of the United States* [121st ed., p. 73]. Washington, DC: Bureau of the Census.)

held about the elderly must be discarded; if anything, greater diversity rather than homogeneity will be evident.

GEOGRAPHIC DISTRIBUTION

Older adults live in a variety of settings throughout the country, with the greatest numbers found in California, New York, Florida, Pennsylvania, and Texas. In terms of the percentage of a state's population older than 65 years of age, Florida takes the lead, followed by Rhode Island, West Virginia, Iowa, and Arkansas. In the past decade, the most dramatic increases in the percentage of elderly residents have occurred in Nevada, Alaska, Hawaii, and Arizona. States with the lowest percentage of total population being over age 65 years are Alaska, Utah, and Georgia.

> ✔ **Point to Ponder**
> *A higher proportion of elders in our society means that younger age groups will be carrying a greater tax burden to support the older population. Should young families sacrifice to support services for elders? Why or why not?*

TABLE 1-3 ● *Increase in the Elderly Population From 1960-2000 (in Millions)*

Age	1960	1970	1980	1991	2000
65++	16.7	20.1	25.7	31.7	34.8
65–69	6.3	7.0	8.8	10.0	9.4
70–74	4.8	5.5	6.8	8.2	8.7
75–79	3.1	3.9	4.8	6.5	7.4
80–84	1.6	2.3	3.0	4.0	4.8
85+	0.9	1.4	2.3	3.1	4.2

(From U.S. Department of Commerce. [2001]. *Statistical abstract of the United States* [121st ed., p. 74]. Washington, DC: Bureau of the Census.)

Race and Gender Differences

Table 1-4 depicts the differences in life expectancy between races and genders. From the late 1980s to the present, the gap in life expectancy between white people and black people has widened because the life expectancy of the black population has declined. The

TABLE 1-4 ● *Race and Gender Differences in Life Expectancy (in Years)*

Year	Total Population	Men		Women	
		White	Black	White	Black
1999	77.0	74.7	68.7	80.0	75.4
2010 (projected)	78.5	76.1	70.9	81.8	77.8

(From U.S. Department of Commerce. [2001]. *Statistical abstract of the United States* [121st ed., p. 73]. Washington, DC: Bureau of the Census.)

U.S. Department of Health and Human Services attributes the declining life expectancy of black people to an increase in deaths from homicide and acquired immunodeficiency syndrome. This reality underscores the need for nurses to be concerned with health and social issues of persons of all ages because these impact a population's aging process.

Throughout the 20th century, the ratio of men to women had steadily declined to the point where there are fewer than 7 older men for every 10 older women (Table 1-5). The ratio declined with each advanced decade. However, this trend is changing and the ratio of men to women is increasing. The higher survival rates of women, along with the practice of women marrying men older than themselves, make it no surprise that more than half of women older than 65 years of age are widowed, and a majority of their male contemporaries are married (Table 1-6).

KEY CONCEPT
Women are more likely to be widowed and living alone in old age than their male counterparts.

Most older adults live in a household with a spouse or other family member, although more than twice the number of women than men live alone in later life (Table 1-7). Most elderly people have contact with their families and are not forgotten or neglected. Realities of the aging family are discussed in greater detail in Chapter 39.

Income and Employment

The percentage of older people below the poverty level has been declining concurrently, with less than

TABLE 1-5 ● *Gender Ratio in the Population 65 Years of Age and Older*

Year	Number of Men Per 100 Women
1910	101.1
1920	101.3
1930	100.5
1940	95.5
1950	89.6
1960	82.8
1970	72.1
1980	67.6
1985	67.9
1990	67.2
1995	69.1
2000	70.4
2025 (projected)	82.9

(From U.S. Department of Commerce. [2001]. *Statistical abstract of the United States* [121st ed., p. 16]. Washington, DC: Bureau of the Census.)

TABLE 1-6 ● *Marital Status of the Population 65 Years of Age and Older (% Distribution)*

Marital Status	Men	Women
Never married	4.2	3.6
Married	72.2	43.8
Spouse present	72.6	41.3
Spouse absent	2.6	2.5
Widowed	14.4	45.3
Divorced	6.1	7.2

(From U.S. Department of Commerce. [2001]. *Statistical abstract of the United States* [121st ed., p. 42]. Washington, DC: Bureau of the Census.)

TABLE 1-7 ● *People 65 Years of Age and Older Living Alone (in Percentages)*

Total	Men	Women
30.1	17.0	39.6

(From U.S. Department of Commerce. [2001]. *Statistical abstract of the United States* [121st ed., p. 42]. Washington, DC: Bureau of the Census.)

15% now falling into this category. However, the elderly still do possess financial problems. Most older people depend on Social Security for more than half of their income (Display 1-1). Women and minority groups have considerably less income than white men. Although the median net worth of older households is nearly twice the national average because of the high prevalence of home ownership by elders, many older adults are "asset rich and cash poor." That is, they may live in a house that has appreciated in value over the years, but they barely have sufficient monthly income to meet basic expenses.

While the percentage of the total population that the elderly represent is growing, they constitute a steadily declining percentage of workers in the labor force. The withdrawal of men from the workforce at earlier ages has been one of the most significant labor force trends since World War II. On the other hand, there has been a significant rise in the percentage of middle-aged women who are employed, although there has been little change in the labor force participation of women 65 years of age and older. Most Baby Boomers are expressing a desire to continue working as they enter retirement age (AARP, 2000).

KEY CONCEPT
Although Social Security was intended to be a supplement to other sources of income for the elderly, it is the main source of income for more than half of all older adults.

Education

The United States continues to witness a trend toward a more educated senior citizen group because of the significant increase in the number of persons completing high school during and since the 1940s (Table 1-8). Elderly people with advanced degrees are and will continue to be more prevalent than in the past. As is true for other age groups, older adults with advanced degrees have higher incomes.

KEY CONCEPT
Future generations of elderly people will have achieved higher levels of formal education than today's older population and will be more informed health care consumers.

Health Status

The elderly experience fewer acute illnesses than younger age groups and have a lower death rate from these problems (Table 1-9). However, elderly people who do develop acute illnesses usually require longer periods of recovery and have more complications from these conditions.

DISPLAY 1-1

Social Security and Supplemental Security Income

Social Security: a benefit check paid to retired workers of specific minimum age (eg, 65 years), disabled workers of any age, and spouses and minor children of those workers. Benefits are not dependent on financial need. It is intended to serve as supplement to other sources of income in retirement.

Supplemental Security Income (SSI): a benefit check paid to persons over age 65 and/or persons with disabilities based on financial need.

TABLE 1-8 ● *Years of School Completed by Age (in Percentages)*

Education	55–64 years	65–74 years	75 years and older
Not a high school graduate	18.3	26.4	35.4
High school graduate	35.7	37.4	34.1
Some college, no degree	16.3	14.2	13.2
Associate's degree	6.2	4.5	3.9
Bachelor's degree	13.1	10.4	8.7
Advanced degree	10.4	7.1	4.7

(From U.S. Department of Commerce. [2001]. *Statistical abstract of the United States* [121st ed., p. 140]. Washington, DC: Bureau of the Census.)

TABLE 1-9 ● *Rates of Acute Illness in Adults by Age (per 100 Population)*

	25–44 years	45–64 years	65 years and older
Infections and parasites	12.2	11.0	6.5
Common cold	18.7	16.4	15.7
Influenza	38.1	26.1	18.6
Digestive system	5.1	5.3	6.6
Injuries	24.9	14.6	17.2

(From U.S. National Center for Health Statistics. (2003). *Vital health statistics* [Series 10, No. 200].)

Chronic illness is a major problem for the older population. Most elderly people have at least one chronic disease, and typically they have several chronic conditions that must be managed simultaneously (Display 1-2). Chronic illness causes some activity limitations for personal care in 49% of all older individuals, and 27% have difficulty with home management activities. The older the age, the greater the likelihood of difficulty with self-care activities and independent living.

DISPLAY 1-2

Ten leading Chronic Conditions Affecting Population Age 65 and Older

Arthritis	Deformities or orthopedic impairments
High blood pressure	Diabetes
Hearing impairments	Chronic sinusitis
Heart conditions	Hay fever, allergic rhinitis (without asthma)
Visual impairments (including cataracts)	Varicose veins

Source: U.S. National Center for Health Statistics. [2003]. *Vital and health statistics.* www.cdc.gov/nchs/data/hus/tables/2002, accessed 5/15/03.

> **KEY CONCEPT**
> The chronic disorders most prevalent in the older population are ones that can have a significant impact on independence and the quality of daily life.

Chronic diseases are not only major sources of disability, but they are also the leading causes of death (Table 1-10). A shift in death rates from various causes of death has occurred over the past three decades; deaths from heart disease have declined, whereas those from cancer have increased.

Use of Resources

The growing number of persons older than 65 years of age has had an impact on the health and social service agencies that serve this group and, consequently, on the government that is the source of payment for most of these services. The elderly have higher rates of hospitalization, surgery, and physician visits than other age groups, and this care is more likely to be paid by federal dollars than private insurers or the elderly themselves (Tables 1-11 and 1-12).

TABLE 1-10 ● *Leading Causes of Death for Persons 65 Years of Age and Older*

Cause of Death	Number of Deaths
All causes	1,753,220
Heart disease	605,673
Malignant neoplasms (cancer)	384,186
Cerebrovascular (stroke)	139,144
Chronic obstructive pulmonary disease	97,896
Pneumonia and influenza	82,989
Diabetes	48,974
Accidents	32,975
Alzheimer's disease	22,416
Nephritis, nephrotic syndrome, nephrosis	22,640
Septicemia	19,012

(From U.S. Department of Commerce. [2001]. *Statistical abstract of the United States* [121st ed., p. 82]. Washington, DC: Bureau of the Census.)

TABLE 1-11 ● *Average Length of Hospital Stay (in Days)*

	65–74 years	75 years and older
Male	5.8	6.3
Female	5.9	6.2

(From U.S. Department of Commerce. [2001]. *Statistical abstract of the United States* [121st ed., p. 113]. Washington, DC: Bureau of the Census.)

Less than 5% of the older population is institutionalized at any given time, although approximately one in four older adults will spend some time in a nursing home during the last years of their lives. Most people who enter nursing homes as private-pay residents spend their assets by the end of 1 year and require government support for their care; most of the Medicaid budget is spent on long-term care.

> **KEY CONCEPT**
> Gerontological nurses need to be advocates in ensuring that cost-containment efforts do not jeopardize the welfare of the elderly.

Impact of the Baby Boomers

In anticipating needs and services for future generations of elders, gerontological nurses must consider the realities of the baby boomers who will be the next wave of senior citizens. Baby boomers are those individuals born between 1946 and 1964 who will be entering their senior years between 2008 and 2030 (Fig. 1-2). They are a highly diverse group, representing people as different as Bill Clinton, Bill Gates, and Cher, although they do have some clearly defined characteristics that set them apart from other groups.

- Most have children, but their low birth rate means that they will have fewer biologic children available to assist them in old age.
- They are the best-educated generation society has ever had.
- Their income tends to be higher than other groups, partly due to two incomes (three in four baby boomer women are in the labor force).

TABLE 1-12 ● *Health Insurance Coverage for Persons Aged 65 Years and Older (Percentages)*

Total	Private/Group Health	Medicare	Medicaid	Not Covered
63.1	35.6	26.7	7.6	1.1

Note: Some older adults with Medicare coverage also carry private supplemental health insurance.
(From U.S. Department of Commerce. [2002]. *Statistical abstract of the United States* [122nd ed., Table 130]. Washington, DC: Bureau of the Census.)

- They favor a more casual dress code than previous generations.
- They are enamored with "high-tech" products and are more likely than younger or older persons to own and use a home computer.

- Their leisure time is scarcer than other adults, and they are more likely to report feeling stressed at the end of the day.
- As inventors of the fitness movement, they exercise more frequently than other adults.

Some predictions can be made concerning this population when they become elders. They will be informed consumers and desire a highly active role in their health care; their ability to access information may enable them to have as much knowledge as their health care providers on some health issues. They will not be satisfied with the conditions of today's nursing homes and will demand that their long-term care facilities be equipped with computer stations, gymnasiums, juice bars, pools, and alternative therapies. Their blended families may need special assistance because of the caregiving demands of potentially several sets of step-parents and step-grandparents. Plans for services and architectural designs must take these types of realities into consideration.

As the percentage of the population who is elderly grows, society will face an increasing demand for the provision of and payment for services to this group. In this era of budget deficits, shrinking revenue, and increased competition for funding of other special interests, questions may arise about the ongoing ability of the government to provide a wide range of services for older adults. There may be concern that the elderly are using a disproportionate amount of tax dollars and that limits should be set. Gerontological nurses must be actively involved in discussions and decisions pertaining to the rationing of services so that the rights of the elderly are expressed and protected. Likewise, gerontological nurses must assume leadership in developing cost-effective methods of care delivery that do not compromise the quality of services to older adults.

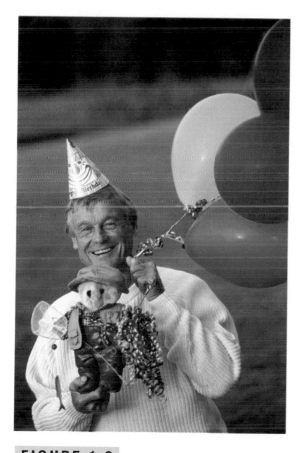

FIGURE 1-2

The first wave of the 76 million baby boomers turns 65 years of age in 2011.

Critical Thinking Exercises

1. Consider the factors influencing a society's willingness to provide assistance to and display a positive attitude toward the elderly (eg, general economic conditions for all age groups).
2. List the anticipated changes in the characteristics of the older population of the future and implications for nursing.
3. What problems may older women experience in life expectancy and income as a result of gender differences?
4. What are some of the differences between older white and black Americans?

Web Connect

Review trends in health and aging at the National Center for Health Statistics website at www.cdc.gov/nchs

● Reference

American Association of Retired Persons. (2000). Boomers look toward retirement. Washington, DC: Author.

● Recommended Readings

American Association of Retired Persons and Public Policy Institute. (1998). Boomers approaching midlife: How secure a future? Washington, DC: Author.

Binstock, R. H., Cluff, L. E., & von Mering, O. (1996). The future of long-term care. Social and policy issues. Baltimore: Johns Hopkins University Press.

Bosworth, B., & Burtless, G. T. (1998). Aging societies: The global dimension. Washington, DC: Brookings Institute Press.

Eisner, R. (1998). Social security: More, not less. New York: Century Foundation Press.

Gruber, J., & Wise, D. A. (1999). Social security and retirement around the world. Chicago: University of Chicago Press.

Jackson, W. A. (1998). The political economy of population aging. Northampton, MA: Elgar.

Kassner, E., & Bectel, R. (1998). Midlife and older Americans with disabilities: Who gets help? A chartbook. Washington, DC: American Association of Retired Persons.

Weissert, C. A., & Weissert, W. G. (1996). Governing health. Politics and policy. Baltimore: Johns Hopkins University Press.

Wise, D. A. (1998). Frontiers in the economics of aging. Chicago: University of Chicago Press.

Wu, K. B. (1998). Income and poverty in the United States in 1995: A chartbook. Washington, DC: Public Policy Institute of the American Association of Retired Persons.

Theories of Aging

■ Learning Objectives

After reading this chapter, you should be able to:

- discuss the change in focus regarding learning about factors influencing aging
- list the major biological theories of aging
- describe the major psychosocial theories of aging
- identify factors that promote a healthy aging process

For centuries people have been intrigued by the mystery of aging, some in hopes of achieving everlasting youth, others of discovering the key to immortality. Throughout history there have been numerous searches for a fountain of youth, the most famous being that of Ponce de León. Ancient Egyptian and Chinese relics show evidence of concoctions designed to prolong life or achieve immortality, and various other cultures have proposed specific dietary regimens, herbal mixtures, and rituals for similar ends. Ancient life expanders, such as extracts prepared from tiger testicles, may seem ludicrous until they are compared with more modern measures such as injections of embryonic tissue and Botox. Even persons who would not condone such peculiar practices may indulge in nutritional supplements, cosmetic creams, and exotic spas that promise to maintain youth and delay the onset of old age.

No single known factor causes or prevents aging; it is unrealistic to think that one theory can explain the complexities of this process. Explorations into biological, psychological, and social aging continue, and although some of this interest focuses on achieving eternal youth, most sound research efforts aim toward a better understanding of this process so that people can age in a healthier fashion and postpone some of the negative consequences associated with growing old. In fact, recent research has concentrated on learning about keeping people healthy and active for a longer period of time rather than extending their lives in a state of long-term disability (Hubert , Bloch, Oehlert, & Fries, 2002). Recognizing that aging theories offer varying degrees of universality, validity, and reliability, nurses can use this information to better understand the factors that may positively and negatively influence the health and well-being of persons of all ages.

Biological Theories

The process of biological aging differs not only from species to species but also from one human being to another. Some general statements can be made concerning anticipated organ changes, as described in Chapter 5; however, no two individuals age identically (Fig. 2-1). Varying degrees of physiologic changes, capacities, and limitations will be found among peers of a given age group. Further, the rate of aging among different body systems within one individual may vary, with one system showing marked decline while another demonstrates no significant change. To explain biological aging, theorists have explored many factors, both internal and external to the human body.

> 🔑 **KEY CONCEPT**
> The aging process varies not only among individuals, but also within different systems of the same person.

GENETIC PROGRAMMING AND ERRORS

Some theorists believe that people inherit a genetic program that determines their specific life expectancy. In the 1960s, the program theory of aging was advanced that claimed that animals and humans are born with a genetic program or biological clock that predetermines life span (Hayflick, 1965). Various studies that have shown a positive relationship between parental age and filial life span support a predetermined genetic program. Studies of in-vitro cell proliferation have demonstrated that various species have a finite number of cell divisions. Fibroblasts from embryonic tissue experienced a greater number of cell divisions than those de-

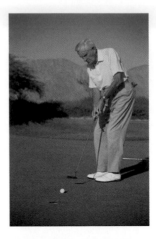

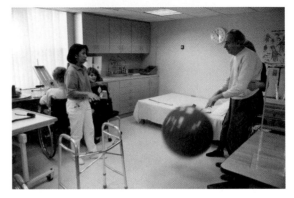

FIGURE 2·1

Aging is a highly individualized process, demonstrated by the differences between persons of similar ages.

rived from adult tissue, and among various species, the longer the life span, the greater the number of cell divisions. These studies support the belief that senescence is under genetic control and occurs at the cellular level (Harvard Gazette Archives, 2001; University of Illinois at Urbana-Champaign, 2002).

Genetic mutations, described under the *error theory*, also are thought to be responsible for aging by causing organ decline as a result of self-perpetuating cellular mutations:

Mutation of DNA
↓
Perpetuation of mutation during cell division
↓

Increasing number of mutant cells in body

↓

Malfunction of tissues, organs, and systems

↓

Decline in body functions

Some theorists think that a growth substance fails to be produced, which results in the cessation of cell growth and reproduction. Others hypothesize that an aging factor responsible for development and cellular maturity throughout life is excessively produced, thereby hastening aging. Cross-linking of DNA strands is hypothesized by some to impair the cell's ability to function and divide. Although minimal research has been done to support this theory, aging may be a result of a decreased ability of RNA to synthesize and translate messages.

> ✔ **Point to Ponder**
> *What patterns of aging are apparent in your biological family? What can you do to influence these?*

CROSS-LINKING

This theory proposes that cellular division is threatened as a result of radiation or a chemical reaction in which a cross-linking agent attaches itself to a DNA strand and prevents normal parting of the strands during mitosis. Over time, as these cross-linking agents accumulate, they form dense aggregates that impede intracellular transport; ultimately, the body's organs and systems fail. An effect of cross-linking on collagen (an important connective tissue in the lungs, heart, blood vessels, and muscle) is the reduction in tissue elasticity associated with many age-related changes.

FREE RADICALS

Free radicals are highly reactive molecules containing an extra electrical charge that are generated from oxygen metabolism. They can result from normal metabolism, reactions with other free radicals, or oxidation of ozone, pesticides, and other pollutants. These molecules can damage proteins, enzymes, and DNA by replacing molecules that contain useful biological information with faulty molecules that create genetic disorder. It is believed that these free radicals are self-perpetuating; that is, they generate other free radicals. Physical decline of the body occurs as the damage from these molecules accumulates over time. However, the body has natural antioxidants that can counteract the effects of free radicals to an extent. Also, β-carotene and vitamins C and E are antioxidants that can offer protection against free radicals.

There has been considerable interest in the role of lipofuscin "age pigments," a lipoprotein by-product of oxidation that can be seen only under a fluorescent microscope, in the aging process. Because lipofuscin is associated with the oxidation of unsaturated lipids, it is believed to have a role similar to that of free radicals in the aging process. As lipofuscin accumulates, it interferes with the diffusion and transport of essential metabolites and information-bearing molecules in the cells. A positive relationship exists between an individual's age and the amount of lipofuscin in the body. Investigators have discovered the presence of lipofuscin in other species in amounts proportionate to the life span of the species (eg, an animal with one tenth the life span of a human being accumulates lipofuscin at a rate approximately 10 times greater than human beings).

AUTOIMMUNE REACTIONS

The primary organs of the immune system, the thymus and bone marrow, are believed to be affected by the aging process. The immune response declines after young adulthood. The weight of the thymus decreases throughout adulthood, as does the ability to produce T-cell differentiation. The level of thymus hormone declines after age 30 and is undetectable in the blood of persons older than age 60 years (Goya Console, Herenu, Brown, & Rimoldi, 2002; Williams, 1995). Related to this is a decline in the humoral immune response, a delay in the skin allograft rejection time, reduction in intensity of delayed hypersensitivity, and a decrease in the resistance to tumor cell challenge. The bone marrow stem cells perform less efficiently. The reduction in immunologic functions is evidenced by an increase in the incidence of infections and many cancers with age. Some theorists believe that the reduction in immunologic activities also leads to an increase in autoimmune response with age. One hypothesis regarding the role of autoimmune reactions in the aging process is that the body misidentifies aged, irregular cells as foreign agents and attacks them:

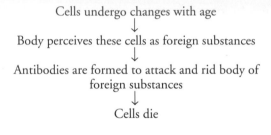

Cells undergo changes with age
↓
Body perceives these cells as foreign substances
↓
Antibodies are formed to attack and rid body of foreign substances
↓
Cells die

Another reason for this reaction could be related to the breakdown of the body's immunochemical memory system, which causes it to misinterpret normal body constituents:

Cells are normal
↓
Immunochemical memory system malfunctions and perceives cells as foreign substances
↓
Antibodies are formed to attack and rid body of foreign substances
↓
Cells die

WEAR AND TEAR

Wear and tear theories attribute aging to the repeated use and injury of the body over time as it performs its highly specialized functions. Like any complicated machine, the body will function less efficiently with prolonged use and numerous insults.

STRESS

In recent years, the effects of stress on physical and psychological health have been widely discussed. Stresses to the body can have adverse effects and lead to conditions such as gastric ulcers, heart attacks, thyroiditis, and inflammatory dermatoses. However, this theory is limited in its universality because individuals react differently to life's stresses—one person may be overwhelmed by a moderately busy schedule, whereas another may become frustrated when faced with a slow, dull pace.

DISEASE

Bacteria, fungi, viruses, and other organisms are thought to be responsible for certain physiologic changes during the aging process. In some cases, these pathogens may be present in the body for decades before they begin to affect body systems. The connection between aging and disease processes has been termed *biogerontology* (Miller, 1997). Although no conclusive evidence exists to link these pathogens with the body's decline, interest in this theory has been stimulated by the fact that human beings and animals have enjoyed longer life expectancies with the control or elimination of certain pathogens through immunization and the use of antimicrobial drugs.

NEUROENDOCRINES AND NEUROCHEMICALS

This group of theories suggests that aging is the result of changes in the brain and endocrine glands. Some theorists claim that specific anterior pituitary hormones promote aging. Others believe that an imbalance of chemicals in the brain impairs healthy cell division throughout the body.

RADIATION

The relationship of radiation and age continues to be explored. Research using rats, mice, and dogs has shown that a decreased life span results from nonlethal doses of radiation. In human beings, repeated exposure to ultraviolet light is known to cause solar elastosis, the "old age" type of skin wrinkling that results from the replacement of collagen by elastin. Ultraviolet light is also a factor in the development of skin cancer. Radiation may induce cellular mutations that promote aging.

NUTRIENTS

The importance of good nutrition throughout life is a theme hard to escape in our nutrition-conscious society. It is no mystery that diet impacts health and aging. Obesity is shown to increase the risk of many diseases and shorten life (NIDDK, 2001; Taylor & Ostbye, 2001).

The quality of diet is as important as the quantity. Deficiencies of vitamins and other nutrients and excesses of nutrients such as cholesterol may cause various disease processes. Recently, increased attention has been given to the influence of nutritional supplements on the aging process; vitamin E, bee pollen, ginseng, gotu kola, peppermint, and kelp are among the nutrients believed to promote a healthy, long life (Margolis, 2000; Smeeding, 2001) Although the complete relationship between diet and aging is not well understood, enough is known to suggest that a good diet may minimize or eliminate some of the ill effects of the aging process.

> **KEY CONCEPT**
> It is beneficial for nurses to advise aging persons to scrutinize products that claim to cause, stop, or reverse the aging process.

ENVIRONMENT

Several environmental factors are known to threaten health and are thought to be associated with the aging process. The ingestion of mercury, lead, arsenic, radioactive isotopes, certain pesticides, and other substances can produce pathologic changes in human beings. Smoking and breathing tobacco smoke and other air pollutants also have adverse effects. Finally, crowded living conditions, high noise levels, and other factors are thought to influence how we age.

> **Point to Ponder**
> *Do you believe nurses have a responsibility to protect and improve the environment? Why or why not?*

The number, diversity, and complexity of factors that potentially influence the aging process show that no one biological theory can adequately explain the cause of this phenomenon. Even when studies have been done with populations known to have a high life expectancy, such as the people of the Caucasus region in southern Russia, longevity has not been attributable to any single factor. These theories are significant to nursing. Nurses can adapt these theories by identifying elements known to influence aging and using them as a foundation to promote positive practices.

Psychosocial Theories

Psychological theories of aging explore the mental processes, behavior, and feelings of persons through-

out the life span, along with some of the mechanisms people use to meet the challenges they face in old age. Sociologic theories address the impact of society and the elderly on each other.

DISENGAGEMENT THEORY

Developed by Elaine Cumming and William Henry, the disengagement theory (Cumming, 1964; Cumming & Henry, 1961) is one of the earliest, most controversial, and widely discussed theories of aging. It views aging as a process in which society and the individual gradually withdraw, or disengage, from each other, to the mutual satisfaction and benefit of both. The benefit to individuals is that they can reflect and be centered on themselves, having been freed from societal roles. The value of disengagement to society is that some orderly means is established for the transfer of power from the old to the young, making it possible for society to continue functioning after its individual members die. The theory does not indicate whether society or the individual initiates the disengagement process.

Several difficulties with this concept are obvious. Many older persons desire to remain engaged and do not want their primary satisfaction to be derived from reflection on younger years. Senators, Supreme Court justices, college professors, and many senior volunteers are among those who commonly derive satisfaction and provide a valuable service to society by not disengaging. Because the health of the individual, cultural practices, societal norms, and other factors influence the degree to which a person will participate in society during his or her later years, some critics of this theory claim that disengagement would not be necessary if society improved the health care and financial means of elders and increased the acceptance, opportunities, and respect afforded them.

A careful examination of the population studied in the development of the disengagement theory hints at its limitations. The disengagement pattern that Cumming and Henry described was based on a study of 172 middle-class persons between 48 and 68 years of age. This group was wealthier, better educated, and of higher occupational and residential prestige than the general aged population. No black people or chronically ill people were involved in the study. Caution is advisable in generalizing findings for the entire aged population based on fewer than

200 persons who are generally not representative of the average aged person. (This study exemplifies some of the limitations of gerontological research before the 1970s.) Although nurses should appreciate that some older individuals may wish to disengage from the mainstream of society, this is not necessarily a process to be expected from all aged persons.

ACTIVITY THEORY

At the opposite pole from the disengagement theory, the activity theory proclaims that an older person should continue a middle-aged lifestyle, denying the existence of old age as long as possible, and that society should apply the same norms to old age as it does to middle age and not advocate diminishing activity, interest, and involvement as its members grow old (Havighurst, 1963). This theory suggests ways of maintaining activity in the presence of multiple losses associated with the aging process, including substituting intellectual activities for physical activities when physical capacity is reduced, replacing the work role with other roles when retirement occurs, and establishing new friendships when old ones are lost. Declining health, loss of roles, reduced income, a shrinking circle of friends, and other obstacles to maintaining an active life are to be resisted and overcome instead of being accepted.

This theory has some merit. Activity is generally assumed to be more desirable than inactivity because it facilitates physical, mental, and social well-being. Like a self-fulfilling prophecy, the expectation of a continued active state during old age may be realized to the benefit of elders and society. Because of society's negative view of inactivity and acting old, encouraging an active lifestyle among the aged is consistent with societal values. Also supportive of the activity theory is the reluctance of many older persons to accept themselves as old. A problem with this theory is the assumption that most older people desire and are able to maintain a middle-aged lifestyle. Some aging persons want their world to shrink to accommodate their decreasing capacities or their preference for less active roles. Many elderly people lack the physical, emotional, social, or economic resources to maintain active roles in society. Aged people who are expected to maintain an active middle-aged lifestyle on an income of less than half that of middle-aged people may wonder if society is giving them conflicting messages. More insights are needed regarding the effects on the elderly of not being able to fulfill expectations to remain active.

CONTINUITY THEORY

The continuity theory of aging, also referred to as the developmental theory, relates personality and predisposition toward certain actions in old age to similar factors during other phases of the life cycle (Neugarten, 1964). Personality and basic patterns of behavior are said to remain unchanged as the individual ages. For instance, activists at 20 years of age will most likely be activists at 70 years of age, whereas young recluses will probably not be active in the mainstream of society when they age. Patterns developed over a lifetime will determine whether individuals remain engaged and active or become disengaged and inactive. The recognition that the unique features of each individual allow for multiple adaptations to aging and that the potential exists for a variety of reactions give this theory validity and support. Aging is a complex process, and the continuity theory considers these complexities to a greater extent than most other theories. Although the full implications and impact of this promising theory are at the stage of research, it offers a reasonable perspective. Also, it encourages the young to consider that their current activities are laying a foundation for their own future old age.

> **KEY CONCEPT**
> Basic psychological patterns are consistent throughout the life span.

DEVELOPMENTAL TASKS

Some theorists have described the process of healthy psychological aging as the result of the successful fulfillment of developmental tasks. Developmental tasks are the challenges that must be met and adjustments that must be made in response to life experiences that are part of an adult's continued growth through the life span.

Erik Erikson described eight stages through which human beings progress from infancy to old age and the challenges, or tasks, that confront individuals during each of these stages (Table 2-1) (Erikson,

TABLE 2-1 ● *Erikson's Developmental Tasks*

Stage	Satisfactorily Fulfilled	Unsatisfactorily Fulfilled
Infancy	Trust	Mistrust
Toddler	Autonomy	Shame
Early childhood	Initiative	Guilt
Middle childhood	Industry	Inferiority
Adolescence	Identity	Identity diffusion
Adulthood	Intimacy	Isolation
Middle age	Generativity	Self-absorption
Old age	Integrity	Despair

1963). The challenge of old age is to accept and find meaning in the life the person has lived; this gives the individual ego integrity that aids in adjusting and coping with the reality of aging and mortality. Feelings of anger, bitterness, depression, and inadequacy can result in inadequate ego integrity (eg, despair).

Refining Erikson's description of old age tasks, Robert Peck detailed three specific challenges facing the elderly that influence the outcome of ego integrity or despair (Peck, 1968):

- *ego differentiation versus role preoccupation:* to develop satisfactions from oneself as a person rather than through parental or occupational roles
- *body transcendence versus body preoccupation:* to find psychological pleasures rather than become absorbed with health problems or physical limitations imposed by aging
- *ego transcendence versus ego preoccupation:* to achieve satisfaction through reflection on one's past life and accomplishments rather than be preoccupied with the finite number of years left to live

Robert Butler and Myrna Lewis outlined the major tasks of later life as the following (Butler & Lewis, 1982):

- adjusting to one's infirmities
- developing a sense of satisfaction with the life that has been lived
- preparing for death

Gerotranscendence is a recent theory that suggests aging entails a transition from a rational, materialistic meta-perspective to a cosmic and transcendent vision (Torn-stam, 1994). As they age, people are less concerned with material possessions, meaningless relationships, and self-interests and instead desire a life of more significance and a greater connection with others.

> ✔ **Point to Ponder**
> *How do you see examples of gerotranscendence in the lives of others and yourself?*

Nursing Implications

Gerontological nurses play a significant role in helping aging persons experience health, fulfillment, and a sense of well-being. In addition to specific measures that can assist the elderly in meeting their psychosocial challenges (Display 2-1), nurses must be sensitive to the tremendous impact their own attitudes toward aging can have on patients. Nurses who consider aging as a progressive decline ending in death may view old age as a depressing, useless period and foster hopelessness and helplessness in older patients. On the other hand, nurses who view aging as a process of continued development may appreciate old age as an opportunity to gain new satisfaction and understanding, thereby promoting joy and a sense of purpose in patients.

> 🔑 **KEY CONCEPT**
> Nurses can promote joy and a sense of purpose in the elderly by viewing old age as an opportunity for continued development and satisfaction rather than a depressing, useless period of life.

The biological, psychological, and social processes of aging are interrelated and interdependent. Frequently, loss of a social role affects an individual's sense of purpose and speeds physical decline. Poor health may force retirement from work, promoting social isolation and the development of a weakened self-concept. Although certain changes occur independently as separate events, most are closely associated with other age-related factors. It is impractical, therefore, to subscribe solely to one theory of aging. Wise nurses will be open-minded in choosing the

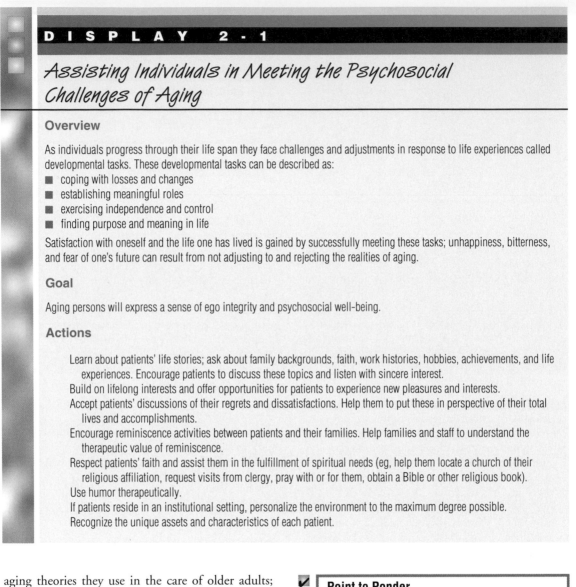

DISPLAY 2-1

Assisting Individuals in Meeting the Psychosocial Challenges of Aging

Overview

As individuals progress through their life span they face challenges and adjustments in response to life experiences called developmental tasks. These developmental tasks can be described as:
- coping with losses and changes
- establishing meaningful roles
- exercising independence and control
- finding purpose and meaning in life

Satisfaction with oneself and the life one has lived is gained by successfully meeting these tasks; unhappiness, bitterness, and fear of one's future can result from not adjusting to and rejecting the realities of aging.

Goal

Aging persons will express a sense of ego integrity and psychosocial well-being.

Actions

Learn about patients' life stories; ask about family backgrounds, faith, work histories, hobbies, achievements, and life experiences. Encourage patients to discuss these topics and listen with sincere interest.

Build on lifelong interests and offer opportunities for patients to experience new pleasures and interests.

Accept patients' discussions of their regrets and dissatisfactions. Help them to put these in perspective of their total lives and accomplishments.

Encourage reminiscence activities between patients and their families. Help families and staff to understand the therapeutic value of reminiscence.

Respect patients' faith and assist them in the fulfillment of spiritual needs (eg, help them locate a church of their religious affiliation, request visits from clergy, pray with or for them, obtain a Bible or other religious book).

Use humor therapeutically.

If patients reside in an institutional setting, personalize the environment to the maximum degree possible.

Recognize the unique assets and characteristics of each patient.

---

aging theories they use in the care of older adults; they will also be cognizant of the limitations of these theories. Display 2-2 highlights some factors to consider in promoting a healthy aging process.

> **✔ Point to Ponder**
> *How would you evaluate the quality of the factors that promote longevity in your own life?*

DISPLAY 2 - 2

Factors Contributing to a Long and Healthy Life

Diet. A positive health state that can contribute to longevity is supported by reducing saturated fats in the diet, limiting daily fat consumption to less than 30% of caloric intake, avoiding obesity, decreasing the amount of animal foods eaten, substituting natural complex carbohydrates for refined sugars, and increasing the consumption of whole grains, vegetables, and fruits.

Activity. Exercise is an important ingredient to good health. It increases strength and endurance, promotes cardiopulmonary function, and has other beneficial effects that can affect a healthy aging process.

Play and laughter. Laughter causes a release of endorphins, stimulates the immune system, and reduces stress. Finding humor in daily routines and experiencing joy despite problems contributes to good health. It has been suggested since the time of Solomon that "a cheerful heart is good medicine, but a crushed spirit dries up the bones" (Proverbs 17:22).

Faith. A strong faith, church attendance, and prayer are directly related to lower rates of physical and mental illness. Religion and spirituality can have a positive effect on the length and quality of life.

Empowerment. Losing control over one's life can threaten self-confidence and diminish self-care independence. Maximum control and decision-making can have a positive effect on morbidity and mortality.

Stress management. It is the rare individual who is unaware of the negative consequences of stress. The unique stresses that may accompany aging, such as the onset of chronic conditions, retirement, deaths of significant others, and change in body appearance, can have significantly detrimental effects. Minimizing stress when possible and using effective stress management techniques are useful interventions.

Critical Thinking Exercises

1. What disease processes are caused by or related to factors believed to influence aging?
2. You are asked to speak to a community group regarding environmental issues. What recommendations could you make for promoting a healthy environment?
3. Think about everyday life in your community. What examples do you see of opportunities to engage and disengage the elderly?
4. What specific methods could you use to assist an older adult in achieving ego integrity?

Web Connect

Conduct a search of the word "antiaging" and explore how currently marketed products and services relate to theories of aging.

●References

Butler, R. N., & Lewis. M. I. (1982). *Aging and mental health* (3rd ed., pp. 142, 376). St. Louis: Mosby.

Cumming, E. (1964). New thoughts on the theory of disengagement. In R. Kastenbaum (Ed.). *New thoughts on old age.* New York: Springer-Verlag.

Cumming, E., & Henry, E. (1961). *Growing old: The process of disengagement.* New York: Basic Books.

Erikson, E. (1963). *Childhood and society* (2nd ed.). New York: Norton.

Goya, R.G., Console, G. M., Herenu, C. B., Brown, O. A., & Rimoldi, O. J. (2002). Thymus and aging: Potential of gene therapy for restoration of endocrine thymic function in thymus-deficient animal models. *Gerontology* 48(5):325–328.

Harvard Gazette Archives (2001). Scientists identify chromosome location of genes associated with long life. *Harvard University Gazette.* Retrieved August 28, 2001, from www.news.harvard.edu/gazette/2001/08.16/chromosomes.html.

Havighurst, J. (1963). Successful aging. In R. H. Williams, C. Tibbitts, & W. Donahue (Eds.). *Processes of aging* (Vol. 1, p. 299). New York: Atherton Press.

Hayflick, L. (1965). The limited in vitro lifetime of human diploid cell strains. *Experimental Cell Research, 37,* 614–636.

Hubert H. B., Bloch D. A., Oehlert J. W., & Fries J. F. (2002). Lifestyle habits and compression of morbidity. *Journals of Gerontology Series A. Biological Sciences and Medical Sciences, 57*(6): M347–M351.

Margolis, S.(Ed.). (2000). Vitamin E recommendations. *The Johns Hopkins Medical Letter: Health After 50, 12*(1): 8.

Miller, R. A. (1997). When will the biology of aging become useful? Future landmarks in biomedical gerontology. *Journal of the American Geriatrics Society, 45,* 1258–1267.

Neugarten, L. (1964). *Personality in middle and late life.* New York: Atherton Press.

NIDDK. (2001). *Understanding adult obesity.* Bethesda, MD: National Institute of Diabetes and Digestive and Kidney Diseases of the National Institutes of Health, NIH Publication No. 01-3680.

Peck, R. (1968). Psychological developments in the second half of life. In B. Neugarten (Ed.). *Middle age and aging* (p. 88). Chicago: University of Chicago.

Smeeding, S. J. W. (2001). Nutrition, supplements, and aging. *Geriatric Nursing* 22(4): 219–224.

Taylor, D. H. & Ostbye, T. (2001). The effect of middle- and old-age body mass index on short-term mortality in older people. *Journal of the American Geriatrics Society, 49*(10):1319–1326.

Tornstam, L. (1994). Gerotranscendence: A theoretical and empirical exploration. In L. E. Thomas & S. A. Eisenhandler (Eds.). *Aging and the religious dimension.* Westport, CT: Greenwood.

University of Illinois at Urbana-Champaign. (2002). Study backs theory that accumulating mutations of "quiet" genes foster aging. *Science News Daily.* Retrieved October 15, 2002, from www.sciencedaily.com/releases/2002/10/021015073143.htm

Williams, M. E. (1995). *The American Geriatrics Society's complete guide to aging and health* (p. 13). New York: Harmony Books.

●Recommended Readings

Arking, R. (1998). *Biology of aging: Observations and principles* (2nd ed.). Sunderland, MA: Sinauer Associations.

Bergeman, C. S. (1997). *Aging: Genetic and environmental influences.* Thousand Oaks, CA: Sage.

Birren, J. E. (Ed.). (1996). *Encyclopedia of gerontology: Age, aging, and the aged.*

The Gerontologist, 36, 737–741.

Crose, R. (1997). *Why women live longer than men and what men can learn from them.* San Francisco: Jossey-Bass.

Gutmann, D. L. (1997). *The human elder in nature, culture and society.* Boulder, CO: Westview Press.

Hillman, J. (1999). *The force of character and the lasting life.* New York: Random House.

Johnson, C. L. (1997). *Life beyond 85 years: The aura of survivorship.*

Matcha, D. A. (1997). *Sociology of aging: A social problems perspective.* Boston: Allyn & Bacon.

Mendes de Leon, C. F., Seeman, T. E., Baker, D. I., Richardson, E. D., & Tinetti, M. E. (1996). Self-efficacy, physical decline, and change in functioning in community-living elders: A prospective study. *Journal of Gerontology: Social Sciences, 51B*(4), S183–S190.

Olshansky, S. J., & Carnes. B. A. (2001). *The quest for immortality: Science at the frontiers of aging.* New York: W. W. Norton & Co.

Whitbourne, S. K. (1997). *Aging individual: Physical and psychological perspectives.* New York: Springer.

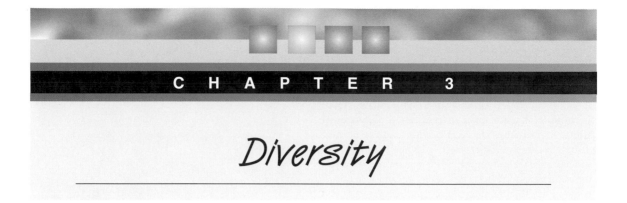

CHAPTER 3

Diversity

■ *Learning Objectives*

After reading this chapter, you should be able to:

- describe unique views of health and healing among major ethnic groups
- identify ways in which nursing care may need to be modified to accommodate persons of diverse ethnic backgrounds

People from a variety of countries have ventured to America to seek a better life in a new land. To an extent, they assimilated and adopted the American way of life; however, the values and customs instilled in them by their native cultures were too deeply ingrained to be erased, and their language and biological differences were often obvious. The unique backgrounds of these newcomers to America influenced the way they reacted to the world around them and the manner in which that world reacted to them. To understand the uniqueness of each older adult encountered, consideration must be given to the influences of ethnic origin.

Members of an ethnic group share similar history, language, customs, and characteristics; they also hold distinct beliefs about aging and the elderly. Ethnic norms can influence diet, response to pain, compliance with self-care activities and medical treatments, trust in health care providers, and other factors. The traditional responsibilities assigned to the old of some ethnic groups can afford the elderly opportunities for meaningful roles and high status.

Studies of cultural influences on aging and effects on the elderly have been sparse but are growing. Experiences and observations can provide insight into the unique characteristics of specific ethnic groups. Although individual differences within a given ethnic group exist and stereotypes should not be made, an understanding of the general characteristics of various ethnic groups can assist nurses in providing more individualized and culturally sensitive care.

Black Americans

Although 13% of the entire U.S. population is black, they represent only 8% of the older population. Most of this group are of African descent. It is believed that a free black man, Pedro Alonso Nino, accompanied Christopher Columbus on his 1492 voyage to America; however, most of the early experiences of black people in this country occurred in the form of slavery. Displacement from families and tribes as they were sold into slavery, insults suffered through discrimination, and strong religious beliefs were major factors influencing the black population's deep commitment to the family and aged relatives. The family could be depended on to aid and comfort its members in the face of the prejudices and hardships of society.

Historically, black Americans have experienced a lower standard of living and less access to health care than their white counterparts. This is reflected in the lower life expectancy of black Americans (see demographics in Chapter 1). For black men, life expectancy has slightly decreased in recent years. However, once a black individual reaches the seventh decade of life, survival begins to equal that of similarly aged white people.

> **KEY CONCEPT**
> After reaching their seventh decade of life, black elderly can hope to enjoy a life expectancy equal to their white cohorts.

To survive to old age is considered a major accomplishment that reflects strength, resourcefulness, and faith for this ethnic group; thus, old age is a personal triumph to black people, not a dreaded curse

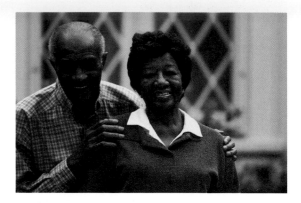

FIGURE 3-1

Although they have a lower life expectancy than white Americans, black Americans can survive as long as their white peers once they reach their senior years.

(Figure 3-1). Considering their history, it should not be surprising to find that black elderly:

- possess many health problems that have accumulated over a lifetime due to a poor standard of living and limited access to health care services
- hold health beliefs and practices that may be unconventional, to stay healthy and treat illness
- look to family members for decision-making and care rather than using formal service agencies
- may have a degree of caution in interacting with and using health services, as a defense against prejudice

Diverse subgroups within the black population, such as Africans, Haitians, Tahitians, and Jamaicans, each possess their own unique customs and beliefs. Differences can be apparent even among black Americans from various regions of the United States. Nurses should be sensitive to the fact that the lack of awareness and respect for these differences can be interpreted as a demeaning or prejudicial sign.

Black skin color is the result of a high melanin content and can complicate the use of skin color for the assessment of health problems. To diagnose cyanosis effectively, for instance, examine the nailbeds, palms, soles, gums, and under the tongue. The absence of a red tone or glow to the skin can indicate pallor. Petechiae are best detected on the conjunctiva, abdomen, and buccal mucosa.

Hypertension is a prevalent health problem among black Americans and occurs at a higher rate than in the white population. One of the factors responsible for this problem is blunted nocturnal response. Only a minor decline in blood pressure occurs during sleep, which increases the strain on the heart and vessels; this is found to occur in the black population more than any other group. Blood pressure monitoring is an important preventive measure for black clients.

In addition to hypertension, other health conditions are more prevalent in the black population than in the white population. For instance, as compared with the white population (National Center for Health Statistics, 2002), the black population has a higher prevalence of heart disease, cancer, and diabetes, and a higher death rate from these diseases.

In recent years, HIV and AIDS have become the third leading cause of death among African American males (U.S. Centers for Disease Control and Prevention, 2002). The obvious high prevalence of these diseases among black males suggests the need for education and counseling of younger adults in order to promote a healthy age and longevity.

Many causes of morbidity and mortality among black Americans can be prevented and effectively controlled by lifestyle changes (eg, good nutrition, regular exercise, effective stress management) and regular health screening and supervision. These are important considerations in planning health services to communities.

Despite the health problems of aged blacks, their rate of institutionalization is lower than that of the white population: only 12% of elderly black people experience institutional care in their lifetimes compared with 23% of elderly white people.

Native Americans

Native Americans inhabited North America for centuries before Columbus explored the New World. An estimated 1 to 1.5 million Native Americans populated America at the time of the arrival of Columbus; many battles with the new settlers during the next four centuries reduced the Native American population to a quarter million. The Native American population has been steadily increasing, with the U.S. Census Bureau now showing approximately 2.4 million Native American people who belong to more

than 500 recognized tribes, nations, and villages in the United States. Less than half of all Native American people live on reservations, with the highest populations found in Arizona, Oklahoma, California, New Mexico, and Alaska. The Indian Health Service, a division of the United States Public Health Service, provides free, universal access to health care to American Indians who reside on reservations. More than half live in urban areas where access to health care is inferior to that on reservations. An estimated 250 different Native American languages are spoken, although most Native American people claim English to be their first language. Less than 7% of the Native American population is older than 65 years of age, representing less than 1% of all older adults.

Native American people have a strong reverence for the Great Creator. They often link their state of health to good or evil forces or to punishment for their acts. Native American medicine promotes the belief that a person must be balanced with nature for good health and that illness results from imbalance. Spiritual rituals, medicine men, herbs, homemade drugs, and mechanical interventions such as suction cups may be used for the treatment of illness.

> **KEY CONCEPT**
> Spiritual rituals, medicine men, herbs, homemade drugs, and mechanical interventions can be used by Native American people to treat illness.

Close family bonds are typical among the Native American population. Family members may address each other by their family relationship rather than by name (eg, cousin, son, uncle, grandfather). The term *elder* is used to denote social or physical status, not just age. Elders are respected and viewed as leaders, teachers, and advisors to the young, although younger and more "Americanized" members are starting to feel that the advice of their elders is not as relevant in today's world and are breaking with this tradition. Native American people strongly believe that individuals have the right to make decisions affecting their lives. The typical nursing assessment process may be offensive to the Native American patient, who may view probing questions, validation of findings, and documentation of responses as inappropriate and disrespectful behaviors during the verbal exchange. A

Native American patient may be ambivalent about accepting services from agencies and professionals. Such assistance has provided many social, health, and economic benefits to improve the life of Native Americans, but it also conflicts with Native American beliefs of being useful, doing for oneself, and relying on spiritual powers to chart the course of life. Native American patients often remain calm and controlled, even in the most difficult circumstances; it is important that providers not mistake this behavior for the absence of feeling, caring, or discomfort.

Various tribes may have specific rituals that are performed at death, such as burying certain personal possessions with the individual. Consulting with members of the specific tribe to gain insight into special rituals during sickness and at death would be advantageous for nurses working with Native American populations.

Point to Ponder

To what attitudes toward people of different cultures were you exposed as a child and how has this molded your current attitudes?

The last part of the 20th century saw a rise in certain preventable diseases among American Indians, attributable to their exposure to new risks, such as a poor diet, insufficient exercise, and unhealthy lifestyle choices. For example, diabetes, a disease uncommon among American Indians at the start of the 20th century, now affects about one in five older American Indians (compared with about one in ten of all elderly Americans). The relatively recent high prevalence of rheumatoid diseases among American Indians as compared to white elders may be related to a genetic predisposition to autoimmune rheumatic disease. The cancer survival rate among Native Americans is lowest than for any U.S. population. Nurses must promote health education and early screening to aid this population in reducing risks and identifying health conditions early.

Jewish Americans

In the sense that they come from a variety of nations, with different customs and cultures, Jewish people are not an ethnic group per se. However, the strength of the Jewish faith forms a bond that crosses national origin and gives this group a strong sense of identity and shared beliefs.

Luis de Torres, a Jewish man, accompanied Columbus on his voyage to America; however, it was not until 1654 that a group of Sephardic Jews settled in New Amsterdam to formally develop the first Jewish community in America. Immigration continued after that time, with large numbers of German Jews entering America after the revolution of 1848, followed by even greater numbers of Yiddish-speaking Eastern European Jews arriving after the pogroms of 1881. Early life in America was not easy for these Jewish immigrants. They often were faced with employment in factories and homes in tenements, as well as prejudice from several quarters. Despite these rough beginnings, Jewish Americans have demonstrated profound leadership in business, arts, and sciences and have made positive contributions to American life. Scholarship is important in the Jewish culture; more than 80% of all Jewish Americans have attended college. Approximately 6 million Jewish people reside in the United States, representing 2.2% of the total population, with most living in urban areas of the Middle Atlantic states. It is estimated that half of the world's Jewish population resides in America.

Religious traditions are important to most Jewish people (Figure 3-2). Sundown Friday to sundown Saturday is the Sabbath, and medical procedures may be opposed during that time (exceptions may be made for seriously ill individuals). A belief that the head and feet should always be covered may be displayed by the desire to wear a skullcap and socks at all times. Orthodox Jews may oppose shaving. The Kosher diet (eg, exclusion of pork and shellfish, prohibition of serving milk and meat products at the same meal or from the same dishes) is a significant aspect of Jewish religion and may be strictly adhered to by some. Fasting on holy days, such as Yom Kippur and Tisha Bav, and the replacement of matzo for leavened bread during Passover may occur.

Modern medical care is encouraged. Rabbinical consultation may be desired for decisions involving organ transplantation or life-sustaining measures. Certain rituals may be practiced at death, such as members of the religious group washing the body and sitting with it until burial. Autopsy is usually opposed.

Family bonds are strong among Jewish Americans; they have strong and positive feelings for the

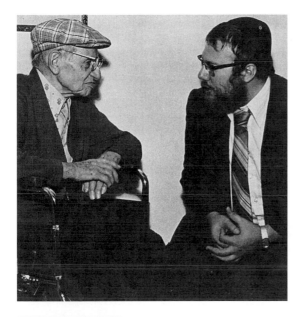

FIGURE 3-2

The rabbi's visit is important for this resident of a geriatric center. (Taylor C., Lillis C., & LeMone P. [2001]. *Fundamentals of nursing: The art & Science of Nursing Care* [4th ed., p. 820]. Philadelphia: Lippincott Williams & Wilkins)

elderly. Illness often draws Jewish families together. Jewish communities throughout the country have shown leadership in developing a network of community and institutional services for their aged, geared toward providing service while preserving Jewish tradition.

Asian Americans

CHINESE AMERICANS

More than 10 million Asian Americans reside in the United States, representing approximately 4% of the population. Although Chinese laborers probably lived in America for centuries before the mid-1800s, it was not until then that large-scale Chinese immigration occurred. During that time, more than 40,000 Chinese people left their homes to escape the horrible drought that China was experiencing and to become part of the gold rush. They were welcomed as cheap labor for the transcontinental railroad construction; at that time 9 of every 10 railroad laborers were "coolies." Most of these Chinese laborers planned to earn large sums of money and then return home or send for their families to join them. Few were able to attain this goal, and they found that the poor economic conditions toward the end of the 19th century made them easy targets for prejudice by persons afraid that these "foreigners" were stealing their jobs; they were left in their new land alone and poor. This immigration pattern explains why older Chinese men in America outnumbered older Chinese women. Prejudice and cultural differences promoted the development of "Chinatowns," which were a comfortable refuge for Chinese people in this country. The largest American Chinese populations are in San Francisco, New York, Los Angeles, Honolulu, and Chicago.

Care of the body and health are of utmost importance to Chinese people, although their approach may be vastly different from that of conventional Western medicine (Display 3-1).

Chinese medicine is based on the belief of the balance of yin and yang; yin is the female negative energy that protects the inner body and yang is the male positive energy that protects the body from external forces. Traditionally, Chinese people have used the senses for assessing medical problems (touching, listening to sounds, detecting odors) rather than machinery or invasive procedures. Herbs, acupuncture, acupressure, and other treatment modalities, which are just being recognized by the Western world, continue to be treatments of choice for many Chinese individuals. These traditional treatments may be selected as alternatives or adjuncts to the use of modern treatment modalities. Ivory figurines of reclining women, now collectors' items, were used by female patients to point to the area of their problems because it was inappropriate for the male physician to touch a woman; although modern Chinese women may have forfeited this practice, they still may be embarrassed to receive a physical examination or care from a man. Typically, disagreement or discomfort is not aggressively or openly displayed by Chinese persons. Nurses may need to observe more closely and ask specific questions (eg, Can you describe your pain? How do you feel about the procedure you are planning to have done? Do you have any questions?) to ensure that the quiet nature of the patient is not misinterpreted to imply that no problems exist.

DISPLAY 3 - 1

Chinese Medicine

For thousands of years the Chinese have practiced a form of medicine that appears very different from what we have come to know in the Western world. It is based on a system of balance; illness is seen as an imbalance and disharmony of the body. One of the theories that explains this balance is that of *yin* and *yang*. *Yin* is the negative, female energy that is represented by that which is soft, dark, cold, and wet. Organs associated with yin qualities include the lungs, kidneys, liver, heart, and spleen. *Yang* is the positive, male energy that is represented by that which is hard, bright, hot, and dry. The gallbladder, small intestine, stomach, colon, and bladder are yang organs. Daytime activity is considered more of a yang state, whereas sleep is more of a yin state.

Chinese medicine also considers the body's balance in relation to the five elements or phases: wood (spring), fire (summer), earth (long summer), metal (autumn), and water (winter).

Qi is the life force that circulates throughout the body in invisible pathways called meridians. A deficiency or blockage of qi can cause symptoms of illnesses. Acupuncture and acupressure can be applied to various points along the meridians to stimulate the flow of qi.

In addition to acupuncture and acupressure, traditional Chinese medicine uses herbs, massage, and therapeutic exercises (such as t'ai chi) to promote a free flow of chi and achieve balance and harmony. These modalities are gaining increasing acceptance in the United States, and research supporting their effectiveness is rapidly increasing.

KEY CONCEPT
Chinese people believe that the female negative energy (yin) and male positive energy (yang) must be in balance.

To Chinese people, achieving old age is a blessing, and the elderly are held in high esteem. They are respected and sought for advice. The family unit is expected to take care of its elder members; thus, there may be a reluctance to use service agencies for the elderly.

JAPANESE AMERICANS

Like the Chinese, Japanese immigration significantly began in the mid-1800s. By the 1890s, more than 25,000 Japanese immigrants lived in America, and American workers' fear of losing their jobs to these newcomers resulted in prejudicial treatment and a restrictive immigration quota at the turn of the last century. The prejudice continued with laws that forbade Japanese Americans to own property and discouraged

the marriage of Japanese people to native-born Americans. Perhaps the worst indignity suffered by this group occurred during World War II, when more than 70,000 American-born Japanese people were confined to "relocation camps"; during this time Japanese people were barred from entering the United States (a restriction that was lifted in 1950). Despite this treatment, Japanese Americans patiently struggled to improve their lives in this country. Traditionally, many Japanese Americans have held jobs as gardeners and farmers, and they, like Chinese Americans, have a lower unemployment rate and higher percentage of professionals than the national average. Today, there are approximately 750,000 Japanese Americans, most of whom live in California and Hawaii.

Although Japanese Americans have not tended to live in isolated pockets to the same extent as Chinese Americans, they have preserved many of their traditions, feel a close bond with one another, and highly value the family. The following terms describe each generation of Japanese American: Issei, first generation (immigrant to America); Nisei, second generation (first American born); Sansei, third generation;

and Yonsei, fourth generation. It is expected that families will take care of their elder members. As in the Chinese culture, the aged are viewed with respect.

The fact that Japanese men were discouraged from marrying American-born women led them to send for brides, often considerably younger than themselves, from their home country. Thus, we see a higher proportion of older Japanese widows in this country.

Similar to the Chinese, Japanese Americans may subscribe to traditional health practices and reject modern technology. They may not express their feelings openly or challenge the health professional; therefore, nursing sensitivity to covert needs is crucial.

OTHER ASIAN GROUPS

In the early 1700s Filipino people began immigrating to America, but most Filipino immigrants arrived in the early 1900s to work as farm laborers. In 1934, an annual immigration quota of 50 was enacted; this quota stayed in place until 1965.

In the early 1900s, Korean people immigrated to America to work on plantations. Many of these individuals settled in Hawaii. Another large influx of Koreans, many of whom were wives of servicemen, immigrated after the Korean War.

The most recent Asian American immigrants have been from Vietnam and Cambodia. Most of these individuals came to the United States to seek political refuge after the Vietnam War.

Although differences among various Asian American groups exist, some similarities are strong family networks and the expectation that family members will care for their elders at home.

> ### ☑ Point to Ponder
> *In what ways do you honor and celebrate your unique heritage?*

Hispanic Americans

The term Hispanic encompasses a variety of Spanish-speaking persons in America, including Spaniards, Mexicans, Cubans, and Puerto Ricans. Hispanic people now represent approximately 6% of the older pop-ulation. The peak immigration periods for each Hispanic subgroup differ. In 1513, Ponce de León discovered and claimed Florida for the King of Spain; in 1565, the Spanish founded the first permanent European colony in America in St. Augustine, Florida. The Spanish held claim to Florida for nearly two centuries, until they traded it for Cuba and the Philippines. Most Spanish immigrants settled in Florida and the southwest. Today, there are approximately 250,000 Spanish Americans living in the United States.

Although Mexican people inhabited the Southwest for decades before the arrival of the Pilgrims, most Mexican immigration occurred during the 20th century as a result of the Mexican Revolution and the poor economic conditions in Mexico. The Mexican population in this country totals more than 8 million, plus an estimated 3 to 5 million illegal immigrants; the majority reside in California and Texas.

Most Puerto Rican immigration occurred after the United States granted citizenship to all Puerto Ricans. After World War II, nearly one third of all Puerto Rico's inhabitants immigrated to America; in the 1970s "reverse immigration" began as growing numbers of Puerto Rican people left the United States to return to their home island. An estimated 1 million Puerto Ricans live in New York City, where most of them have settled.

Most Cuban immigrants are recent newcomers to America; the majority of the greater than 1 million Cuban Americans fled Cuba after Castro seized power. More than 25% of the Cuban American population resides in Florida, with other large groups in New York and New Jersey. Among all Hispanics, Cuban people are the most highly educated and have the highest earnings.

Many Hispanic people view states of health and illness as the actions of God; by treating one's body with respect, living a good life, and praying, one will be rewarded by God with good health. Illness results when one has violated good practices of living or is being punished by God. Medals and crosses may be worn at all times to facilitate well-being, and prayer plays an important part in the healing process. Illness may be viewed as a family affair, with multiple family members involved with the care of the sick individual. Rather than using practitioners of Western medicine to treat their health problems, some Hispanic persons may prefer traditional practitioners, such as:

- Curranderos: women who have special knowledge and charismatic qualities
- Sobadoras: persons who give massages and manipulate bones and muscles
- Espiritualistas: persons who analyze dreams, cards, and premonitions
- Brujos: women who control witchcraft
- Senoras: older women who have learned special healing measures

The Hispanic population holds older relatives in high esteem. Old age is viewed as a positive time in which the aged person can reap the harvest of his or her life. Hispanic people expect that children will take care of their elder parents, and families try to avoid institutionalization at all costs. Indeed, this group has a lower rate of nursing home use than the general population.

Nurses may find that English is a second language to Hispanic people, which becomes particularly apparent during periods of illness when stress causes a retreat to the native tongue.

Elderly Prisoners

In addition to belonging to various ethnic groups, older adults can be part of unique subcultures that set them apart from society, as is the case with prison inmates. It is estimated that inmates age 50 and older make up 11% of the prison population (Pfeffer, 2002). Prison inmates in general tend to have poorer health status than their cohorts in the community, attributable to poor socioeconomic status and inaccessibility to health care. The stress of imprisonment adds to their poor health status. These realities, combined with the increased prevalence of chronic conditions with advanced age, result in a significant health challenges for elderly prisoners. Unfortunately, the quality of diet, physical environment, and medical care within prisons is not the same as that found in the community. Professionals with expertise in geriatrics and health care settings to address the unique needs of disabled elders are lacking within the prison setting.

Gerontological nurses are challenged to address the growing needs of nursing care of imprisoned elders. Proactive actions could include offering expertise to local prison health units in the form of educational programs and consultation, mobilization of nurse and other types of volunteers to assist elder prisoners, and advocacy for adequate standards of gerontological nursing care in these settings.

Nursing Considerations

Numerous ethnic groups that have not been mentioned also possess unique histories, beliefs, and practices. Rather than viewing ethnic differences as odd and forcing patients to conform to "American" traditions, nurses should respect the beauty of this diversity and make every effort to preserve it. Dietary preferences should be accommodated, adaptations made for special practices, and unique ways of managing illness understood. If nurses are unfamiliar with a particular ethnic group, they should invite family members to educate them or contact churches or ethnic associations (eg, Polish American Alliance, Celtic League, Jewish Family and Children's Society, Slovak League of America) for interpreters or persons who can serve as cultural resources. One powerful means to learn about cultural influences for individual patients is to ask them to describe their life stories (see Chapter 4). Nurses convey sensitivity and caring when they try to recognize and support patients' ethnic backgrounds. Nurses also will become enriched by gaining an appreciation and understanding of the many various interesting ethnic groups.

The U.S. Department of Health and Human Services has developed standards for culturally and linguistically appropriate services that can guide clinical settings in working with diverse populations that can be accessed on their website at http://www.omhrc.gov/CLAS/indexfinal.htm.

> **KEY CONCEPT**
> In the future, the percentage of white elders will decrease as society experiences a growth in minority seniors.

Population projections support the continued ethnic diversity of the group over age 60. As the percentage of white elders decreases, there will be a rise in minority seniors, particularly among Hispanics, black Americans, and Asians. Greater differences will be seen among future aged populations and will affect services in a variety of ways. Among the needs that could present are:

- institutional meal planning that incorporates ethnic foods
- multilingual health education literature
- readily available translators

- provisions for celebration of holidays (eg, Chinese New Year, St. Patrick's Day, Black History Month, Greek Orthodox Easter)
- special-interest groups for residents of long-term care facilities

Nurses need to ensure that cultural differences of elders are understood, appreciated, and respected.

Critical Thinking Exercises

1. What are some reasons for the elderly of minority groups to be suspicious or distrustful of health care services in this country?
2. What would you do if faced with a situation in which an older client refused to allow you to provide nursing care for him because you are of a different ethnic or racial group?
3. Mrs. Chang is a very traditional Chinese woman who began living with her son and daughter-in-law 3 years ago, after her husband's death. Mrs. Chang and her husband had lived in a "Chinatown" part of the city where they could freely communicate in Chinese and interact with other Chinese individuals. She never developed fluency in English and had experienced considerable difficulty communicating with neighbors since moving into her son's suburban community. Mrs. Chang's son has assimilated American values and practices and has been critical of his mother for her traditional ways; he would not acknowledge her when she spoke in Chinese and refused to allow her to cook Chinese foods. His wife is not Chinese but has been sympathetic to the elder Mrs. Chang.

   Last week Mrs. Chang suffered a stroke that left her with weakness and some aphasia. She will require care and supervision. Mrs. Chang's son states that he does not want his mother in a nursing home, but that he is not sure he can manage her; his wife says she is willing to take a leave of absence from work and help care for her mother-in-law, if that is what her husband wants.

   What problems do you anticipate for each of the Chang family members? What can be arranged to assist this family? How could you assist Mrs. Chang in preserving her ethnic practices?

Web Connect

Select your own ethnic group or another one in which you are interested and explore the issues relevant to its older population by conducing a search for "_____ elderly" (eg, Greek elderly, French elderly)

● Resources

Bureau of Indian Affairs
www.doi.gov/bureau-indian-affairs.html
National Asian Pacific Center on Aging
1511 Third Avenue
Suite 914
Seattle, WA 98101
(800)33-NACPA
www.nacpa.org

National Association for Hispanic Elderly
234 East Colorado Boulevard
Suite 300
Pasadena, CA 91101
(800) 953-8553
www.aoa.dhhs.gov/directory/139.html

National Center on Black Aged
1220 L Street NW
Suite 800
Washington, DC 20005
(202) 637-8400
www.ncba-aged.org

National Hispanic Council on Aging
2713 Ontario Road NW
Washington, DC 20009
(202) 265-1288
www.nhcoa.org

National Indian Council on Aging
6400 Uptown Boulevard NE
Suite 510W
Albuquerque, NM 87110
(505) 888-3276
www.nicoa.org

National Resource Center on Native American Aging
P.O. Box 7090
Grand Forks, ND 58202
(800) 896-7628
www.und.nodak.edu/dept/nrcnaa

Office of Minority Health Resource Center
P.O. Box 37337
Washington, DC 20013
(800) 444-6472
www.omhrc.gov

Organization of Chinese Americans
1001 Connecticut Avenue NW
Washington, DC 20036
(202) 223-5500
www.ocanatl.org

● References

Keegan , L. (2000). A comparison of the use of alternative therapies among Mexican americans and Anglo-Americans in the Texas Rio Grande Valley. *Journal of Holistic Nursing, 18*(3), 280–293.

National Center for Health Statistics. (2002). Rates of illness by age, sex, and race. Data Warehouse on *Trends in Aging.* http://www.cdc.gov/nchs/agingact.htm.

Pfeffer, S. (2002). One strike against the elderly: Growing old in prison, *Medill News Service,* August 2002. Retrieved May 25, 2003, from www.journalism.medill.northwestern.edu/docket/01-1127aging.html

U.S. Centers for Disease Control and Prevention. (2002). Table No. 176, AIDS cases reported by patient characteristics, 1981–2001. *HIV/AIDS Surveillance Report, Volume 13, No. 2.*

● Recommended Readings

American Association of Homes and Services for the Aging. (1995). Diversity outlook. *Currents, 10*(9), A–D.

Armer , J. M., & Conn, S. C. (2001). Exploration of spirituality and health among diverse rural elderly individuals. *Journal of Gerontological Nursing, 27*(6), 28–37.

Baker , D. P. (1999) *Virginia opens special prison for aging inmates* (web page). Retrieved August 8, 2000, from http://www.dallasnews.com/national/0703nat4prison.htm

Barsa, B. R. N. (1998). *The independence of urban Hispanic elderly: The growing need for social support networks.* New York: Garland.

Burggraf, V. (2000). The older woman: Witchnicity and health. *Geriatric Nursing, 21*(4), 183–187.

Burlingame, V. S. (1999). *Ethnogerocounseling: Counseling ethnic elders and their families.* New York: Springer.

Chinn, S. L. (2000). Culturally competent health care. *Public Health Reports, 115,* 25–33.

Chow, R.K. (2002). Initiating a long-term care nursing service for aging inmates. *Geriatric Nursing, 23*(1), 24–27.

Delgado, M. (1998). *Latino elders and the Twenty-First Century: Issues and challenges for culturally competent research and practice.* New York: Haworth Press.

Enslein, J., Tripp-Reimer, T., Kelley, L. S., & McCarty, L. (2002). Evidence-based protocol. Interpreter facilitation for individuals with limited English proficiency. *Journal of Gerontological Nursing, 28*(7), 5–13.

Good , M., Picot, B. L., & Salem, S. G., et al. (2000). Cultural differences in music chosen for pain relief. *Journal of Holistic Nursing, 18*(3), 245–260.

Johnson , R. A. and Tripp-Reimer, T. (2001a). Aging, ethnicity, and social support: A review. *Journal of Gerontological Nursing, 27*(6), 15–21.

Johnson, R. A., & Tripp-Reimer, T. (2001b). Relocation among ethnic elders: A review. *Journal of Gerontological Nursing, 27*(6), 22–27.

Leininger, M. (1995). *Transcultural nursing: Concepts, theories, research and practices.* New York: McGraw-Hill.

Lipson, J. G., Dibble, S. L., & Minarik, P. A. (1996). *Culture and nursing care: A pocket guide.* San Francisco: UCSF Nursing Press.

Litwin, H. (Ed.). (1996). *Social networks of older people: A cross-national analysis.* Westport, CT: Praeger.

Lyons, B. P. (1997). *Sociocultural differences between American-born and West Indian-born elderly blacks: A comparative study of health and social service use.* New York: Garland.

Stegbauer, C. C., Engle, V. F., & Graney, M. J. (1995). Admission health status differences of black and white indigent nursing home residents. *Journal of the American Geriatric Society, 43*(10), 1103–1106.

St. Clair, A., & McKenry, L. (1999). Preparing culturally competent practitioners. *Journal of Nursing Education, 38*(5), 228–234.

Sterritt, P. F., & Pokorny, M. E. (1998). African-American caregiving for a relative with Alzheimer's disease. *Geriatric Nursing, 19,* 127–134.

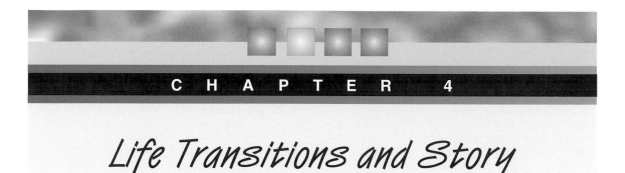

CHAPTER 4

Life Transitions and Story

■ Chapter Outline

Role changes
Adjustments faced as children become independent
Shift in roles and responsibilities
Ageism
Societal prejudice
Advocating for realistic understanding of aged and aging
Grandparenting
Impact of changing family structures and lifestyles
Grandparenthood as a learned behavior
Widowhood
New responsibilities faced
Adjustments
Retirement
Impact of loss of work on status, roles, and identity
Multiple losses faced with retirement
Phases of retirement
Awareness of mortality
Reality of mortality with advancing age
Significance of life review and reminiscence
Increasing health risks
Adjustments related to body image and roles
Variation in acceptance among individuals
Reduced income
Lack of financial security

Readjustments in lifestyle
Importance of pre-retirement planning
Shrinking social world
Death and relocation of significant others
Geographic or self-imposed isolation
Loneliness versus solitude
Life story

■ Learning Objectives

After reading this chapter, you should be able to:

- discuss changes that occur in aging families
- list challenges faced by widows
- outline the phases of retirement
- discuss the impact of age-related changes on roles
- describe changes in one's social world with aging
- list nursing measures to assist individuals in adjusting to the challenges of aging

Growing old is not easy. Various changes during the aging process demand multiple adjustments that require stamina, ability, and flexibility. Frequently, more simultaneous changes are experienced in old age than during any other

35

period of life. Many young adults find it exhausting to keep pace with technological advances, societal changes, cost-of-living fluctuations, and labor market trends. Imagine how complex and complicated life can be for older individuals, who must also face retirement, reduced income, possible housing changes, frequent losses through deaths of significant persons, and a declining ability to function. Further, each of these life events can be accompanied by role changes that can influence behavior, attitudes, status, and psychological integrity. To promote awareness and appreciation of the complex and arduous adjustments involved, this chapter considers some of the factors that affect the successful coping with the multiple changes associated with aging and the achievement of satisfaction and well-being during the later years.

Role Changes

The dynamic parental role frequently changes to meet the growth and development needs of both parent and child. During middle and later life, parents must adjust to the independence of their children as they become responsible adult citizens and leave home. The first child usually leaves home and establishes an independent unit 22 to 25 years after the parents married. For persons who have invested most of their adult lives nurturing and providing for their offspring, a child's independence may have significant impact. Although parents who are freed from the responsibilities and worries of rearing children have more time to pursue their own interests, they are also freed from the meaningful, purposeful, and satisfying activities associated with childrearing, and this frequently results in a profound sense of loss.

Today's older woman has been influenced by a historical period that emphasized the role of wife and mother. For instance, to provide job opportunities for men returning from World War II, women were encouraged to focus their interests on raising a family and to forfeit the scarce jobs to men. Unlike many of today's younger women, who combine (and sometimes equally value) employment and motherhood, these women centered their lives on their families, from which they derived their sense of fulfillment. Having developed few roles from which to achieve satisfaction other than that of wife and mother, many of these older women feel a void when their children

are grown and gone. Compounding this problem, the highly mobile lifestyle of many young persons limits the degree of direct contact she has with her adult children and with her grandchildren.

The older man shares many of the same feelings as his wife. Throughout the years, he feels he has performed useful functions that made him a valuable member of society. He may have fought for his country in indisputably honorable wars. Most likely, he worked hard to support his wife and children, and his masculinity was reinforced with proof of his ability to beget and provide for offspring. With his children grown, he is no longer required to provide—a mixed blessing in which he may find both relief and purposelessness (Fig. 4-1). In addition, he learns that the rules have changed—his pride in being a war hero may have been shattered by antiwar advocates, his ability to support a family without the need for his wife to work is now viewed by some as oppressive, his efforts to replenish the earth are scorned by today's zero-population proponents, and his attempt to fill the masculine role for which he was socialized is considered macho or inane by today's standards.

The emergence of today's nuclear family units changed the roles and functions of the individuals in a family. The elderly are expected to have limited input into the lives of their adult children. Children are not required to meet the needs of their aging parents

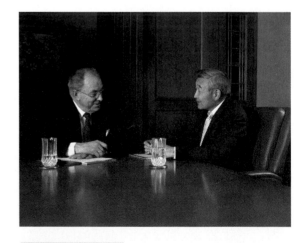

FIGURE 4-1

People who defined self by their work role may have difficulty adjusting to retirement.

for financial support, health services, or housing. Moreover, parents increasingly do not depend on their children for their needs, and the belief that children are the best insurance for old age is fading. In addition, grandparenting, although satisfying, is not usually an active role, especially because grandchildren may be scattered throughout the country. These changes in family structure and function are not necessarily negative. Most children do not abandon or neglect their aging parents; they maintain regular contact. Separate family units may help the parent–child relationship develop on a more adult-to-adult basis, to the mutual satisfaction of young and old. Although the advantages of nuclear family living are often seen primarily as a benefit to younger adults, older adults also enjoy the independence and freedom from responsibilities that nuclear family life offers.

> ✔ **Point to Ponder**
> *List at least three ways that your life is different from the lives of your parents and grandparents.*

Ageism

Ageism is a concept introduced several decades ago and is defined as "the prejudices and stereotypes that are applied to older people sheerly on the basis of their age . . . " (Butler, Lewis, & Sutherland, 1991). It is not difficult to detect overt ageism in our society. Rather than showing appreciation for the vast contributions of the aged and their wealth of resources, society is beset with prejudices and lacks adequate provisions for them, thus derogating their dignity. The same members of society who object to providing sufficient income and health care benefits for the elderly enjoy an affluence and standard of living that was the result of the efforts of those older persons.

Although the elderly constitute the most diverse and individualized age group within the entire population, they continue to be stereotyped by the following misconceptions:

- Old people are sick and disabled.
- Most old people are in nursing homes.
- Senility comes with old age.
- People either get very tranquil or very cranky as they age.

- Old people have lower intelligence and are resistant to change.
- Old people are not able to have sexual intercourse and are not interested in sex anyhow
- There are few satisfactions in old age.

For a majority of older persons, the above statements are not true. Increased efforts are necessary to heighten societal awareness of the realities of aging. Groups such as the Gray Panthers have done an outstanding job of informing the public about the facts regarding aging and the problems and rights of older adults. More advocates for the elderly are needed.

Ageism carries several consequences. By separating the elderly from themselves, people are less likely to see the similarities between themselves and older adults. This not only leads to a lack of understanding of the elderly, but also reduces the opportunities for the young to gain realistic insights into aging. Further, separating the elderly from the rest of society makes it easier to minimize the socioeconomic challenges of the older population. Unfortunately, systematically stereotyping and discriminating against the elderly won't prevent individuals from growing old themselves and experiencing the challenges of old age.

Chapter 2 outlines Erikson's (1963) stages of life in which he describes the last stage of the life cycle as concerned with achieving integrity versus despair. Integrity results when the older individual derives satisfaction from an evaluation of his or her life. Disappointment with life and the lack of opportunities to alter the past bring despair. The experiences of our entire lifetime determine whether our old age will be an opportunity for freedom, growth, and contentment or a miserable imprisonment of our human potential.

Grandparenting

Americans' extended life expectancy enables more people to experience the role of grandparent and spend more years in that role than previous generations. More than 90 million Americans, one in three individuals, is a grandparent (AARP, 2002).

Grandchildren can bring considerable joy and meaning to the lives of elders. (Fig. 4-2). In turn, grandparents who are not burdened with the same daily childrearing responsibilities of parents can offer love, guidance, and enjoyment to the family's young.

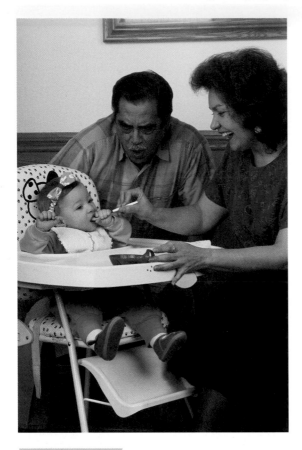

FIGURE 4-2

Grandparenting offers new roles and joys for many elders.

They can share lessons learned from their life experiences and family history and traditions that help the young understand their roots. There can be as many grandparenting styles as there are personalities; there is no single model of grandparenthood. (**Visit the Connection website to learn more about grandparent's gifts to grandchildren.**)

Changes in family structure and activities present new challenges to today's grandparents. Most mothers are employed outside of the home. As a result, grandparents may assume childcare responsibilities to a greater extent than previous generations did. This is compounded by the fact that approximately one-third of children are being raised by one parent. In addition to childcare, grandparents may provide a home

for their children and grandchilren. Also, some elders' grandchildren are being raised in a homosexual household, because an estimated 8 to 10 million children have gay and lesbian parents (Spock, 2002). New family compositions can arise through remarriages: more than one third of minor children live in blended households. As a result of their child's marriage, elders may find themselves becoming step-grandparents, a role for which few are prepared. Conscious choices will be needed to love and accept these new family members.

In addition to elders having to adapt to new family lifestyles and structures, children and grandchildren may need to adapt to grandparents who have different lifestyles from previous generations. Rather than the stay-at-home grandma who cooked elaborate family dinners and welcomed grandchildren whenever they needed a sitter, today's grandmother may have an active career and social calendar and not want to be burdened with frequent babysitting responsibilities or hosting of family functions. Grandparents may be divorced, causing their children and grandchildren to face issues such as grandmother's weekend trips with her new male friend or grandpop's new, much younger wife. The family may need to be referred for counseling to help them address these issues.

More than 4.5 million children are being raised by their grandparents, representing more than 6% of all children, and many more live with their grandparents off and on; a grandparent is raising a grandchild in an estimated 1 in 20 households (AARP, 2003). Caregiving often arises out of crises with the child's parents, such as substance abuse, teen pregnancy, or incarceration. Elders may need help thinking through the implications of deciding to raise a grandchild; some questions that nurses can raise with grandparents contemplating this decision include:

- How will raising this child affect your own health, marriage, and lifestyle?
- Have you any health conditions that could interfere with this responsibility?
- What is your back-up plan in the event that you become ill or disabled?
- Do you have the energy and physical health required to care for an active child?
- Can you afford to care for the child, pay medical and educational expenses, and the like?

- What rights and responsibilities will the child's parent(s) have?
- Do you have the legal right to serve as a surrogate parent (eg, to give consent for medical procedures)? Have you consulted with an attorney?

Organizations exist to assist grandparents who are raising grandchildren. Such organizations are listed at the end of this chapter.

Grandparenthood is a learned role and some elders may need guidance to become effective grandparents. Elders may need to be guided in thinking through issues such as:

- respecting their children as parents and not interfering in the parent–child relationship
- calling before visiting
- establishing rules for babysitting
- allowing their children to establish their own traditions within their family and not expecting them to adhere to the grandparent's traditions

Nurses can help families locate resources that can assist in meeting the challenges of grandparenting. Also, nurses can suggest activities that can help grandparents be connected with their grandchildren, particularly if they are not geographically close; these can include audio and video tapes, e-mails, faxes, and handwritten letters. (In addition to offering a means of communication, these can provide lasting memories that can be passed from one generation to another.) Elders can be encouraged to keep diaries, scrapbooks, and notebooks of family recipes and customs that can help their grandchildren and future generations have special insights into their ancestors.

Widowhood

The death of a spouse is a common event that alters family life for many older persons. The loss of that individual with whom one has shared more love and life experiences and more joys and sorrows than anyone else may be intolerable. How, after many decades of living with another human being, does one adjust to the sudden absence of that person? How does one adjust to setting the table for one, to coming home to an empty house, or to not touching that warm, familiar body in bed? Adjustment to this significant loss is coupled with the demand to learn the new task of living alone.

The death of a spouse affects more women than men because most older men are married and most older women become widows—a situation that is expected to continue in the future (Fig. 4-3). In fact, most women will be widowed by the time they reach their eighth decade of life. Unlike many of today's younger women, who have greater independence through careers and changed norms, most of today's older women have led family-oriented lives and have been dependent on their husbands. Their age, limited education, lack of skills, and long period of unemployment while raising their families are handicaps in a competitive job market. If these women can find employment, adjusting to the new demands of work may be difficult and stressful. On the other hand, the unemployed widow may learn that pensions or other sources of income may be reduced or discontinued when the husband dies, necessitating an adjustment to an extremely limited budget. In addition to financial dependence, the woman may have depended on her husband's achievements to provide her with gratification and identity. Frequently, the achievements of children serve this same purpose. Sexual desires may be unfulfilled because of lack of opportunity, religious beliefs regarding sex outside marriage, fear of

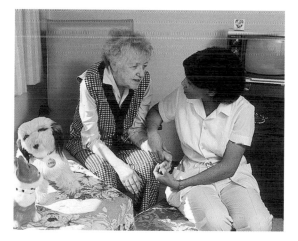

FIGURE 4-3

Death of a spouse affects more women than men. (Taylor C., Lillis C., & LeMone P. [2001]. *Fundamentals of nursing: The art & Science of Nursing Care* [4th ed., p. 201]. Philadelphia: Lippincott Williams & Wilkins)

repercussion from children and society, or residual attitudes from early teachings about sexual mores. If a woman's marriage promoted friendships with other married couples and only inactive relationships with single friends, the new widow may find that her number of single female friends is small.

For the most part, when the initial grief of the husband's death passes, most widows adjust quite well. The high proportion of older women who are widowed provides an availability of friends who share similar problems and lifestyles, especially in urban areas. Old friendships may be revived to provide sources of activity and enjoyment. Some widows may discover that the loss of certain responsibilities associated with their partner's death, such as cooking and laundering, brings them a new, pleasant freedom. With alternative roles to develop, sufficient income, and choice over lifestyle, many women are able to make a successful adjustment to widowhood. Nurses may facilitate this adjustment by identifying sources of friendships and activities such as clubs, volunteer organizations, or groups of widows in the community, and by helping the widow understand and obtain all the benefits to which she is entitled. This may require reassuring her that enjoying her new freedom and desiring relationships with other men is no reason to feel guilty and supporting her as she learns to adjust to the loss of her husband and the new role of widow. (See Chapter 41 for more information on death and dying.)

> **KEY CONCEPT**
> The high prevalence of widows provides a pool of friends who share similar challenges and lifestyles.

Retirement

One of the major adjustments of an aging individual is the loss of a work role through retirement. For many, this role transition is the first experience of the impact of aging. Retirement is especially difficult in our society, in which worth is commonly judged by an individual's productivity. Work is often viewed as the dues required for active membership in a productive society. The attitude that unemployment, for whatever reason, is an undesirable state is adhered to by many of today's older persons, who were raised under the omnipresent cloud of the Puritan work ethic.

> **KEY CONCEPT**
> Work is often viewed as the dues required for active membership in a productive society.

Occupational identity is largely responsible for an individual's social position and for the social role attached to that position. Although individuals function differently in similar roles, some behaviors continue to be associated with certain roles, which promote stereotypes. Certain stereotypes continue to be heard frequently—the tough construction worker, the wild exotic dancer, the fair judge, the righteous clergyman, the learned lawyer, and the eccentric artist. The realization that these associations are not consistently valid does not prevent their propagation. Too frequently, individuals are described in terms of their work role rather than their personal characteristics, for example, "the nurse who lives down the road" or "my son the doctor." Considering the extent to which social identity and behavioral expectations are derived from the work role, it is not surprising that an individual's identity is threatened when retirement occurs. During childhood and adolescence we are guided toward an independent, responsible adult role, and in academic settings we are prepared for our professional roles, but where and when are we prepared for the role of retiree?

> **Point to Ponder**
> *What do you derive, or think you will derive, from being a nurse in terms of purpose, identity, values, relationships, activities, and so on? What similar gains are you achieving from other roles in your life?*

Gerontological nursing is concerned with the welfare of both the current aged population and future ones. A lifetime of poor health care practices is a handicap that cannot be remedied in old age. Assisting aging individuals with their retirement preparations is preventive intervention that enhances the potential for health and well-being in old age. As a part of such intervention, aging individuals should be encouraged to establish and practice good health habits such as following a proper diet; avoiding alcohol, drug, and tobacco abuse; and having regular physical examinations.

When one's work is one's primary interest, activity, and source of social contacts, separation from work leaves a significant void in one's life. Aging individuals should be urged to develop interests unrelated to work. Retirement is facilitated by learning how to use, appreciate, and gain satisfaction from leisure time throughout an employed lifetime. In addition, enjoying leisure time is a therapeutic outlet for life stresses throughout the aging process.

> 🔑 **KEY CONCEPT**
> When work is one's primary interest, activity, and source of social contacts, separation from work leaves a significant void in one's life.

Gerontological nurses must understand the realities and reactions encountered when working with retired persons. Although the experience of retirement is unique for each individual, some reactions and experiences tend to be fairly common. The phases of retirement described by Robert Atchley decades ago continue to offer insight into this complicated process (Atchley, 1975):

- *Remote phase.* Early in the occupational career, future retirement is anticipated, but rational preparation is seldom done.
- *Near phase.* When the reality of retirement is evident, preparation for leaving one's job begins, as does fantasy regarding the retirement role.
- *Honeymoon phase.* Following the retirement event, a somewhat euphoric period begins, in which fantasies from the preretirement phase are tested. Retirees attempt to do everything they never had time for simultaneously. A variety of factors (eg, finances, health) limit this, leading to the development of a stable lifestyle.
- *Disenchantment phase.* As life begins to stabilize, a letdown, sometimes a depression, is experienced. The more unrealistic the preretirement fantasy, the greater the degree of disenchantment.
- *Reorientation phase.* As realistic choices and alternative sources of satisfaction are considered, the disenchantment with the new retirement routine can be replaced by developing a lifestyle that provides some satisfaction.
- *Stability phase.* An understanding of the retirement role is achieved, and this provides a framework for concern, involvement, and action in the elderly person's life. Some enter this phase directly after the honeymoon phase, and some never reach it at all.
- *Termination phase.* The retirement role is lost as a result of either the resumption of a work role or dependency due to illness or disability.

It is obvious that different nursing interventions may be required during each phase. Some of the preretirement planning recommendations discussed earlier can be used during the remote phase. Counseling regarding the realities of retirement may be part of the near phase, whereas helping retirees place their newfound freedom into proper perspective may be warranted during the honeymoon phase. Being supportive of retirees during the disenchantment phase without fostering self-pity and helping them identify new sources of satisfaction may facilitate the reorientation process. Appreciating and promoting the strengths of the stability phase may reinforce an adjustment to retirement. When the retirement phase is terminated due to disease or disability, the tactful management of dependency and the respectful appreciation of losses are extremely important.

Nurses' evaluations of their own attitudes toward retirement are beneficial. Does the nurse see retirement as a period of freedom, opportunity, and growth or as one of loneliness, dependency, and meaninglessness? Is the nurse intelligently planning for her own retirement or denying it by avoiding encounters with retirement realities? Nurses' views of retirement affect the retiree–nurse relationship. Gerontological nurses can provide especially good models of constructive retirement practices and attitudes.

Awareness of Mortality

Widowhood, the death of friends, and the recognition of declining functions heighten older persons' awareness of the reality of their own death. During their early years, individuals intellectually understand they will not live forever, but their behaviors often deny this reality. The lack of a will and burial plans may be indications of this denial. As the reality of mortality becomes acute with advancing age, interest in fulfilling dreams, deepening religious convictions, strengthening family ties, providing for the ongoing welfare of family, and leaving a legacy are often apparent signs.

The significance of a life review in interpreting and refining our past experiences as they relate to our self-concept and help us understand and accept our life history has been well discussed (Butler & Lewis, 1982; Webster & Haight, 2002). Rather than being a pathologic behavior, discussing the past is therapeutic and important for the elderly. The thought of impending death may be more tolerable if people understand that their life has had depth and meaning. Unresolved guilt, unachieved aspirations, perceived failures, and other multitudinous aspects of "unfinished business" may be better understood and perhaps resolved. Although the condition of old age may provide limited opportunities for excitement and achievement, satisfaction may be gained in knowing that there were achievements and excitements in other periods of life (Fig. 4-4). The old woman may be frail and wrinkled, but she can still delight in remembering how she once drove young men wild. The retired old man may feel that he is useless to society now, but he realizes his worth through the memory of wars he fought to protect his country and the pride he feels in knowing he supported his family through a depression.

The young can benefit from the reminiscences of the aged by gaining a new perspective on life as they learn about their ancestry. Imagine the impact of hearing about slavery, immigration, epidemics, industrialization, or wars from an older relative who has been part of that history. What history book's description of the Great Depression can compare with hearing a grandparent describe events one's own family experienced, such as going to bed hungry at night? In addition to their place in the future, the young can fully realize their link with the past when the desire of the elderly to reminisce is appreciated and fostered.

> **KEY CONCEPT**
> Reminiscence is not only therapeutic for the elderly, but connects the young listener with the past.

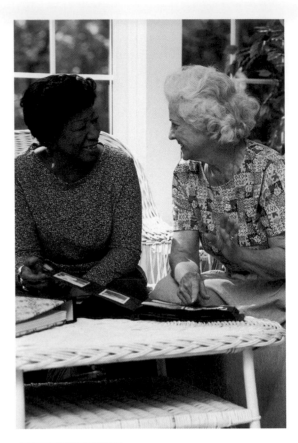

FIGURE 4-4

Reminiscing is a culturally universal phenomenon of aging. It is a way for the older adult to reassess life experiences and further develop a sense of accomplishment, fulfillment, and reward in life.

Older persons should be encouraged to discuss and analyze the dynamics of their lives, and listeners should be receptive and accepting. Poems and autobiographies, as unsophisticated as they may be, should be recognized as significant legacies from the old to the young. One 71-year-old man started a family scrapbook for each of his children. Any photograph, newspaper article, or announcement pertaining to any family member was reproduced and included in every album. The family patiently tolerated this activity and reluctantly sent him copies of graduation programs and photographs for every scrapbook. The family viewed the main value of this activity as providing something benign to keep him occupied. It was not until years after his death that the significance of this great task was appreciated as a priceless gift. Such tangible items may serve as an assurance to both young and old that the impact of an aged relative's life will not cease at death.

Increasing Health Risks

The obvious changes in appearance and bodily function that occur during the aging process make it necessary for the aging individual to adjust to a new body image. Colorful soft hair turns gray and dry, flexible straight fingers become bent and painful, body contours are altered, and height decreases. Stairs once climbed several times daily demand more time and energy to negotiate as the years accumulate. As subtle, gradual, and natural as these changes may be, they are recognized and, consequently, body image and self-concept are affected.

The manner in which individuals perceive themselves and function can determine the roles they play. A construction worker who has reduced strength and energy may forfeit his work role; a club member who cannot hear conversations may cease attending meetings; fashion models may stop seeking jobs when they perceive themselves as old. Interestingly, some persons well into their seventh and eighth decades refuse to join a senior citizen club and accept the role associated with being a member of such a club because they do not perceive themselves as being old. The nurse will gain insight into the self-concept of older persons by evaluating what roles they are willing to accept and what roles they reject.

> **🔑 KEY CONCEPT**
> Insights into an elder's self-concept can be gained by examining the roles that are accepted and rejected.

It is sometimes difficult for the aging person to accept the body's declining efficiency. Poor memory, slow response, easy fatigue, and altered appearance are among the many frustrating results of declining function, and they are dealt with in various ways. Some older people deny them and often demonstrate poor judgment in an attempt to make the same demands on their bodies as they did when younger. Others try to resist these changes by investing in cosmetic surgery, beauty treatments, miracle drugs, and other expensive endeavors that diminish the budget but not the normal aging process. Still others exaggerate these effects and impose an unnecessarily restricted lifestyle on themselves. Societal expectations frequently determine the adjustment individuals make to declining function.

Common results of declining function are illness and disability. As described in Chapter 1, most older people have one or more chronic diseases, and more than one third have a serious disability that limits major activities such as work and housekeeping. The elderly often fear that their illness or disability may cause them to lose their independence. Becoming a burden to their family, being unable to meet the demands of daily living, and having to enter a nursing home are some of the fears associated with dependency. Children and parents may have difficulty exchanging dependent-independent roles. The physical pain arising from an illness may not be as intolerable as the dependency it causes.

Nurses should help aging persons understand and face the common changes associated with advanced age. Factors that promote optimum function should be encouraged, including proper diet; paced activity; regular physical examination; early correction of health problems; effective stress management; and avoidance of alcohol, tobacco, and drug abuse. Assistance should be offered, with attention to preserving as much of the individual's independence and dignity as possible.

Reduced Income

Financial resources are important at any age because they affect our diet, health, housing, safety, and independence, and influence many of our choices in life. The economic profile of many older persons is poor. Retirement income is less than half the income earned while fully employed. For a majority of the elderly, Social Security income, originally intended as a supplement, is actually the primary source of retirement income—and even it has not kept pace with inflation.

Only a minority of the older population has income from a private pension plan, and those who do often discover that the fixed benefits established when the plan was subscribed are meager by today's standards because of inflation. Of the workers who are currently active in the labor force, more than half will not have pension plans when they retire. More than one in six of all older adults live in poverty; only a minority are fully employed or financially comfortable. Few elderly persons have accumulated enough assets during their lifetime to provide financial security in old age.

A reduction in income is a significant adjustment for many older persons because it triggers other adjustments. For instance, an active social life and leisure pursuits may have to be markedly reduced or eliminated. Relocation to less expensive housing may be necessary, possibly forcing the aged to break many family and community ties. Dietary practices may be severely altered, and health care may be viewed as a luxury over which other basic expenses, such as food and rent, take priority. If the older parent has to depend on children for supplemental income, an additional adjustment may be necessary.

The importance of making financial preparations for old age many years before retirement is clear. Nurses should encourage aging working people to determine whether their retirement income plans are keeping pace with inflation (Table 4-1). Also, older individuals need assistance in obtaining all the benefits they are entitled to and in learning how to manage their income wisely. Nurses should be aware of the impact of economic welfare on health status and should actively involve themselves in political issues that promote adequate income for all individuals.

> ☑ **Point to Ponder**
>
> *What are you doing to prepare for your own retirement?*

Shrinking Social World

Loneliness and desolation emphasize all the misfortunes of people who are growing old. Children are grown and gone, friends and spouse may be deceased, and others who could allay the loneliness may avoid the older individual because they find it difficult to accept the changes they see or to face the fact that they too will be old some day. Location in a sparsely populated rural area can geographically isolate older persons, and when they live in an urban area, they may be fearful of crime and venture from home infrequently.

Hearing and speech deficits and language differences can also foster loneliness. Insecurity resulting from multiple losses can cause suspiciousness of others and lead to a self-imposed isolation. At a time of many losses and adjustments, personal contact, love, extra support, and attention—not isolation—are needed. These are essential human needs. It is likely that a failure to thrive will occur in adults who feel unwanted and unloved just as it does in infants, who display anxiety, depression, anorexia, and behavioral and other difficulties when they perceive love and attention to be inadequate.

Nurses should attempt to intervene when they detect isolation and loneliness in an elderly person. Various programs provide telephone reassurance or home visits as a source of daily human contact. The person's faith community may also provide assistance. Nurses can help the elder locate and join social groups and perhaps even accompany the individual to the first meeting. A change in housing may be necessary to provide a safe environment conducive to social interaction. If the older person speaks a foreign language, relocation to an area in which members of the same ethnic group live can often remedy loneliness. Frequently, pets serve as significant and effective companions for the elderly.

It should be emphasized that being alone is not synonymous with being lonely. Periods of solitude are essential at all ages and provide us with the opportunity to reflect, analyze, and better understand the dynamics of our lives. Older individuals may want periods of solitude to reminisce and review their lives. Some individuals, young and old, prefer and choose to be alone and do not feel isolated or lonely in any way. Of course, attention should also be paid to the correction of hearing, vision, and other health problems that may be the cause of social isolation.

KEY CONCEPT
Periods of solitude are essential to reflect, analyze, and better understand the dynamics of life.

TABLE 4-1 ● *Retirement Budget*

Income Sources	Current Monthly Income	Income After Retirement
Salary		
Pension		
Second job		
Social security		
Spouse's income		
Other (*eg,* savings, rents, IRAs, investments)		
Total		

Living Requirements	Current Monthly Expenses	Expenses After Retirement
Living accommodations		
Mortgages or rent		
Utilities (*eg,* gas, electricity, water)		
Taxes		
Maintenance		
Telephone		
Food and other necessities		
Clothing		
Medical (*eg,* doctor, dentist, medicine)		
Prescriptions		
Insurance		
Life		
Health		
Automobile		
Automobile maintenance (*eg,* gas, oil, repairs)		
Loans and other credit		
Entertainment		
Donations		
Subtotal		
Other expenses (10% of subtotal)		
Total		
Net (income minus expenses)	Current	After retirement

Life Story

Rich threads of life experience are accumulated with aging that create the unique fabric of one's life. When seen in isolation, some of these threads may seem to have little value or make little sense, much like a network of threads on the undersurface of a tapestry. However, when the threads are woven together and the tapestry can be viewed as a whole, a person can see the special purpose of individual life experiences—good and bad. Weaving the threads of life experiences into the tapestry of a life story can be highly beneficial to the elderly person and others. Successes can be appreciated and the value of trials and failures can be realized. Others are able to gain insight into the person's life in totality rather than have their understanding limited by what may be an unrepresentative segment of life that now presents. Customs, knowledge, and wisdom can be recognized, preserved, and passed to younger generations.

> ✔ **Point to Ponder**
> *What are the major threads that have woven your life tapestry thus far?*

DISPLAY 4 - 1

Eliciting Life Stories

Elders possess rich life histories that have accrued during the many years they have lived. These unique histories contribute to the identity and individuality of older adults. Learning about life histories aids nurses in understanding elders' preferences and activities, facilitating self-actualization, and preserving identity and continuity of life experiences. Knowledge of life histories also enables caregivers to see their patients in a larger context, connected to a past full of varied roles and experiences.

A basic requisite to eliciting life stories is a willingness to listen. Often, a direct request will be sufficient to open the door to a life history. There also are some aids to facilitate this process, including:

Tree of Life

Ask the elder to write significant events (graduation, first job, relocations, marriages, deaths, childbirths, etc.) from the past on each branch and then discuss each.

Time Line

Ask the elder to write significant events on or near the year when they occurred and then discuss each.

Life Map

Ask the elder to write significant events on the map and discuss each.

Oral History

Ask the elder to start with his or her earliest memory and tell the story of his or her life into a tape recorder. (Suggest that the elder make this recording as a gift for younger family members.)

A variety of approaches can be used to elicit life stories (Display 4-1). Guiding older adults through this experience provides not only a therapeutic exercise for the elderly and an invaluable legacy for loved ones, but also, offers the gerontological nurse the gift of sharing and honoring the unique life journeys of elders.

NURSING DIAGNOSIS HIGHLIGHT

INEFFECTIVE ROLE PERFORMANCE

Overview

Ineffectiveness in role performance exists when there is a change in the perception or performance of a role. This can be associated with a physical, emotional, intellectual, motivational, educational, or socioeconomic limitation in the ability to fill the role, or restrictions in role performance imposed by others. There can be considerable distress, depression, or anger at not fulfilling the accustomed role and its associated responsibilities.

Causative or contributing factors

Illness, fatigue, pain, declining function, altered cognition, depression, anxiety, knowledge deficit, limited finances, retirement, lack of transportation, loss of significant other, ageism, restrictions imposed by others

Goals

The client realistically appraises role performance, adjusts to changes in role performance, and learns to perform responsibilities associated with roles.

Interventions

- Assess client's roles and responsibilities; identify deficits in role performance and reasons for deficits; review client's perception of role and feelings associated with altered role performance
- Assist client in realistically evaluating cause of altered role performance and potential for improvement in role performance
- Identify specific strategies to improve role performance (eg, instructing, negotiating with family members to allow client to perform role, counseling client to accept real limitations, referring to community resources, improving health problem, encouraging client to seek help with responsibilities, advising for stress management)
- Encourage client to discuss concerns with family members; assist client in arranging family conference
- Refer client to assistive resources, as appropriate, such as support groups, occupational therapist, financial counselor, Over-60 Employment Service, visiting nurse, and social services

Critical Thinking Exercises

1. How will the life experiences of today's 30-year-old woman affect her ability to adapt to old age? What factors will enable her to cope more or less as well than her grandmother's generation of women?
2. Cite examples of how society defines an individual's worth through the work role.
3. Describe actions nurses can take to help aging individuals prepare for retirement.
4. How can you determine if an older individual's time alone is reflective of needed solitude or social isolation?
5. What examples of ageism can be found in television programs, advertisements, and other vehicles of communication?
6. List specific measures nurses can take to help older persons adjust to the multiple changes faced in late life.
7. How can the geronotological nurse elicit life stories from older adults in the midst of caregiving demands during a busy shift?

Web Connect

Determine your personal financial health in your later years by using AARP's *Retirement Calculator* at
http://partners.financenter.com/aarp/calculate/us-eng/ retire02a.fcs

● Resources

AARP Grandparent Information Center
www. aarp.org/getans/consumer/grandparents.html

Grandparents Raising Grandchildren
P.O. Box 104
Colleyville, TX 76034
(817) 577-0435
www.uwex.edu/ces/gprg/gprg.htm

International Society for Reminiscence and Life Review
Center for Continuing Education/Extension
University of Wisconsin-Superior
Main 230
1800 Grand Ave.
Superior, WI 54880
(715) 394-8469
lweiland@staff.uwsuper.edu

National Grandparent Information Center
AARP
601 E Street NW
Washington, DC 20049
(202) 434-2296
www.aarp.org

● References

AARP. (2002). *The grandparent survey 2002 report. Executive summary.* Washington, DC: Author.

AARP. (2003). *Grandparent information center.* [On-line] Available: www.aarp.org/confacts/programs/gic.html

Atchley, R. C. (1975). *The sociology of retirement.* Cambridge, MA: Schenkman.

Butler, R. H., & Lewis, M. I. (1982). *Aging and mental health* (3rd ed., p. 58). St. Louis: Mosby.

Butler, R. H., Lewis, M. I., & Sutherland, T. (1991). *Aging and mental health* (4th ed.). New York: Merrill/MacMillan.

Erikson, E. (1963). *Childhood and society* (2nd ed.). New York: Norton.

Spock, B. (2002). Gay and lesbian parents. *Dr.Spock.com.* Retrieved May 25, 2003, from www.drspock.com/article/0,1510,4028+AgeM2_12+cbx_families,00.html.

Webster, J. D., & Haight, B. K. (2002). *Critical advances in reminiscence work: From theory to application.* New York: Springer.

● Recommended Readings

Alford-Cooper, F. (1998). *For keeps: Marriages that last a lifetime.* Armonk, NY: Sharpe.

Astor, B. (1998). *Baby boomers guide to caring for aging parents.* New York: Macmillan.

Battle, C. W. (1998). *The retirement handbook: How to maximize your assets and protect your quality of life.* New York: Allworth Press.

Bender, M., Bauchham, P., & Norris, A. (1999). *The therapeutic purpose of reminiscence.* Thousand Oaks, CA: Sage.

Bouvard, M. G. (1998). *Grandmothers: Granddaughters remember.* Syracuse, NY: Syracuse University Press.

Browne, C. V. (1998). *Women, feminism, and aging.* New York: Springer.

Cadidhizar, R., Bechtel, G. A., & Woodring, B. C. (2000). The changing role of grandparenthood. *Journal of Gerontological Nursing, 26*(1), 24–29.

Carson, L. (1996). *The essential grandparent: A guide to making a difference.* Deerfield Beach, FL: Health Communications.

Clarfield, A. M. (2001). "Of a certain age": Wisdom through the eyes of fascinating older people. *Clinical Geriatrics, 9*(9), 15–16.

Conway, J. (1997). *Men in midlife crisis.* Colorado Springs, CO: Chariot Victor Publishers.

Costa, D. L. (1998). *Evolution of retirement: An American economic history,* 1880–1990. Chicago: University of Chicago Press.

Davidhizar, R., Bechtel, G. A., Woodring, B. C. (2000). The changing role of grandparenthood. *Journal of Gerontological Nursing, 26*(1), 24–29.

Dean, A. (1997). *Growing older, growing better: Daily meditations for celebrating aging.* Carlsbad, CA: Hay House.

Ebersole, P. (2000). Ageism is a women's issue. *Geriatric Nursing, 21*(4), 174.

Guse, L., Inglis, J., Chicoine, J., et al. (2000). Life albums in long-term care: Residents, family, and staff perceptions. *Geriatric Nursing, 21*(1), 34–37.

Hartt, W., & Hartt, M. (1998). *The complete idiot's guide to grandparenting.* New York: Alpha Books.

Hegge, M., & Fischer, C. (2000). Grief responses of senior and elderly widows: Practice implications. *Journal of Gerontological Nursing, 26*(2), 35–43.

Heston, C. (1997). *To be a man: Letters to my grandson.* New York: Simon and Schuster.

Hillman, J. (1999). *The force of character and the lasting life.* New York: Random House.

Hirst, S. P., & Raffin, S. (2001). "I hate those darn chickens…": The power in stories for older adults and nurses. *Journal of Gerontological Nursing, 27*(9), 24–29.

Jowell, B. T., & Schwisow, D. (1997). *After he's gone: A guide for widowed and divorced women.* Secaucus, NJ: Carol Publishing Group.

Kitzinger, S. (1996). *Becoming a grandmother: A life in transition.* New York: Simon and Schuster.

Korte, J. N., & Hall, E. (1997). *Seasons of life: The dramatic journey from birth to death.* Ann Arbor, MI: University of Michigan Press.

Lee, G. (1997). *On the way to over the hill: A guide to aging gracefully.* Seattle, WA: Educare Press.

Lemme, B. H. (1999). *Development in adulthood* (2nd ed.). Boston: Allyn & Bacon.

Logan, J. R., & Spitze, G. D. (1996). *Family ties: Enduring relations between parents and their grown children.* Philadelphia: Temple University Press.

Moore, S. L. (2000). Aging and meaning in life: Examining the concept. *Geriatric Nursing, 21*(1), 2729.

Morse, S., & Robbins, D. Q. (1998). *Moving mom and dad: Why, where, how, and when to help parents relocate* (2nd ed.). Berkeley, CA: Lanier Publishing.

Puentes, W. J. (2000) Using social reminiscence to teach therapeutic communication skills. *Geriatric Nursing, 21*(3), 318–320.

Quadagno, J. S.(1999). *Aging and the life course: An introduction to social gerontology.* Boston: McGraw-Hill College.

Redburn, D. E. (Ed.). (1998). *Social gerontology.* New York: Auburn House.

Rippier, W. H. (1997). *Women and aging: A guide to literature.* Boulder, CO: Lynne Rienner.

Rybarczyk, B., & Bellg, A. (1997). *Listening to life stories: A new approach to stress intervention in health care.* New York: Springer.

Scott, L. (1997). *Wise choices beyond midlife: Women mapping the journey ahead.* Watsonville, CA: Papier-Mache Press.

Szinovacz, M. E. (1997). *Grandparenthood: Profiles, supports, transitions.* Norfolk, VA: Old Dominion University.

Szinovacz, M. E. (1998). *Handbook on grandparenthood.* Westport, CT: Greenwood Press.

Wall, G., & Collins, V. F. (1997). *Your next fifty years: A completely new way to look at how, when, and if you should retire.* New York: Henry Holt.

Westheimer, R. K., & Kaplan, S. (1998). *Grandparenthood.* New York: Routledge.

Wicks, R. J. (1997). *After 50: Spiritually embracing your own wisdom years.* New York: Paulist.

Yeaworth, R. C. (2002). Long-term care and insurance. *Journal of Gerontological Nursing, 28*(11), 45–51.

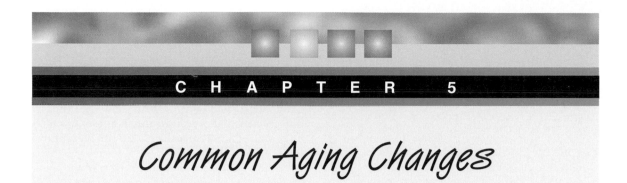

Common Aging Changes

■ Chapter Outline

*L*iving is a process of continual change. Infants become toddlers, pubescent children blossom into young men and women, and dependent adolescents develop into responsible adult citizens. The continuation of change into later life is natural and expected.

The type, rate, and degree of physical, emotional, psychological, and social changes experienced during life are highly individualized; such changes are influenced by genetic factors, environment, diet, health, stress, lifestyle choices, and numerous other elements. The result is not only individual variations among aged persons, but also differences in the pattern of aging of various body systems within the same individual. Although some similar elements in the pattern of aging can be identified among individuals, it must be recognized that the pattern of aging is unique in each person.

Changes to the Body

GENERAL CHANGES

Organ and system changes can be traced to changes at the basic cellular level. The number of cells is gradually reduced, leaving fewer functional cells in the body. Lean body mass is reduced, whereas fat tissue increases until the sixth decade of life. Total body fat as a proportion of the body's composition increases (Harris, Vasser, Everhart, Tylavsky, Fuerst, et al., 2000). Cellular solids and bone mass are decreased. Extracellular fluid remains fairly constant, although intracellular fluid is decreased, resulting in less total body fluid. This makes dehydration a significant risk to the elderly.

Some of the more noticeable effects of the aging process begin to appear after the fourth decade of life. It is then that men experience hair loss, and both sexes develop gray hair and wrinkles. As body fat atrophies, the body's contours gain a bony appearance along with a deepening of the hollows of the intercostal and supraclavicular spaces, orbits, and axillae. Elongated ears, a double chin, and baggy eyelids are among the more obvious manifestations of the loss of tissue elasticity throughout the body. Skin-fold thickness is significantly reduced in the forearm and on the back of the hands. The loss of subcutaneous fat content, responsible for the decrease in skin-fold thickness, also is responsible for a decline in the body's natural insulation, making older adults more sensitive to cold temperatures.

Stature decreases, resulting in a loss of approximately 2 inches in height by 80 years of age. Body shrinkage is due to reduced hydration, loss of cartilage, and thinning of the vertebrae, causing the long bones of the body, which do not shrink, to appear disproportionately long. Reduction in height can be further exaggerated by any curvature of the spine, hips, and knees that may be present.

These changes are gradual and subtle. Further differences in structure and function can arise from changes to specific body systems (Fig. 5-1).

CARDIOVASCULAR SYSTEM

Heart size does not change significantly with age; enlarged hearts are associated with cardiac disease, and marked inactivity can cause cardiac atrophy. There is a slight left ventricular hypertrophy, and the aorta becomes dilated and elongated. Atrioventricular valves become thick and rigid as a result of sclerosis and fibrosis, compounding the dysfunction associated with any cardiac disease that may be present.

Physiologic changes in the cardiovascular system appear in a variety of ways. Throughout the adult years, the heart muscle loses its efficiency and con-

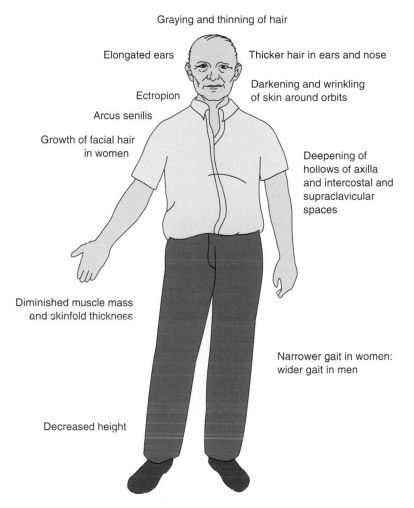

Graying and thinning of hair

Elongated ears

Thicker hair in ears and nose

Ectropion

Darkening and wrinkling of skin around orbits

Arcus senilis

Growth of facial hair in women

Deepening of hollows of axilla and intercostal and supraclavicular spaces

Diminished muscle mass and skinfold thickness

Narrower gait in women: wider gait in men

Decreased height

FIGURE 5-1

Age-related changes noticeable upon inspection.

tractile strength, resulting in a reduction in cardiac output under conditions of physiologic stress. There is increased irregularity and a decrease in the number of pacemaker cells and a thickening of the shell surrounding the sinus node. The isometric contraction phase and relaxation time of the left ventricle are prolonged; more time is required for the cycle of diastolic filling and systolic emptying to be completed. Usually, adults adjust to this change quite well; they learn that it is easier and more comfortable for them to take an elevator rather than the stairs, to drive instead of walking a long distance, and to pace their activities. When unusual demands are placed on the heart (eg, shoveling snow for the first time of the sea-

son, receiving bad news, running to catch a bus), the changes are realized. The same holds true for the elderly, who are not severely affected by less cardiac efficiency under nonstressful conditions. When older persons are faced with an added demand on their hearts, the difference is noted. Although the peak rate of the stressed heart may not reach the levels experienced by younger persons, tachycardia in the elderly will last for a longer time. Stroke volume may increase to compensate for this situation, which results in elevated blood pressure, although the blood pressure can remain stable as tachycardia progresses to heart failure in the elderly. The resting heart rate is unchanged.

> **KEY CONCEPT**
> Age-related cardiovascular changes are most apparent when unusual demands are placed on the heart.

There is variation among older adults in maximum exercise capacity and maximum oxygen consumption. Older adults in good physical condition have comparable cardiac function to younger persons who are in poor condition.

The vessels consist of three layers, each of which is affected differently by the aging process. The tunica intima is the innermost layer and experiences the most direct changes, including fibrosis, calcium and lipid accumulation, and cellular proliferation. These changes contribute to the development of atherosclerosis. The middle layer, the tunica media, experiences a thinning and calcification of elastin fibers and an increase in collagen, which cause a stiffening of the vessels. Impaired baroreceptor function and increased peripheral resistance, leading to a rise in systolic blood pressure, result. The outermost layer, the tunica ad-

ventitia, is not affected by the aging process. Decreased elasticity of the arteries is responsible for vascular changes to the heart, kidney, and pituitary gland (Fig. 5-2). Reduced sensitivity of the blood pressure-regulating baroreceptors increases problems with postural hypotension and postprandial hypotension (blood pressure reduction of at least 20 mm Hg within 1 hour of eating). The reduced elasticity of the vessels, coupled with thinner skin and less subcutaneous fat, causes the vessels in the head, neck, and extremities to become more prominent.

RESPIRATORY SYSTEM

Various structural changes in the chest reduce respiratory activity. The calcification of costal cartilage makes the trachea and rib cage more rigid; the anterior-posterior chest diameter increases, often demonstrated by kyphosis; and thoracic inspiratory and expiratory muscles are weaker. There is a blunting of the cough and laryngeal reflexes. Cilia are reduced in number and there is hypertrophy of the bronchial mucous gland, further complicating the ability to expel mucus and debris. Alveoli are reduced in number and

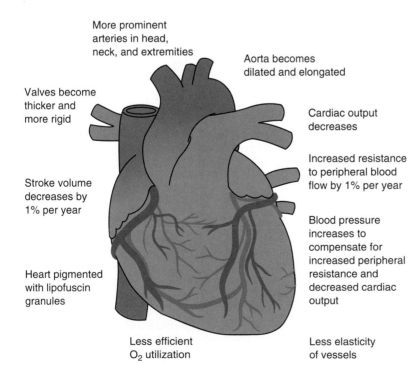

More prominent arteries in head, neck, and extremities

Aorta becomes dilated and elongated

Valves become thicker and more rigid

Cardiac output decreases

Increased resistance to peripheral blood flow by 1% per year

Stroke volume decreases by 1% per year

Blood pressure increases to compensate for increased peripheral resistance and decreased cardiac output

Heart pigmented with lipofuscin granules

Less efficient O_2 utilization

Less elasticity of vessels

FIGURE 5-2

Cardiovascular changes that occur with aging.

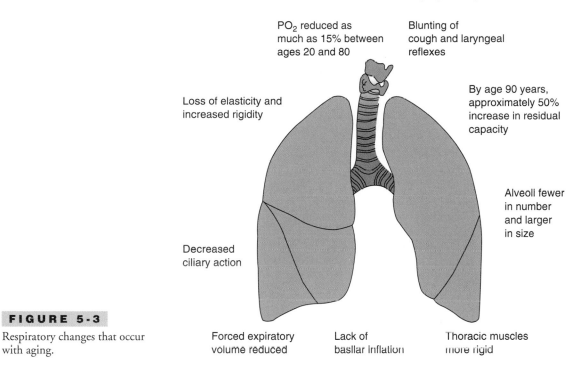

PO$_2$ reduced as much as 15% between ages 20 and 80

Blunting of cough and laryngeal reflexes

Loss of elasticity and increased rigidity

By age 90 years, approximately 50% increase in residual capacity

Alveoli fewer in number and larger in size

Decreased ciliary action

FIGURE 5-3

Respiratory changes that occur with aging.

Forced expiratory volume reduced

Lack of basilar inflation

Thoracic muscles more rigid

stretched due to a progressive loss of elasticity—a process that begins by the 6th decade of life. The lungs become smaller and more rigid and have less recoil (Fig. 5-3). These changes cause less lung expansion, insufficient basilar inflation, and decreased ability to expel foreign or accumulated matter. The lungs exhale less effectively, thereby increasing the residual volume. As the residual volume increases, the vital capacity is reduced; maximum breathing capacity also decreases. If respiratory activity is reduced under normal circumstances, one can imagine the profound effects of immobility on the respiratory system. With less effective gas exchange and lack of basilar inflation, the elderly are at high risk for developing respiratory infections. Endurance training can produce a significant increase in lung capacity of older adults.

> **KEY CONCEPT**
> The reduced respiratory activity associated with advanced age enables pneumonia to develop very easily in older adults, especially when they are immobile.

GASTROINTESTINAL SYSTEM

Although not as life-threatening as cardiovascular or respiratory problems, gastrointestinal symptoms are of more bother and concern to older persons. This system is altered by the aging process at all points. Tooth loss is not a normal consequence of growing old, but poor dental care, diet, and environmental influences have contributed to most of today's older population being edentulous. Increasing numbers of root cavities and cavities around existing dental work occur. After 30 years of age, periodontal disease is the major reason for tooth loss. Tooth enamel becomes harder and more brittle. Dentin, the layer beneath the enamel, becomes more fibrous and its production is decreased. The root pulp experiences shrinkage and fibrosis, the gingiva retracts, and bone density in the alveolar ridge is lost. Flattening of the chewing cusps is common. The bones that support the teeth decrease in density and height, contributing to tooth loss. Most of the elderly must rely on dentures, which may not be worn regularly because of discomfort or poor fit. If natural teeth are present, they often are in poor condition, having flatter surfaces, stains, and varying degrees of erosion and abrasion of the crown and root structure. The tooth brittleness of some older people creates the possibility of aspiration of tooth fragments.

Taste sensations become less acute with age because the tongue atrophies, affecting the taste buds; chronic irritation (as from pipe smoking) can reduce taste efficiency to a greater degree than that experienced through aging alone. The sweet sensations on the tip of the tongue tend to suffer a greater loss than the sensations for sour, salt, and bitter flavors. Excessive seasoning of foods may be used to compensate for taste alterations and could lead to health problems for the elderly. Loss of papillae and sublingual varicosities on the tongue are common findings.

Approximately one third of the amount of saliva produced in younger years is produced in old age. Saliva often is diminished in quantity and is of increased viscosity as a result of some of the medications commonly used to treat geriatric conditions. Salivary ptyalin is decreased, interfering with the breakdown of starches. Because of subtle changes in the swallowing mechanism, swallowing can take twice as long (Shaker, Ren, Bardan, Easterling, Dua, Xie, et al., 2003)

Esophageal motility is affected by age. Presbyesophagus occurs, a condition characterized by a decreased intensity of propulsive waves and an increased frequency of nonpropulsive waves. The esophagus tends to become slightly dilated and esophageal emptying is slower, which can cause discomfort because food remains in the esophagus for a longer time. Relaxation of the lower esophageal sphincter may occur; when combined with the elderly person's weaker gag reflex and delayed esophageal emptying, aspiration becomes a risk.

The stomach is believed to have reduced motility in old age, along with decreases in hunger contractions. Studies regarding changes in gastric emptying time have been inconclusive, with some claiming delayed gastric emptying to occur with normal aging and others attributing it to other factors. The gastric mucosa atrophies. Hydrochloric acid and pepsin decline with age; the higher pH of the stomach contributes to an increased incidence of gastric irritation in the elderly.

Some atrophy occurs throughout the small and large intestines, and fewer cells are present on the absorbing surface of intestinal walls. Functionally, there is no significant change in mean small bowel transit time with age. Fat absorption is slower, and dextrose and xylose are more difficult to absorb. Absorption of vitamin B, vitamin B_{12}, vitamin D, calcium, and iron is faulty. The large intestine has reductions in mucous secretions and elasticity of the rectal wall. Normal aging does not interfere with the motility of feces through the bowel, although other factors that are highly prevalent in late life do contribute to constipation. Bowel elimination can be affected by an age-related loss of tone of the internal sphincter; awareness of the need to evacuate the bowels is reduced by slower transmission of neural impulses to the lower bowel.

With advancing age, the liver has reduced weight and volume but this seems to produce no ill effects. The older liver is less able to regenerate damaged cells. Liver function tests remain within a normal range. Less efficient cholesterol stabilization and absorption cause an increased incidence of gallstones (Fig. 5-4). The pancreatic ducts become dilated and distended, and often the entire gland prolapses.

GENITOURINARY SYSTEM

The renal mass becomes smaller with age, which is attributable to a cortical loss rather than a loss of the renal medulla. Renal tissue growth declines, and atherosclerosis may promote atrophy of the kidney. These changes can have a profound effect on renal function, reducing renal blood flow and the glomerular filtration rate by approximately one-half between the ages of 20 and 90 years (Kielstein, Body-Boger, Frolich, Ritz, Haller, et al., 2003).

Tubular function decreases. There is less efficient tubular exchange of substances, conservation of water and sodium, and suppression of antidiuretic hormone secretion in the presence of hypo-osmolality. Although these changes can contribute to hyponatremia and nocturia, they do not affect specific gravity to any significant extent. The decrease in tubular function also causes decreased reabsorption of glucose from the filtrate, which can cause 1+ proteinurias and glycosurias not to be of major diagnostic significance.

Urinary frequency, urgency, and nocturia accompany bladder changes with age. Bladder muscles weaken and bladder capacity decreases. Emptying of the bladder is more difficult; retention of large volumes of urine may result. The micturition reflex is delayed. Although urinary incontinence is not a normal outcome of aging, some stress incontinence may oc-

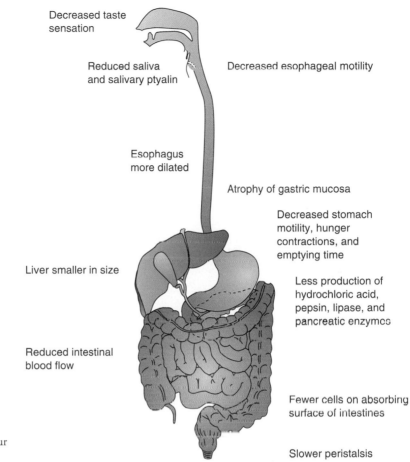

Decreased taste sensation

Reduced saliva and salivary ptyalin

Decreased esophageal motility

Esophagus more dilated

Atrophy of gastric mucosa

Decreased stomach motility, hunger contractions, and emptying time

Liver smaller in size

Less production of hydrochloric acid, pepsin, lipase, and pancreatic enzymes

Reduced intestinal blood flow

Fewer cells on absorbing surface of intestines

Slower peristalsis

FIGURE 5-4

Gastrointestinal changes that occur with aging.

cur because of a weakening of the pelvic diaphragm, particularly in multiparous women (Fig. 5-5).

The seminal vesicles are affected by age by a smoothing of the mucosa, thinning of the epithelium, replacement of muscle tissue with connective tissue, and reduction of fluid-retaining capacity. The seminiferous tubules experience increased fibrosis, thinning of the epithelium, thickening of the basement membrane, and narrowing of the lumen. The structural changes can cause a reduction in sperm count in some men. Venous and arterial sclerosis and fibroelastosis of the corpus spongiosum can affect the penis with age. The older man does not lose the physical capacity to achieve erections or ejaculations. No conclusive evidence exists regarding age-related changes to the testes.

Prostatic enlargement occurs in most elderly men. The rate and type vary among individuals. Three fourths of men aged 65 years and older have some degree of prostatism, which causes problems with urinary frequency. Although most prostatic enlargement is benign, it does pose a greater risk of malignancy and requires regular evaluation.

The female genitalia demonstrate many changes with age, including atrophy of the vulva from hormonal changes, accompanied by the loss of subcutaneous fat and hair and a flattening of the labia. The vagina of the older woman appears pink and dry with a smooth, shiny canal because of the loss of elastic tissue and rugae. The vaginal epithelium becomes thin and avascular. The vaginal environment is more alkaline in older women and is accompanied by a

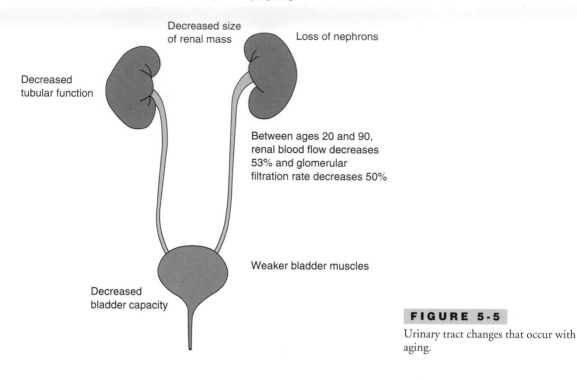

Decreased size
of renal mass

Loss of nephrons

Decreased
tubular function

Between ages 20 and 90,
renal blood flow decreases
53% and glomerular
filtration rate decreases 50%

Weaker bladder muscles

Decreased
bladder capacity

FIGURE 5-5

Urinary tract changes that occur with
aging.

change in the type of flora and a reduction in secretions. The cervix atrophies and becomes smaller; the endocervical epithelium also atrophies. The uterus shrinks and the endometrium atrophies; however, the endometrium continues to respond to hormonal stimulation, which can be responsible for incidents of postmenopausal bleeding in older women on estrogen therapy. The fallopian tubes atrophy and shorten with age, and the ovaries atrophy and become thicker and smaller (Fig. 5-6). Despite these changes, the older woman does not lose the ability to engage in and enjoy intercourse or other forms of sexual pleasure. Estrogen depletion also causes a weakening of pelvic floor muscles, which can lead to an involuntary release of urine when there is an increase in intra-abdominal pressure.

MUSCULOSKELETAL SYSTEM

The kyphosis, enlarged joints, flabby muscles, and decreased height of many elderly persons announce the variety of musculoskeletal changes occurring with age. Along with other body tissue, muscle fibers atrophy and decrease in number, with fibrous tissue gradually replacing muscle tissue. Overall muscle mass,

muscle strength, and muscle movements are decreased; the arm and leg muscles, which become particularly flabby and weak, display these changes well. Because the variability in the rate of these changes could suggest they result from inactivity rather than aging, the importance of exercise to minimize the loss of muscle tone and strength cannot be emphasized enough. Muscle tremors may be present and are believed to be associated with degeneration of the extrapyramidal system. The tendons shrink and harden, which causes a decrease in tendon jerks. Reflexes are lessened in the arms, are nearly totally lost in the abdomen, but are maintained in the knee. For various reasons, muscle cramping frequently occurs.

> **KEY CONCEPT**
> Regular exercise helps maintain muscle strength and tone and reduces some of the negative functional consequences of aging.

Bone mineral and mass are reduced, contributing to the brittleness of the bones of older people, espe-

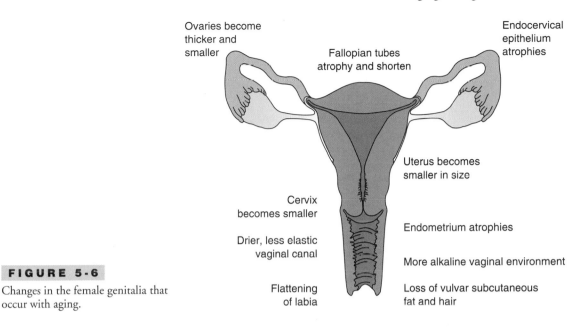

Ovaries become thicker and smaller

Fallopian tubes atrophy and shorten

Endocervical epithelium atrophies

Uterus becomes smaller in size

Cervix becomes smaller

Endometrium atrophies

Drier, less elastic vaginal canal

More alkaline vaginal environment

Flattening of labia

Loss of vulvar subcutaneous fat and hair

FIGURE 5-6

Changes in the female genitalia that occur with aging.

cially older women. There is diminished calcium absorption, a gradual resorption of the interior surface of the long bones, and a slower production of new bone on the outside surface. These changes make fractures a serious risk to the elderly. Although long bones do not significantly shorten with age, thinning disks and shortening vertebrae reduce the length of the spinal column, causing a reduction in height with age. Height may be further shortened because of varying degrees of kyphosis, a backward tilting of the head, and some flexion at the hips and knees. A deterioration of the cartilage surface of joints and the formation of points and spurs may limit joint activity and motion (Fig. 5-7).

NERVOUS SYSTEM

It is difficult to identify with accuracy the exact impact of aging on the nervous system because of the dependence of this system's function on other body systems. For instance, cardiovascular problems can reduce cerebral circulation and be responsible for cerebral dysfunction. There is a decline in brain weight and a reduction in blood flow to the brain; however, these structural changes do not appear to affect thinking and behavior. Declining nervous system function may be unnoticed because changes are often

nonspecific and slowly progressing. A reduction in nerve cells and cerebral blood flow and metabolism are known to occur. The nerve conduction velocity is lower. These changes are manifested by slower reflexes and delayed response to multiple stimuli. Kinesthetic sense lessens. There is a slower response to changes in balance, a factor contributing to falls. Because the brain affects the sleep–wake cycle, changes in the sleep pattern occur, with stages III and IV of sleep becoming less prominent. Frequent awakening during sleep is not unusual, although only a minimal amount of sleep is actually lost (Fig. 5-8).

SENSORY ORGANS

Vision

Each of the five senses becomes less efficient with advanced age, interfering in varying degrees with safety, normal activities of daily living, and general well-being. Perhaps the greatest of such interferences results from changes in vision. Presbyopia, the inability to focus or accommodate properly due to reduced elasticity of the lens, is characteristic of older eyes and begins in the fourth decade of life. This vision problem causes most middle-aged and older adults to need corrective lenses to accommodate close and detailed

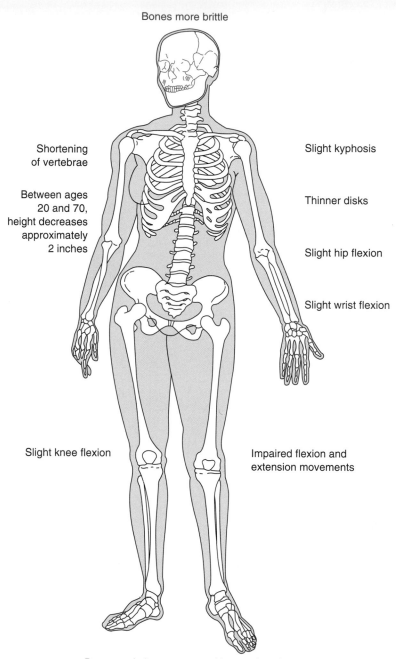

Bones more brittle

Shortening
of vertebrae

Between ages
20 and 70,
height decreases
approximately
2 inches

Slight knee flexion

Slight kyphosis

Thinner disks

Slight hip flexion

Slight wrist flexion

Impaired flexion and
extension movements

Decrease in bone mass and bone mineral

FIGURE 5-7

Skeletal changes that occur with aging.

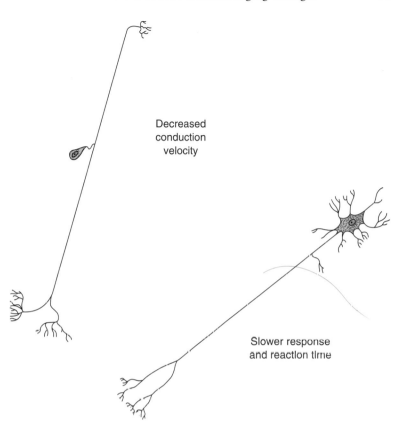

Decreased
conduction
velocity

Slower response
and reaction time

FIGURE 5-8

Neurologic changes that occur with
aging.

work. The visual field narrows, making peripheral vision more difficult. The pupil is less responsive to light because the pupil sphincter hardens, the pupil size decreases, and rhodopsin content in the rods decreases. As a result, the light perception threshold increases and vision in dim areas or at night is difficult; older individuals require more light than younger persons to see adequately.

Alterations in blood supply of the retina and retinal pigmented epithelium can cause macular degeneration, a condition in which there is a loss in central vision. Changes in the retina and retinal pathway interfere with critical flicker fusion (the point at which a flickering light is perceived as continuous rather than intermittent).

The density and size of the lens increases, causing the lens to become stiffer and more opaque. Opacification of the lens leads to the development of cataracts, which increases sensitivity to glare, blurs vision, and interferes with night vision. Exposure to the ultraviolet rays of the sun contribute to cataract development. Yellowing of the lens (possibly related to a chemical reaction involving sunlight with amino acids) and alterations in the retina that affect color perception make the elderly less able to differentiate the low tone colors of the blues, greens, and violets.

Depth perception becomes distorted, causing problems in correctly judging the height of curbs and steps. Dark and light adaptation takes longer, as does the processing of visual information. Less efficient reabsorption of intraocular fluid increases the older person's risk for developing glaucoma. The ciliary muscle gradually atrophies and is replaced with connective tissue.

The appearance of the eye may be altered; reduced lacrimal secretions can cause the eyes to look dry and dull, and fat deposits can cause a partial or complete glossy white circle to develop around the periphery of the cornea (arcus senilis). Corneal sensitivity is diminished, which can increase the risk of injury to the cornea. The accumulation of lipid deposits in the cornea can cause a scattering of light rays, which blurs vision. In the posterior cavity, bits of debris and condensation become visible and may float across the visual field; these are commonly called floaters. Vitreous decreases and the proportion of liquid increases, causing the vitreous body to pull away from the retina; blurred vision, distorted images, and floaters may result. Visual acuity progressively declines with age due to decreased pupil size, scatter in the cornea and lens, opacification of the lens and vitreous, and loss of photoreceptor cells in the retina.

Hearing

Presbycusis is progressive hearing loss that occurs as a result of age-related changes to the inner ear, including loss of hair cells, decreased blood supply, reduced flexibility of basilar membrane, degeneration of spiral ganglion cells, and reduced production of endolymph. This degenerative hearing impairment is the most serious problem affecting the inner ear and retrocochlea. High-frequency sounds of 2000 Hz and above are the first to be lost; middle and low frequencies may also be lost as the condition progresses. A variety of factors, including continued exposure to loud noise, may contribute to the occurrence of presbycusis. This problem causes speech to sound distorted as some of the high-pitched sounds (s, sh, f, ph, ch) are filtered from normal speech. This change is so gradual and subtle that affected persons may not realize the extent of their hearing impairment. Hearing can be further jeopardized by an accumulation of cerumen in the middle ear; the higher keratin content of cerumen as one ages contributes to this problem. The acoustic reflex, which protects the inner ear and filters auditory distractions from sounds made by one's own body and voice, is diminished due to a weakening and stiffening of the middle ear muscles and ligaments. In addition to hearing problems, equilibrium can be altered because of degeneration of the vestibular structures and atrophy of the cochlea, organ of Corti, and stria vascularis.

Taste and Smell

Approximately half of all elderly persons have experienced some loss of their ability to smell. The sense of smell is reduced with age because of a decrease in the number of sensory cells in the nasal lining and fewer cells in the olfactory bulb of the brain. By age 80, detection of scent is almost half as sensitive as it was at its peak. As most of taste acuity is dependent on smell, the reduction in the sense of smell alters the sense of taste. There is atrophy of the tongue with age that can diminish taste sensations, although there is not conclusive evidence that the number or responsiveness of taste buds decreases. Reduced saliva production, poor oral hygiene, medications, and conditions such as sinusitis can affect taste.

Touch

Tactile sensation is reduced, as observed in the elderly's reduced ability to sense pressure and pain and differentiate temperatures. These sensory changes can cause misperceptions of the environment and, as a result, profound safety risks (Fig. 5-9).

ENDOCRINE SYSTEM

With age, the thyroid gland undergoes fibrosis, cellular infiltration, and increased nodularity. The resulting decreased thyroid gland activity causes a lower basal metabolic rate, reduced radioactive iodine uptake, and less thyrotropin secretion and release. Protein-bound iodine levels in the blood do not change, although total serum iodide is reduced. The release of thyroidal iodide decreases with age, and excretion of the 17-ketosteroids declines. The thyroid gland progressively atrophies, and the loss of adrenal function can further decrease thyroid activity. Secretion of thyroid-stimulating hormone (TSH) and the serum concentration of thyroxine (T_4) do not change, although there is a significant reduction in triiodothyronine (T_3), believed to be a result of the reduced conversion of T_4 to T_3. Overall, thyroid function remains adequate.

Much of the secretory activity of the adrenal cortex is regulated by adrenocorticotropic hormone (ACTH), a pituitary hormone. As ACTH secretion decreases with age, secretory activity of the adrenal gland decreases also. Although the secretion of ACTH does not affect aldosterone secretion, it has been shown that less aldosterone is produced and excreted in the urine of older persons. The secretion of glucocorticoids, 17-ketosteroids, progesterone, androgen, and estrogen, also influenced by the adrenal gland, are reduced as well.

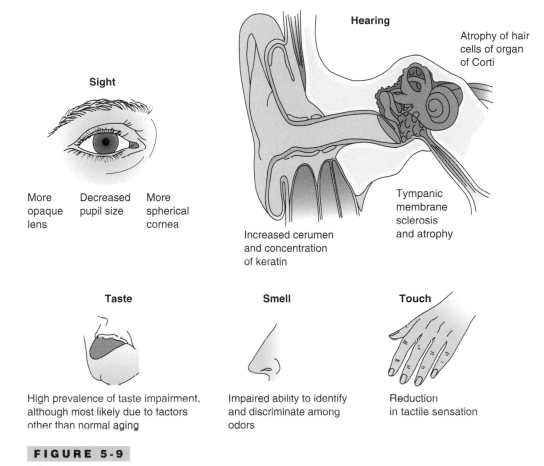

Sight

More opaque lens   Decreased pupil size   More spherical cornea

Hearing

Atrophy of hair cells of organ of Corti

Tympanic membrane sclerosis and atrophy

Increased cerumen and concentration of keratin

Taste

High prevalence of taste impairment, although most likely due to factors other than normal aging

Smell

Impaired ability to identify and discriminate among odors

Touch

Reduction in tactile sensation

FIGURE 5-9

Effects of sensory changes.

The pituitary gland decreases in volume by approximately 20% in older persons. Somatotropic growth hormone remains present in similar amounts, although the blood level may be reduced with age. Decreases are seen in ACTH, TSH, follicle-stimulating hormone, luteinizing hormone, and luteotropic hormone to varying degrees. Gonadal secretion declines with age, including gradual decreases in testosterone, estrogen, and progesterone. With the exception of alterations associated with changes in plasma calcium level or dysfunction of other glands, the parathyroid glands maintain their function throughout life.

There is a delayed and insufficient release of insulin by the beta cells of the pancreas in the elderly, and there is believed to be a decreased tissue sensitivity to circulating insulin. The older person's ability to metabolize glucose is reduced, and sudden concentrations of glucose cause higher and more prolonged hyperglycemia levels; therefore, it is not unusual to detect higher blood glucose levels in nondiabetic older persons.

KEY CONCEPT
Higher blood glucose levels than are normal in the general adult population are not unusual in nondiabetic elderly people.

IMMUNE SYSTEM

The depressed immune response of older adults causes infections to be a significant risk for this age group. After midlife, thymic mass is lost steadily, to the point that serum activity of thymic hormones is almost undetectable in the aged. T-cell activity declines, and more immature T cells are present in the thymus. A significant decline in cell-mediated immunity occurs, and T lymphocytes are less able to proliferate in response to mitogens. Changes in the T cells contribute to the reactivation of varicella-zoster and *Mycobacterium tuberculosis,* infections that are witnessed in many older individuals. Serum immunoglobulin concentration is not significantly altered; the concentration of IgM is lower, whereas the concentrations of IgA and IgG are higher. Responses to influenza, parainfluenza, pneumococcus, and tetanus vaccines are less effective (although vaccination is recommended for the elderly). Inflammatory defenses decline and, often, inflammation presents atypically in the elderly (eg, low-grade fever, minimal pain).

THERMOREGULATION

Normal body temperatures are lower in later life than in younger years. Mean body temperature ranges from 96.9° to 98.3°F orally and 98° to 99°F rectally. Rectal and auditory canal temperatures are the most accurate and reliable indicators of body temperature in older adults.

There is a reduced ability to respond to cold temperatures due to inefficient vasoconstriction, decreased cardiac output, diminished shivering, and reduced muscle mass and subcutaneous tissue. At the other extreme, differences in response to heat are related to impaired sweating mechanisms and decreased cardiac output.

INTEGUMENTARY SYSTEM

Diet, general health, activity, exposure, and hereditary factors influence the normal course of aging of the skin. This system's changes are often the most bothersome because they are obvious and clearly reflect advancing years. Flattening of the dermal-epidermal junction, reduced thickness and vascularity of the dermis, slowing of epidermal proliferation, and an increased quantity and degeneration of elastin fibers occur. Collagen fibers become coarser and more random, reducing skin elasticity. The dermis becomes more avascular and thinner. As the skin becomes less elastic and more dry and fragile, and as subcutaneous fat is lost, lines, wrinkles, and sagging become evident. Skin becomes irritated and breaks down more easily. There is a reduction in the number of melanocytes, and those present cluster, causing skin pigmentation, commonly referred to as age spots; these are more prevalent in areas of the body exposed to the sun. The reduction in melanocytes cause older adults to tan more slowly and less deeply. Skin immune response declines causing the elderly to be more prone to skin infections. Benign and malignant skin neoplasms occur more with age.

Scalp, pubic, and axillary hair thins and grays due to a progressive loss of pigment cells and atrophy and fibrosis of hair bulbs; hair in the nose and ears becomes thicker. By age 50, most white men have some degree of baldness and about half of all people have evidence of gray hair. Growth rate of scalp, pubic, and axillary hair declines; the growth of facial hair may occur in older women. An increased growth of eyebrow, ear, and nostril hair occurs in older men. Fingernails grow more slowly, are fragile and brittle, develop longitudinal striations, and experience a decrease in lunula size. Perspiration is slightly reduced because the number and function of the sweat glands are lessened.

☑ **Point to Ponder**
In the past 10 years, what changes have you experienced in regard to appearance, behaviors, and attitudes? How do you feel about these?

Changes to the Mind

Psychological changes can be influenced by general health status, genetic factors, educational achievement, activity, and physical and social changes. Sensory organ impairment can impede interaction with the environment and other people, thus influencing psychological status. Feeling useless and socially isolated may obstruct optimum psychological function. Recognizing the variety of factors potentially affecting psychological status and the range of individual responses to those factors, some generalizations can be discussed.

PERSONALITY

Drastic changes in basic personality normally do not occur as one ages. The kind and gentle old person was most likely that way when young; likewise, the cantankerous old person probably was not mild and meek in earlier years. Excluding pathologic processes, the personality will be consistent with that of earlier years; possibly, it will be more openly and honestly expressed. The alleged rigidity of older persons is more a result of physical and mental limitations than a personality change. An older person's insistence that her furniture not be rearranged may be interpreted as rigidity, but it may be a sound safety practice for someone coping with poor memory and visual deficits. Changes in personality traits may occur in response to events that alter self-attitude, such as retirement, death of a spouse, loss of independence, income reduction, and disability. No personality type describes all older adults. Morale, attitude, and self-esteem tend to be stable throughout the life span.

> **KEY CONCEPT**
> Personality in late life is a reflection of lifelong personality.

MEMORY

The three types of memory are short-term, lasting from 30 seconds to 30 minutes; long-term, involving that learned long ago; and sensory, which is obtained through the sensory organs and lasts only a few seconds. Retrieval of information from long-term memory can be slowed, particularly if the information is not used or needed on a daily basis. The ability to retain information in the consciousness while manipulating other information—working memory function—is reduced. Some age-related forgetfulness can be improved by the use of memory aids (mnemonic devices) such as associating a name with an image, making notes or lists, and placing objects in consistent location. Memory deficits can result from a variety of factors other than normal aging. **(Visit the Connection website for helpful hints to enhance memory in elders.)**

INTELLIGENCE

In general, it is wise to interpret the findings related to intelligence and the elderly with much caution because results may be biased from the measurement tool or method of evaluation used. Early gerontological research on intelligence and aging was guilty of such biases. Sick old people cannot be compared with healthy persons; people with different educational or cultural backgrounds cannot be compared; and one group of individuals who are skilled and capable of taking an IQ test cannot be compared with those who have sensory deficits and may not have ever taken this type of test. Longitudinal studies that measure changes in a specific generation as it ages and that compensate for sensory, health, and educational deficits are relatively recent, and they serve as the most accurate way of determining intellectual changes with age.

Basic intelligence is maintained; one does not become more or less intelligent with age. The abilities for verbal comprehension and arithmetic operations are unchanged. Crystallized intelligence, which arises from the dominant hemisphere of the brain, is maintained through the adult years; this form of intelligence enables the individual to use past learning and experiences for problem-solving. Fluid intelligence, emanating from the nondominant hemisphere, controls emotions, retention of nonintellectual information, creative capacities, spatial perceptions, and aesthetic appreciation; this is believed to decline in later life. Some decline in intellectual function occurs in the moments preceding death.

LEARNING

Although learning ability is not seriously altered with age, other factors can interfere with the older person's ability to learn, including motivation, attention span, delayed transmission of information to the brain, perceptual deficits, and illness. Older persons may display less readiness to learn and depend on previous experience for solutions to problems rather than experiment with new problem-solving techniques. Differences in the intensity and duration of the elderly person's physiologic arousal may make it more difficult to extinguish previous responses and acquire new material. The early phases of the learning process tend to be more difficult for older persons than younger individuals; however, after a longer early phase, they are then able to keep equal pace. Learning occurs best when the information is related to previously learned information. Although little difference is apparent between the old and young in verbal or abstract ability, older persons do show some difficulty with perceptual motor tasks. Some evidence indicates a tendency toward simple association rather than analysis. Because it is generally a greater problem to learn new habits when old habits exist and must be unlearned, relearned, or modified, elderly persons with many years of history will have difficulty in this area. **(Visit the Connection website for helpful hints to enhance learning in elders.)**

> **KEY CONCEPT**
> Older adults maintain the capacity to learn, although a variety of factors can easily interfere with the learning process.

ATTENTION SPAN

Older adults demonstrate a decrease in vigilance performance (ie, the ability to retain attention longer than 45 minutes). They are more easily distracted by irrelevant information and stimuli and are less able to perform tasks that are complicated or require simultaneous performance.

Nursing Implications

An understanding of common aging changes is essential to ensure competent gerontological nursing practice. Such knowledge can aid in promoting practices that enhance wellness, reducing risks to health and well-being, and identifying pathology in a timely manner. Table 5-1 lists some nursing actions related to age-related changes.

> **KEY CONCEPT**
> By promoting good health practices in persons of all ages, gerontological nurses can help greater numbers of individuals enter late life with positive health states.

Gerontological nurses must realize that, despite the numerous changes commonly experienced with age, most older adults function admirably well and live normal, satisfying lives. Although nurses need to acknowledge factors that can alter function with aging, they should also emphasize the capabilities and assets possessed by older adults and assist persons of all ages in achieving a healthy aging process.

TABLE 5-1 ● *Nursing Actions Related to Age-Related Changes*

Age-related Change	Nursing Action
Reduction in intracellular fluid	Prevent dehydration by ensuring fluid intake of at least 1,500 mL daily
Decrease in subcutaneous fat content, decline in natural insulation	Ensure adequate clothing is worn to maintain body warmth; maintain room temperatures between 70°F (21°C) and 75°F (24°C)
Lower oral temperatures	Use thermometers that register low temperatures; assess baseline norm for body temperature when patient is well to be able to identify unique manifestations of fever
Decreased cardiac output and stroke volume; increased peripheral resistance	Allow rest between activities, procedures; recognize the longer time period required for heart rate to return to normal following a stress on the heart, and evaluate presence of tachycardia accordingly; ensure blood pressure level is adequate to meet circulatory demands by assessing physical and mental function at various blood-pressure levels
Decreased lung expansion, activity, and recoil; lack of basilar inflation; increased rigidity of lungs and thoracic cage; less effective gas exchange and cough response	Encourage respiratory activity; recognize that atypical symptoms and signs can accompany respiratory infection; monitor oxygen administration closely, keep oxygen infusion rate under 4 mL, unless otherwise prescribed

(continued)

TABLE 5-1 ● *Nursing Actions Related to Age-Related Changes (Continued)*

Age-related Change	Nursing Action
Brittleness of teeth; retraction of gingiva	Encourage daily flossing and brushing; ensure patient visits dentist annually; inspect oral cavity for periodontal disease, jagged-edged teeth, other pathologies
Reduced acuity of taste sensations	Observe for overconsumption of sweets and salt; be sure foods are served attractively; season food healthfully
Drier oral cavity	Offer fluids during meals; have patient drink before swallowing tablets and capsules, and examine oral cavity after administration to ensure drugs have been swallowed
Decreased esophageal and gastric motility; decreased gastric acid	Assess for indigestion; encourage 5–6 small meals rather than 3 large ones; advise patient not to lie down for at least 1 hour following meals
Decreased colonic peristalsis; duller neural impulses to lower bowel	Encourage toileting schedule to provide adequate time for bowel elimination; monitor frequency, consistency, and amount of bowel movements
Decreased size of renal mass, number of nephrons, renal blood flow, glomerular filtration rate, tubular function	Ensure age-adjusted drug dosages are prescribed; observe for adverse responses to drugs; recognize that urine testing for glucose can be unreliable, urinary creatinine excretion and creatinine clearance are decreased, and blood urea nitrogen level is higher
Decreased bladder capacity	Assist patient with need for frequent toileting; ensure safety for visits to bathroom during the night
Weaker bladder muscles	Observe for signs of urinary tract infection; assist patient to void in upright position
Enlargement of prostate gland	Ensure patient has prostate examined annually
Drier, more fragile vagina	Advise patient in safe use of lubricants for comfort during intercourse
Increased alkalinity of vaginal canal	Observe for signs of vaginitis
Atrophy of muscle; reduction in muscle strength and mass	Encourage regular exercise; advise patient to avoid straining or overusing muscles
Decreased bone mass and mineral content	Instruct patient in safety measures to prevent falls and fractures; encourage good calcium intake and exercise
Less prominent stages III and IV of sleep	Avoid interruptions at night; assess quantity and quality of sleep
Decreased visual accommodation; reduced peripheral vision; less effective vision in dark and dimly lit areas	Ensure patient has ophthalmologic exam annually; use night lights; avoid drastic changes in level of lighting; ensure objects used by patient are within visual field
Yellowing of lens	Avoid using shades of greens, blues, and violets together
Decreased corneal sensitivity	Advise patient to protect eyes
Presbycusis	Ensure patient has audiometric exam if problem exists; speak to patient in loud, low-pitched voice
Reduced capacity to sense pain and pressure	Ensure patient changes positions before tissue reddens, inspect body for problems that patient may not sense; recognize unique responses to pain
Reduced immunity	Prevent persons who have infectious diseases from infection early; recommend pneumococcal, tetanus, and annual influenza vaccinations; promote good nutritional status to improve host defenses
Slower metabolic rate	Advise patient to avoid excess calorie consumption
Altered secretion of insulin and metabolism of glucose	Advise patient to avoid high carbohydrate intake; observe for unique manifestations of hyper- or hypoglycemia.
Flattening of dermal–epidermal junction; reduced thickness and vascularity of dermis; degeneration of elastin fibers	Use principles of pressure ulcer prevention
Skin drier	Recognize need for less frequent bathing; avoid use of harsh soaps; use skin softeners
Slower response and reaction time	Allow adequate time for patient to respond, process information, perform tasks

Critical Thinking Exercises

Mr. Gaskin is a 72-year-old retired truck driver admitted to the hospital for treatment of acute glomerulonephritis. His height is 5 feet 11 inches and his weight is 180 pounds. You note from the record that he weighed 220 pounds last year and has experienced a reduction in weight at each of his monthly physician's visits. Although he has a moderate degree of chronic obstructive pulmonary disease, he continues to smoke one pack of cigarettes daily. He has varicosities on both lower extremities and hemorrhoids. Mr. Gaskin is coherent and responds appropriately. His wife comments that he always has had a sharp mind, although in the past few years he has become considerably quieter and less gregarious. As you observe Mr. Gaskin throughout the day you note that he:

- becomes short of breath with minimal exertion
- develops edema
- has urinary hesitancy and scanty urine output
- adds considerable salt to his food before tasting it
- has difficulty hearing normal conversation
- moves very little when in bed

1. Based on the information provided, answer the following questions:
   Which signs and observations are related to normal aging and which can you attribute to pathology?
   What factors contributed to the health conditions possessed by Mr. Gaskin?
   Describe the risks that are high for Mr. Gaskin and list nursing measures that could minimize them.
2. What age-related changes can you identify in yourself and in your parents?
3. Consider recommendations that you would give young adults for promotion of a healthy aging process.

Web Connect

Sign up for the National Center for Chronic Disease Prevention and Health Promotion's *Public Health and Aging E-Mail Forum* and access current information about healthy aging at www.cdc.gov/aging

●References

Harris, T. B., Visser, M., Everhart, J., Tylavsky, F., Fuerst, T., et al. (2000). Waist circumference and sagittal diameter reflect total body fat better than visceral fat in older men and women. *The Health, Aging, And Body Composition Study Research Group, Annals of New York Academy of Science*, *904*(1), 462–473.

Shaker, R., Ren, J., Bardan, E., Easterling, C., Dua, K., Xie, P., & Kern, M. (2003). Pharyngoglottal closure reflex: Characterization in healthy young, elderly and dysphagic patients with redeglutitive aspiration. *Gerontology, 49*(1), 12–20.

Kielstein, J. T., Body-Boger, S. M., Frolich, J. C., Ritz, E., Haller, H., & Fliser, D. (2003). Asymmetric dimethylarginine, blood pressure, and renal perfusion in elderly subjects. *Circulation, 107*(14),1891–1895.

●Recommended Readings

Arking, R. (1998). *Biology of aging: Observations and principles* (2nd ed.). Sunderland, MA: Sinauer Associates.

Belsky, J. (1999). *The psychology of aging: Theory, research, and interventions* (3rd ed.). Pacific Grove, CA: Brooks/Cole Publishers.

Creagan, E. T. (Ed.). (2001). *Mayo Clinic on healthy aging.* Rochester, MN: Mayo Clinic.

Feinsilver, S. H. (2003). Sleep in the elderly. What is normal? *Clinical Geriatric Medicine, 19*(1),177–88.

Finkelstein, J. A., & Schiffman, S. S. (1999). Workshop on taste and smell in the elderly: An overview. *Physiology and Behavior, 66*(2), 173–176.

Hamilton, H. E. (1999). *Language and communication in old age: Multidisciplinary perspectives.* New York: Garland.

Howieson, D. B., Camicioli, R., Quinn, J., Silbert, L. C., Care, B., Moore, M. M., Dame, A., Sexton, G., & Kaye, J. A. (2003). Natural history of cognitive decline in the old old. *Neurology, 60*(9),1489–1494.

Hultsch, D. F. (1998). *Memory change in the aged.* Cambridge, UK: Cambridge University Press.

Mobbs, C. V., & Hof, P. R. (1998). *Functional endocrinology of aging.* Basel: Karger.

Salerno, J. A. (2002). Living longer, living better: The promise of aging research. *Caring, 21*(8), 8–10.

Schultz-Aellen, M. F. (1997). *Aging and human longevity.* Boston: Birkhauser.

Shephard, R. J. (1997). *Aging, physical activity, and health.* Champaign, IL: Human Kinetics.

Skelton, D. A., Young, A., Greig, C. A., & Malbut, K. E. (1995). Effects of resistance training on strength, power, and selected functional abilities of women aged 75 and older. *Journal of the American Geriatric Society, 43*(10), 1081–1086.

Smyer, M. A., & Qualls, S. H. (1999). *Aging and mental health.* Malden, MA: Blackwell.

Wang, E., & Snyder, S. (1998). *Handbook of the aging brain.* San Diego: Academic Press.

Zeleznik, J. (2003). Normative aging of the respiratory system. *Clinical Geriatric Medicine, 19*(1), 1–18.

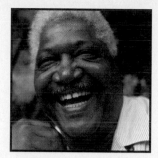

Foundations of Gerontological Nursing

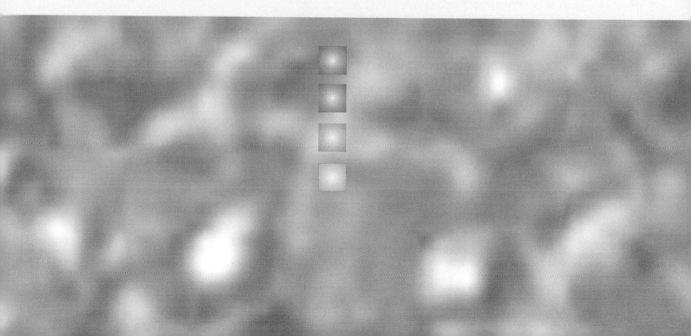

The Specialty of Gerontological Nursing

■ Chapter Outline

Development of gerontological nursing
Nursing's long history of caring for elderly
Landmarks in development of
gerontological nursing
Gerontological nursing roles
Healer
Caregiver
Educator
Advocate
Innovator
Advanced practice nursing
Significance to gerontological care
Geriatric nurse practitioner, clinical
specialists
Standards
Purpose of standards
Various standards for gerontological
nursing practice
Evidence-based practice
Use of research for clinical decision-
making
Meta-analysis, cost analysis
Principles guiding gerontological nursing
practice
Aging is natural process
Variety of factors influence aging
Unique data and knowledge used
Elderly possess same universal self-care
demands as others
Focus of gerontological nursing is to help
elderly achieve personhood
Holistic gerontological care
Use of knowledge and skills from various
disciplines
Consideration of physical, mental, social,
and spiritual health
Balance of mind, body, and spirit

■ Learning Objectives

After reading this chapter, you should be
able to:

- list landmarks that affected the
  development of gerontological nursing

- discuss major roles in gerontological
  nursing

- identify standards used in
  gerontological nursing practice

- list principles guiding gerontological
  nursing practice

- explain holistic gerontological nursing
  care

Development of Gerontological Nursing

Nurses, long interested in the care of the aged, seem to have assumed more responsibility than other professional disciplines for this segment of the population. In 1904, the *American Journal of Nursing* printed the first nursing article on the care of the aged, presenting many principles that continue to guide gerontological nursing practice today (Bishop, 1904): "You must not treat a young child as you would a grown person, nor must you treat an old person as you would one in the prime of life." Interestingly, this same journal featured an article entitled "The Old Nurse," which emphasized the value of the aging nurse's years of experience (DeWitt, 1904).

After the Federal Old Age Insurance Law (better known as Social Security) was passed in 1935, many older persons had an alternative to alms houses and could independently purchase room and board (Figure 6-1). Because many of the homes that offered these services for the aged were operated by women who called themselves nurses, it is not coincidental that such residences later became known as nursing homes.

For many years, care of the aged was an unpopular branch of nursing practice. Geriatric nurses were thought to be somewhat inferior in capabilities, neither good enough for acute settings nor ready to "go to pasture." Geriatric facilities may have further discouraged many competent nurses from working in these settings by paying low salaries. Little existed to counter the negativism in educational programs, where experiences with older persons were inadequate in both quantity and quality and attention focused on the sick rather than the well, who were more representative of the older population. Although nurses were among the few professionals involved with the aged, gerontology was missing from most nursing curriculums until recently.

Frustration over the lack of value placed on geriatric nursing led to an appeal to the American Nurses Association (ANA) for assistance in promoting the status of this area of practice. After years of study, in 1961 the ANA recommended that a specialty group for geriatric nurses be formed. In 1962, the ANA's Conference Group on Geriatric Nursing Practice held its first national meeting. This group became the Division of Geriatric Nursing in 1966, gaining full recognition as a nursing specialty. An important contribution by this group was the development in 1969 of *Standards for Geriatric Nursing Practice*, first published in 1970. Certification of nurses for excellence in geriatric nursing practice followed, with the first 74 nurses achieving this recognition in 1975. The birth of the *Journal of Gerontological Nursing*, the first professional journal to meet the specific needs and interests of gerontological nurses, also occurred in 1975.

Through the 1970s, nurses began to become increasingly aware of their role in promoting a healthy aging experience for all individuals and ensuring the wellness of older adults. As a result, they expressed interest in changing the name of the specialty from geriatric to gerontological nursing to reflect a broader scope than the care of the ill aged. In 1976, the Geriatric Nursing Division became the Gerontological Nursing Division. Table 6-1 lists landmarks in the growth of gerontological nursing.

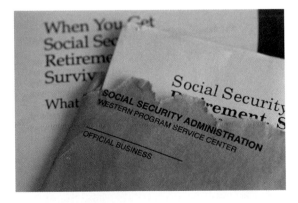

FIGURE 6-1

Social Security provided a means for many elders to be independent.

KEY CONCEPT
Gerontological nursing involves the care of aging people and emphasizes the promotion of the highest possible quality of life and wellness. Geriatric nursing focuses on the care of the sick aged.

TABLE 6-1 ● *Landmarks in the Growth of Gerontological Nursing*

1902	First article on care of aged in *American Journal of Nursing* written by a physician
1904	First article on care of aged in *American Journal of Nursing* written by a nurse
1950	First gerontological nursing text published (*Geriatric Nursing*, K. Newton)
	First master's thesis on care of aged (Eleanor Pingrey)
	Geriatrics recognized as an area of specialization in nursing
1952	First nursing study on care of aged published in *Nursing Research*
1961	American Nurses Association recommends specialty group for geriatric nurses
1962	First national meeting of American Nurses Association Conference on Geriatric Nursing Practice
1966	Formation of Geriatric Nursing Division of American Nurses Association
	First gerontological nursing clinical specialist nursing program (Duke University)
1968	First nurse makes presentation at International Congress of Gerontology (Laurie Gunter)
1969	Development of standards for geriatric nursing practice
1970	First publication of *ANA Standards of Gerontological Nursing Practice*
1975	First offering of *ANA Certification in Gerontological Nursing* (74 nurses certified)
	First specialty publication for gerontological nurses, *Journal of Gerontological Nursing*
	First nursing conference at International Congress of Gerontology
1976	ANA changes name from Geriatric Nursing Division to Gerontological Nursing Division
1976	Publication of *ANA Standards of Gerontological Nursing*
	ANA Certification of Geriatric Nurse Practitioners initiated
1980	*Geriatric Nursing* journal launched by *American Journal of Nursing Company*
1981	First International Conference on Gerontological Nursing
	ANA Division of Gerontological Nursing develops statement on scope of practice
1982	Development of Robert Wood Johnson Teaching Home Nursing Program
1983	First university chair in gerontological nursing in the United States (Case Western Reserve)
1984	National Gerontological Nursing Association (NGNA) formed
	ANA Division of Gerontological Nursing Practice becomes Council on Gerontological Nursing
1986	National Association for Directors of Nursing Administration in Long-Term Care (NADONA/LTC) formed
1989	ANA Certification of Gerontological Clinical Specialists first offered
1990	Division of Long-Term Care established within ANA Council of Gerontological Nursing
1996	Hartford Gerontological Nursing Initiatives funding launched by John A. Hartford Foundation

In the past few decades, the specialty of gerontological nursing has experienced profound growth. Whereas only 32 articles on the topic of the nursing care of the aged were listed in the *Cumulative Index to Nursing Literature* in 1956, and only twice that number appeared a decade later, the number of articles published yearly more than doubled thereafter. Gerontological nursing texts grew from a few in the 1960s to a few dozen in the 1970s, and the quantity and quality of this literature has been rising since. Growing numbers of nursing schools are including gerontological nursing courses in their undergraduate programs and offering advanced degrees with a major in this area. To date, thousands of nurses have become certified in various aspects of gerontological practice. (For information on certification, please see the Resource listing for the American Nurses' Credentialing Center at the end of this chapter.) Nursing administration in long-term care, geropsychiatric nursing, geriatric rehabilitation, and other areas of subspecialization have evolved. The specialty has indeed advanced rapidly, and all indications are that this growth will continue.

Along with the growth of the specialty there has been a heightened awareness of the complexity of gerontological nursing. Elderly people exhibit great diversity in terms of health status, cultural background, lifestyle, living arrangement, socioeconomic status, and other variables. Most have chronic conditions that uniquely affect acute illnesses, reactions to treatments, and quality of life. Symptoms of illness can be atypical. Multiple health conditions can coexist and muddle the ability to chart the course of a single disease or identify the underlying cause of symptoms. The conditions that older adults experience can cut across many clinical specialties, thereby challenging gerontological nurses to have a broad knowledge base. The risk for complications is high. Other factors, such as limited finances or social isolation, affect the state of health and well-being. Also, the elective status of geriatrics in many medical and nursing schools can limit the pool of colleagues who are knowledgeable about the unique aspects of caring for the elderly.

Gerontological Nursing Roles

In their activities with older adults, nurses function in a variety of roles, most of which fall under the following categories (Display 6-1).

HEALER

Early nursing practice was based on the Christian concept of the intertwining of the flesh and spirit. In the mid-1800s, nursing's role as a healing art was recognized; this is apparent through Florence Nightingale's writings that nursing "put the patient in the best condition for nature to act upon him" (Nightingale, 1946). Although the early emphasis on nurturance, comfort, empathy, and intuition was replaced by detachment, objectivity, and scientific approaches as medical knowledge and technology grew more sophisticated, the revival of the holistic approach to health care has enabled nurses to again recognize the interdependency of body, mind, and spirit in health and healing. Nursing plays a significant role in helping individuals stay well, overcome or cope with disease, restore function, find meaning and purpose in life, and mobilize internal and external resources. In the healer role, the gerontological nurse recognizes that most human beings value health, are responsible and active participants in their health maintenance and illness management, and desire harmony and wholeness with their environment. A holistic approach is essential, recognizing that older individuals must be viewed in the context of their biological, emotional, social, cultural, and spiritual elements. (Information on holistic nursing can be obtained from the American Holistic Nurses' Association, listed under Resources at the end of this chapter.)

> ✔ **Point to Ponder**
> *Henri Nouwen (1990) spoke of the "wounded healer" who uses his or her own wounds as a means to assist in the healing of others. What life experiences or "wounds" do you possess that enable you to assist others in their healing journeys?*

CAREGIVER

The major role filled by nurses is that of caregiver. In this role, gerontological nurses use gerontological theory in the conscientious application of the nursing process to the care of elders. Inherent in this role is the active participation of older adults and their significant others and promotion of the highest degree of self-care of the elderly. This is especially significant in that there is a risk that elders who are ill and disabled can have decisions made and actions taken for them—in the interest of "providing care," "efficiency," and "best interest"—that rob them of their existing independence.

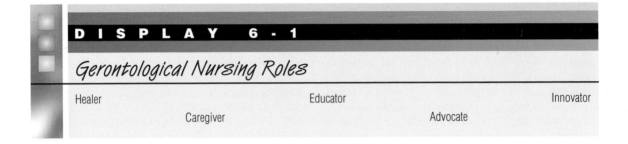

DISPLAY 6-1

Gerontological Nursing Roles

Healer		Educator		Innovator
	Caregiver		Advocate	

Although the body of knowledge of geriatrics and gerontological care has grown considerably, many practitioners are lacking in this information. Gerontological nurses are challenged to ensure that the care of older adults is based on sound knowledge that reflects the unique characteristics, needs, and responses of the elderly by disseminating gerontological principles and practices. Nurses working in this specialty area are challenged to gain the knowledge and skills that will enable them to meet the unique needs of elders.

EDUCATOR

Gerontological nurses must be prepared to take advantage of formal and informal opportunities to share knowledge and skills related to the care of older adults. This education extends beyond professionals to the general public. Areas in which gerontological nurses can educate others include normal aging, pathophysiology, geriatric pharmacology, and resources. Essential to this role is effective communication involving listening, interacting, clarifying, coaching, validating, and evaluating.

> **KEY CONCEPT**
> For healing to be a dynamic process, nurses need to identify their own weaknesses, vulnerabilities, and need for continued self healing. This belief is consistent with the concept of the wounded healer and suggests that by recognizing the wounds of all human beings, including themselves, nurses can provide services within a loving, compassionate framework.

ADVOCATE

The gerontological nurse can function in this role in several ways. First and foremost, advocacy for individual clients is essential and can include aiding older adults in asserting their rights and obtaining required services, facilitating a community's or other group's efforts to affect change and achieve benefits for older adults, and promoting gerontological nursing, including new and expanded roles of nurses in this specialty.

INNOVATOR

Gerontological nursing continues to be an evolving specialty; therefore, opportunities exist to develop new technologies and different modalities of care delivery. As an innovator, the gerontological nurse assumes an inquisitive style, making conscious decisions and efforts to experiment for an end result of improved gerontological practice. This requires the nurse to be willing to think "out of the box" and take risks associated with traveling down new roads, transforming visions into reality.

These roles can be actualized in a variety of practice settings, discussed in Chapter 10, and offer opportunities for gerontological nurses to demonstrate significant creativity and leadership.

Advanced Practice Nursing

To competently and effectively care for the clinical complexities of older adults, nurses need preparation in the unique principles and best practices of geriatric care. This requires the broad knowledge base, capacity for independent practice and leadership, and complex clinical problem-solving ability that is possible by nurses prepared for advanced practice roles. Advance practice roles include geriatric nurse practitioners, geriatric nurse clinical specialists, and geropsychiatric nurse clinician. Most of these roles require the completion of a master's degree at minimum.

There is strong evidence that nurses in advanced practice roles make a significant difference to the care of elders. Geriatric nurse practitioners have been shown to improve the quality and reduce the cost of care for elderly persons in hospitals, nursing homes, and ambulatory care settings (Paier and Strumpf, 1999; Bagley, Chan-Tack, Hicks, Rayburn, Nasir, Willems, Kim, Poplin, et al., 2000). Gerontological clinical nurse specialists in acute hospitals have been found to reduce complications, shorten length of stay, and reduce complications and the need for readmission post-discharge (Paier and Strumpf, 1999). The clear positive impact on the health and well-being of the elderly should encourage gerontological nurses to pursue these types of advanced practice roles and to encourage the employment of these advanced practitioners in their clinical settings.

Standards

Professional nursing practice is guided by standards. Standards reflect the level and expectations of care that are desired and serve as a model against which practice can be judged. Thus, standards serve to both guide and evaluate nursing practice.

Standards arise from a variety of sources. State and federal regulations outline minimum standards of practice for various health care workers (eg, nurse practice acts) and agencies (eg, nursing homes). The Joint Commission on Accreditation of Healthcare Organizations has developed standards for various clinical settings that strive to describe the maximum attainable performance levels. The ANA Standards of the Gerontological Nurse, as listed in Display 6-2, are unique in that they are the only standards developed by and for gerontological nurses. Nurses must regularly evaluate their actual practices against all standards governing their practice areas to ensure their actions reflect the highest quality care possible.

Evidence-Based Practice

There was a time when nursing care was guided more by trial and error than sound research and knowledge. Fortunately, that has changed and nursing now uses a systematic approach that uses existing research for clinical decision-making—a process known as evidence-based practice (Westhoff, 2000). Among the more popular ways to report the synthesis and analysis of information are the meta-analysis and cost-analysis (Agency for Healthcare Research and Quality, 2001). *Meta-analysis* is a process in which published research studies on a specific topic are analyzed and their results compiled. This allows the results of many small studies to be combined to allow more significant conclusions to be made.

With *cost-analysis* reporting, data is gathered on outcomes to make comparisons. For instance, the rate of pressure ulcers in one facility may be compared to another facility that has similar characteristics. (This process is called benchmarking.) The data can be used to stimulate improvements.

KEY CONCEPT
Best practices are built on evidence-based practice and the expertise of the nurse.

Principles Guiding Gerontological Nursing Practice

Scientific data regarding theories, life adjustments, normal aging, and pathophysiology of aging are combined with selected information from psychology, sociology, biology, and other physical and social sciences to provide specialized care to the older population. Professional nurses are responsible for using these scientific data as the foundation for nursing practice and ensuring through educational and managerial means that other caregivers use a sound knowledge base.

Data from a variety of disciplines are incorporated in the development of nursing principles, or those proven facts or theories that are accepted by society and guide nursing actions. In addition to the basic principles that direct the delivery of care to persons in general, specific and unique principles are used in caring for individuals of certain age groups or those who possess particular health problems. Some of the principles guiding gerontological nursing practice are listed in Display 6-3 and are discussed below.

AGING: A NATURAL PROCESS

Every living organism begins aging from the time of conception. The process of maturing or aging helps the individual achieve the level of cellular, organ, and system function necessary for the accomplishment of life tasks. Constantly and continuously, every cell of every organism ages. Despite the normality and naturalness of this experience, many people approach aging as though it were a pathologic experience, witnessed by comments that associate aging with:

- "looking gray and wrinkled"
- "losing one's mind"
- "becoming sick and frail"
- "obtaining little satisfaction from life"
- "returning to childlike behavior"
- "being useless"

D I S P L A Y   6 - 2

ANA Standards of Gerontological Nursing Practice

Standards of Clinical Gerontological Nursing Care

Standard I. Assessment

The gerontological nurse collects patient health data.

Standard II. Diagnosis

The gerontological nurse analyzes the assessment data in determining diagnoses.

Standard III. Outcome Identification

The gerontological nurse identifies expected outcomes individualized to the older adult.

Standard IV. Planning

The gerontological nurse develops a plan of care that prescribes interventions to attain expected outcomes.

Standard V. Implementation

The gerontological nurse implements the interventions identified in the plan of care.

Standard VI. Evaluation

The gerontological nurse evaluates the older adult's progress toward attainment of expected outcomes.

Standards of Professional Gerontological Nursing Performance

Standard I. Quality of Care

The gerontological nurse systematically evaluates the quality of care and effectiveness of nursing practice.

Standard II. Performance Appraisal

The gerontological nurse evaluates his or her own nursing practice in relation to professional practice standards and relevant statutes and regulations.

Standard III. Education

The gerontological nurse acquires and maintains current knowledge in nursing practice.

Standard IV. Collegiality

The gerontological nurse contributes to the professional development of peers, colleagues, and others.

Standard V. Ethics

The gerontological nurse's decisions and actions on behalf of older adults are determined in an ethical manner.

Standard VI. Collaboration

The gerontological nurse collaborates with the older adult, the older adult's caregivers, and all members of the interdiciplinary team to provide comprehensive care.

Standard VII. Research

The gerontological nurse interprets, applies, and evaluates research findings to inform and improve gerontological nursing practice.

Standard VIII. Resource Utilization

The gerontological nurse considers the factors related to safety, effectiveness, and cost in planning and delivering patient care.

(From American Nurses Association. [2001]. *Scope and standards of gerontological nursing practice*. Washington, DC: American Nurses Association. [A full copy of the standards including the accompanying rationale and measurement criteria can be obtained from American Nurses Publishing, 600 Maryland Avenue, SW, Suite 100 West, Washington, D.C. 20024.)]

DISPLAY 6-3

Principles of Gerontological Nursing Practice

- Aging is a natural process common to all living organisms.
- Various factors influence the aging process.
- Unique data and knowledge are used in applying the nursing process to the older population.
- The elderly share similar self-care and human needs with all other human beings.
- Gerontological nursing strives to help older adults achieve optimum levels of physical, psychological, social, and spiritual health so that they can achieve wholeness.

These are hardly valid descriptions of the outcomes of aging for most people. Aging is not a crippling disease; even with limitations that could be imposed by pathologies of late life, opportunities for usefulness, fulfillment, and joy are readily present. A realistic understanding of the aging process can promote a positive attitude toward old age.

> **KEY CONCEPT**
> Aging is a natural experience, not a pathologic process.

FACTORS INFLUENCING THE AGING PROCESS

Heredity, nutrition, health status, life experiences, environment, activity, and stress produce unique effects in each individual. Among the variety of factors either known or hypothesized to affect the usual pattern of aging, inherited factors are believed by some researchers to determine the rate of aging. Malnourishment can hasten the ill effects of the aging process, as can exposure to environmental toxins, diseases, and stress. On the other hand, mental, physical, and social activity can reduce the rate and degree of declining function with age. These factors are examined in more detail in Chapter 2.

Every person ages in an individualized manner, although some general characteristics are evident among most people in a given age category. Just as we would not assume that all 30-year-old people are identical and would evaluate, approach, and communicate with each person in an individualized manner, we must recognize that no two persons 60, 70, or 80 years of age are alike. Nurses must understand the multitude of factors that influence the aging process and recognize the unique outcomes for each individual.

ADJUSTING THE NURSING PROCESS

In nursing the elderly, scientific data related to normal aging and the unique psychological, biological, social, and spiritual characteristics of the older person are integrated with a general knowledge of nursing. The nursing process provides a systematic approach to the delivery of nursing service and integrates a wide range of knowledge and skills. The scope of nursing includes more than following a medical order or performing an isolated task; the nursing process involves a holistic approach to individuals and the care they require. The unique physiologic, psychological, social, and spiritual challenges of the elderly are considered in every phase of the nursing process.

COMMON NEEDS

Core needs that promote health and optimum quality of life are:

- *Physiological balance:* respiration, circulation, nutrition, hydration, elimination, movement, rest, comfort, immunity, and risk reduction

- *Connection:* familial, societal, cultural, environmental, spiritual, and to self
- *Gratification:* purpose, pleasure, dignity

Through self-care practices, people usually perform activities independently and voluntarily to meet these life requirements. When an unusual circumstance interferes with an individual's ability to meet these demands, nursing intervention could be warranted. The requirements for these needs and specific problems that the elderly may experience in fulfilling them are discussed in Unit III.

ACHIEVING OPTIMAL HEALTH

One can view aging as the process of realizing one's humanness, wholeness, and unique identity in an ever-changing world. In late life, people achieve a sense of personhood that allows them to demonstrate individuality and move toward self-actualization. By doing so, they are able to experience harmony with their inner and external environment, realize their self-worth, enjoy full and deep social relationships, achieve a sense of purpose, and develop the many facets of their being. Gerontological nurses play an important role in helping people achieve wholeness. Within the framework of the self-care theory, nursing actions toward this goal are:

- strengthening the individual's self-care capacity
- eliminating or minimizing self-care limitations
- providing direct services by acting for, doing for, or assisting the individual when demands cannot be met independently

The thread woven throughout the above nursing actions is the promotion of maximum independence. Although it may be more time-consuming and difficult, allowing older persons to do as much for themselves as possible produces many positive outcomes for their biopsychosocial health.

✔ | **Point to Ponder**
What self-care practices are a routine part of your life? What is lacking?

Holistic Gerontological Care

Holism refers to the integration of the biologic, psychological, social, and spiritual dimensions of an individual to form a sum that is greater than its parts (Dossey, 1997). Holistic gerontological care incorporates knowledge and skills from a variety of disciplines (Fig. 6-2) to address the physical, mental, social, and spiritual health of individuals. Holistic gerontological care is concerned with:

- facilitating growth toward wholeness
- promoting recovery and learning from an illness
- maximizing quality of life when one possesses an incurable illness or disability
- providing peace, comfort, and dignity as death is approached

In holistic care, the goal is not to treat diseases but to serve the needs of the total person through the healing of the body, mind, and spirit.

> 🔑 **KEY CONCEPT**
> Gerontological nurses help older individuals achieve a sense of wholeness by guiding them in understanding and finding meaning and purpose in life; facilitating harmony of the mind, body, and spirit; mobilizing their internal and external resources; and promoting self-care behaviors.

Health promotion and healing through a balance of the body, mind, and spirit of individuals are at the core of holistic care. This concern has relevance for gerontological care. The impact of age-related changes and the effects of the highly prevalent chronic conditions easily can threaten the well-being of the body, mind, and spirit; therefore, nursing interventions to reduce such threats are essential. Because chronic diseases and the effects of advanced age cannot be eliminated, healing rather than curative efforts will be those most beneficial in gerontological nursing practice. Equally significant is assisting older adults toward self-discovery in their final phase of life so that they find meaning, connectedness with others, and an understanding of their place in the universe.

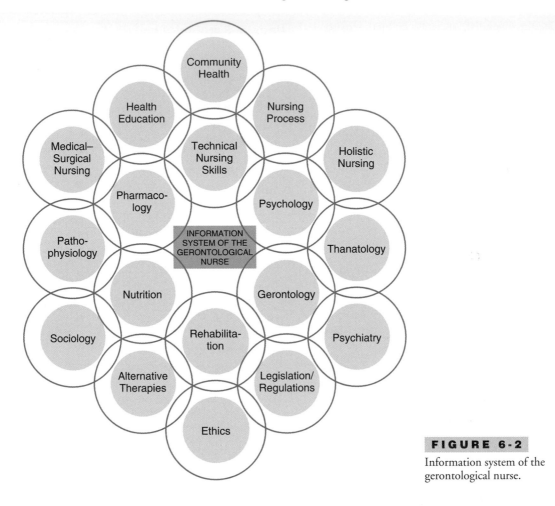

FIGURE 6-2

Information system of the gerontological nurse.

Critical Thinking Exercises

1. What were some of the reasons for the poor status of gerontological nursing in the past?
2. Why is the nursing role of healer particularly meaningful to gerontological practice?
3. What theme regarding the involvement of the older adult is apparent in the ANA Standards of the Gerontological Nurse?
4. Discuss the characteristics that make gerontological nursing a unique specialty.
5. What are some of the ways that nurses who do not choose to pursue advanced degrees themselves, can promote advanced practice roles?
6. What does wholeness mean to you?

Web Connect

Learn about the efforts of the John A. Hartford Foundation to enhance gerontological nursing at www.gerontologicalnursing.info

● Resources

American Holistic Nurses Association
P.O. Box 2130
Flagstaff, AZ 86004
800-278-AHNA
www.ahna.org

American Nurses' Credentialing Center
600 Maryland Avenue SW
Suite 100 W
Washington, DC 20024
800-284-CERT
www.nursingworld.org/ancc

● References

Agency for Healthcare Research and Quality (2001). Evidence-based practice centers. Rockville, MD: Agency for Healthcare Research and Quality.

Bagley, B., Chan-Tack, K. M., Hicks, P., Rayburn, K., Nasir, L., Willems, J. P., Kim, C., Poplin, C. M., et al. (2000). Health outcomes among patients treated by nurse practitioners or physicians. *Journal of the American Medical Association, 283*(1), 2521–2524.

Bishop, L. F. (1904). Relation of old age to disease with illustrative cases. *American Journal of Nursing, 4*(4), 674.

DeWitt, K. (1904). The old nurse. *American Journal of Nursing, 4*(4), 177.

Dossey, B. M. (1997). Holistic nursing practice, In B. M. Dossey (Ed.). *Core curriculum for holistic nursing* (p. 5). Gaithersburg, MD: Aspen.

Nightingale, F. (1946). *Notes on nursing: What it is, and what it is not.* Philadelphia: Lippincott.

Nouwen, H. J. M. (1990). *The wounded healer.* New York: Doubleday.

Paier, G. S., & Strumpf, N.E. (1999). Meeting the needs of older adults for primary health care. In M. Mezey & D.O. McGivern (Eds.), *Nurses, nurse practitioners: Evolution to practice* (3rd ed., pp. 300–315). New York: Springer Publishing Company.

Westhoff, C. I. (2000). Evidence-based medicine: An overview. *International Journal of Fertility, 45*(Suppl. 2), 105–112.

● Recommended Readings

Dossey, B. M., Keegan, L., & Guzzetta, C. E. (2000). *Holistic nursing: A handbook for practice* (3rd ed.). Gaithersburg, MD: Aspen.

Edmunds, M. S., Hoff, L. A., Kaylor, L., Mower, L., & Sorrell, S. (1999). Bridging gaps between mind, body, and spirit: Healing the whole person. *Journal of Psychosocial Nursing and Mental Health Services, 37*(10), 35–38.

Eliopoulos, C. (1999). *Integrating conventional and alternative therapies. Holistic care of chronic conditions.* St Louis: Mosby.

Guildner, S. (1995). Gerontological nursing issues and demands beyond the year 2005. *Journal of Gerontological Nursing, 21*(6), 6–9.

Johnson, P., & Thane, P. (1998). *Old age from antiquity to post-modernity.* New York: Routledge/LSE.

Luggen, A. S., & Travis, S. S. (1998). *NGNA core curriculum for gerontological advanced practice nurses.* Thousand Oaks, CA: Sage.

Rempusheski, V. F. (1996). Historical and futuristic perspectives on aging and gerontological nursing. In L. Rew (Ed.). *Awareness in healing.* Albany, NY: International Thomson Publishing.

Swanson, E. A., & Tripp-Reimer, T. (1996). *Advances in gerontological nursing.* New York: Springer.

Holistic Model for Gerontological Care

Chapter Outline

Health promotion-related needs
The meaning of health
Physiological balance
Connection
Gratification
Wholeness
Health challenges-related needs
Education
Counseling
Coaching
Monitoring
Coordination
Therapies
Requisites to meet needs
Physical, mental, socioeconomic abilities
Knowledge, experience, skill
Desire and decision to take action
Gerontological nursing interventions
Examples of application
Case example in assessment: The Case of Mr. R
Case example in application of the holistic model: The Case of Mrs. D

Learning Objectives

After reading this chapter, you should be able to:

• describe needs of elders pertaining to the promotion of health and the management of health challenges

• list the requisites that influence elders' abilities to meet self-care needs

• describe the general types of nursing interventions that are employed when elders present self-care deficits

Surviving to old age is a tremendous accomplishment. Basic life requirements such as obtaining adequate nutrition, keeping oneself relatively safe, and maintaining the body's normal functions have been met with some success to survive to this time. The hurdles of coping with crises, adjusting to change, and learning new skills have been confronted and overcome to varying degrees. Throughout their lives, the elderly have faced many important decisions, such as should they:

- leave the "old country" to make a fresh start in America?
- stay in the family business or seek a job in the local factory?
- risk their lives to fight for a cause in which they believe?
- encourage their children to fight in an unpopular war?
- invest their entire savings in a business of their own?
- allow their children to continue their education when the children's employment would ease a serious financial hardship?

Too often, nurses seek interventions to meet the needs of the elderly that come from external sources rather than recognizing that the elderly have considerable inner resources for self-care and empowering them to use these strengths. Older adults then become passive recipients of care rather than active participants. This seems unreasonable because most elders have had a lifetime of taking care of themselves and others, making their own decisions, and meeting life's most trying challenges. They may become angry or depressed at being forced to forfeit their decision-making functions to others. They may unnecessarily develop feelings of dependency, uselessness, and powerlessness. Gerontological nurses must recognize and mobilize the strengths and capabilities of older people so that they can be responsible and active participants in, rather than objects of care. Tapping the resources of elders in their own care promotes normalcy, independence, and individuality; it aids in reducing risks of secondary problems related to the reactions of older adults to an unnecessarily imposed dependent role; and it honors their wisdom, experience, and capabilities.

> **KEY CONCEPT**
> Our elders have had to be strong and resourceful to navigate the stormy waters of life.

Health Promotion-Related Needs

The concept of health seems simple yet it is quite complex. Viewing health as the *absence of disease* offers little more clarity than defining cold as the absence of hot and creates an image that begs for a more positive, broad understanding. In regard to older adults, most of whom are living with chronic conditions, this definition would relegate a majority of them to the ranks of the unhealthy.

When asked to describe the factors that contribute to health, most people would be likely to list the basic life-sustaining needs such as breathing, eating, eliminating, resting, being active, and protecting oneself from risks (Fig. 7-1). These are essential to maintaining the physiological balance that sustains life. However, the reality that we can have all of our physiological needs satisfied, yet still not feel well, demonstrates that physiological balance is but one component of overall health. Connection with ourselves, others, a higher being, and nature are important factors influencing health (Fig. 7-2). The fulfillment of physiological needs and a sense of being connected promote well-being of the body, mind, and spirit that enables us to experience gratification through achieving purpose, pleasure, and dignity (Fig. 7-3). This holistic model demonstrates that optimal health includes those activities that not only enable us to exist, but also help us to realize effective, enriched lives (Fig. 7-4).

> ✔ **Point to Ponder**
> *What does it mean to you to be healthy and whole?*

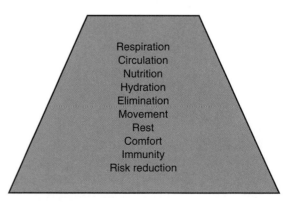

Respiration
Circulation
Nutrition
Hydration
Elimination
Movement
Rest
Comfort
Immunity
Risk reduction

FIGURE 7-1

Components of physiological balance.

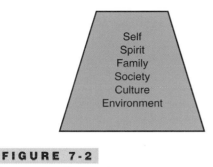

Self
Spirit
Family
Society
Culture
Environment

FIGURE 7-2

Components of connection.

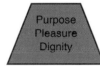

Purpose
Pleasure
Dignity

FIGURE 7-3

Components of gratification.

An improved definition of health arises when we consider the root meaning of the word health: *whole*. Using this foundation, health becomes *a state of wholeness . . . an integration of body, mind, and spirit to achieve the highest possible quality of life each day*

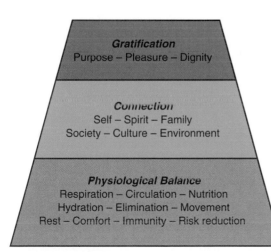

Gratification
Purpose – Pleasure – Dignity

Connection
Self – Spirit – Family
Society – Culture – Environment

Physiological Balance
Respiration – Circulation – Nutrition
Hydration – Elimination – Movement
Rest – Comfort – Immunity – Risk reduction

FIGURE 7-4

Health promotion-related needs.

(Fig. 7-5). For some individuals, this can mean exercising at the gym, engaging in challenging work, and having a personal relationship with God; for others, it can represent propelling oneself in a wheelchair to a porch, enjoying the beauty of nature, and connecting with a universal energy.

Views of health cannot only differ from individual to individual, but within the same individual from one time to another. Health priorities and expectations in a 70-year-old person may not resemble what they were when that individual was half that age. Cultural and religious influences can also affect one's view of health.

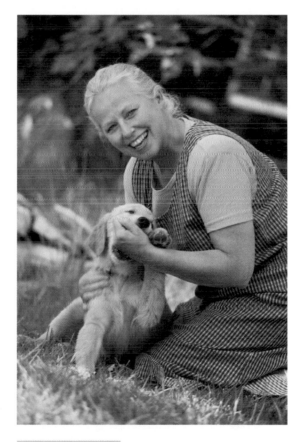

FIGURE 7-5

Rather than being limited to meaning the absence of disease, health implies a wholeness and harmony of body, mind, and spirit.

Optimal health of older adults rests on the degree to which the needs for physiological balance, connection, and gratification are satified. There is the risk that in busy clinical settings, the less tangible needs of gratification and connection can be overlooked; as advocates for the elderly, gerontological nurses must assure that comprehensive care is provided by not omitting these important needs.

Health Challenges-Related Needs

An unfortunate reality is that most older adults live with at least one chronic condition that challenges their health status. In fact, most involvement that nurses have with older adults typically involves assisting them with the demands imposed by health challenges. Older adults with acute or chronic conditions have the same basic health needs as healthy individuals (ie, physiological balance, connection, gratification); however, their conditions may create new needs such as:

- *Education:* As individuals face a new diagnosis they need to understand the condition and its care.
- *Counseling:* A health condition can trigger a variety of feelings and impose lifestyle adjustments.
- *Coaching:* Just as athletes and musicians require the skills of a professional who can bring out the best in them, patients, too, can benefit from efforts to improve compliance and motivation.
- *Monitoring:* The complexities of health care and the changing status of aging people warrant oversight from the nurse who can track progress and needs.
- *Coordination:* Older adults with a health condition often visit several health care providers; assistance with scheduling appointments, following multiple instructions, keeping all members of the team informed, and preventing conflicting treatments often is needed.
- *Therapies:* Often, health conditions are accompanied by the need for medications, exercises, special diets, and procedures. These therapies can include conventional ones that are commonly used in mainstream practice or complementary ones, such as biofeedback, herbal remedies, acupressure, and yoga. Patients may need partial or total assistance as they implement these treatments.

The assessment process considers patients' effectiveness in meeting the needs arising from health challenges. When deficits are evident, further exploration is necessary to determine which of the requisites to meet needs are deficient, similar to the process used in assessing health promotion-related needs. Figure 7-6 outlines this process.

Requisites to Meet Needs

As straightforward and clear as the health promotion and health challenges-related needs may seem, these needs are met with varying degrees of success because they are dependent on several factors:

Physical, mental, and socioeconomic abilities. An individual relies on several factors to meet even the most basic life demands. For example, to normally fulfill nutritional needs, a person must have the ability to experience hunger sensations; proper cognition to adequately select, prepare, and consume food; good dental status to chew food; a functional digestive tract to utilize ingested food; energy to shop and prepare food; and the funds to purchase food. Deficits in any of these areas can create risks to nutritional status. A variety of nursing interventions can be used to reduce or eliminate physical, mental, and socioecomonic deficits.

Knowledge, experience, and skills. Limitations exist when the knowledge, experience, or skills required for a given self-care action are inadequate or nonexistent. An individual with a wealth of social skills is capable of a normal, active life that includes friendships and other social interaction. People who have knowledge of the hazards of cigarette smoking will be more capable of protecting themselves from health risks associated with this habit. On the other hand, an older man who is widowed may not be able to cook and provide an adequate diet for himself, having always depended on his wife for meal preparation. The person who has diabetes and cannot self-inject the necessary insulin may not be able to meet the therapeutic demand for insulin administration. Specific nursing considerations for enhancing self-care capacities are offered in other chapters.

Desire and decision to take action. The value a person sees in performing the action, as well as the

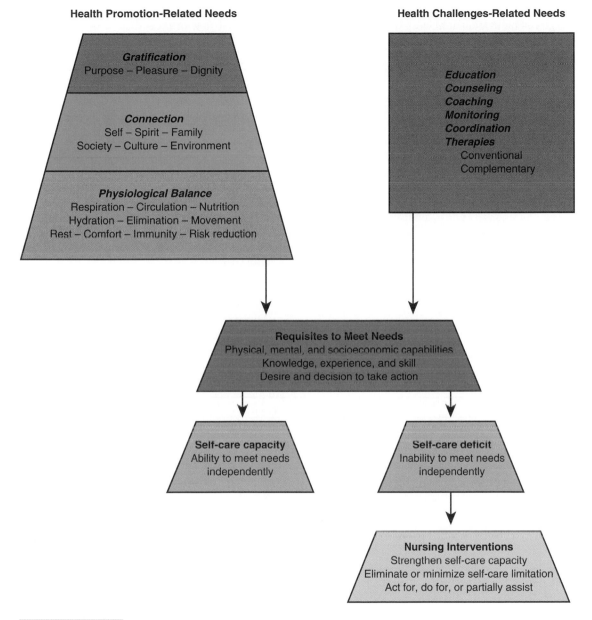

FIGURE 7-6

Gerontological nursing interventions for health promotion and health challenges-related needs.

person's knowledge, attitudes, beliefs, and degree of motivation, influences the desire and decision for action. Limitations result if a person lacks desire or decides against action. If an individual is not interested in preparing and eating meals because of social isolation and loneliness, a dietary deficiency may develop. A hypertensive individual's lack of desire and decision to forfeit potato chips and pork products in the diet because of a belief that it is not worth the effort may create a real health threat. The person who is not informed of the importance of physical activity may not realize the need to arise from bed during an illness and consequently may develop complications. Dying individuals, viewing death as a natural process, may decide against medical intervention to sustain life and may not comply with prescribed therapies.

Values, attitudes, and beliefs are deeply established and not easily altered. Although the nurse should respect the right of individuals to make decisions affecting their lives, if limitations restrict their ability to meet self-care demands, the nurse can help by explaining the benefit of a particular action, providing information, and motivating. In some circumstances, as with an emotionally ill or mentally incompetent person, desires and decisions may have to be superseded by professional judgments.

> **KEY CONCEPT**
> There can be vastly different reasons for elders to have a deficit in meeting a similar need. This challenges the gerontological nurse to explore the unique and sometimes subtle dynamics of each older person's life.

Gerontological Nursing Interventions

If the individual is successful in fulfilling needs, there is no need for nursing intervention except to reinforce the capability for self-care. However, the inability to meet needs independently creates a need for nursing intervention. Nursing interventions are directed toward empowering the elder by strengthening self-care capacities, eliminating or minimizing self-care limita-

tions, and providing direct services by acting for, doing for, or assisting the individual when requirements cannot be independently fulfilled (Fig. 7-7).

Examples of Application

Frequently, nursing's involvement with the elderly is associated with intervening when health conditions exist. When individuals face health challenges, new needs frequently arise, such as administering medications, observing for symptoms, and performing special treatments. In geriatric nursing, consideration must be given to assessing the impact of the health challenge on the individual's self-care capacity and identifying appropriate nursing interventions to ensure that the needs related to both health promotion and the management of health challenges are adequately met. During the assessment, the nurse identifies the specific health challenges-related needs that are present and the requisites (eg, physical capability, knowledge, desire) that need to be addressed to strengthen self-care capacity.

It is signficant that interventions include those actions that can empower the elder to achieve maximum self-care in regard to health challenges-related needs. Figure 7-6 demonstrates how the holistic self-care model becomes operational in geriatric nursing practice. The cases that follow demonstrate the application of this model.

> **KEY CONCEPT**
> More effort may be needed to instruct and coach an elder to perform a self-care task independently, and more time may be taken for the person to perform the task independently than would be necessary if a caregiver did the task; however, the benefits of independence to the elder's body, mind, and spirit are worth the investment.

CASE EXAMPLE IN ASSESSMENT—THE CASE OF MR. R

Mr. R, who has lived with diabetes for a long time, administers insulin daily and follows a diabetic diet. Because of a recent urologic problem, he may now need to take antibiotics daily and perform intermittent self-

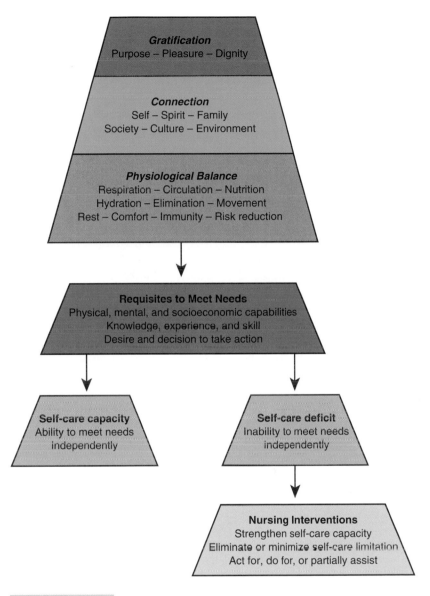

FIGURE 7-7

Gerontological nursing interventions for health promotion-related needs

catheterization. *During the assessment, the nurse identifies the presence of these illness-imposed needs.*

After the primary assessment has revealed the presence of needs related to health challenges, the nurse will evaluate how well these needs are met.

The nurse finds that Mr. R performs self-catheterization according to procedure and is administering his antibiotics as prescribed, but is not adhering to his diabetic diet and alters his insulin dosage based on "how he feels that day."

The next level of assessment must seek the reasons for deficits in meeting the health challenges-related needs.

Mr. R has knowledge of the diabetic diet and wants to comply, but had depended on his wife to prepare meals and now that she is deceased, he has difficulty cooking nutritious meals independently. He denies ever being informed of the need for regular doses of his insulin and states that he has relied on the advice of his brother-in-law, also a diabetic, who told him "to take an extra shot of insulin when he eats a lot of sweets."

Once the shortcomings in skills and knowledge behind the patient's deficits in meeting these health challenges-related needs are identified, specific nursing care plan actions can be developed.

CASE EXAMPLE IN APPLYING THE HOLISTIC MODEL—THE CASE OF MRS. D

The following case demonstrates how this model can work.

Mrs. D, 78 years of age, was admitted to a hospital service for acute conditions with the identified problems of a fractured neck of the femur, malnutrition, and a need for a different living arrangement. Initial observation revealed a small-framed, frail-looking lady, with obvious signs of malnutrition and dehydration. She was well oriented to person, place, and time and was able to converse and answer questions coherently. Although her memory for recent events was poor, she seldom forgot to inform anyone who was interested that she neither liked nor wanted to be in the hospital. Her previous and only other hospitalization had been 55 years earlier.

Mrs. D had been living with her husband and an unmarried sister for more than 50 years when her husband died. For the 5 years following his death, she depended heavily on her sister for emotional support and guidance. Then her sister died, which promoted feelings of anxiety, insecurity, loneliness, and depression. For the year since her sister's death she has lived alone, caring for her six-room home in the county with no assistance other than that from a neighbor who did the marketing for Mrs. D and occasionally provided her with transportation. On the day of her admission to the hospital, Mrs. D had fallen on her kitchen floor, weak from her malnourished state. Discovering her hours later, her neighbor called an ambulance, which transported Mrs. D to the hospital. Once the diagnosis of fractured femur was established, plans were made to perform a nailing procedure, to correct her malnourished state, and to find a new living arrangement because her home demanded more energy and attention than she was capable of providing.

Based on Mrs. D's self-care capacities and limitations, the nursing diagnoses described in Display 7-1 that arose from her holistic needs, were identified and related actions planned.

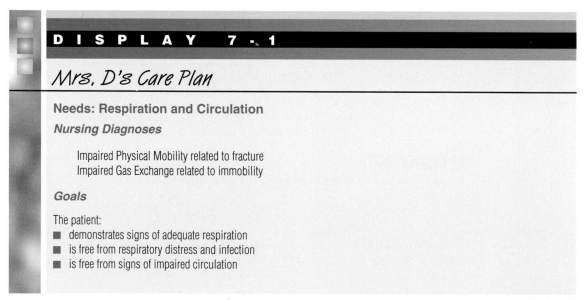

DISPLAY 7-1

Mrs. D's Care Plan

Needs: Respiration and Circulation

Nursing Diagnoses

Impaired Physical Mobility related to fracture
Impaired Gas Exchange related to immobility

Goals

The patient:
- demonstrates signs of adequate respiration
- is free from respiratory distress and infection
- is free from signs of impaired circulation

(Continued)

Related Nursing Intervention	*Type of Intervention*
1. Maintain normal respirations	
Prevent blockage of airway or any other interference with normal breathing	Partially assisting
Observe for and detect respiratory problems early	Partially assisting
2. Promote active and passive exercises	
Teach and encourage turning, coughing, and deep-breathing exercises	Strengthening self-care capacity
Encourage active exercises, such as using blow bottles and deep breathing	Strengthening self-care capacity
Perform passive range-of-motion exercise	Doing for
3. Avoid external interferences with respiration	
Provide good room ventilation	Doing for
Avoid restrictive clothing, linens, or equipment	Doing for
Position in manner conducive to best respiration	Partially assisting
Prevent anxiety-producing situations, such as delays in answering call bell	Doing for

Needs: Nutrition and Hydration

Nursing Diagnoses

Imbalanced Nutrition: Less than Body Requirements related to depression and loneliness

Goals

The patient:
- consumes at least 1500 mL of fluids and 1800 calories of nutrients daily
- increases weight to 125 lb

Related Nursing Intervention	*Type of Intervention*
1. Stimulate appetite	
Plan diet according to person's preferences, consistent with therapeutic requirements	Partially assisting
Provide a quiet, pleasant environment that allows for socialization with others	Doing for
Stimulate appetite through appearance and seasoning of foods	Minimizing self-care limitation
2. Plan meals	
Read menu selection to patient	Partially assisting
Guide choice of high-protein, carbohydrate, and vitamin- and mineral-rich foods	Minimizing self-care limitation
Access food preferences and include them in menu selections	Acting for
3. Assist with feeding	

(Continued)

Conserve energy and promote adequate intake by preparing food tray, encouraging rest periods, and feeding when necessary	Strengthening self-care capacity, doing for, and partially assisting
4. Prevent complications	Acting for
Do not leave solutions, medications, or harmful agents in location where they may be mistakenly ingested (especially when assessment indicates visual limitations)	
Check temperature of foods and drinks to prevent burns (especially when assessment indicates decreased cutaneous sensation)	Acting for
Assist in the selection of foods conducive to bone healing and correction of malnutrition	Partially assisting
Observe fluid intake and output for early detection of imbalances	Minimizing self-care limitation
Assess general health status frequently to detect new problems or improvements that have resulted from changes in nutritional status (eg, weight changes, skin turgor, mental status, strength)	Acting for and minimizing self-care limitation

Need: Elimination

Nursing Diagnoses

   Constipation related to immobility
   Risk for Infection related to malnutrition and interferences with normal bathing

Goals

The patient:
- is free from infection
- establishes a regular bowel elimination schedule
- is free from constipation
- is clean and odor free

Related Nursing Intervention	*Type of Intervention*
1. Promote regular elimination of bladder and bowels	Partially assisting
Guide the selection of a diet high in roughage and fluids	
Observe and record elimination pattern	Acting for and minimizing self-care limitation
Assist with exercises to promote peristalsis and urination	Partially assisting
Arrange schedule to provide regular time periods for elimination	Acting for
Assist with hygienic care of body surfaces	Partially assisting
Provide privacy when bedpan is used	Acting for and minimizing self-care limitation

(Continued)

2. Develop good hygienic practices
   Teach importance and method of cleansing   Strengthening self-care
      perineal region after elimination
3. Prevent social isolation
   Prevent, detect, and correct body odors   Acting for and minimizing self-care limitation
      resulting from poor hygienic practices

Need: Movement

Nursing Diagnoses

Activity Intolerance related to malnutrition and fracture
Impaired Physical Mobility related to fracture

Goals

The patient:
- maintains/achieves sufficient range of joint motion to engage in activities of daily living (ADL)
- is free from complications secondary to immobility

Related Nursing Intervention	*Type of Intervention*
1. Adjust hospital routines to individual's pace	Strengthening self-care capacity
Space procedures and other activities	Acting for
Allow longer periods for self-care activities	Minimizing self-care limitation
2. Provide for energy conservation	
Promote security and relaxation through the	Acting for
avoidance of frequent changes of personnel	
Prevent complications associated with immobility (such	Minimizing self-care limitation
as decubiti, constipation, renal calculi, contractures,	
hypostatic pneumonia, thrombi, edema, and lethargy)	
Encourage frequent change of position	Minimizing self-care limitation
Motivate and reward activity	Strengthening self-care capacity
Teach simple exercises to prevent complications	
and improve motor dexterity	Strengthening self-care capacity
Plan activities to increase independence progressively	Acting for and strengthening self-care capacity

Need: Rest

Nursing Diagnosis

Disturbed Sleep Pattern related to hospital environment and movement limitations associated with fracture

Goals

The patient:
- obtains sufficient sleep to be free from fatigue
- learns measures to facilitate sleep and rest

(Continued)

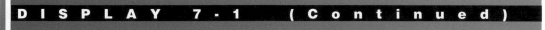

DISPLAY 7-1 (Continued)

Related Nursing Intervention	Type of Intervention
1. Control environmental stimuli	Acting for
Schedule rest periods between procedures	Acting for
2. Instruct in progressive relaxation	Strengthening self-care capacity

Need: Comfort

Nursing Diagnosis

Acute Pain related to fracture

Goals

The patient:
- is free from pain
- is able to participate in activities of daily living without pain-related restrictions

Related Nursing Intervention	Type of Intervention
1. Monitor for signs of pain	Minimizing self-care limitation
	Strengthening self-care capacity
2. Assist with positioning and exercises to reduce discomfort	Partially assist
3. Plan analgesic administration in collaboration with health care team	Minimizing self-care limitation

Need: Immunity

Nursing Diagnosis

Ineffective Health Maintenance
Risk for Infection

Goals

The patient:
is free from infection

Related Nursing Intervention	Type of Intervention
1. Encourage good food and fluid intake	Strengthening self-care capacity
2. Teach client to include foods in diet that positively affect immune system, such as milk, yogurt, nonfat cottage cheese, eggs, fresh fruits and vegetables, garlic	Strengthening self-care capacity
3. Instruct in and assist with immune-enhancing exercises such as yoga and t'ai chi	Strengthening self-care capacity
4. Review immunization history and arrange for immunizations as needed	Strengthening self-care capacity

(Continued)

DISPLAY 7-1 **(Continued)**

5. Instruct in stress management techniques	Strengthening self-care capacity

Need: Risk Reduction

Nursing Diagnoses

Disturbed Sensory Perception (visual, auditory, olfactory, tactile) related to advanced age
Risk for Injury related to sensory deficits
Risk for Impaired Skin Integrity related to immobility, malnutrition, and decreased sensations
Impaired Home Maintenance related to altered health state, convalescence

Goals

The patient:
- is free from injury
- possesses intact skin
- effectively and correctly uses assistive devices, eyeglasses, hearing aids (as prescribed) to compensate for sensory deficits
- has safe, acceptable living arrangements after discharge

Related Nursing Intervention	*Type of Intervention*
1. Compensate for poor vision	
Read to person	Doing for and minimizing self-care limitation
Write information and label with large letters and color coding when possible	Minimizing self-care limitation
Remove obstacles that could cause accidents such as foreign objects in bed, clutter on floor, and solutions that could be mistaken as water	Minimizing self-care limitation and acting for
Communicate this problem to other personnel	Acting for
Initiate an ophthalmology referral	Acting for
2. Compensate for decreased ability to smell	
Prevent and correct odors resulting from poor hygienic practices	Partially assisting and minimizing self-care limitation
Detect unusual odors early (may be symptomatic of infection)	Acting for
3. Compensate for hearing loss	
Speak clearly and loudly while facing person	Minimizing self-care limitation
Use feedback techniques to make sure person has heard and understood	Minimizing self-care limitation
Initiate referral to ear, nose, and throat clinic	Acting for
4. Maintain good skin condition	
Inspect for rashes, reddened areas, and sores	Doing for
Assist with hygienic practices	Partially assisting
Give back rubs, change person's position frequently, and keep person's skin soft and dry	Doing for, partially assisting, and minimizing self-care limitation

(Continued)

D I S P L A Y   7 - 1   (C o n t i n u e d)

5. Prevent falls	Partially assisting
Support person who is ambulating or being transported	Partially assisting
Maintain muscle tone	Strengthening self-care capacity
Keep bed rails up and support person in wheelchair	Doing for
Provide rest periods between activities	Strengthening self-care capacity and minimizing self-care limitation
Place frequently used objects within easy reach	Partially assisting
6. Maintain proper body alignment	
Use sandbags, trochanter rolls, and pillows	Minimizing self-care limitation and partially assisting
Support person's affected limb when it is lifted or moved	Partially assisting and minimizing self-care limitation
7. Seek safe living arrangements in preparation for person's discharge	Acting for and partially assisting
Evaluate patient's preferences, capacities, and limitations to suggest appropriate arrangements	Acting for and partially assisting
Initiate referral to social worker	Acting for

Need: Connection

Nursing Diagnoses

Spiritual Distress, Hopelessness, and Powerlessness related to hospitalization, health state, and lifestyle changes
Impaired Social Interaction related to hospitalization and health state

Goals

The patient:
- expresses satisfaction with the amount of social interaction
- identifies means for fulfilling spiritual needs
- is free from signs of emotional distress

Related Nursing Intervention	Type of Intervention
1. Control environmental stimuli	Acting for
Schedule the same personnel for caregiving	Acting for
Maintain a regular daily schedule	Strengthening self-care capacity
Arrange for a roommate with similar interests and background	Acting for and strengthening self-care capacity
2. Promote meaningful social interactions	Strengthening self-care capacity
Instruct others to speak clearly and sufficiently loud while facing the person	Strengthening self-care capacity
Plan meaningful activities	Strengthening self-care capacity

(Continued)

Promote and maintain an oriented state	Strengthening self-care capacity and minimizing self-care limitation
Display interest in person's social interactions and encourage their continuation	Strengthening self-care capacity
Initiate contacts with community agencies to develop relationships that can continue after discharge	Acting for and minimizing self-care limitation
Assist with grooming and dressing	Partially assisting and minimizing self-care limitation
3. Learn about patient's spirituality and religious beliefs and incorporate this into care	Strengthening self-care capacity
4. Arrange for pastoral/spiritual counseling	Acting for and strengthening self-care capacity
Encourage verbalization of feelings concerning meaning of health state and life changes	Strengthening self-care capacity
Provide opportunities for prayer	Strengthening self-care capacity

Need: Gratification

Nursing Diagnoses

Anxiety, Fear, Hopelessness, and Powerlessness related to hospitalization and health state
Impaired Social Interaction related to hospitalization
Chronic Low Self-Esteem related to health problems and life situation

Goals

The patient:
■ demonstrates preinjury level of physical activity
■ performs self-care activities to maximum level of independence
■ expresses satisfaction with the amount of solitude
■ is free from signs of emotional distress

Related Nursing Action	*Type of Action*
1. Control environmental stimuli	Acting for
Respect privacy	Strengthening self-care capacity
2. Provide opportunities for solitude	Acting for and strengthening self-care capacity
Provide several preplanned time periods during the day in which person can be alone	Acting for and strengthening self-care capacity
Provide privacy by pulling curtains around bed and making use of facilities such as chapel	Minimizing self-care limitations
3. Improve physical limitations where possible	
Assist with reeducation for ambulation	Partially assisting and strengthening self-care capacity
Exercise body parts to maintain function	Partially assisting and minimizing self-care limitation
Encourage patient to consume an adequate diet	Strengthening self-care capacity

(Continued)

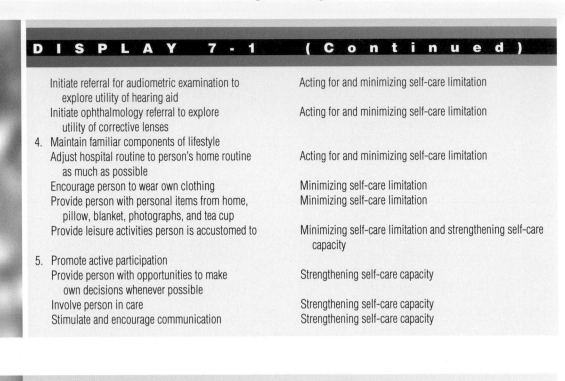

Initiate referral for audiometric examination to explore utility of hearing aid	Acting for and minimizing self-care limitation
Initiate ophthalmology referral to explore utility of corrective lenses	Acting for and minimizing self-care limitation
4. Maintain familiar components of lifestyle	
Adjust hospital routine to person's home routine as much as possible	Acting for and minimizing self-care limitation
Encourage person to wear own clothing	Minimizing self-care limitation
Provide person with personal items from home, pillow, blanket, photographs, and tea cup	Minimizing self-care limitation
Provide leisure activities person is accustomed to	Minimizing self-care limitation and strengthening self-care capacity
5. Promote active participation	
Provide person with opportunities to make own decisions whenever possible	Strengthening self-care capacity
Involve person in care	Strengthening self-care capacity
Stimulate and encourage communication	Strengthening self-care capacity

Critical Thinking Exercises

1. Identify life experiences that have been unique to today's older population and that have prepared them to cope with some of the challenges of old age.
2. List age-related changes that could affect each of the health promotion-related needs.
3. What are some reasons for older adults not wanting to function independently in self-care activities?
4. Why is it important to identify actions that strengthen self-care capacity rather than acting or doing for the patient?
5. Describe some situations in which older adults are at risk of losing independence as a result of nurses doing for them rather than promoting independence.

Web Connect

Review various perspectives on the meaning of holistic health at the websites of the American Holistic Medicine Association, www.holisticmedicine.org; the American Holistic Nurses Association, www.ahna.org; and American Holistic Health Association www.ahha.org.

● Recommended Readings

Aminbzadeh, F., Amos, S., Byszewski, A., & Dalziel, W. B. (2002). Comprehensive geriatric assessment: Exploring clients' and caregivers' perceptions of the assessment process and outcomes. *Journal of Gerontological Nursing, 28*(6), 6–13.

Creagan, E. T. (Ed.). (2001). *Mayo Clinic on healthy aging.* Rochester, NY: Mayo Clinic.

Eason, L. E. (2003). Concepts in health promotion: Perceived self-efficacy and barriers in older adults. *Journal of Gerontological Nursing, 29*(5), 11–19.

Eliopoulos, C. (1999). *Manual of gerontologic nursing* (2nd ed.). St. Louis: Mosby.

Felten, B. S., & Hall, J. M. (2001). Conceptualizing resilience in women older than 85: Overcoming adversity from illness or loss. *Journal of Gerontological Nursing, 27*(11), 35–42.

Grando, V. T., Mehr, D., Popejoy, L., Maas, M., Rantz, M, et al. (2002). Why older adults with light care needs enter and remain in nursing homes. *Journal of Gerontological Nursing, 28*(7), 47–53.

Hertz, J. E., & Anschutz, C. A. (2002). Relationships among perceived enactment of autonomy, self-care, and holistic health in community-dwelling older adults. *Journal of Holistic Nursing, 20*(2), 166–186.

Lewis, M., Hepburn, K., Corcoran-Perry, S., Narayan, S., & Lally, R. M. (1999). Options, outcomes, values, likelihoods. Decision-making guide for patients and their families. *Journal of Gerontological Nursing, 25*(12), 19–25.

Lindgren, C. L., & Murphy, A. M. (2002). Nurses' and family members perceptions of nursing home residents' needs. *Journal of Gerontological Nursing, 28*(4), 45–53.

Maddox, M. (1999). Older women and the meaning of health. *Journal of Gerontological Nursing, 25*(12), 26–33.

Moore, S. L., Metcalf, B., & Schow, E. (2000). Aging and meaning in life: Examining the concept. *Geritaric Nursing, 21*(1), 27–29.

Powers, P. H., Goldstein, C., Plank, G., Thomas, K., & Conkright, L. (2000). The value of patient- and family-centered care. *American Journal of Nursing, 100*(5), 84–89.

Resnick, B., & Fleishell, A. (2002). Developing a restorative care program. *American Journal of Nursing, 102*(7), 91–93.

Wu, A. W., Young, Y., Dawson, N. V., Brant, L., Galanos, A. N., et al. (2002). Estimates of future physical functioning by seriously ill hospitalized patients, their families, and their physicians. *Journal of the American Geriatrics Society, 50*(2), 230–237.

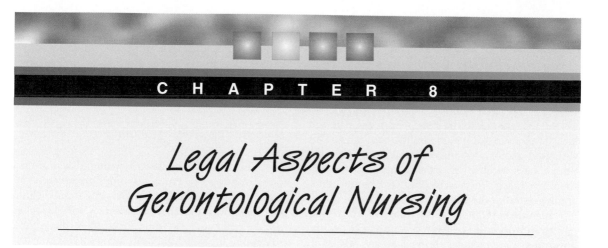

CHAPTER 8

Legal Aspects of Gerontological Nursing

■ Learning Objectives

After reading this chapter, you should be able to:

• list legal risks in gerontological nursing practice and ways to minimize them

• discuss ways to protect the legal rights of older adults

Nurses in every specialty must be cognizant of the legal aspects of their practice, and gerontological nurses are no exception. In fact, legal risks can intensify and legal questions can often arise when working in geriatric care settings. Frequently, gerontological nurses are in highly independent and responsible positions in which they must make decisions without an abundance of professionals with whom to confer. They are also often responsible for supervising nonprofessional staff and ultimately are accountable for the actions of these subordinates. In addition, gerontological nurses are likely to face difficult situations in which their advice or guidance may be requested by patients and families; they may be asked questions regarding how to protect the assets of the wife of a patient with Alzheimer's disease, how to write a will, what can be done to cease life-sustaining measures, and who can give consent for a patient. Also, the multiple problems faced by older adults, their high prevalence of frailty, and their lack of familiarity with laws and regulations, may make them easy victims of unscrupulous practices. Advocacy, then, is an integral part of gerontological nursing; nurses need to be concerned about protecting the rights of their elderly patients. To fully protect themselves, their patients, and their employers, nurses must have knowledge of basic laws and ensure that their practice falls within legally sound boundaries.

103

Laws Governing Gerontological Nursing Practice

Laws are generated from several sources (Display 8-1). Because many laws are developed at the state and local levels, variation exists among the states. This variation necessitates nurses' familiarity with the unique laws within their specific states, particularly those governing professional practice, labor relations, and regulation of health care agencies.

There are both public and private laws. *Public law* governs relationships between private parties and the government and includes criminal law and regulation of organizations and individuals engaged in certain practices. The scope of nursing practice and the requirements for being licensed as a home health agency fall under the enforcement of public law. *Private law* governs relationships between individuals and organizations and involves contracts and torts (ie, wrongful acts against another party, including assault, battery, false imprisonment, and invasion of privacy).

These laws set standards of conduct, which, if violated, can result in liability of the wrongdoer. Display 8-2 reviews some of the general acts that could make nurses liable for violating the law.

Legal Risks Facing Nurses

Most nurses do not commit wrongful acts intentionally; however, certain situations can increase the nurse's risk of liability. Such situations include working without sufficient resources, not checking agency policy or procedure, bending a rule, giving someone a break, taking shortcuts, or trying to work when physically or emotionally exhausted. Not only repeated episodes of carelessness, but also the chance that is taken just one time can result in serious legal problems. Nurses must assess all the potential legal risks in their practice and make a conscious effort to minimize them. Some of the issues that could present legal risks for nurses are presented below.

DISPLAY 8-1

Sources of Laws

Constitutions

State basic rights, grant powers, and place limits on government agencies that guide laws development by those agencies (eg, the right to freedom of speech)

Court Decisions

Establish precedents from cases heard in state or federal courts (eg, the right to discontinue life-support measures)

Statutes

Laws established by local, state, and federal legislation (eg, nurse practice acts)

Regulations

Laws enacted by state and federal administrative agencies that specifically define the methods to achieve goals and objectives of statutes (eg, conditions of participation for agencies to receive reimbursement from Medicare or Medicaid)

Attorney General Opinions

Laws derived from the opinions of the chief attorney for the state or federal government (eg, decisions regarding whether or not a case reflects a violation of law prior to filing a lawsuit for that case)

Acts That Could Result in Legal Liability for Nurses

Assault

A deliberate threat or attempt to harm another person that the person believes could be carried through (eg, telling a patient that he will be locked in a room without food for the entire day if he does not stop being disruptive).

Battery

Unconsented touching of another person in a socially impermissible manner or carrying through an assault. Even a touching act done to help a person can be interpreted as battery (eg, performing a procedure without consent).

Defamation of Character

An oral or written communication to a third party that damages a person's reputation. Libel is the written form of defamation; slander is the spoken form. With slander, actual damage must be proven, expect when:

■ accusing someone of a crime
■ accusing someone of having a loathsome disease
■ making a statement that affects a person's professional or business activity
■ calling a woman unchaste

Defamation does not exist if the statement is true and made in good faith to persons with a legitimate reason to receive the information. Stating on a reference that an employee was fired from your agency for physically abusing patients is not defamation if, in fact, the employee was found guilty of those charges. On the other hand, stating on a reference that an employee was a thief because narcotics were missing every time she was on duty can be considered defamation if the employee was never proved guilty of those charges.

False Imprisonment

Unlawful restraint or detention of a person. Preventing a patient from leaving a facility is an example of false imprisonment, unless it is shown that the patient has a contagious disease or could harm himself or herself or others. Actual physical restraint need not be used for false imprisonment to occur: telling a patient that he will be tied to his bed if he tries to leave can be considered false imprisonment.

Fraud

Willful and intentional misrepresentation that could cause harm or cause a loss to a person or property (eg, selling a patient a ring with the claim that memory will be improved when it is worn).

Invasion of Privacy

Invading the right of an individual to personal privacy. Can include unwanted publicity, releasing a medical record to unauthorized persons, giving patient information to an improper source, or having one's private affairs made public. (The only exceptions are reporting communicable diseases, gunshot wounds, and abuse.) Allowing a visiting student to look at a patient's pressure ulcers without permission can be an invasion of privacy.

Larceny

Unlawful taking of another person's possession (eg, assuming that a patient will not be using her personally owned wheelchair anymore and giving it away to another patient without permission).

Negligence

Omission or commission of an act that departs from acceptable and reasonable standards, which can take several forms:

■ *Malfeasance:* committing an unlawful or improper act (eg, a nurse performing a surgical procedure)
■ *Misfeasance:* performing an act improperly (eg, including the patient in a research project without obtaining consent)
■ *Nonfeasance:* failure to take proper action (eg, not notifying the physician of a serious change in the patient's status)
■ *Malpractice:* failure to abide by the standards of one's profession (eg, not checking that a nasogastric tube is in the stomach before administering a tube feeding)
■ *Criminal negligence:* disregard to protecting the safety of another person (eg, allowing a confused patient, known to have a history of starting fires, to have matches in an unsupervised situation)

> **KEY CONCEPT**
> Situations that increase the risk of liability include working with insufficient resources, failing to follow policies and procedures, taking shortcuts, or working when feeling highly stressed.

MALPRACTICE

Nurses are expected to provide services to patients in a careful, competent manner according to a standard of care. The *standard of care* is considered the norm for what a reasonable individual in a similar circumstance would do. When performance deviates from the standard of care, negligence, or malpractice, can be charged. Examples of situations that could lead to malpractice include:

- administering the incorrect dosage of a medication to a patient, thereby causing the patient to experience an adverse reaction
- identifying respiratory distress in a patient, but not informing the physician in a timely manner
- leaving an irrigating solution at the bedside of a confused patient, who then drinks that solution
- forgetting to turn an immobile patient during the entire shift, resulting in the patient developing a pressure ulcer
- having a patient fall because one staff member attempted to lift the patient when two were needed

The fact that a negligent act occurred in itself does not warrant that damages be recovered; instead, it must be demonstrated that the following conditions were present:

Duty: a relationship between the nurse and the patient in which the nurse has assumed responsibility for the care of the patient

Negligence: failure to conform to the standard of care (ie, malpractice)

Injury: physical or mental harm to the patient, or violation of the patient's rights resulting from the negligent act

> **KEY CONCEPT**
> Duty, negligence, and injury must be present for malpractice to exist.

The complexities involved in caring for older adults, the need to delegate responsibilities to others, and the many competing demands on the nurse contribute to the risk of malpractice. As the responsibilities assumed by nurses increase, so will the risk of malpractice. Nurses should be aware of the risks in their practice and be proactive in preventing malpractice (Display 8-3). Also, it is advisable for nurses to carry their own malpractice insurance and not rely only on the insurance provided by their employers. Employers may refuse to cover nurses under their policy if it is believed they acted outside of their job descriptions; further, jury awards can exceed the limits of employers' policies.

> ✔ **Point to Ponder**
> *In addition to the time and money involved in defending a lawsuit, what are some consequences of being accused of malpractice?*

CONSENT

Patients are entitled to know the full implications of procedures and make an independent decision as to whether or not they choose to have them performed. This may sound simple enough, but it is easy for consent to be overlooked or improperly obtained by health care providers. For instance, certain procedures may become so routine to staff that they fail to realize patient permission must be granted, or a staff member may obtain a signature from a patient who has a fluctuating level of mental competency and who does not fully understand what is being signed. In the interest of helping patients and delivering care efficiently, or from a lack of knowledge concerning consent, staff members can subject themselves to considerable legal headaches.

> **KEY CONCEPT**
> Patients who do not fully comprehend or who have fluctuating levels of mental function are incapable of granting legally sound consent.

Consent must be obtained before performing any medical or surgical procedure; performing procedures without consent can be considered battery. Usually

D I S P L A Y   8 - 3

Recommendations for Reducing the Risk of Malpractice

Be familiar with and follow the nurse practice act that governs nursing practice in the specific state.

Keep current of and adhere to policies and procedures of the employing agency.

Ensure that policies and procedures are revised as necessary.

Do not discuss a patient's condition, share patient information, or allow access to a patient's medical record to anyone unless the patient has provided written consent.

Consult with the physician when an order is unclear or inappropriate.

Know the patients' normal status and promptly report changes in status.

Assess patients carefully and develop realistic care plans.

Read patients' care plans and relevant nursing documentation before giving care.

Identify patients before administering medications or treatments.

Document observations about patients' status, care given, and significant occurrences.

Assure that documentation by self and subordinates is accurate and that documentation reflects care that actually was provided.

Know the credentials and assure competency of all subordinate staff.

Discuss with supervisory staff assignments that cannot be completed due to insufficient staff or supplies.

Do not accept responsibilities that are beyond your capabilities to perform and do not delegate assignments to others unless you are certain that they are competent to perform the delegated tasks.

Report broken equipment and other safety hazards.

Report or file an incident report when unusual situations occur.

Promptly report all actual or suspected abuse to the appropriate state and local agencies.

Attend continuing education programs and keep current of knowledge and skills pertaining to your practice.

(Adapted from Eliopoulos, C. [2002]. *Legal risks management guidelines and principles for long-term care facilities* [p. 28]. Glen Arm, MD: Health Education Network.)

when patients enter a health care facility they sign consent forms that authorize the staff to perform certain routine measures (eg, bathing, examination, care-related treatments, and emergency interventions). These forms, however, do not qualify as *carte blanche* consent for all procedures. Even blanket consent forms that patients may sign, authorizing staff to do anything required for treatment and care, are not valid safeguards and may not be upheld in a court of law. Consent should be obtained for anything that exceeds basic, routine care measures. Particular procedures for which consent definitely should be sought include any entry into the body, either by incision or through natural body openings; any use of anesthesia, cobalt or radiation therapy, electroshock therapy, or experimental procedures; any type of research participation, invasive or not; and any procedure, diagnostic or treatment, that carries more than a slight risk. Whenever there is doubt regarding whether consent is necessary, it is best to err on the safe side.

Consent must be *informed*. It is unfair to the patient and legally unsound to obtain the patient's signature for a myelogram without telling the patient what that procedure entails. Ideally, a written consent that describes the procedure, its purpose, alternatives to the procedure, expected consequences, and risks should be signed by the patient, witnessed, and dated. It is best that the person performing the procedure (eg, the physician or researcher) be the one to explain the procedure and obtain the consent. Nurses or other staff members should not be in the position of obtaining consent for the physician because they may not be able to answer some of the medical questions posed by the patient. Nurses can play an important role in the consent process by ensuring that it is properly obtained, answering questions, reinforcing information, and making the physician aware of any misunderstanding or change in the desire of the patient. Finally, nurses should not influence the patient's decision in any way.

Every conscious and mentally competent adult has the right to refuse consent for a procedure. To protect the agency and staff, it is useful to have the patient sign a release stating that consent is denied and that the patient understands the risks associated with refusing consent. If the patient refuses to sign the release, this should be witnessed, and both the professional seeking consent and the witness should sign a statement that documents the patient's refusal for the medical record.

COMPETENCY

Increasingly, particularly in long-term care facilities, nurses are confronting patients who are confused, demented, or otherwise mentally impaired. Persons who are mentally incompetent are unable to give legal consent. Often in these circumstances, staff will turn to the next of kin to obtain consent for procedures; however, the appointment of a guardian to grant consent for the incompetent individual is the responsibility of the court. When the patient's competency is questionable, staff should encourage family members to seek legal guardianship of the patient or request the assistance of the state agency on aging in petitioning the court for appointment of a guardian.

Various forms of guardianship can be granted (Display 8-4), each with its own restrictions. The guardian is monitored by the court to ensure that he or she is acting in the best interests of the incompetent individual. In the case of a guardian of property, the guardian must file financial reports with the court.

Guardianship differs from power of attorney in that the latter is a mechanism used by competent individuals to appoint someone to make decisions for them. Usually, a power of attorney becomes invalid if the individual granting it becomes incompetent, except in the case of a durable power of attorney. A durable power of attorney allows competent individuals to appoint someone to make decisions on their behalf in the event that they become incompetent; this is a recommended procedure for individuals with dementias and other disorders in which competency can be anticipated to decline. To ensure protection of patients' rights, nurses should recommend that patients and their families seek legal counsel for guardianship and power of attorney issues, and when such appointment has been made, clarify the type of decision-making authority that the appointed parties possess.

> **KEY CONCEPT**
> A durable power of attorney can be useful for patients with Alzheimer's disease because they can appoint someone to make decisions on their behalf at a time when they may be incompetent to do so.

STAFF SUPERVISION

In many settings, gerontological nurses are responsible for supervising other staff, many of whom may be nonprofessional. In these situations, nurses are responsible not only for their own actions but also for the actions of the staff they are supervising. This falls under the doctrine of *respondent superior,* the old master–servant rule. Nurses must understand that if a patient is injured by one of their subordinates while their employee is working within the scope of the applicable job description, they can be liable. Various types of situations can create risks for nurses:

- permitting unqualified or incompetent persons to deliver care
- failing to follow up on delegated tasks
- assigning tasks to staff members for which they are not qualified or competent
- allowing staff to work under conditions with known risks (eg, short staffed, improperly functioning equipment)

These are considerations that nurses need to keep in mind when they accept responsibility for covering the house, sending an aide into a home to deliver care without knowing the aide's competency, or allowing registry or other employees to work without fully orienting them to agency policies and procedures.

DISPLAY 8 - 4

Kinds of Decision-Making Authority That Individuals can Legally Possess Over Patients

Guardianship

Court appointment of an individual or organization to have the authority to make decisions for an incompetent person. Guardians can be granted decision-making authority for specific types of issues:

- Guardian of property (conservatorship): this limited guardianship allows the guardian to take care of financial matters but not make decisions concerning medical treatment.
- Guardian of person: decisions pertaining to the consent or refusal for care and treatments can be made by persons granted this type of guardianship.
- Plenary guardianship (committeeship): all types of decisions pertaining to person and property can be made by guardians under this form.

Power of Attorney

Legal mechanism by which competent individuals appoint parties to make decisions for them; this can take the form of:

- Limited power of attorney: decisions are limited to certain matters (eg, financial affairs) and power of attorney becomes invalid if the individual becomes incompetent.
- Durable power of attorney: provides a mechanism for continuing or initiating power of attorney in the event the individual becomes incompetent.

DRUGS

Nurses are responsible for the safe administration of prescribed medications. Preparing, compounding, dispensing, and retailing medications fall within the practice of pharmacy, not nursing, and, when performed by nurses, can be interpreted as functioning outside their licensed scope of practice. An act as seemingly benign as going into the agency's pharmacy after hours, pouring some tablets into a container, labeling that container, and taking it to the unit so that a patient can receive the drug that is urgently needed is illegal.

 KEY CONCEPT
A nurse pouring drugs from the central pharmacy's supply into a container for use by a patient can be viewed as illegally practicing pharmacy.

RESTRAINTS

The Omnibus Budget Reconciliation Act (OBRA) heightened awareness of the serious impact of restraints by imposing strict standards on their use in long-term care facilities. This increased concern regarding and sensitivity to the use of chemical and physical restraints has had a ripple effect on other practice settings.

Anything that restricts a patient's movement (eg, protective vests, trays on wheelchairs, safety belts, geriatric chairs, side rails) can be considered a restraint. Improperly used restraining devices can not only violate regulations concerning their use, but also result in litigation for false imprisonment and negligence.

Alternatives to restraints should be used whenever possible. Measures to help manage behavioral problems and protect the patient include alarmed doors, wristband alarms, bed alarm pads, beds and chairs close to the floor level, and increased staff supervision and contact. Specific patient behavior that creates risks to the patient and others should be documented. Assessment of the risk posed by the patient not being restrained and the effectiveness of alternatives should be included.

When restraints are deemed absolutely necessary, a physician's order for the restraints must be obtained, stating the specific conditions for which the restraints are to be used, the type of restraints, and the duration of use. Agency policies should exist for the use of restraints and should be followed strictly. At no time should restraints be used for the convenience of staff. Detailed documentation should include the times for initiation and release of the restraints, their effectiveness, and the patient's response. The patient requires close observation while restrained.

KEY CONCEPT

At no time should restraints be used for the convenience of staff.

At times, staff may assess that restraint use is required, but the patient or family objects and refuses to have a restraint used. If counseling does not help the patient and family understand the risks involved in not using the restraint, the agency may wish to have the patient and family sign a release of liability that states the risks of not using a restraint and the patient's or family's opposition. Although this may not free the nurse or agency from all responsibility, some limited protection may be afforded and, by signing the release, the patient and family may realize the severity of the situation.

TELEPHONE ORDERS

In home health and long-term care settings, nurses often do not have the benefit of an on-site physician. Changes in the patient's condition and requests for new or altered treatments may be communicated over the telephone, and, in response, physicians may prescribe orders accordingly. Accepting telephone orders predisposes nurses to considerable risks because the order can be heard or written incorrectly or the physician can deny that the order was given. It may not be realistic or advantageous to patient care to totally eliminate telephone orders, but nurses should mini-

mize their risks in every way possible by using the following precautions:

- Try to have the physician immediately fax the written order, if possible.
- Do not involve third parties in the order (eg, do not have the order communicated by a secretary or other staff member for the nurse or the physician).
- Communicate all relevant information to the physician, such as vital signs, general status, and medications administered.
- Do not offer diagnostic interpretations or a medical diagnosis of the patient's problem.
- Write down the order as it is given and immediately read it back to the physician in its entirety.
- Place the order on the physician's order sheet, indicating it was a telephone order, the physician who gave it, time, date, and the nurse's signature.
- Obtain the physician's signature within 24 hours.

Tape-recorded telephone orders may be a helpful way for nurses to validate what they have heard, but they may not offer much protection in the event of a lawsuit unless the physician is informed that the conversation is being recorded or unless special equipment with a 15-second tone sound is used.

NO-CODE ORDERS

The caseloads of many gerontological nurses contain a high prevalence of terminally ill patients. It may be understood by all parties involved that these patients are going to die and that resuscitation attempts would be inappropriate; however, unless an order specifically states that the patient should not be resuscitated, failure to attempt to save that person's life could be viewed as negligence. Nurses must ensure that no-code orders are legally sound, remembering several points. First, no-code orders are medical orders and must be written and signed on the physician's order sheet to be valid. DNR (ie, do not resuscitate) placed on the care plan or a special symbol at the patient's bedside is not legal without the medical order. Next, unless it is detrimental to the patient's well-being or the patient is incompetent, consent for the no-code decision should be obtained; if the patient is unable to consent, family consent should be sought. Finally, every agency should develop a no-code policy to guide staff in these situations; this could be an excellent item for an ethics committee to review.

ADVANCE DIRECTIVES AND ISSUES RELATED TO DEATH AND DYING

A variety of issues surrounding patients' deaths pose legal concern for nurses. Some of these issues arise long before death occurs, when patients choose to execute an advance directive or a living will. *Advance directives* express the desires of competent adults regarding terminal care, life-sustaining measures, and other issues pertaining to their dying and death. In 1990, Congress passed the Patient Self-Determination Act (which went into effect December 1, 1991), which requires all health care institutions receiving Medicare or Medicaid funds to ask patients on admission if they possess a living will or durable power of attorney for health care. The patient's response must be recorded in the medical record. States vary in their acceptance of living wills; there may even be variation among agencies regarding the conditions under which this document will be entered into the medical record. Nurses can aid by making physicians and other staff aware of the presence of a patient's living will, informing patients of any special measures they must take to have the document be accepted into the medical record, and, unless contraindicated, following the patient's wishes (Fig. 8-1). Readers are advised to check the status of living will legislation in their individual states.

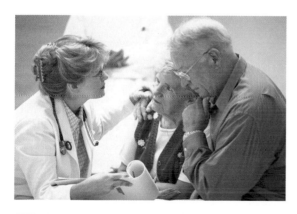

FIGURE 8-1

Gerontological nurses guide elders as they consider advance directives.

> **KEY CONCEPT**
> An advance directive can spare the family the burden of making significant decisions for the patient at a very difficult time.

Other issues arise when patients are terminally ill and dying; one such issue involves wills. *Wills* are statements of individuals' desires for the management of their affairs after their death. For a will to be valid, the person making it must be of sound mind, legal age, and not coerced or influenced into making it. The will should be written—although under certain conditions, some states recognize oral, or nuncupative, wills—signed, dated, and witnessed by persons not named in the will. The required number of witnesses may vary among the states.

To avoid problems, such as family accusations that the patient was influenced by the nurse because of his dependency on her, nurses should avoid witnessing a will. Nurses should, however, help patients obtain legal counsel when they wish to execute or change a will. Legal aid agencies and local schools of law are also sources of assistance for older adults wishing to write their wills. If a patient is dying and wishes to dictate a will to the nurse, the nurse may write it exactly as stated, sign and date it, have the patient sign it if possible, and forward it to the agency's administrative offices for handling. It is useful for gerontological nurses to encourage persons of all ages to develop a will to avoid having the state determine how their property will be distributed in the event of their deaths.

The pronouncement of death is another area of concern. Nurses often are placed in the position and are capable of determining when a patient has died and notifying the family and funeral home. The physician is then notified of the death by telephone and signs the death certificate at a later time. This rather common and benign procedure actually is illegal for nurses because the act of pronouncing a patient dead falls within the scope of medical practice, not nursing. Nurses should safeguard their licenses by either holding physicians responsible for the pronouncement of death or lobbying to have the law changed so that they are protected in these situations.

Postmortem examinations of deceased persons are useful in learning more about the cause of death.

They also contribute to medical education. In some circumstances, such as when the cause of death is suspected to be associated with a criminal act, malpractice, or an occupational disease, the death may be considered a medical examiner's case and an autopsy may be mandatory. Unless it is a medical examiner's case, consent for autopsy must be obtained from the next of kin, usually in the order of spouse, children, parents, siblings, grandparents, aunts, uncles, and cousins.

ABUSE

Elder abuse can occur in patients' homes or in health care facilities by loved ones, caregivers, or strangers. Particularly in long-term caregiving relationships, in which family members or staff "burn out," abuse may be an unfortunate consequence.

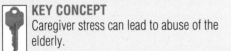

> **KEY CONCEPT**
> Caregiver stress can lead to abuse of the elderly.

Abuse can assume many forms, including inflicting pain or injury; stealing; mismanaging funds; misusing medications; causing psychological distress; withholding food or care; or sexually abusing, exploiting, or confining a person. Even threatening to commit any of these acts is considered abuse. Gerontological nurses must be alert to indications of possible neglect during routine interactions with elders; signs could include:

- delay in seeking necessary medical care
- malnutrition
- dehydration
- skin breaks, bruises
- poor hygiene and grooming
- urine odor, urine-stained clothing/linens
- excoriation or abrasions of genitalia
- inappropriate administration of medications
- repeated infections, injuries, or preventable complications from existing diseases
- elder's evasivenss in describing condition, symptoms, problems, home life
- unsafe living environment
- social isolation
- anxiety, suspiciousness, depression

All cases of known or suspected abuse should be reported. States vary regarding reporting mechanisms; nurses should thus consult specific state laws. The Resource listing includes organizations that can provide information on elder abuse and guidance on finding attorneys to assist an elder who is the victim of abuse.

OTHER ISSUES

Other situations can cause nurses to be liable for negligence, including the following:

- failing to take action (eg, not reporting a change in the patient's condition or not notifying the administration of a physician's incompetent acts)
- contributing to patient injury (eg, not providing appropriate supervision of confused patients or leaving side rails down)
- failing to report a hazardous situation (eg, not letting anyone know that the fire alarm system is inoperable or not informing anyone that a physician is performing procedures under the influence of alcohol)
- handling patient's possessions irresponsibly
- failing to follow established policies and procedures

> ✔ **Point to Ponder**
> *Are you familiar with your state's nurse practice act and the regulations governing the area in which you practice or will practice?*

Legal Safeguards

Common sense can be the best ally of sound nursing practice. It never should be forgotten that patients, visitors, and employees do not forfeit their legal rights or responsibilities when they are within the health care environment. Laws and regulations impose additional rights and responsibilities in patient—provider and employee—employer relationships. Nurses can and should protect themselves in the following ways:

- familiarize themselves with the laws and rules governing their specific care agency/facility, their state's nurse practice act, and labor relations

- become knowledgeable about their agency's policies and procedures and adhere to them strictly
- function within the scope of nursing practice
- determine for themselves the competency of employees for whom they are responsible
- check the work of employees under their supervision
- obtain administrative or legal guidance when in doubt about the legal ramifications of a situation
- report and document any unusual occurrence
- refuse to work under circumstances that create a risk to safe patient care
- carry liability insurance

Critical Thinking Exercises

1. Discuss the reasons why gerontological nursing is a high-risk specialty for legal liability.
2. Identify the process you would follow in your community to obtain guardianship for an incompetent older adult who has no family.
3. Describe the approach you would use to discuss the development of an advance directive with an older adult.
4. Discuss the actions you would take if faced with the following situations:

   A nurse whom you supervise makes repeated errors and does not seem competent to do his job. You begin documenting your observations but are told by your immediate supervisor to "just bite your tongue and live with it because he is the administrator's son."

   A patient confides in you that her son is forging her name on checks and gradually emptying out her bank accounts.

   The facility in which you work is attempting to be restraint free and strongly discourages the use of these devices; however, a resident's daughter insists that her mother be restrained because she has fallen twice within the past month.

Web Connect

Learn about your state's requirements for reporting abuse and sanctions for failing to do so in the American Bar Association's *Factbook on the Law and the Elderly* at their website www.abanet.org/media/factbooks/eldtoc.html

●Resources

American Association of Retired Persons (AARP)
Elder Law Forum
www.aarp.org/litigation/elf.html

American Bar Association
Senior Lawyers Division
750 North Lake Shore Drive
Chicago, IL 60611
(312) 988-5000
www.abanet.org/srlawyers/home.html

National Academy of Elder Law Attorneys
1604 North Country Club Road
Tucson, AZ 85716
(520) 881-4005
www.naela.com

National Center on Elder Abuse
c/o American Public Welfare Association
810 First Street NE
Suite 500
Washington, DC 20002
www.gwjapan.com/NCEA

Black Elderly Legal Assistance Support Project
National Bar Association
1225 11th Street NW
Washington, DC 20001
(202) 842-3900
www.kenyada.com/senior.htm

National Senior Citizens Law Center
1101 14th Street NW
Suite 400
Washington, DC 20005
(202) 289-6976
www.nsclc.org

Nursing Home Abuse/Elder Abuse Attorneys
Referral Network
www.nursing-home-abuse-elderly-abuse-attorneys.com

● Recommended Readings

Dunlap, R. K. (1997). Teaching advance directives: The why, when and how. *Journal of Gerontological Nursing, 23*(12), 11–16.

Eliopoulos, C. (2002). *Legal risks management guidelines and principles for long-term care facilities.* Glen Arm, MD: Health Education Network.

Gillick, M., Berkman, S., & Cullen, L. (1999). A patient-centered approach to advance medical planning in the nursing home. *Journal of the American Geriatrics Society, 47*(2), 227–230.

Heeschen, S. J. (2000) Making the most of quality indicator information. *Geriatric Nursing, 21*(4), 206–209.

Hirst, S. P. (2000). Resident abuse: An insider's perspective. *Geriatric Nursing, 21*(1), 38–42.

Hogstel, M. O., & Curry, L. C. (1999). Elder abuse revisited. *Journal of Gerontological Nursing, 25*(7), 10–18.

Mezey, M., Mitty, E., & Ramsey, G. (1997). Assessment of decision-making capacity: Nursing's role. *Journal of Gerontological Nursing, 23*(3), 28–35.

Middleton, H., Johnson, C., Elkins, A. D., & Lee, A. E. (1999). Physical and pharmacologic restraints in long-term care facilities. *Journal of Gerontological Nursing, 25*(7), 26–32.

Monarch, K. (2002). *Nursing and the law.* Washington, DC: American Nurses Publishing.

Pearlman, R. A. (1997). Determination of decision-making capacity. In C. K. Cassel, H. J. Cohen, & E. B. Larson, et al. (Eds.), *Geriatric medicine* (3rd ed.). New York: Springer.

Perrin, K. O. (1997). Giving voice to the wishes of elders for end-of-life care. *Journal of Gerontological Nursing, 23*(3), 18–27.

Peterson, A.M. (2002). Overview of the nursing home litigation process. *Geriatric Nursing, 23*(1), 37–42.

Quinn, M. J. (2002). Undue influence and elder abuse: Recognition and intervention strategies. *Geriatric Nursing, 23*(1), 11–16.

Rempusheski, V. F., & Hurley, A. C. (2000). Advance directives and dementia. *Journal of Gerontological Nursing, 26*(10), 27–34.

Valente, S. M. (2001). End-of-life issues. *Geriatric Nursing, 22*(6), 294–297.

Voelker, R. (2002). Elder abuse and neglect: A new research topic. *Journal of the American Medical Association, 288,* 2254–2256.

Zimny, G. H. (Ed.). (1998). *Guardianship of the elderly: Psychiatry and judicial aspects.* New York: Springer.

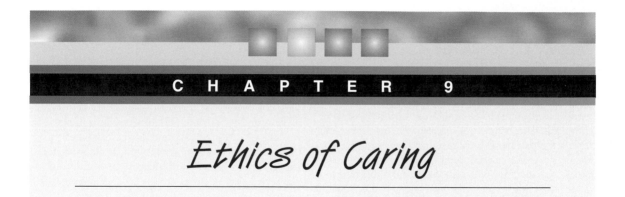

Ethics of Caring

■ Chapter Outline

■ Learning Objectives

After reading this chapter, you should be able to:

- list factors that have increased ethical dilemmas for nurses

- discuss various philosophies regarding right and wrong

- describe ethical principles guiding nursing practice

- identify measures to help nurses make ethical decisions

Changes Increasing Ethical Dilemmas for Nurses

Professional ethics has become a popular phrase in nursing circles. The concept of principles guiding right and wrong conduct is not new to nursing; in fact, gerontological nurses face significant ethical decisions in their daily practice. However, changes within the profession and the entire health care delivery system have heightened the significance of ethics to nursing practice.

EXPANDED ROLE OF NURSES

Nurses have gone beyond the confines of simply following doctors' orders and providing basic comfort and care. They now perform sophisticated assessments, diagnose nursing problems, monitor and give complicated treatments, use alternative modalities of care, and, particularly in geriatric care settings, increasingly make independent judgments about patients' status. This wider scope of functions, combined with higher salaries and greater status, has increased the accountability and responsibility of nurses for the care of patients (Fig. 9-1).

MEDICAL TECHNOLOGY

Artificial organs, genetic screening, new drugs, computers, lasers, ultrasound, and other innovations have increased the medical community's ability to diagnose and treat problems and to save lives that once would have been given no hope. However, new problems have accompanied these advances, such as determining on whom, when, and how this technology should be used.

NEW FISCAL CONSTRAINTS

In the past, the major concern of health care providers and agencies was to provide quality services to help

people maintain and restore health. Now, competing with and sometimes overriding this concern, are those regarding being cost effective, minimizing bad debts, and developing alternate sources of revenue. Patients' needs are weighed against economic survival, resulting in some difficult decisions. Further, in this era of rationed care and scarce resources, questions are raised regarding the right of older adults to expect a high quality and quantity of health and social services while other groups lack basic assistance.

> **KEY CONCEPT**
> Increasingly, questions are raised regarding the right of elders to expect benefits that other members of society do not enjoy.

GREATER NUMBERS OF OLDER ADULTS

The impact of entitlement programs and services for older persons was felt less severely when only a small portion of the population was old, but with growing numbers of people spending more years in old age and the ratio of dependent individuals to productive workers increasing, society is beginning to feel burdened. Although the elderly's problems and needs are more evident, the ability and responsibility of society to support these needs are in question.

> **Point to Ponder**
> *Do you believe that gerontological nurses have an ethical responsibility to advocate for elders by objecting to and bringing public attention to policy and reimbursement decisions that are not in elders' best interests?*

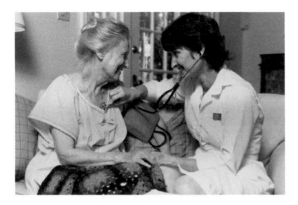

FIGURE 9-1

Nurses follow the principles of doing good, treating people equally, honoring their word, and respecting elders' rights.

Philosophies Guiding Ethical Thinking

The word *ethics* originated in ancient Greece—*ethos* means those beliefs that guide life. Most current definitions of ethics revolve around the concept of accepted standards of conduct and moral judgment. Basically, ethics help us determine right and wrong courses of action. As simple as this sounds, different philosophies disagree about what constitutes right and wrong:

Utilitarianism. This philosophy holds that good acts are those from which the greatest number of people will benefit and gain happiness.

Egoism. At the opposite pole from utilitarianism, egoism proposes that an act is morally acceptable if it is of the greatest benefit to oneself and that there is no reason to perform an act that benefits others unless one will personally benefit from it as well.

Relativism. This philosophy can be referred to as situational ethics, in that right and wrong are relative to the situation. Within relativism are several subgroups of thinking. Some relativists believe that there can be individual variation in what is ethically correct, whereas others feel that the individual's beliefs should conform to the overall beliefs of society for the given time and situation.

Naturalism. There are two schools of thought among naturalists. One holds that something is good if there are positive attitudes or interests in it. The other theorizes that something is good if the ideal, objective person has a positive attitude or interest in it.

To illustrate the application of these four different philosophies, consider the hypothetical situation of four poor old men who share a household. One day, one of these men finds a lottery ticket in the mailbox while checking the household's mail. The ticket holds the winning number for a million dollars. Ethically, does he owe his housemates any of the winnings?

A *utilitarian* would propose that he split the winnings with his housemates because that would bring good to the greatest number of people. An *egoist* would encourage him to keep the winnings because that would do him the most good personally. A *relativist* might say that normally he should keep the winnings, but because in this situation he will have more money than he will need, he should share the winnings. A *naturalist* would say that he should share the money only if his housemates consider this the right thing to do.

Now consider the application of the philosophical approaches to the issue of federal subsidies to older adults.

A *utilitarian* could say that 12% of the population should not use one third of the gross national prod-uct and that the money instead should be equally allocated on a per capita basis. An *egoist* would say that the individual old person should take whatever he feels he needs, regardless of the impact on others. A *relativist* could say that the elderly can use this proportion of the budget unless more is needed for dependent children or defense, at which point it would no longer be right to do so. A *naturalist* would say that as long as most of society and its leadership felt positive about spending so much of the budget on the elderly, it is right to do so.

Obviously other philosophies exist, but the few that have been briefly described demonstrate the diversity of approaches to ethical thinking and reinforce the fact that determining right and wrong actions can be a complicated endeavor.

🔑 **KEY CONCEPT**
Individuals can be guided by a wide range of ethical philosophies that cause them to view the same situation in vastly different ways.

Ethics in Nursing

EXTERNAL AND INTERNAL INFLUENCES ON ETHICS

Professions such as nursing require a code of ethics on which practice can be based and evaluated. A professional code of ethics is accepted by those who practice the profession as the formal guidelines for their actions. The American Nurses Association (ANA) Code of Ethics for Nurses (Display 9-1) outlines the broad values of the profession. The American Holistic Nurses' Association has developed the *Code of Ethics for Holistic Nursing* that provides guidance for nurses' actions and responsibilities for self, others, and the environment (you can review the full document on their website at www.ahna.org). These are not the only values that direct nursing practice, though. Federal, state, and local standards, in the form of regulations, also guide practice. In addition, standards for specific practitioners and care settings have been developed by various organizations such as the Joint Commission for the Accreditation of Healthcare Organizations. Individual agencies, too, have philosophies, goals, and objectives that support

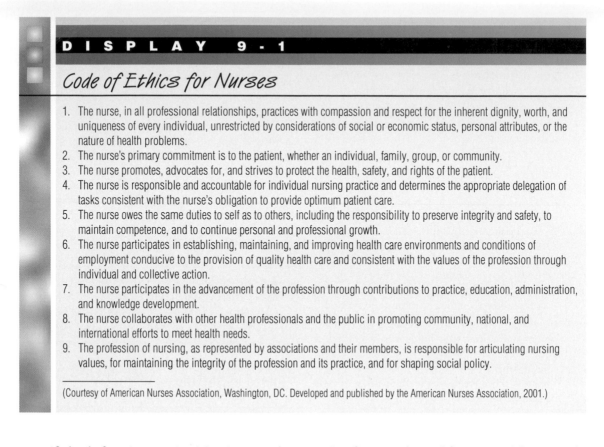

(Courtesy of American Nurses Association, Washington, DC. Developed and published by the American Nurses Association, 2001.)

a specific level of nursing practice. Most importantly, individual nurses possess values that they have developed throughout their lives that will largely influence ethical thinking. Ideally, a nurse's individual value system meshes with that of the profession, society, and employer; conflict can arise when value systems are incompatible.

KEY CONCEPT

The American Nurses Association (ANA) Code for Nurses and various standards of practice supplement the nurse's personal value system to influence ethical decision making.

ETHICAL PRINCIPLES

Several ethical principles are used to guide health care, including the following:

Beneficence: to do good for patients. This principle is based on the belief that the education and experience of nurses enable them to make sound decisions that serve patients' best interests. Nurses are challenged to take actions that are good for patients while not ignoring patients' desires. To override patients' decisions and invoke professional authority to take actions that nurses view as in patients' best interests is viewed as *paternalism* and interferes with the freedom and rights of patients.

Nonmaleficence: to prevent harm to patients. This principle could be viewed as a subset of beneficence because the intent is ultimately to take action that is good for patients.

Justice: to be fair, treat people equally, and give patients the service they need. At the foundation of this principle is the belief that patients are entitled to services based on need, regardless of ability to pay. Scarce resources have challenged this concept of unrestricted access and use of health care services.

Fidelity and Veracity: fidelity means to respect our words and duty to patients; veracity is truthfulness. This principle is central to all nurse–patient interactions because the quality of this relationship depends on trust and integrity. Older patients may have higher degrees of vulnerability than younger adults and may be particularly dependent on the truthfulness of their caregivers.

Autonomy: to respect patients' freedoms, preferences, and rights. Ensuring and protecting older patients' right to provide informed consent are consistent with this principle.

Few nurses would argue with the value of these principles. In fact, practices that reinforce these principles are widely promoted, such as ensuring that patients receive the care they need, respecting the rights of patients to consent to or deny consent for treatment, preventing incompetent staff from caring for patients, and following acceptable standards of practice. Actual nursing practice is seldom simple, however, and situations emerge that add new considerations to the application of moral principles to patient care. Ethical dilemmas can emerge when other circumstances interfere with the clear, basic application of ethical principles.

> ☑ **Point to Ponder**
>
> *How do you respond to and try to solve ethical dilemmas? If you are in practice, do you accept different standards in practice from what you would accept in your personal life? If so, why?*

Ethical Dilemmas Facing Nurses

Nursing practice involves many situations that could produce conflicts—conflicts between nurses' values and external systems affecting their decisions and conflicts between the rights of patients and nurses' responsibilities to those patients. Display 9-2 presents examples of such dilemmas. These examples are typical of the decisions facing nurses every day and for which there are no simple answers. (**Visit the Con-**

nection website for additional examples of dilemmas that nurses face.)

It is easy to say that nurses should always follow the regulations, adhere to principles, and do what is best for the patient. But can nurses be expected to follow these guidelines 100% of the time? What if following the rules means they may lose the income on which their families depend, violate the rights of individuals to decide their own destinies, cause problems for coworkers or their employers, or be labeled as troublemakers? Is it alright to knowingly violate a regulation or law if no real harm will result? Do nurses need to limit how much of an advocacy role they can assume? Should nurses base their decisions on what is right for themselves, their patients, or their employers? To whom are nurses really most responsible and accountable?

> 🔑 **KEY CONCEPT**
> Most clinical situations do not lend themselves to simple, clear-cut ethical decisions.

Measures to Help Nurses Make Ethical Decisions

Although guidelines exist, no solid answers can solve all of the ethical dilemmas that nurses face. Nurses should, however, minimize their struggles in making ethical decisions by using critical thinking and employing the following measures:

Encourage patients' expressions of desires. Advise patients to express their desires in advance directives, wills, and other legally binding documents and advocate compliance with patients' wishes.

Identify significant others who impact and are impacted. Consider family members, friends, and caregivers who are involved with the patient and the situation, and their concerns and preferences.

Know thyself. The nurse should review his or her personal value system. The influences of religion, cultural beliefs, and personal experiences should be explored to understand one's unique comfort zone with specific ethical issues.

Read. Review the medical literature for discussions and case experiences of other nurses to gain a

Ethical Dilemmas in Gerontological Nursing Practice

While working in an outreach program to bring services to community-based elderly, you meet Mr. Brooks, a 68-year-old homeless man. Mr. Brooks asks your opinion about respiratory symptoms that he has been experiencing over the past several months. He reports a chronic cough, hemoptysis, and dyspnea. He appears thin and admits to having lost weight. He states he has smoked at least one pack of cigarettes daily for over 50 years and has no intention of changing his smoking habit. Although he is not cognitively impaired, he strongly resists efforts to find him housing and arrange for medical evaluation and treatment. You are convinced that without intervention, Mr. Brooks will not survive much longer.

Do you respect Mr. Brooks' right to make his own decisions about his life, even if those decisions run contrary to what is best for his health and well-being?

You are the new director of nursing for a nursing home and were pleased to get the job because yours has become the sole source of income for your family. Ten cases of diarrhea develop among the residents and you know that the regulations require that you report five cases or more. You bring this to the attention of the medical director and administrator, who direct you not to "cause trouble by putting the health department on their backs." The medical director assures you that the problem is not serious and will pass in a few days. You know you should notify the health department, but you also know that the administrator fired the last nursing director for opposing him on a similar issue.

Do you allow a regulation to be violated or risk losing a job that you may badly need?

Insurance coverage expires tomorrow for 76-year-old Mrs. Brady, and the physician has written an order for her discharge. Because Mrs. Brady continued to be weak and slightly confused, she was not able to be instructed in the safe use of home oxygen and medication administration during her hospitalization. Her 80-year-old husband, who is expected to be her primary caregiver, is weak and in poor health himself. The social worker tells you that arrangements have been made for a nurse to visit the home daily but that the couple does not qualify for 24-hour home care assistance. You and other nursing staff members firmly believe that Mrs. Brady's health will be in jeopardy if she is discharged tomorrow. The physician tells you that you are probably right, but "the hospital cannot be expected to eat the bills that Medicare does not want to pay."

Do you increase the hospital's financial risks by insisting that nonreimbursed care be provided?

Seventy-nine-year-old Mr. Adams lies in his bed in a fetal position, unresponsive except to deep painful stimuli. He has multiple pressure ulcers, recurrent infections, and must be fed with a nasogastric tube. His wife and children express concern over the quality of his life and state that Mr. Adams would never have wanted to survive in this state. The children privately tell the multidisciplinary team that if their father's care expenses continue, their mother will be destitute, and they beg the staff to remove the tube. The family expresses that they do not have the emotional or financial resources to take the issue to court. The physician is sympathetic, but states he feels compelled to continue the feedings and antibiotics because he does not condone euthanasia; however, privately, the physician tells you that he will close his eyes and keep quiet if you want to pull the tube without anyone knowing.

Do you exceed your authority and discontinue a life-sustaining measure to grant the family's request?

Mrs. Smith is dying of cancer and being cared for at home by her husband. The couple has been married for 63 years and has never been apart during that time. They are highly interdependent and each one's world revolves around the other's. During your home nursing visit, the couple openly discusses their plans with you. They tell you that they have agreed that when Mrs. Smith's pain becomes too severe to tolerate, they will both ingest sufficient medication, which they have accumulated, to kill themselves, and die peacefully in each other's arms.

Do you ignore your responsibility to report suicidal intent to respect a couple's wish to end their lives together?

wider perspective into the types of ethical problems confronted within nursing and strategies for managing them. Literature outside the field of nursing can help add new facets to one's thinking.

Discuss. In formal education programs or informal coffee breaks, talk about issues with other health team members. Members of the clergy, attorneys, ethicists, and others also can provide interesting perspectives.

Form an ethics committee. Bring together various members of the health team, clergy, attorneys, and lay persons to study ethical problems within the specific care setting, clarify legal and regulatory boundaries, develop policies, discuss ethical problems that surface, and investigate charges of ethical misconduct.

Consult. Clinical ethics consultation emerged in the 1970s and has grown since. It takes the form of an ethics committee, or consultation provided by expert individuals or groups (eg, lawyers, philosophers, or clinicans who specialize in bioethics). Clinical ethics consultants provide education, mediate moral conflict, facilitate moral reflection, and advocate for patients (American Society for Bioethics and the Humanities, 2001). (For information on the competencies and practice of Health Care Ethics Consultants, visit the website of the American Society for Bioethics and the Humanities at www.asbh.org/papers.)

Share. When faced with a difficult ethical decision, talk with others and seek guidance and support.

Evaluate decisions. Assess the outcomes of the actions and whether or not the same courses of action would be chosen in a similar situation in the future. Even the worst decision holds some lessons.

🔑 **KEY CONCEPT**
Knowing one's own value system is beneficial in facing ethical decisions.

Gerontological nursing holds its share of ethical questions. Should resources be spent for a heart transplant for an octogenarian? Should an affluent child rather than public funds pay for a parent's care? How much sacrifice must a family endure to care for a relative at home? How much compromise in care can nurses accept to keep an agency's budget healthy? Nurses must be active participants in the process of developing ethically sound policies and practices affecting the care of the elderly. The choice between being a leader or an ostrich in this arena can significantly determine the future status of gerontological nursing practice.

Critical Thinking Exercises

1. What factors have influenced your personal ethics?
2. Discuss the dilemmas arising from the following situations:
   - having a terminally ill patient confide plans to commit suicide
   - being instructed to discharge a patient whose care is no longer being reimbursed while knowing that the patient is not ready for discharge
   - having to terminate a nursing assistant for attendance problems, knowing that she is the sole wage earner for her family
   - being asked by a senior citizen group to support their position of converting a local playground into a senior citizen center
   - learning of an insurer's proposed policy of not reimbursing for dialysis and organ transplants for persons over 75 years of age

Web Connect

Discover what nurses are doing to have a voice in bioethics by visiting the website of the Nursing Ethics Network at www.nursingethicsnetwork.org

● Reference

American Society for Bioethics and the Humanities. (2001). *Core competencies for health care ethics consultation.* Glenview, IL: American Society for Bioethics and the Humanities. (also accessible via website: www.acgme.org/outcome/comp/ compFull.asp)

● Recommended Readings

Ali, N. S. (1999). Promotion of advance care planning in the nonhospitalized elderly. *Geriatric Nursing, 20*(5), 260–265.

Ankrom, M., Zelesnick, L., Barofsky, I., Georas, S., Finucane, T. E., & Greenough, W. B. (2001). Elective discontinuation of life-sustaining mechanical ventilation on a chronic ventilator unit. *Journal of the American Geriatrics Society, 49*(11), 1549–1554.

Baer, C. A. (1997). *Elders' views on the right to die: Facilitating decisions about life-sustaining treatment.* New York: Garland.

Baggs, J. G., & Mick, D. J. (2000). Collaboration: A tool addressing ehtical issues for elderly patients near the end of life in intesive care units. *Journal of Gerontological Nursing, 26*(9), 41–47.

Burgener, S. C. (1999). Care decisions in irreversible dementia: Who speaks for the patient? *Journal of Gerontological Nursing, 25*(8), 53–55.

Gordon, M. (2001). When swallowing is dangerous, who decides? *Annals of Long-Term Care, 9*(6), 76–79.

Gordon, M. (2001). Whose life is it and who decides? A dilemma in long-term care. *Annals of Long-Term Care, 9*(11), 32–36.

Kayser-Jones, J. (2000). A case study of the death of an older woman in a nursing home: Are nursing care practices in compliance with ethical guidelines? *Journal of Gerontological Nursing, 26*(9), 48–50.

Manning, M. (1998). *Euthanasia and physician-assisted suicide: Killing or caring?* New York: Paulist Press.

Mullins, L. C., & Hartley, T. M. (2002). Residents' autonomy: Nursing home personnel's perceptions. *Journal of Gerontological Nursing, 28*(2), 35–44.

Nusbaum, N. J. (2001). Feeding tubes: Ethical decision making in theory and practice. *Annals of Long-Term Care, 9*(11), 20.

Nusbaum, N. J. (2001). The refusal of medically indicated therapy. *Annals of Long-Term Care, 9*(1), 63–64.

Sieger, C. E., Arnold, J. F., & Ahronheim, J. C. (2002). Refusing artificial nutrition and hydration: Does statutory law send the wrong message? *Journal of the American Geriatrics Society, 50* (3), 544–550.

Smith, G. P. (1996). *Legal and healthcare ethics for the elderly.* Washington, DC: Taylor and Francis.

Valente, S.M. (2001). End-of-life issues. *Geriatric Nursing, 22*(6), 294–298.

Gerontological Nursing Practice Settings

■ Chapter Outline

Role of gerontological nurses in diverse
   care settings
Practice settings for gerontological
   nurses
Preventive and ancillary services
   Banking
   Burial
   Consumer affairs
   Counseling
   Education
   Employment
   Financial aid
   Food, health, transportation, and housing
   Information and referral
   Legal and tax
   Recreation
   Religion
   Shopping at home
   Transportation
   Volunteer work
Supportive services
   Assisted living
   Care and case management
   Chores
   Day care
   Foster care and group homes
   Home-delivered meals
   Home monitoring

   Telephone reassurance
Partial and intermittent care services
   Day treatment and day hospital programs
   Home health care
   Hospice
Complete and continuous care services
   Hospital care
   Long-term care facilities
Nonconventional services
Matching services to needs
   Physical, emotional, social, and spiritual
      factors
   Individual differences
   Flexibility
   Matching needs to services

■ Learning Objectives

After reading this chapter, you should be
able to:

- list major functions of gerontological
  nurses

- describe various practice settings for
  gerontological nurses

- describe the continuum of services
  available to older adults

- discuss factors that influence service
  selection for older adults

Role of Gerontological Nurses in Diverse Care Settings

The effects of a graying population are all around us. The media report the spiraling costs of Medicare and Social Security. Banks advertise reverse annuity mortgage programs aimed at helping aging persons remain in their homes. A new retirement community is constructed. A major corporation initiates an adult day-care program. A family leave law is passed. The local hospital issues a circular informing the community of new services for senior citizens. A nearby church sponsors a caregiver support group.

Even if we were not nurses and nursing students, we could not help but notice the impact of older adults on all segments of society. As nurses and nursing students, we are increasingly aware that the elderly are major users of virtually all health care services. Consider the following:

- Growing numbers of Americans are interested in wellness programs that help them stay youthful, active, and healthy.
- More than one third of all surgical patients are over 65 years of age (U.S. Dept. of Commerce, 1999).
- The prevalence of mental health problems increases with age.
- Chronic diseases occur at a rate four times greater in old age than at other ages (U.S. National Center for Health Statistics, 2002).
- Approximately 40% of all older persons will spend some time in a nursing home during their lives (Center for Medicare and Medicaid Services, 2001).
- Most beds in acute medical hospitals are filled by elderly patients.
- Older adults are the most significant users of home health services.

Whether working in nursing homes, health maintenance organizations (HMOs), outpatient surgical centers, hospice programs, rehabilitation units, or private practice, nurses are likely to be involved in gerontological nursing.

The diversity of the aging population and the complexity of needs it presents demands a wide range of nursing services. The functions of the gerontological nurse (Display 10-1) are varied and multifaceted and address the following goals:

- Educate persons of all ages in practices that promote a positive aging experience.
- Assess and provide interventions for nursing diagnoses.
- Identify and reduce risks.
- Promote self-care capacity and independence.
- Collaborate with other health care providers in the delivery of services.
- Maintain health and integrity of the aging family.
- Advocate and protect the rights of older adults.
- Promote the use of ethics and standards in the care of older adults.
- Help the elderly face the transition to death with peace, comfort, and dignity.

As the presence of older adults in diverse health care settings continues to increase, there will be a crucial need in such settings for nurses with gerontological nursing expertise. These nurses must understand normal aging, unique presentations and management of geriatric health problems, pharmacodynamics and pharmacokinetics in later life, psychological challenges, socioeconomic issues, spirituality, family dynamics, unique risks to health and well-being, and available resources. By possessing gerontological nursing knowledge and skills, nurses can promote efficient, effective, and appropriate health care services to older adults in a variety of settings.

Practice Settings for Gerontological Nurses

One exciting aspect of gerontological nursing is the diversity of settings in which nurses can practice. Some of these settings, such as long-term care facilities and home health agencies, have a long history of nursing participation. Others, such as senior housing complexes and adult day-care centers, offer new opportunities for nurses to demonstrate creativity and leadership.

A *continuum of care,* including services for the most independent and well elderly at one end and the most dependent and ill at the other, is essential to meet the complex and changing needs presented by the older population (Fig. 10-1). The continuum of care provides opportunities for community-based services, institutionally based services, or a combination of both. Nurses' roles and responsibilities can

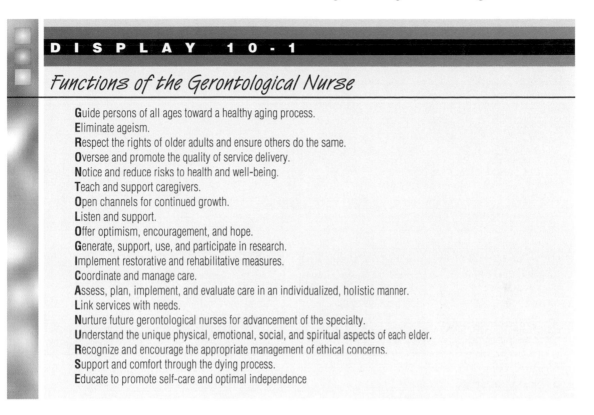

DISPLAY 10-1

Functions of the Gerontological Nurse

Guide persons of all ages toward a healthy aging process.
Eliminate ageism.
Respect the rights of older adults and ensure others do the same.
Oversee and promote the quality of service delivery.
Notice and reduce risks to health and well-being.
Teach and support caregivers.
Open channels for continued growth.
Listen and support.
Offer optimism, encouragement, and hope.
Generate, support, use, and participate in research.
Implement restorative and rehabilitative measures.
Coordinate and manage care.
Assess, plan, implement, and evaluate care in an individualized, holistic manner.
Link services with needs.
Nurture future gerontological nurses for advancement of the specialty.
Understand the unique physical, emotional, social, and spiritual aspects of each elder.
Recognize and encourage the appropriate management of ethical concerns.
Support and comfort through the dying process.
Educate to promote self-care and optimal independence

differ vastly in each of these settings. To plan care for elders effectively, nurses must be familiar with the various forms of care available. In fact, visiting various agencies to learn about their services firsthand can prove beneficial for the gerontological nurse. Although services can vary from one area to another, some general examples are described below.

Preventive and Ancillary Services

Most older adults reside in the community and function with minimal or no formal assistance. Many of them adjust their lives to accommodate changes commonly experienced with aging; some manage complex care demands. Nurses are challenged to help older adults maintain independence, prevent risks to health and well-being, establish meaningful lifestyles, and develop self-care strategies for health and medical needs.

KEY CONCEPT
When working with community-based older adults, nurses focus on maintaining independence, preventing risks to health and well-being, establishing meaningful lifestyles, and developing self-care strategies for health and medical needs.

The services in this category support independent individuals in maintaining their self-care capacity so that they can avoid physical, emotional, social, and spiritual problems. In this category of services, nurses most likely will be involved with the following:

- identifying service needs
- referring elders to appropriate services
- supporting and coordinating services

Various services in this category are described below.

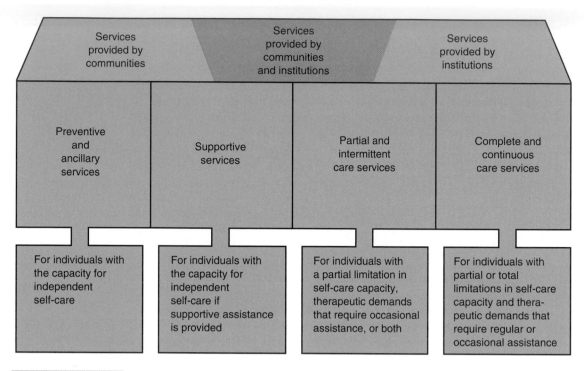

Services provided by communities	Services provided by communities and institutions	Services provided by institutions
Preventive and ancillary services	Supportive services	Partial and intermittent care services	Complete and continuous care services
For individuals with the capacity for independent self-care	For individuals with the capacity for independent self-care if supportive assistance is provided	For individuals with a partial limitation in self-care capacity, therapeutic demands that require occasional assistance, or both	For individuals with partial or total limitations in self-care capacity and therapeutic demands that require regular or occasional assistance

FIGURE 10-1

Continuum of care services for older adults.

BANKING

Many banks offer free checking accounts and other special services to senior citizens. By completing a direct deposit form at their bank, older adults can have the Social Security Administration mail Social Security and Supplemental Security Income checks directly to the bank; likewise, pension checks can be deposited directly into checking accounts. This service saves older adults from having to travel to the bank and serves as a protection from crime. Reverse annuity mortgages can be arranged through banking institutions to allow older adults to use the equity in their homes to remain in the community. It is advisable for older persons to explore details of such services with their individual financial institution.

BURIAL

Various agencies provide financial assistance for burial and funeral expenses. For instance, wartime veter-ans are eligible for some assistance from the Veterans Administration (VA). Also, the Social Security Administration provides a small payment for burial expenses to those who have been insured by that program. Local offices of these administrations can be contacted for information; funeral directors are also a good source of information about these benefits. Finally, social service agencies and religious organizations often provide assistance for persons with insufficient funds to pay for burial expenses.

CONSUMER AFFAIRS

The elderly are frequent victims of unscrupulous people who profit by making convincing but invalid promises. It is important for older adults to investigate cure-alls, vacation programs, and get-rich-quick schemes before investing their funds. Local offices of the Better Business Bureau and consumer protection agencies provide useful information to prevent fraud and deception and offer counseling if problems do arise.

COUNSELING

Financial problems, the need to locate new housing, strained family relationships, widowhood, adjustment to a chronic illness, and retirement are among the situations that may necessitate professional counseling. Local social service agencies, religious organizations, and private therapists are among the resources that offer assistance.

EDUCATION

Some public schools offer literacy, high school equivalency, vocational, and personal interest courses for older adults. Many colleges have free tuition for the elderly. Individual schools should be contacted for more details.

EMPLOYMENT

State employment services and the Over-60 Employment Counseling Service conduct programs that provide employment counseling and job placement. Various states also have foster grandparent programs, older businessperson associations, and senior aide projects. Local offices on aging can direct older persons to employment programs and opportunities in their community.

FINANCIAL AID

The Social Security Administration may be able to help older persons obtain retirement income, disability benefits, supplemental security income, and Medicare or other health insurances. The district office of the Social Security Administration can provide direct assistance and information. The VA can provide financial aid to older veterans and their families; interested persons should be directed to the local VA office. Finally, various communities offer discounts to senior citizens at department stores, pharmacies, theaters, concerts, restaurants, and transportation services. Lists of discounts may be obtained from local offices on aging.

FOOD, HEALTH, TRANSPORTATION, AND HOUSING

Departments of social services can supply information about and applications for food stamps to help elderly persons purchase food within the constraints of their budget. These departments may also provide grocery shopping services and nutrition classes. Many senior citizen clubs and religious organizations offer lunch programs that combine socialization with nutritious meals. The local office on aging or the health department can direct persons to the sites of such programs.

Older adults should be encouraged to engage in preventive health practices to avoid illness and detect health problems at an early stage. Health services for the elderly are provided by health departments, HMOs, private practitioners, and hospital outpatient services. In addition to health services, these providers may help older adults obtain transportation and financial assistance for their health care. Elders should inquire about such services at their nearest health care office.

Local social service agencies and departments of housing and community development can assist older persons in locating adequate housing at an affordable cost. These agencies also may be able to direct the older homeowner to resources to assist in home repairs and provide information regarding property tax discounts. A variety of life-care communities, villages, mobile home parks, and apartment complexes, specifically designed for older persons, are available throughout the country. Some of these housing complexes include special security patrols, transportation services, health programs, recreational activities, and architectural adjustments (eg, low cabinets, grab bars in bathrooms, tinted windows, slopes instead of stairs, and emergency call bells). Some of these housing options require a "buy-in fee" or purchase price or a monthly fee or both. The older person exploring retirement housing should be advised that sound facts are more important to decision-making than exciting promises. Visits to the housing complex and a full investigation of benefits and costs prior to a contractual commitment are essential.

INFORMATION AND REFERRAL

Local offices on aging, commissions on retirement education, libraries, and health departments usually provide assistance to the elderly in learning about available services. Older persons should be encouraged to use these resources for any questions and assistance needed. The Silver Pages telephone directory for older adults is also a useful resource. In addition, the Administration on Aging hosts a website that is a gateway to a wide range of information and services for older adults; this can be accessed through www.oa.dhhs.gov/practice/default.htm.

LEGAL AND TAX

Local legal aid bureaus and lawyer referral services of the Bar Association may help older adults obtain competent legal assistance at a nominal cost. The Internal Revenue Service can help older people prepare federal tax returns, and the state comptroller's office can assist with state tax returns; local offices should be contacted for additional information. Various colleges and law schools should be investigated for free legal and tax services offered to senior citizens.

RECREATION

Bureaus of recreation, religious organizations, and other groups may sponsor clubs and activities expressly for senior citizens. Local commissions or offices on aging can provide information related to the availability of such programs, their activities, schedules, and persons to contact for details. Local chapters of the American Association of Retired Persons (AARP) can provide valuable information on services that keep older persons active and independent, ranging from creative leisure endeavors at home to discount travel opportunities. Information about leisure pursuits is just one of the many services the AARP provides. Finally, art museums, libraries, theaters, concert halls, restaurants, and travel agencies should be contacted for special programs offered to senior citizens.

RELIGION

Churches, synagogues, and mosques offer not only a place of worship, but also a community that can provide tremendous fellowship, support, and assistance to persons of all ages. Many religious groups offer health and social services such as congregate eating programs, nursing homes, home visitation, and chore assistance. In many circumstances, recipients of services need not be members of the religious group. Individual churches and synagogues or the mother organization (eg, Associated Jewish Charities, Catholic Charities) should be contacted for information.

SHOPPING AT HOME

Persons who are homebound, geographically isolated from services, or who have busy schedules may find it useful to shop at home through mail-order catalogs, home-shopping services on television, and the Internet. Shopping by mail has a long tradition and reduces the inconveniences and risks associated with traveling to a shopping district, maneuvering in stores, handling large sums of money in public, and carrying packages. The shipping and handling charges may be no greater than transportation costs, not to mention the energy expended in direct shopping.

Additionally, many libraries have a service in which books and tapes can be borrowed by mail; the elderly should be encouraged to inquire about such services at their local branch. The U.S. Postal Service provides a service for a nominal fee in which stamps can be ordered by mail; order blanks for stamps by mail can be obtained by contacting the local postal station or postal carrier.

TRANSPORTATION

Older persons often are given discounts for bus, taxi-cab, subway, and train services; individual agencies should be contacted for more information. Commissions or offices on aging, health and social services departments, and local chapters of the American Red Cross may be able to direct persons to services accommodating wheelchairs and other special needs. Various health and medical facilities provide transportation for persons using their services; individual facilities should be explored for specific details.

VOLUNTEER WORK

The wealth of knowledge and experience possessed by older persons makes them especially good at volunteer work. Not only do older volunteers provide valuable services to others, but they may also achieve a sense of self-worth from their contributions to society. Communities offer numerous opportunities for senior volunteers in hospitals, nursing homes, organizations, schools, and other sites. Older persons should be encouraged to inquire about volunteer opportunities at the agency in which they are interested in serving. Frequently, agencies without a formal volunteer program are able to use a volunteer's service if contacted. National programs also provide meaningful volunteer services in which older persons can participate. The American National Red Cross, Service Corps of Retired Executives, and Retired Senior Volunteer Program are a few such programs. Local offices of these programs should be consulted for details.

Supportive Services

The services in this category offer assistance to individuals who are capable of self-care if aided, but who are at risk for physical, emotional, and social problems without some planned intervention. These services can be provided in community or institutional settings.

ASSISTED LIVING

Assisted living supplements independent living with special services that maximize an individual's capacity for self-care. Terminology used to describe assisted living can fall under the categories of residential care facilities, personal care, and boarding homes; different states use different regulatory designations. The housing complex is adjusted to meet the needs of older or disabled persons (eg, wide doorways, low cabinets, grab bars in bathroom, call-for-help light). A guard, hostess, or resident screens and greets visitors in the lobby. Various degrees of personal care assistance may be provided. Residents are encouraged to develop mutual support systems; one example is a system in which residents check on one another every morning to see if anyone needs help. Tenant councils may determine policies for the facility. Some facilities have a health professional on call or on duty during certain hours; social programs and communal meals may also be available. State health department regulatory agencies and the local office of the Department of Housing and Urban Development may be able to direct interested persons to such facilities.

CARE AND CASE MANAGEMENT

The identification of needs, location and coordination of services, and maintenance of an independent lifestyle can be tremendous challenges for elderly persons with chronic health problems. In response to this, the field of geriatric care and case management has developed.

Care and case managers most often are registered nurses or social workers who assess an individual's needs, identify service needs, and help the person obtain and coordinate these services. Such services include medical care, home health services, socialization programs, financial planning and management, and housing. By coordinating care and services, geriatric care and case managers assist elders in remaining independent in the community for as long as possible. The services of care and case managers often provide peace of mind to family members who are unable to be involved with their older family members on a daily basis.

As a system of credentials within this field has surfaced, there is greater distinction between care management and case management. Both of these disciplines perform some type of assessment, develop plans, help people implement and coordinate services, and evaluate care. A distinguishing difference between the two, however, is that care management is a long-term relationship that could endure through multiple episodes of care (eg, when a family contracts with a care manager to oversee the care of a relative on a long-term basis), whereas case management usually focuses on needs during a specific episode of care (eg, from hospitalization through rehabilitation for a hip fracture). Case management is viewed as a means to control health care costs and may emphasize services for cost containment; care management may include case management in addition to services unrelated to health care.

Social workers, local information and referral services, and the National Association of Professional Geriatric Care Managers (1604 North Country Club Road; Tucson, AZ 85716; [520] 881-8008; www.caremanager.org) can be contacted for assistance in locating care and case managers.

> **KEY CONCEPT**
> The American Nurses Association has found professional nurses to be excellent case managers because of their knowledge and skills training, their ability to deliver care that includes both physical and sociocultural components, their familiarity with the process of services referral, and the parallels between the nursing process and the process of case management.

CHORES

Social service agencies, health departments, private homemaker agencies, and religious organizations have services for older persons that help them remain in their homes and maintain independence. These services include light housekeeping, minor repairs, errands, and shopping. Local agencies should be contacted for specific information.

DAY CARE

Adult day-care programs are the fastest growing component of community-based long-term care, currently numbering over 3500 centers in the United States (National Adult Day Services Association, 2003). These centers provide health and social services to persons with moderate physical or mental disabilities and give respite to their caregivers. Participants attend the program for a portion of the day and enjoy a safe, pleasant, therapeutic environment under the supervision of qualified personnel (Fig. 10-2). The programs attempt to maximize the existing self-care capacity of participants while preventing further limitations. Although the primary focus is social and recreational, there usu-

ally is some health component to these programs, such as health screening, supervision of medication administration, and monitoring of health conditions. Rest periods and meals accompany the planned therapeutic activities. Transportation to the site is provided, usually by vehicles equipped to accommodate wheelchairs and persons with other special needs.

In addition to helping older persons avoid further limitations and institutionalization, day-care programs are extremely beneficial to the families of participants. Families interested in caring for their older relatives may be able to continue their routine lifestyle (eg, maintaining a job, raising small children), knowing that they can have respite from their caregiving responsibilities for a portion of the day while the older person is cared for and safe.

Adult day-care programs are sponsored by public agencies, religious organizations, and private groups, with one-third being freestanding and the remaining ones affiliated with a larger parent organization; each varies in schedule, activities, costs, and program focus. The local telephone directory or information and referral service, as well as the National Adult Day Services Association, can provide information on programs in specific communities.

FOSTER CARE AND GROUP HOMES

Adult foster care and group home programs offer services to individuals who are capable of self-care but who require supervision to protect them from harm. Older persons placed in these homes may need someone to direct their self-care activities (eg, remind them to bathe and dress, encourage and provide good nutrition); they may also need someone to oversee their judgments (eg, financial management). Foster care and group living serve as short- or long-term alternatives to institutionalization for older persons unable to manage independently in the community. The local department of social services can supply details about these programs.

HOME-DELIVERED MEALS

Persons unable to shop and prepare meals independently may benefit from having meals delivered to their homes. Such a service not only facilitates good nutrition but also provides an opportunity for social contact. Meals on Wheels is the most popularly

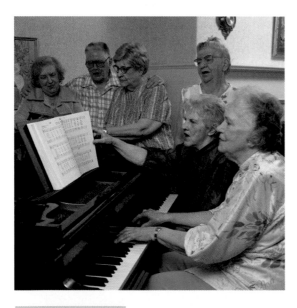

FIGURE 10-2

Adult day care centers provide opportunities for a variety of recreational activities.

known program for home delivery of meals, although various community groups provide a similar service. If a local Meals on Wheels is unavailable, departments of social services, health departments, and commissions or offices on aging should be consulted for alternative programs.

HOME MONITORING

Some hospitals, nursing homes, and commercial agencies provide home monitoring systems, whereby the older adult wears a small remote alarm that can be pressed in the event of a fall or other emergency. The alarm triggers a central monitoring station to call designated contact persons or the police to assist the individual. This type of service can be located by calling the local agency on aging or looking in the telephone directory under listings such as Medical Alarms.

TELEPHONE REASSURANCE

Older adults who are homebound, disabled, or lonely may benefit from a telephone reassurance program. Those who participate in the program receive a daily telephone call—usually at a mutually agreed on time—to provide them with social contact and ensure that they are safe and well. Local chapters of the American Red Cross and other health or social service agencies should be consulted for telephone reassurance programs that they may conduct.

Partial and Intermittent Care Services

The services in this category provide assistance to individuals with a partial limitation in self-care capacity and a therapeutic demand that requires occasional assistance. Either because of the degree of the self-care limitation or the complexity of the therapeutic action required, the individual would be at risk of institutionalization if some assistance were not provided at periodic intervals.

DAY TREATMENT AND DAY HOSPITAL PROGRAMS

Day treatment and day hospital programs offer social and health services with a primary focus on the latter.

Assistance is provided with self-care activities (eg, bathing, feeding) and therapeutic needs (eg, medication administration, wound dressing, physical therapy). Physicians, nurses, occupational therapists, and physical therapists are among the care providers affiliated with programs for day treatment. Like adult day-care programs, geriatric day treatment or day hospital programs usually provide transportation to and from the program. Sponsored by hospitals, nursing homes, or other agencies, these programs can be used as alternatives to hospitalization and nursing home placement and can facilitate earlier discharge from these care settings. The local commission or office on aging can guide persons to programs for day treatment or day hospitals in their community.

HOME HEALTH CARE

Home health care provides nursing and other therapies in individuals' homes. Visiting nurse associations have a long reputation of providing care in the home and are able to help many older persons remain in their homes rather than enter an institution. Programs vary, and services can include bedside nursing, home health aides, physical therapy, health education, family counseling, and medical services. The VA, Medicare, and Medicaid, as well as private insurers, provide reimbursement for home health services, although the conditions and length of coverage vary; specific coverage should be reviewed with the insurer. These programs can be found through health departments, in telephone directories, or through social workers who assist with discharge planning.

HOSPICE

Although hospice care is listed here under partial and intermittent care services, it can also be included under complete and continuous care services. This is because the nature of the patient's needs determines the level at which this service will be provided.

Rather than a site of care, hospice is a philosophy of caring for dying individuals. Hospice provides support and palliative care to patients and their families. Typically, an interdisciplinary team helps patients and families meet physical, emotional, social, and spiritual needs. The focus is on the quality of remaining life rather than life extension. Survivor support is also an important component of hospice care. Although hospice programs can exist within an institutional setting, most hospice care is provided in the home. Insurers vary in the conditions that must be met for reimbursement of hospice services; individual insurers should be consulted for specific information. Health care and social service agencies can be consulted for information about hospice programs in specific communities.

Complete and Continuous Care Services

The services in this category provide regular or continuous assistance to individuals with some limitation in self-care capacity whose therapeutic needs require 24-hour supervision by a health care professional.

HOSPITAL CARE

Hospital care for older persons may be required when diagnostic procedures and therapeutic actions indicate a need for specialized technologies or frequent monitoring. Older adults can be patients of virtually all acute hospital services, except, of course, pediatrics and obstetrics (and here they may be encountered as relatives of the primary patients). Although the procedure or diagnostic problem for which they are hospitalized will dictate many of their service needs, there are some basic measures that can enhance the quality of the hospital experience, as described in Display 10-2.

Increasingly, hospitals are establishing special services for older adults, such as geriatric assessment centers, hot lines, and long-term care units. Local medical societies and state hospital associations can answer inquiries about specific hospitals.

Two issues that gerontological nurses need to consider regarding the hospital care of older adults are abbreviated stays and the move toward same-day, outpatient services for procedures that once would have required hospitalization. Although shortening hospital stays can be effective in lowering costs and perhaps reducing or eliminating a patient's hospital-induced complications, many older patients require a longer recovery time than younger adults and may not have adequate assistance in the home. Nurses must assess older patients' capacity to care for themselves—obtain and prepare food and manage their households—before discharge and arrange assistance as necessary. A telephone call after discharge to check on the patient's status is also useful. (Additional information on hospital care of elders is provided in Chapter 38.)

LONG-TERM CARE FACILITIES

Long-term care facilities, commonly called nursing homes, provide 24-hour supervision and nursing care to persons who are unable to be cared for in the community. Chapter 39 discusses these facilities and related nursing responsibilities.

Nonconventional Services

As the emphasis on holistic health and public awareness of and desire for complementary and alternative therapies grow, older adults may seek new or nonconventional types of services (Fig. 10-3). Examples of nontraditional services include:

- wellness and renewal centers
- alternative therapy education and counseling
- acupuncture, acupressure
- t'ai chi, yoga, and meditation classes
- therapeutic touch
- medicinal herbal prescriptions
- herbal and homeopathic remedies
- guided imagery sessions
- sound, light, and aromatherapy

Nurses possess a wide range of knowledge and skills that, when combined with additional preparation in complementary and alternative therapies, makes them ideal providers of some of these nonconventional services. Even if they are not direct providers of alternative therapies, nurses can advocate for older adults' rights to make informed choices about using such therapies; educate them about the benefits, risks, and limitations of therapies; and help them find reputable providers. Ideally, these therapies are used in concert with conventional ones in an integrative care model to enable patients to use the best of both worlds.

✔ **Point to Ponder**

What types of factors must be considered when establishing a private practice? What do you think prevents more nurses from becoming self-employed nurse entrepreneurs?

DISPLAY 10·2

Measures That Enhance the Quality of Hospital Care for Older Adults

Perform a comprehensive assessment. It is not uncommon for the patient's diagnostic problem to be the primary and sometimes only concern during the hospitalization. However, the patient being treated for a myocardial infarction or hernia also may suffer from depression, caregiver stress, hearing deficit, or other problems that significantly affect health status. By capitalizing on the contact with the patient during the hospitalization and conducting a comprehensive evaluation, nurses can reveal risks and problems that affect health status and that have not been detected before. Broader problems, other than those for which the patient was admitted to the hospital, should be explored.

Recognize differences. Older patients should not be considered in the same way as younger patients: different norms may be used to interpret laboratory tests and clinical findings, the signs and symptoms of disease can appear atypically, more time is needed for care activities, drug dosages must be age-adjusted. The priorities of older patients can differ from those of younger patients. Nurses must be able to differentiate normal pathology from pathology in older adults and understand the modifications that must be made in caring for this population.

Reduce risks. The hospital experience can be traumatic for older patients if special protection is not afforded. The elderly require more time to recover from stress; therefore, procedures and activities must be planned to provide rest. Altered function of major systems and decreased immunity make it easy for infections to develop. Reduced ability of the heart to manage major shifts in fluid load demand close monitoring of intravenous infusion rates. Lower normal body temperature, the lack of shivering, and reduced capacity to adapt to severe changes in environmental temperature require that older patients receive special protection against hypothermia. Differences in pharmacodynamics and pharmacokinetics in the elderly alter their response to medications and heighten the need for close monitoring of drug therapy. The strange environment, sensory deficits, and effects of illness and medications cause falls to occur more easily and make injury prevention a priority. Confusion often emerges as a primary sign of a complication, challenging staff to detect this disorder promptly and identify its cause. Nurses should ensure that measures are taken to reduce patients' risks and recognize complications promptly when they do occur.

Maintain and promote function. Priorities addressing the primary reason for admission usually take the forefront during a patient's hospitalization. For example, the arrhythmia must be corrected, the infection controlled, the fracture realigned. In the midst of diagnostic procedures and treatment activities, there must be consideration of factors that will ensure the older patient's optimal function and independence.

Matching Services to Needs

The needs of the aging population are diverse and multitudinous. In addition, the needs of an individual older adult are dynamic; in other words, needs fluctuate as capacities and life demands change. This aspect of care takes several factors into consideration:

Physical, emotional, social, and spiritual factors. Services must be available to meet the unique needs of the older population in a holistic manner. These services should be planned to address whatever problems or needs older adults are likely to develop and implemented in a manner relevant to the unique characteristics of this group. For instance, a local health department interested in meeting the special

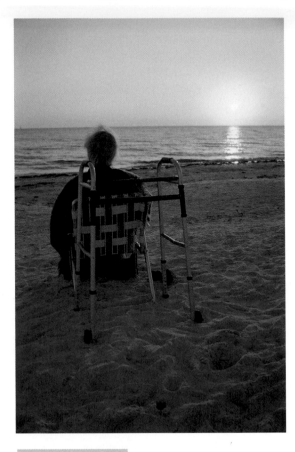

FIGURE 10-3

Increasingly, older adults are turning to yoga, meditation, and other complementary health practices.

needs of older adults could add screening programs for hearing, vision, hypertension, and cancer to their existing services. Likewise, a social service agency with an abundance of programs for younger families may decide that a widow's support group and retirement counseling services are relevant additions. The consideration of physical, emotional, social, and spiritual factors is essential to providing holistic nursing care.

Individual differences. Physical, emotional, social, and spiritual services are based on the individual's needs at a given time, recognizing that priorities are not fixed. An older adult could be seen in an outpatient medical service for hypertension control and during that visit express concern regarding a recent rent increase. Unless assistance is obtained to provide additional income or lower-cost housing, the potential effects of this social problem, such as stress and dietary sacrifices, may exacerbate the individual's hypertension. Ignoring this individual's need for particular social services, then, can minimize the effectiveness of the health services provided.

Flexibility. Opportunities must exist for the older individual to move along the continuum of care, depending on his or her capacities and limitations at different times. Perhaps an elderly woman lives with her children and attends a senior citizen recreational program during the day. If this woman fractures her hip, she may move along the continuum to hospitalization for acute care and then to a nursing home for convalescence. As her condition improves and she becomes more independent, she moves along the continuum to home care and then possibly adult day care until she regains full independence.

Matching needs to services. Individualization must be practiced to match the unique needs of the individual with specific services. Just as it is inappropriate to assume that all persons over 65 years of age require nursing home placement, it is equally inappropriate to assume that all older persons would benefit from counseling, sheltered housing, home-delivered meals, adult day care, or any other service. Older individuals' unique capacities and limitations and, most importantly, their preferences should be assessed to identify the most appropriate services for them.

The listing of resources at the end of the chapter can help gerontological nurses and nursing students locate and perhaps stimulate services for older adults. Nurses are encouraged to contact their local agencies on aging and information and referral services for the location of services within specific communities.

Critical Thinking Exercises

1. How would you defend the position that professional nurses are ideal geriatric care managers?
2. Mrs. Johns is a 79-year-old woman who has been admitted to an acute medical hospital for a fractured femur. The orthopedic surgeon anticipates no problem in Mrs. Johns ambulating and eventually returning to the community, provided she is successful in her rehabilitation program. You learn that she lives with her son's family in a large metropolitan area. She has a dementia that requires close supervision and reminders to toilet, dress, and eat; however, with these reminders, she is physically capable of performing activities of daily living.

   Based on the basic information supplied to you in the above vignette, what are the various types of services that can help Mrs. Johns and her family throughout the course of her recovery?
3. What could you do to stimulate the development of services for aging persons in your community? What resources could you mobilize to assist you in this effort?

Web Connect

Locate housing and care options for older adults in your community by searching for your state's "services for the aging" and for specific services (eg, Assisted Living Centers in Pennsylvania, Retirement Communities in Wisconsin)

● Resources

General

Administration on Aging Elder Page
Information for older persons and families
aoa.dhhs.gov/elderpage.html

American Association of Retired Persons
601 E Street NW
Washington, DC 20049
(202) 434-2277
www.aarp.org

American Geriatrics Society
770 Lexington Avenue
Suite 400
New York, NY 10021
(212) 308-1414
www.americangeriatrics.org

American Health Care Association
1200 15th Street, NW
Washington, DC 20005
(202) 833-2050
www.ahca.org

American Holistic Nurses Association
P.O. Box 2130
Flagstaff, AZ 86004
(800) 278-AHNA
www.ahna.org

American Nurses Association, Inc.
Council on Gerontological Nursing
600 Maryland Avenue
Suite 100 West
Washington, DC 20024
(800) 274-4262
www.nursingworld.org

American Society on Aging
833 Market Street
Suite 512
San Francisco, CA 94103
(415) 543-2617
www.asaging.org

Design for Aging
American Institute of Architects
1735 New York Avenue NW
Washington, DC 20006
www.aia.org

Children of Aging Parents
1609 Woodbourne Road
Suite 302-A
Levittown, PA 19057
(800) 277-7294
www.caps4caregivers.org

Gerontological Society of America
1275 K Street NW
Suite 350
Washington, DC 20005
(202) 842-1275
www.geron.org

Gray Panthers
2025 Pennsylvania Avenue
Washington, DC 20006
(202) 466-3132
www.graypanthers.org

Legal Services for the Elderly
130 West 42nd Street
17th Floor
New York, NY 10036
(212) 391-0120
www.aoa.dhhs.gov/directory/125.html

National Association of Area Agencies on Aging
1112 16th Street NW
Suite 100
Washington, DC 20036
(202) 296-8130
www.n4a.org

National Association of Professional Geriatric Care Managers
1604 North Country Club Road
Tucson, AZ 85716
(520) 881-8008
www.caremanager.org

National Association for Spanish-Speaking Elderly
2025 I Street NW
Suite 219
Washington, DC 20006
(202) 293-9329
www.hispanicfederation.org

National Caucus and Center on Black Aged
1424 K Street NW
Suite 500
Washington, DC 20005
(202) 797-8227
www.ncba-aged.org

National Council on the Aging, Inc.
409 Third Street SW
Suite 202
Washington, DC 20024
www.ncoa.org

National Council on Senior Citizens
925 15th Street NW
Washington, DC 20036
(202) 479-1200
www.ncscinc.org

National Eldercare Locator
1112 16th Street NW
Suite 100
Washington, DC 20036
(800) 677-1116
www.aginginfo.org/elderloc

National Gerontological Nursing Association
7250 Parkway Drive
Suite 510
Hanover, MD 21076
(800) 723-0560
www.ngna.org

National Hospice Organization
301 Maple Avenue, West
Suite 506
Vienna, VA 22180
(703) 938-4449
www.nho.org

National Center for Complementary and Alternative Medicine
National Institutes of Health
P.O. Box 8218
Silver Spring, MD 20907
(888) 644-6226
www.nccam.gov

National Institute on Aging
9000 Rockville Pike
Bethesda, MD 21205
(301) 496-1752
www.aoa.dhhs.gov

Nursing Homes

American Association of Homes and Services for the Aging
2519 Connecticut Avenue, NW
Washington, DC 20008
(202) 783-2242
www.aahsa.org

American Nurses Association, Inc.
Council on Nursing Home Nurses
600 Maryland Avenue SW
Suite 100 West
Washington, DC 20024
(800) 274-4262
www.nursingworld.org

National Association of Directors of Nursing Administration in Long-Term Care
10999 Reed Hartman Highway
Suite 234
Cincinnati, OH 45242
(800) 222-0539
www.nadona.org

National Citizens Coalition for Nursing Home Reform
1424 16th Street NW
Washington, DC 20036
(202) 332-2275
www.nccnhr.org

Home Health/Community Health

American Public Health Association
Section on Gerontological Health
1015 18th Street NW
Washington, DC 20036
www.apha.org

Faith in Action
To locate local interfaith volunteer caregiving
programs
(877) 324-8411
www.fiavolunteer.org

Hospice Association of America
228 7th Street SE
Washington, DC 20003
(202) 546-4759
www.hospice-amrica.org

National Association of Home Care
205 C Street NE
Washington, DC 20002
www.nahc.org

Visiting Nurse Associations of America
3801 East Florida Avenue
Suite 900
Denver, CO 80210
(800) 426-2547
www.vnaa.org

Adult Day Care

National Adult Day Services Association
409 Third Street, SW
Suite 200
Washington, DC 20024
(202) 479-6682
www.ncoa.org/nadsa

Support Groups

Please refer to resource listings throughout the book under the specific condition.

● References

Center for Medicare and Medicaid Services. (2001). *Guide to choosing a nursing home.* Rockville, MD: U.S. Department of Health and Human Services.

National Adult Day Services Association. (2003). Website *www.nadsa.org/findacenter.htm* accessed 5/25/03.

U.S. Department of Commerce. (1999). Average length of hospital stay. In *Statistical abstract of the United States* (119th ed., p. 138). Washington, DC: U.S. Bureau of the Census.

U.S. National Center for Health Statistics. (2002). Prevalence of selected chronic conditions by age and sex. *Vital and health statistics.* Retrieved May 15, 2003, from www.cdc.gov/nchs/data/hus/tables/2002.

● Recommended Readings

Bottrell, M. M., O'Sullivan, J. F., Robbins, M. A., Mitty, E. L., & Mezey, M. D. (2001). Transferring dying nursing home residents to the hospital: DON perspectives on the nurse's role in transfer decisions. *Geriatric Nursing 22*(6), 310–317.

Burton, L. C., Weiner, J. P., Stevens, G. D., & Kasper, J. (2002). Health outcomes and Medicaid costs for frail older individuals: A case study of a managed care organization versus fee-for-service care. *Journal of the American Geriatrics Society, 50*(2), 382–388.

Copeland, M. (2002). E-Community health nursing. *Journal of Holistic Nursing, 20*(2), 152–164.

Donovan, C., & Dupuis, M. (2000). Specialized care unit: Family and staff's perceptions of significant elements. *Geriatric Nursing, 21*(1), 30–33.

Eliopoulos, C. (1999). *Integrating alternative and conventional therapies: Holistic care for chronic conditions.* St. Louis: Mosby.

Eliopoulos, C. (2002). *Nursing administration manual for*

long-term care facilities (6th ed.). Glen Arm, MD: Health Education Network.

Eloniemi-Sulkava, U., Notkola, I. L., Hentinen, M., Kivela, S. L., Sivenius, J., & Sulkava, R. (2001) Effects of supporting community-living demented patients and their caregivers: A randomized trial. *Journal of the American Geriatrics Society, 49*(10),1282–1286.

Gelfand, D. E. (1999). *The aging network: Programs and services* (5th ed.). New York: Springer.

Grando, V. T., Mehr, D., Popejoy, L., Maas, M., Rantz, M, et al. (2002). Why older adults with light care needs enter and remain in nursing homes. *Journal of Gerontological Nursing, 28*(7), 47–52.

Hagen, B. (2001). Nursing home placement: Factors affecting caregivers' decisions to place family members with dementia. *Journal of Gerontological Nursing, 27*(2), 44–47.

Hammer, B. J. (2001). Community-based case management for positive outcomes. *Geriatric Nursing, 22*(5), 271–275.

Hayes, J. M. Respite for caregivers: A community-based model in a rural setting. *Journal of Gerontological Nursing, 25*(1), 22–26.

Hertz, J. E., & Anschutz, C. A. (2002). Relationships among perceived enactment of autonomy, self-care, and holistic health in community-dwelling older adults. *Journal of Holistic Nursing, 20*(2), 166–186.

Johnson, R. A., & Tripp-Reimer, T. (2001). Relocation among ethnic elders: A review. *Journal of Gerontological Nursing, 27*(6), 22–26.

Lewis, M., Hepburn, K., Corcoran-Perry, S., Narayan, S., & Lally, R. M. (1999). Options, outcomes, values, likelihoods. Decision-making guide for patients and their families. *Journal of Gerontological Nursing, 25*(12), 19–25.

Malonbeach, E. E., Royer, M., & Jenkins, C. C. (1999). Is cognitive impairment a guide to use of video respite? Lessons from a special care unit. *Journal of Gerontological Nursing, 25*(5), 17–21.

Penrod, J., & Dellasega, C. (2001). Caregivers' perspectives of placement: Implications for practice. *Journal of Gerontological Nursing, 27*(11), 28–36.

Racher, F. E. (2002). Synergism of frail rural elderly couples: Influencing interdependent independence. *Journal of Gerontological Nursing, 28*(6), 32–39.

Rice, R. (2000). Telecaring in home care: Making a telephone visit. *Geriatric Nursing, 21*(1), 56.

Rosswurm, M. S., Larrabee, J. H., & Zhang, J. (2002). Training family caregivers of dependent elderly adults through on-site and telecommunications programs. *Journal of Gerontological Nursing, 28*(7), 27–38.

Siegler, E. L., Glick, D., & Lee, J. (2002). Optimal staffing for acute care of the elderly (ACE) units. *Geriatric Nursing, 23*(3), 152–154.

Tichawa, U. (2002). Creating a continuum of care for elderly individuals. *Journal of Gerontological Nursing, 28*(1), 46–51.

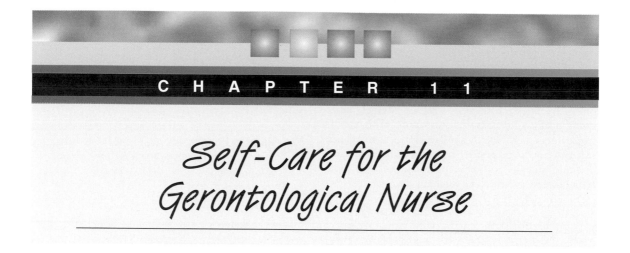

CHAPTER 11

Self-Care for the Gerontological Nurse

■ *Learning Objectives*

After reading this chapter you should be
able to:

• list the attributes of a nurse healer

• describe the meaning of presence

• identify strategies that can be used for
  self-care and nurturing

Gerontological nursing is a unique specialty in the wide range of knowledge and skills that are drawn upon when providing services to aging adults. Orthopedics . . . pharmacology . . . psychiatry . . . sociology . . . gastroenterology . . . There seems to be no limit to the information that nurses need to use as they care for the diverse population of elders.

Gerontological Nurses Create Foundations for Healing

Providing expert gerontological nursing care demands more than possessing knowledge and clinical skills. Nurses bring life experiences, unique personalities, and their very *being* to their relationships with elders as they:

• guide elders with common yet challenging life transitions
• assist individuals in exploring the deeper meaning of the experiences they face
• soothe the physical, emotional, and spiritual pain that frequently invade fragile territory
• provide the care that facilitates individuals in becoming integrated, restored, and balanced

Offering this level of nursing care demands that nurses establish heart-to-heart connections—the kind that differentiate doing a job from authentic caring for another human being. Nurses aren't merely task doers but important instruments of their patients' healing process.

Nurses who support holism and healing do not sit on the sidelines as observers. They are engaged in patients' healing processes. The impact that this level of engagement can make is similar to that of the dance instructor who takes the student by the hand and demonstrates the correct steps instead of merely offering directions from the sidelines.

> **KEY CONCEPT**
> Nurses actively engage in the patient's dance of healing—teaching, guiding, modeling, coaching, encouraging, and helping the patient through the various steps.

Characteristics of Nurse Healers

If completion of tasks was all that constituted nursing care, robots could easily replace nurses. After all, technology exists that could enable a machine to administer a medication, reposition a patient, monitor vital signs, record significant events, and perform other common tasks. Yet, the nursing profession emerged as a *healing art* characterized by its practitioners offering comfort, compassion, support, and caring that were equally (and perhaps sometimes more) important to patients' healing as the procedural tasks of caregiving. The nurse served as a healer whose interactions assisted the patient in returning to wholeness (ie, optimal function and harmony among body, mind, and spirit).

Effective nurse healers are models of holism, which begins with good self-care practices. They not only eat a proper diet, exercise, obtain adequate rest, and follow other positive health practices, but they also are attentive to their emotional and spiritual well-being. Integrity demands that nurses know what they want others to know and behave as they want others to behave.

The ability to be present in the moment also characterizes nurse healers. Despite the many real activities that nurses typically must complete, the "busyness" of the average clinical setting, and the unending "to do" list lingering over them, nurse healers are able to protect their interactions with patients from distractions. When with patients, they are *with* them,

giving their full undivided attention. They listen and *hear* what patients are saying—and not saying—and use their senses to detect subtle clues of needs. Even if the time spent with individual patients is brief, the time fully belongs to their patients.

> ✔ **Point to Ponder**
> *Reflect on an interaction in which the person with whom you were speaking seemed distracted and hurried. How did that influence your communication?*

Availability of body, mind, and spirit is displayed by nurse healers. They provide the time and space for patients to express, explore, and experience. "That's not my job" are words seldom heard from nurse healers. For example, a nurse may be monitoring a patient who is recovering from cataract surgery in an outpatient surgical unit when the patient confides to the nurse that he is distressed at learning that his grandchild was arrested for possession of illegal drugs. A response from the nurse along the lines of "You shouldn't worry about that now" gives the message that the nurse isn't available to discuss the patient's concern and most likely will close the door to further discussion. By contrast, responding "This must be very difficult for you" could be more helpful in conveying openness and interest. Although the nurse in the latter example may not be able to provide all the possible assistance that the patient may require, he or she can allow the patient the safe space to unload this burden on his mind and offer suggestions for follow-up help.

Nurse healers make connections with their patients. They engage with patients in meaningful ways that require openness, respect, acceptance, and a nonjudgmental attitude. They commit to learning about what makes each patient a unique individual...the life journey that has been traveled, the story that has formed. At times, this may require that nurses offer insights from their own journeys and share some of the chapters from their lives.

> **KEY CONCEPT**
> Exploring the unique threads that have been woven into the tapestry of a patient's life facilitates connection.

Self-Care and Nurturing

The depth and intensity of the nurse–patient relationship that results when nurses function as healers creates a highly therapeutic and meaningful experience that reflects the essence of professional nursing. Although the formal educational preparation of nurses offers the foundation for this level of healing relationship, the nurse's self-care influences the potential height and depth that can be realized (Fig. 11-1). Some strategies for self-care include following positive health care practices and strengthening and building connections. Let's look at the ways these strategies are actualized.

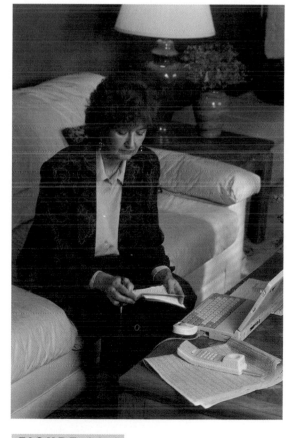

FIGURE 11-1

Nurses compromise their ability to care for others when they do not care for themselves.

FOLLOWING POSITIVE HEALTH CARE PRACTICES

Like all human beings, nurses have basic physiological needs that include:

- respiration
- circulation
- nutrition
- hydration
- elimination
- movement
- rest
- comfort
- immunity
- risk reduction

Most nurses are familiar with the requirements necessary to meet each of these needs (eg, proper diet, exercise plans) but may not be applying this information to their personal lives. Self-care can suffer as a result.

A periodic "check-up" of physical status can prove useful in disclosing problems that could not only minimize the ability to provide optimal services to patients, but also that could threaten personal health and well-being. Table 11-1 provides a form that can be used to guide this self-evaluation. It could prove useful for nurses to allocate a few hours, find a quiet place, and critically review their health status.

After identifying problems, realistic actions can be planned to improve health. Writing the actions on an index card and placing that card in an area that is regularly seen (eg, dresser, desk, or dashboard) can provide regular reminders of intended corrective actions.

 KEY CONCEPT
Efforts to improve self-care practices can be facilitated by partnering with a "buddy" who can offer support, encouragement, and a means for accountability.

STRENGTHENING AND BUILDING CONNECTIONS

Humans are relational beings who are intended to live in community with others. The richness of nurses' connections in their personal lives provides fertile soil to grow meaningful connections with patients. Yet, as basic and common as relationships can be, they can be

TABLE 11-1 ● *Taking Stock of Unhealthy Practices*

Need	Sign/Symptom/ Unhealthy Habit	Cause(s)/ Contributing Factor(s)	Corrective Action
Respiration/ circulation			
Nutrition/ hydration			
Elimination			
Movement			
Rest			
Solitude			
Comfort			
Immunity			
Risk reduction			

quite challenging. Among the major challenges nurses may face are finding and protecting the time and energy to connect with others in meaningful ways. Like many other professionals in helping professions, nurses may find that the physical, emotional, and mental energies exerted in a typical workday leave lit-

tle in reserve to invest in nurturing relationships with friends and family. The reactions to work-related stress can be displaced to significant others, thereby interfering with positive personal relationships. To compound the problems, concern for patients' welfare or employer pressure can lead to excessive overtime work, leaving precious little time and energy for nurses to do anything more in their off hours than attend to basics. Strained personal connections are the weeds of untended relationship gardens.

> ✔ **Point to Ponder**
>
> *List five signficant individuals in your life. Reflect on the amount of quality time you have with each of them and if this time is conducive to a strong relationship.*

The allocation of time and energy requires the same planning as the allocation of any finite resource. Ignoring this reality risks suffering the consequences of poor relationships. Recognizing that there always will be activities to vie for time and energy, nurses need to take control and develop practices that reflect the value of personal relationships. This can involve limiting the amount of overtime worked to no more than "x" hours each week, dedicating every Thursday evening to dining out with the family or blocking out Sunday afternoons to visit or telephone friends. Expressing intentions through understood "personal policies" (eg, informing a supervisor that you will work no more than one double shift per month) and committing time on your calendar (eg, blocking off every Sunday afternoon for "friends' time") increase the likelihood that significant relationships will receive the attention they require.

Time and energy also must be protected to afford ample time for connecting with God or another higher power. The spiritual groundedness resulting from this connection enables nurses to better understand and serve the spiritual needs of patients. Spiritual connection can be enhanced by prayer, fasting, attending church or temple, engaging in Bible studies, taking periodic retreats, and practicing days of solitude and silence.

> ✔ **Point to Ponder**
>
> *What does it mean to you to be connected to self?*

Connection with self is essential to nurses' self-care, and this begins with a realistic self-appraisal. There are a variety of strategies that can be used to facilitate this process, such as:

- *Sharing life stories.* Every adult has a unique and rich storehouse of experiences that have been cemented into the life in which he or she dwells. Oral sharing of life stories with others helps people gain insight into themselves and put experiences into a perspective that affords meaning. As stories are shared, people begin to see that theirs are not the only lives that have been less than ideal, sprinkled with pain, or unfolding in unintended ways. Writing one's life story is a powerful means of reflection that affords a permanent record that can be revisited and reconsidered as deeper wisdom about self and others is gained. Display 11-1 provides some ideas for topics to be included in a life story. The process of sharing life stories can be particularly meaningful for gerontological nurses in their work with elders who often have interesting life histories that they are eager to share—and that frequently can offer rich life lessons.

- *Journaling.* Reflection on one's life can be facilitated by writing personal notes in a journal or diary. These differ from written life stories in that they record current activities and thoughts rather than past ones. An honest written account of feelings, thoughts, conflicts, and behaviors can help people learn about themselves and work through issues.

- *Meditating.* The ancient practice of meditation has helped people sort out thoughts and gain clarity into direction for ages. Many nurses find meditation challenging because the nature of their work consists of *doing*—and multitask doing, at that! However, periods of *being still* enable nurses to offer an optimum healing presence to their patients. There are several techniques that can be used for meditating (see Chap. 14, Display 14-4); individuals vary in their preference for the different forms of meditation. Some people may focus on a word or prayer, whereas others may choose to have no intentional thought and to be open to whatever thoughts drift into their minds. Essential elements to any form of meditation are a quiet environment, comfortable position, and calm and passive attitude. The physiological responses associated with the deep relaxation achieved during meditation have many health benefits (eg, improved immunity, reduced blood pressure, and increased peripheral blood flow). Often, issues that have been struggled with are clarified through meditation.

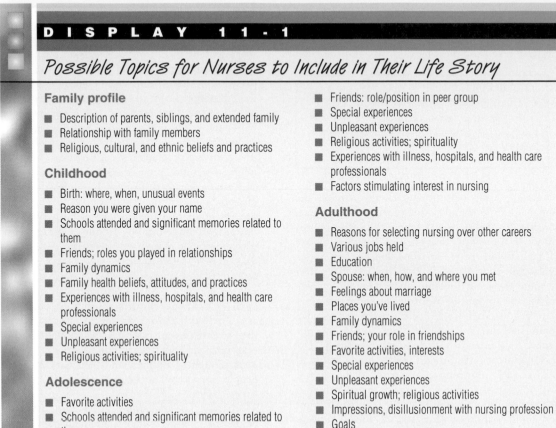

DISPLAY 11-1

Possible Topics for Nurses to Include in Their Life Story

Family profile

- Description of parents, siblings, and extended family
- Relationship with family members
- Religious, cultural, and ethnic beliefs and practices

Childhood

- Birth: where, when, unusual events
- Reason you were given your name
- Schools attended and significant memories related to them
- Friends; roles you played in relationships
- Family dynamics
- Family health beliefs, attitudes, and practices
- Experiences with illness, hospitals, and health care professionals
- Special experiences
- Unpleasant experiences
- Religious activities; spirituality

Adolescence

- Favorite activities
- Schools attended and significant memories related to them

- Friends: role/position in peer group
- Special experiences
- Unpleasant experiences
- Religious activities; spirituality
- Experiences with illness, hospitals, and health care professionals
- Factors stimulating interest in nursing

Adulthood

- Reasons for selecting nursing over other careers
- Various jobs held
- Education
- Spouse: when, how, and where you met
- Feelings about marriage
- Places you've lived
- Family dynamics
- Friends; your role in friendships
- Favorite activities, interests
- Special experiences
- Unpleasant experiences
- Spiritual growth; religious activities
- Impressions, disillusionment with nursing profession
- Goals
- Legacy you'd like to leave

- *Taking retreats.* To many nurses, particularly women, taking a few days off "to do nothing" seems like a luxury that cannot be afforded. After all, there is the house to get in order, shopping that must be done, and overtime that can be worked to gather a few extra dollars for vacation. In addition to the tasks that compete for attention and time, there may be the mental script that insidiously gives the message that it is selfish to forfeit tangibly productive activities to spend time thinking, reflecting, and experiencing. Yet, unless nurses want their interactions with patients to be solely mechanical (ie, task oriented), they must treat themselves as more than machines. Their bodies, minds, and spirits must be restored and refreshed periodically to offer holistic care—and retreats offer an ideal means to achieve

that. A retreat is a withdrawal from normal activities. It can be structured or unstructured, guided by a leader or self-directed, and taken with a group or alone. Although retreats are offered in exotic locations that offer lavish provisions, they needn't be luxurious or expensive. Whatever the location or structure, key elements of the retreat experience are a respite from routine responsibilities, freedom from distractions (telephones, children, and doorbells), no one to care for and worry about other than self, and a quiet place. During the retreat, time is spent on activities that can aid in achieving peace and clarity, such as meditating, journaling, expressing oneself creatively through art, and praying. If life circumstances prevent a multiday or even a full-day retreat from being possible, a partial-day retreat can be planned within one's home by establishing peace and privacy (eg, sending children off, asking roommates to stay away for the morning, unplugging telephones, or placing an out-of-order sign on the doorbell) and allocating time in retreat-type activities. The charge that a retreat provides to one's physical, emotional, and spiritual batteries will more than compensate for the tasks that were postponed.

KEY CONCEPT
When nurses have strong, grounded connections to themselves, they are in a better position to have meaningful connections with patients.

Self-Care Is a Dynamic Process

Self-care is an ongoing process that demands active attention. However, *knowing* the actions that sup-

port self-care is only the beginning. *Committing* to engaging in one's self-care completes the picture. This may mean that limits are set on the amount of overtime worked to adhere to an exercise schedule or that one is willing to face the uncomfortable feelings experienced during the process of reflecting on less than pleasant life experiences. Sacrifices, unpopular decisions, and discomfort can result when one chooses to "work on oneself." Yet, it is this inner work that contributes to nurses being effective healers.

KEY CONCEPT
Life and the attention it requires change; therefore, self-care is dynamic. Areas that seemed to be under control may spring leaks and demand new attention. Strategies that proved successful in the past may become less effective and need replacement.

Critical Thinking Exercises

1. Mindful care of one's body, mind, and spirit is essential to providing holistic gerontological nursing care. What does *mindful care* mean to you?
2. What would hinder you from engaging in self-care practices? What could you do to reduce obstacles to your self-care?
3. What signs, symptoms, or unhealthy habits exist in your life? What types of corrective actions could you commit to improve them?
4. How could you incorporate elements of self-care described in this chapter in an employee health program to aid people in aging well?

Web Connect

Learn about a nursing organization interested in nurturing nurses by visiting the website of the American Holistic Nurses' Association at www.ahna.org

● Resources

American Holistic Nurses' Association
P.O. Box 2130
Flagstaff, AZ 86003
(800) 278-2462
www.ahna.org

● Recommended Readings

Barnum, B. S. (2003). *Spirituality in nursing: From traditional to new age.* New York: Springer Publishing Co.
Cox, A. M., & Albert, D. H. (Eds.). (2003). *The healing heart: Communities.* British Columbia, Canada: New Society Publishers.

Kane, J., & Warner, C. G (1999). *Touched by a nurse: Special moments that transform lives.* Philadelphia: Lippincott Williams & Wilkins.

Kosowski, M. M., & Roberts, V. W. (2003). When protocols are not enough: Intuitive decision making by novice nurse practitioners. *Journal of Holistic Nursing, 21*(1), 52–72.

Sappington, J. Y. (2003). The spirit of holistic nursing. *Journal of Holistic Nursing, 21*(1), 8–19.

Watson, J. (1999). *Postmodern nursing and beyond.* Philadelphia: Churchill Livingstone.

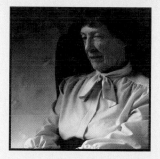

Fostering Connection and Gratification

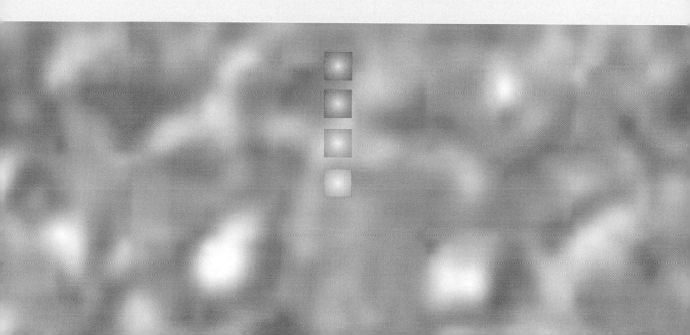

Connecting With Self

■ Learning Objectives

After reading this chapter you should be able to:

- list factors that contribute to an individual's unique body, mind, and spirit

- describe measures that can be used to facilitate self-reflection

- list survivor competencies

- discuss strategies to empower older adults

- differentiate sexuality from sexual function

- identify measures to manage menopausal symptoms

*O*ne of the hallmarks of successful aging is knowledge of self . . . an awareness of the realities of who one is and one's place in the world. From infancy on, we engage in dynamic experiences that mold the unique individuals we are. By adulthood, we have formed the skeleton of our identities. Continued interactions and life experiences as we journey through life further add to the development of our identities.

The self, the personal identity an individual possesses, has several dimensions that basically can be described as body, mind, and spirit. The body includes physical characteristics and functioning; the mind encompasses cognition, perception, and emotions; and the spirit represents meaning and purpose derived from a relationship with God or other higher power. A variety of factors affect the development of body, mind, and spirit, such as genetic makeup, family composition and dynamics, roles, ethnicity, environment, education, religious experiences, relationships, culture, lifestyle, and health practices (Fig. 12-1).

> **Point to Ponder**
> *What are the significant factors of your background that influenced your unique body, mind, and spirit?*

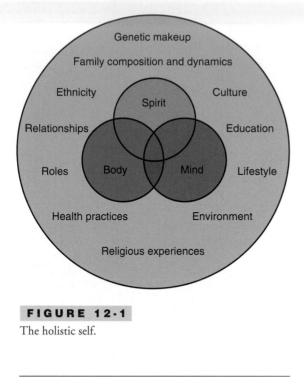

FIGURE 12-1

The holistic self.

Self-Reflection

Although a realistic appraisal of one's identify and place in the world fosters healthy aging, not all persons complete this task successfully. Some people may live with unrealistic expectations or views of themselves, going through life playing parts that are ill-suited for them and wasting time in fruitless or unfulfilling activities. Harry is an example of this:

*H*arry, the eldest of five children, was raised in an inner-city community in which poverty was the norm. His father was an auto mechanic who had difficulty holding jobs. His mother didn't miss an opportunity to voice her dissatisfaction with her husband's meager income nor to emphasize to Harry that he needed to be sure to "make it big and not be like his father."

The message instilled by his mother and his desire for a better life than he enjoyed as a child fueled Harry to be a high achiever. By age 30, Harry owned a small chain of convenience stores, a large home in the suburbs, sev-

eral luxury cars, and most of the possessions that reflected an upper middle-class lifestyle. Harry was proud that he could provide a comfortable life for his wife and expensive education for his children—quite the opposite of what his father achieved. Yet, something was missing. His business demanded most of his time and energy; therefore, he had little left of himself to offer his family. He also rarely had the time for his passion, restoring classic cars. His life seemed to consist of managing his businesses and sleeping, with an occasional social event with his family. Time for relaxation and reflection had no place in Harry's busy life.

In his late 50s, with children grown and his business worth enough to provide a comfortable retirement income, Harry was in a position where he didn't have to work the long days—or at all for that matter. His wife encouraged him to consider selling his business and spend his time "tinkering with cars and taking it easy." Although he was tempted, Harry felt that he just couldn't do this. Unfortunately, the script to "make it big," programmed into Harry's mind as a child, held him prisoner to a role that brought him little joy and fulfillment. Furthermore, he had no idea of what his purpose and identity was other than being an entrepreneur.

Like Harry, many individuals may reach their senior years without having evaluated who they really are, what drives them to behave as they do, or what their true purposes and pleasures are.

> **KEY CONCEPT**
> Some adults may have not invested the time and effort in self-evaluation and, consequently, reach old age with a lack of clarity of their identity.

Exploring and learning about one's true self are significant to holistic health in late life. Examining and coming to terms with thoughts, feelings, beliefs, and behaviors foster elders' reaching a state of integrity rather than feeling despair over the lives they've lived. However, as important a process as it is, self-reflection does not come easily or naturally for some individuals. They may require interventions to facilitate this process; therefore, guiding aging people through self-reflective activities is an important therapeutic measure that gerontological nurses may need to offer. Some of the activities that could be used to facilitate self reflection include:

- *Life review.* Life review is the process of intentionally reflecting on past experiences in an effort to resolve troublesome or traumatic life events and assess one's life in totality. In gerontological care, life review has long been recognized as an important process to facilitate integrity in old age (ie, to help elderly people appreciate that their lives have had meaning). Eliciting life stories from elders is not a difficult process; in fact, many older adults welcome opportunities to share their life histories and life lessons to interested listeners. For those who may require some facilitation, creative activities, such as compiling a scrapbook or dictating a family history, can stimulate the process. Life review can be a positive experience because elders can reflect on the obstacles they've overcome and accomplishments they've made. It can provide the incentive to heal fractured relationships and complete unfinished business. On the other hand, life review can be a painful experience for older adults who realize the mistakes they've made and the lives they've hurt. Rather than conceal and avoid these negative feelings, elders can benefit by discussing them openly and working through them; referrals to therapists and counselors may be indicated to assist with unresolved grief, depression, or anxiety.
- *Journaling.* Whether it's done with pencil and paper or a word-processing program, the process of writing often facilitates self-reflection. There is no one right way to keep a journal or diary; individuals should be encouraged to develop styles that are comfortable for them. Some people may make daily entries that include details about their communications, sleep patterns, mood, and activities, whereas others make periodic entries that address major emotional and spiritual issues. Nurses can assist individuals who have not kept journals and diaries by guiding them in the selection of a blank book and writing instrument. This is an important step, not only because these tools will be used often, but also because the book will be a

tangible compilation of significant thoughts and feelings that could have meaning to others in years to come. Novices to journaling can be encouraged to start by reflecting on their lives and beginning their journals/diaries with a summary of the past. Suggesting that feelings and thoughts be written, in addition to the events of the day, can contribute to the process being one that fosters self-reflection.

- *Writing letters and e-mails.* Letters are another means to reflect and express feelings. Often thoughts and feelings can be expressed in writing that individuals may not feel comfortable verbalizing. For some older adults, letters of explanation and apology to friends and family with whom there have been strained relationships can be a healing exercise. Elders can be encouraged to locate friends and family in other parts of the country (or world) with whom they haven't had contact for a while and initiate communication concerning what has transpired in their lives and current events. Letters to grandchildren and other younger members of the family can provide a means to share relevant family history and offer special attention (many children love to receive their own mail!). Older adults may enjoy communicating by e-mail because of the ease and relatively low cost. If they don't own their own computers, elders can be referred to local senior centers or libraries that offer free or nominal cost access to the Internet.
- *Oral history.* For people unable or unwilling to write, dictating into a tape recorder can be a beneficial alternative. Some people may be able to organize and articulate their thoughts quite well independently, whereas others may be aided by a written outline or questions to guide them. Volunteers can be used as interviewers, guiding the elder through a taped review of life activities and feelings. The recorded history can be a priceless legacy of the person's life for generations to come.
- *Art.* Many people find that painting, sculpting, weaving, and other forms of creative expression facilitate self-reflection and expression. It is important that the *process,* not the finished product, be emphasized. Arts and crafts classes and groups often are offered by local organizations dedicated to specific activities (eg, weavers' guild, arts' council),

schools, and senior centers. Nurses can assist elders in locating such groups in their communities.

These certainly do not exhaust the strategies that can be used to foster self-reflection. Nurses are bound only by their creativity in the approaches used for self-reflective activities.

 KEY CONCEPT
Producing a work of art, discussing literature, and sharing one's life story are among the many interventions that can be used to foster self-reflection.

Strengthening Inner Resources

The declines and dependencies that increasingly are present in late life can cause us to view elders as being fragile and incapable. However, most elderly individuals possess significant inner resources—physical, emotional, and spiritual—that have enabled them to survive to old age. Behaviors that exemplify their survivor capabilities are described in Display 12-1.

KEY CONCEPT
By considering the strengths displayed by the elderly as they navigated the aging process, nurses and others can develop an enlightened perspective of the older population.

Against the backdrop of threats to independence and self-esteem, nurses best serve elders by maintaining and bolstering their inner strengths. Basic to this effort is ensuring physical health and well-being. It is quite challenging for persons of any age to optimally meet intellectual, emotional, socioeconomic, and spiritual challenges when their basic physical needs are not fully satisfied or they are experiencing the symptoms associated with deviations from health. Comprehensive and regular assessment of health status and interventions to promote health provide a solid base from which inner strengths can be nurtured.

☑ **Point to Ponder**
How would you judge your "survivor competencies?" What experiences have contributed to this?

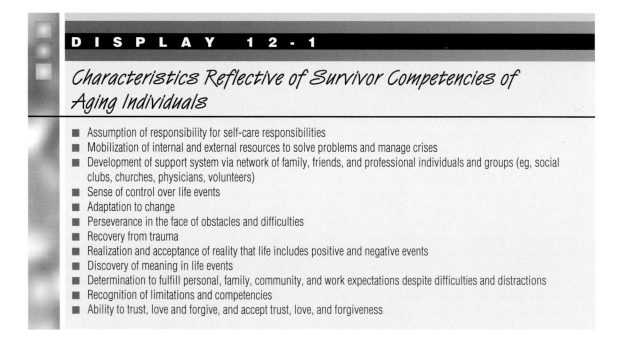

DISPLAY 12-1

Characteristics Reflective of Survivor Competencies of Aging Individuals

- Assumption of responsibility for self-care responsibilities
- Mobilization of internal and external resources to solve problems and manage crises
- Development of support system via network of family, friends, and professional individuals and groups (eg, social clubs, churches, physicians, volunteers)
- Sense of control over life events
- Adaptation to change
- Perseverance in the face of obstacles and difficulties
- Recovery from trauma
- Realization and acceptance of reality that life includes positive and negative events
- Discovery of meaning in life events
- Determination to fulfill personal, family, community, and work expectations despite difficulties and distractions
- Recognition of limitations and competencies
- Ability to trust, love and forgive, and accept trust, love, and forgiveness

By being empowerment facilitators, nurses can support elders' inner strengths. Nurses must begin this process by examining and strengthening their own level of empowerment. When nurses develop a mindset of seeing possibilities despite fiscal and other constraints, they are better able to help elders see possibilities despite potential constraints imposed by age and illness. **(Visit the Connection website to learn more about how nurses can become empowered.)** In addition to role models, nurses can facilitate empowerment by:

• including elders in care planning and caregiving activities to the maximum extent possible
• providing a variety of options to elders and freedom to choose among them
• equipping elders for maximum self-care and self-direction by educating, relating, coaching, sharing, and supporting them
• advocating for elders as they seek information, make decisions, and executive their own selected self-care strategies
• offering feedback, positive reinforcement, encouragement, and support

A sense of hope fosters empowerment and is a thread that reinforces the fabric of inner strengths. Hope is an expectation—that a problem will be resolved, relief will be obtained, and something desired will be obtained. Hope enables people to see beyond the present and make sense of the senseless. It empowers them to take action. Nurses foster hope in elders by honoring the value of their lives despite infirmities and limitations, assisting in establishing goals, supporting the use of coping strategies, building on capabilities, and displaying an optimistic, caring attitude. Spiritual beliefs and practices also provide inner strength that enable the elderly to cope with current challenges and maintain hope and optimism for the future (see Chap. 14); nurses need to support elders in their prayers, devotional readings, church attendance, and other expressions of spirituality.

Sexuality

Adults continue to be sexual beings into their senior years. Sexuality encompasses much more than a physical act. It includes love, warmth, caring, and sharing between individuals; seeing beyond gray hair, wrin-

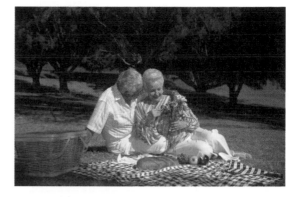

FIGURE 12-2

Stereotypical images of the older adult as narrow minded, forgetful, sexless, and dependent are untrue for most of the older adult population.

kles, and other manifestations of aging; and the intimate exchange of words and touches by sexual human beings. Feeling important to and wanted by another person promotes security, comfort, and emotional well-being (Fig. 12-2). With the multiple losses that the elderly experience, the comfort and satisfaction derived from a meaningful relationship are especially significant. Sexuality also includes expressing oneself as and being perceived as a man or a woman. This can be confusing to elders in light of society's emphasis over the past several decades on eliminating masculine and feminine stereotypes. Today's elders were socialized into masculine and feminine roles—the elderly have had a lifetime of experience with the expectation that men are to be aggressive, independent, and strong and that women are to be pretty, gentle, and dependent on their male counterparts. It is as difficult and unfair to try to alter the roles of older persons as it is to try to convince today's liberated woman that she is limited to the roles of wife and mother. The socialization of today's older population and its role expectations must be recognized and respected.

KEY CONCEPT
Sexuality includes love, warmth, caring, and sharing between people and identification with a sexual role.

Nevertheless, nurses may witness subtle or blatant violations of respect to the elderly's sexual identity. Examples of such a lack of respect include:

- belittling elders' interest in clothing, cosmetics, and hairstyles
- dressing men and women residents of an institution in similar asexual clothing
- denying a woman's request for a female aide to bathe her
- forgetting to button, zip, or fasten clothing when dressing the elderly
- unnecessarily exposing older individuals during examination or care activities
- discussing incontinent episodes when the involved individual's peers are present
- ignoring a man's desire to be cleaned and shaved before his female friend visits
- not recognizing attempts by older adults to look attractive
- joking about two senior citizens' interest in and flirtation with each other

Why is it difficult to understand that a recognition of sexual identity is important to elders? It is not unusual for a 30-year-old to be interested in the latest fashions, for two 35-year-olds to be dating, or for a 20-year-old woman to prefer a female gynecologist. Almost any young woman wouldn't want a new date to see her before she had time to adjust her cosmetics, hair, and clothing. Chances are that no care provider would walk into the room of a 25-year-old in traction and undress and bathe him in full view of other elders in the room. Older adults are entitled to the same dignity and respect and appreciate the same recognition as sexual human beings that is afforded to persons of other ages. The aging process does not rob the older person of sexual identity.

> ☑ **Point to Ponder**
> *What attitudes toward sex and the elderly do you hold? What contributed to the formation of these attitudes?*

The nurse can foster sexuality and intimacy in the elderly in various ways, some of which have already been discussed. Basic education can help the elderly and persons of all ages understand the effects of the aging process on sexuality by providing a realistic framework of sexual functioning. This can be provided when sexual function is discussed during routine health assessments, as part of structured health education classes, and during discharge planning when capabilities and restrictions are reviewed.

A willingness on the nurse's part to discuss sex openly with older people demonstrates recognition, acceptance, and respect for their sexuality. A sexual history as part of the nursing assessment provides an excellent framework for launching such discussions. Physical, emotional, and social threats to the elderly's sexuality and intimacy should be identified and solutions should be sought for problems—whether caused by the disfigurement of surgery, obesity, depression, poor self-concept, fatigue, or lack of privacy. Practices that can enhance sexual function should be promoted, including regular exercise, good nutrition, limited alcohol intake, ample rest, stress management, good hygiene and grooming practices, and enjoyable foreplay.

> 🔑 **KEY CONCEPT**
> The nurse's willingness to discuss sex openly with older adults demonstrates recognition, acceptance, and respect for their sexuality.

Consideration must be given to the sexual needs of older persons in institutional settings. Too often, couples admitted to the same facility are not able to share a double bed, and frequently they are not even able to share the same room if they require different levels of care. It is unnatural, unreal, and unfair to force a person to travel to another wing of a building to visit a spouse who has intimately shared 40, 50, or 60 years of his or her life. There are few or no places in most institutional settings where two such individuals can find a place to share intimacy where they will not be interrupted or are in full view of others. Older people in institutional settings have a right to privacy that goes beyond lip service. They should be able to close and lock a door, feeling secure that this action will be honored. They should not be made to feel guilty or foolish by their expressions of love and sexuality. They should not have to have their sexuality sanctioned, screened, or severed by any other person.

Masturbation often is beneficial for releasing sexual tensions and maintaining continued function of the genitalia. Nurses can convey their acceptance and understanding of the value of this activity by providing privacy and a nonjudgmental attitude. An open viewpoint can prevent the elderly from developing feelings of guilt or abnormality related to masturbation.

On the other hand, nurses must appreciate that sexual satisfaction can have different meaning to elders than to the young. To some older men and women, holding, caressing, and exchanging loving words can be as meaningful as intercourse or sexually explicit conversation.

Nurses must recognize, respect, and encourage sexuality in the elderly. Nurses, as role models, can foster positive attitudes. Improved understanding, increased sensitivity, and humane attitudes can help the older population of today and tomorrow realize the full potential of sexuality in their later years.

Menopause as a Journey to Inner Connection

To some individuals, menopause is viewed as a time of experiencing and managing hormonal changes. In fact, to some extent, menopause has been "medicalized" because it is considered a problem or condition that must be treated. Although there are real physiological concerns to consider, menopause is broader in scope than merely a physiological experience. It is a time of important transition in a woman's life that can result in an awakening of a new wholeness of body, mind, and spirit. By the time the average woman reaches menopause, she has considerable life experience that has afforded her a special wisdom. Many cultures honor the wisdom gleaned from years of living and seek the guidance of elders. Unfortunately, Western society tends to prize the physical beauty of youth over the inner beauty of age. Women in their fifties, sixties, and beyond can feel unattractive, unappreciated, and underused as a result.

KEY CONCEPT
Menopause marks the entry into a new season of life, characterized by wisdom and groundedness.

As a generation of baby boomers—who are redefining the norms for aging—experiences menopause, an enlightened view of menopause is emerging. This generation of assertive, proactive women will not be confined to limited roles based on physical characteristics. They will desire and demand that their talents be used and that they have opportunities for continued growth. The wonder and wisdom of age may receive a long-deserved place of importance.

Effective management of the physical aspects of menopause can enable women to experience this season of life as a positive passage rather than distressing detour. Gerontological nurses can serve aging women well by being knowledgeable about menopause and helping them separate myths from realities about this life transition.

Menopause, the permanent cessation of menses for at least 1 year, occurs for most women around the fifth decade of life when estrogen levels fall and the reduced number of ovarian follicles lose their ability to respond to gonadotropic hormone stimulation. Before menopause, the main source of estrogen is estradiol, which is produced by the ovaries. When the ovaries decline in function, most estrogen is obtained through the conversion of androstenedione to estrone in the skin and adipose tissue. A variety of factors can cause estrogen levels to vary among postmenopausal women. Display 12-2 lists symptoms that may be associated with estrogen loss.

> ☑ **Point to Ponder**
> *Do you view menopause as a time marking the loss of youthfulness and beauty or the beginning of a journey into new creativity and wisdom? What has influenced your opinion?*

Hormone therapy can reduce the symptoms associated with menopause. Before the 1990s, many postmenopausal women used estrogen replacement therapy (using estrogen alone). However, estrogen alone was shown to increase the risk of endometrial cancer, so hormone replacement therapy (HRT), which uses a combination of estrogen and progestin, replaced estrogen therapy alone. Because of the relatively short experience with the prescription of HRT, all of its effects are unknown. Some research has suggested that HRT can improve cognition and prevent

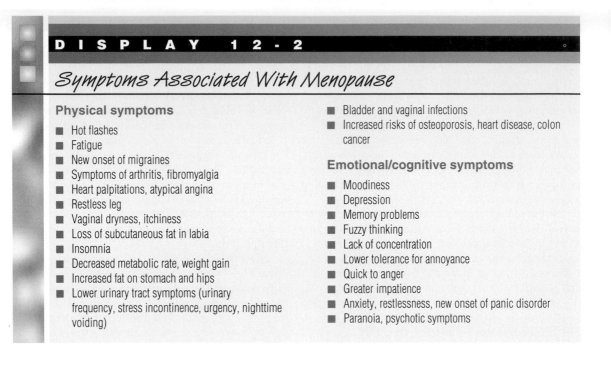

DISPLAY 12-2

Symptoms Associated With Menopause

Physical symptoms

- Hot flashes
- Fatigue
- New onset of migraines
- Symptoms of arthritis, fibromyalgia
- Heart palpitations, atypical angina
- Restless leg
- Vaginal dryness, itchiness
- Loss of subcutaneous fat in labia
- Insomnia
- Decreased metabolic rate, weight gain
- Increased fat on stomach and hips
- Lower urinary tract symptoms (urinary frequency, stress incontinence, urgency, nighttime voiding)

- Bladder and vaginal infections
- Increased risks of osteoporosis, heart disease, colon cancer

Emotional/cognitive symptoms

- Moodiness
- Depression
- Memory problems
- Fuzzy thinking
- Lack of concentration
- Lower tolerance for annoyance
- Quick to anger
- Greater impatience
- Anxiety, restlessness, new onset of panic disorder
- Paranoia, psychotic symptoms

Alzheimer's disease (Gandy, 2003). Long-term (10 or more years) HRT currently is believed to increase the risk of breast cancer, although the risk is influenced by individual risk factors (Grady, 2003). At this point, short-term therapy to manage symptoms is considered safe for most women, although greater understanding of the long-term effects is needed before therapy beyond 5 years is advised (NAMS Report, 2003).

Whether or not to begin HRT is an individual decision that a woman needs to make after careful review of risk factors and discussion with her health care provider. Contraindications to HRT include endometriosis, thrombophlebitis, migraines, neuroophthalmologic disease, liver disease, and estrogen-dependent or endometrial cancer. If HRT is chosen, it should begin with the lowest possible dose that will control symptoms and be reviewed annually, particularly as research continues to yield new findings. Some of the potential side effects of HRT include fluid retention, changes in body weight, irregular bleeding, breast tenderness or swelling, nausea, vomiting, anorexia, skin irritation,

gingival bleeding and tenderness, depression, and insomnia.

Display 12-3 describes some natural and alternative ways to control menopausal symptoms.

KEY CONCEPT
One of the outcomes of the dynamic process of development is the ability to see oneself realistically.

Aging women can benefit from basic education about menopause. Some of the major topics that could be included in a menopausal educational program are outlined in Display 12-4. Nurses can help women appreciate menopause as a time to take stock and rechart their course. Emotions and symptoms can be used as teachers that show areas of oneself that beg for expression. Creative energies can be unleashed and new interests discovered. The significance of caring for and nurturing self can be realized. Whether it is their maturation or a desire to

DISPLAY 12-3

Complementary and Alternative Approaches to Controlling Menopausal Symptoms

Acupuncture

Diet
- Foods rich in plant estrogens: apples, beans, carrots, celery, nuts, seeds, soy products (approximately 100–160 mg/day of soy is needed to obtain significant relief), wheat, and whole grains
- Foods rich in boron to increase estrogen retention: asparagus, beans, broccoli, cabbage, peaches, prunes, strawberries, and tomatoes
- Avoidance of adrenal-stimulating foods: alcohol, caffeine, refined carbohydrates, salt, and sugar

Exercise

Imagery

Herbs
- American ginseng, black cohosh, chickweed, dong quai, motherwort, sage, licorice root

Homeopathic remedies
- Vaginal lubrication: bryonia
- General symptoms: amyl nitrosum, natrum muriaticum, sepia, and sulphur

Meditation

Regular, adequate sleep

Stress management practices

Tai chi

Vaginal moisturizing agents
- Commercial vaginal moisturizing creams (eg, Replens), water-based gels
- Herbal salves made with marshmallow root, calendula blossom, comfrey, licorice root, and wild yam
- St. John's wort oil

Vitamins and minerals
- Calcium, chromium, magnesium, selenium, and vitamins C, D, and E

Yoga

not waste the precious limited time one has remaining in life, older adults tend to understand themselves and their lives. Impossible expectations and pretense can be let go, allowing more meaningful and creative aspects of later life to be unleashed. Elders can live in truth and love as who they truly are. This self-acceptance can provide the security to broaden their perspectives and purposes and deepen their connections with others and a higher power.

DISPLAY 12-4

Topics for Inclusion in a Menopause Education Program

■ Menopause is a naturally occurring process, not a disease. It is characterized by the absence of menstrual periods for at least 12 consecutive months.

■ Menopause is a gradual process. Most women experience *perimenopause* about 3–6 years before menopause when menstrual periods permanently cease. By age 40, most women begin having irregular periods.

■ Menopause is a multihormone process. In addition to estrogen, progesterone declines although not in a direct proportion. In fact, some of the symptoms associated with menopause can be the result of declining progesterone with an estrogen dominance. One outcome of estrogen dominance over progesterone is the blocking of the action of thyroid hormone. Although it does not occur in all menopausal women, some can have declines in testosterone, which affects libido and sexual pleasure. Factors such as stress and obesity affect hormonal secretion.

■ Estrogen affects functions beyond those of reproduction. Estrogen:
  ○ increases the chemical enzyme choline acetyltransferase needed to synthesize the neurotransmitter acetylcholine (which is critical for memory)
  ○ promotes the growth of dendritic spines on neurons
  ○ enhances the availability of the neurotransmitters serotonin, norepinephrine, and dopamine
  ○ acts like an antioxidant to protect nerve cells from free radical damage

■ Many physical, cognitive, and emotional symptoms can be associated with low estrogen levels (see Display 12-3).

■ Diagnostic blood tests should be done to properly assess menopausal state; these include FSH, LH, estradiol (estrogen), testosterone, and free testosterone levels. If sexual dysfunction or low libido is present, evaluate thyroid function (T_3, T_4, free T_4, TSH), platelet MAO, and prolactin.

■ Hormonal replacement therapy (HRT) carries risks and benefits that must be weighed for each individual. HRT can control unpleasant symptoms thus fostering a good quality of life, reduce the risk of colon cancer and heart disease, and, possibly, offer protection against Alzheimer's disease and stroke. Negative aspects of HRT include an increased risk of ovarian, lung, and certain breast cancers; blood clots; and gallbladder disease.
  ○ A variety of estrogens are available, including:
  ○ Premarin, derived from *pre*gnant *mar*es ur*ine*
  ○ Estradiol
  ○ Estrone
  ○ Combinations (usually not advised because the dose of each component is too low to be effective)

■ Progesterone usually is added to estrogen to prevent hyperplasia of the uterine lining.

■ Complementary therapies and practices can assist in controlling symptoms in some women (see Display 12-3).

FSH, follicle-stimulating hormone; LH, luteinizing hormone; TSH, thyroid-stimulating hormone; MAO, monoamine oxidase.

Critical Thinking Exercises

1. In what ways will today's young generation be in a better or worse position than today's elders in developing survivor competencies?

2. What attitudes and actions of health care providers can have a negative effect on the sexuality of older adults? What can have a positive effect?

3. Describe how a positive self-concept could affect total health status

NURSING DIAGNOSIS HIGHLIGHT

SEXUAL DYSFUNCTION

Overview

Sexual dysfunction implies a problem in the ability to derive sexual satisfaction. This condition can be identified through the patient's history (eg, complaints of impotence, dyspareunia, lack of interest in sex, changes in relationship with partner), physical findings (eg, genital infection, prolapsed uterus, diabetes mellitus), or behavior (eg, depression, anxiety, self-deprecation). Sometimes changes in the elder's life can give clues to the presence of sexual dysfunction problems, such as recent widowhood, onset of a new health problem, or moving to a child's home.

Causative or contributing factors

Age-related dryness and fragility of vaginal canal, vaginal infection, venereal disease, neurological disease, cardiovascular disease, diabetes mellitus, decreased hormone production, pulmonary disease, arthritis, pain, prostatitis, prolapsed uterus, cytocele, rectocele, medications, overeating, obesity, fatigue, alcohol consumption, fear of worsening health problem, lack of partner, unwilling or unable partner, boredom with partner, fear of failure, guilt, anxiety, depression, stress, negative self-concept, lack of privacy, religious conflict, altered appearance

Goal

The patient expresses satisfaction with sexual function.

Interventions

- Obtain a sexual history from the elder. Note availability and quality of relationship with partner, lifelong pattern of sexual function, recent changes to sexual function, signs and symptoms of sexual dysfunction, knowledge and attitudes about sex, medical problems, drugs used, mental status, myths and misinformation, feelings about sexual dysfunction.
- If the cause of sexual dysfunction is not readily available through the history, refer elder for comprehensive physical examination.
- Identify causative or contributing factors to sexual dysfunction and plan interventions to correct them.
- Refer to sexual counselor or therapist as needed.
- Clarify misconceptions (eg, cannot have sex after a heart attack).
- Provide education as to normal sexual function, measures to promote sexual function, how to minimize impact of health problems on sexual function (Heart Association, Arthritis Foundation, and other disease-specific organizations provide literature on promoting sexual function in presence of disease).
- Assist elder in having good appearance and improving self-concept as needed.
- Advise in health practices that will promote sexual function, such as regular gynecologic examinations, alcohol use in moderation, good diet, exercise.
- Ensure staff are nonjudgmental about elder's unique means of sexual expression.
- If elder is hospitalized or institutionalized, provide privacy for sexual expression.

Web Connect

Explore the resources and current information on menopause by visiting the website of the North American Menopause Society at www.menopause.org.

● Resources

American Association of Sex Educators, Counselors, and Therapists
P.O. Display 238
Mount Vernon, IA 52314
www.aasect.org

Menstrual Health Foundation
104 Petaluma Street
Sebastopol, CA 95472
(707) 829-3154

Pride Senior Network
1756 Broadway
Suite 11H
New York, NY 10019
(212) 757-3203
www.pridesenior.org

Sexuality Information and Education Council of the United States
130 West 42nd Street
Suite 350
New York, NY 10036
(212) 819-9770
www.siecus.org

● References

Gandy, S. (2003). Estrogen and neurodegeneration. *Neurochemical Research, 28*(7), 1003–1008.

Grady, D. (2003). Postmenopausal hormones. Therapy for symptoms only. *New England Journal of Medicine, 348*(19), 1835–1837.

NAMS Report. (2003). Amended report from the NAMS Advisory Panel on postmenopausal hormone therapy. *Menopause: Journal of the North American Menopause Society, 10*(1), 6–12.

● Recommended Readings

Bauer, M. (1999). Their only privacy is between their sheets: Privacy and sexuality of elderly nursing home residents. *Journal of Gerontological Nursing, 25*(8), 37–41.

Borysenko, J. (1998). *A woman's book of life: The biology, psychology, and spirituality of the feminine life cycle.* New York: Riverhead Books.

Cary, C. (1998). *A foxy old woman's guide to living with friends.* Freedom, CA: Crossing Press.

Conway, J. (1997). *Men in midlife crisis.* Colorado Springs, CO: Chariot Victor Publishers.

Cumming, D. C., & Cumming, C. E. (1998). Hormone replacement therapy: Part I: Should your elder do with—or without—it? *Consultant, 38,* 2417–2420, 2425–2427, 2431.

Cumming, D. C., & Cumming, C. E. (1998). Hormone replacement therapy: Part II: Should your elder do without it? *Consultant, 38,* 2435–2438, 2441–2442.

Felton, B. S., & Hall, J. M. (2001). Conceptualizing resilience in women older than 85: Overcoming adversity from illness or loss. *Journal of Gerontological Nursing, 27*(11), 46–53.

Hertz, J. E., & Anschutz, C. A. (2002). Relationships among perceived enactment of autonomy, self-care, and holistic health in community dwelling older adults. *Journal of Holistic Nursing, 20*(2), 166–186.

Kaiger-Walker, K. (1997). *Positive aging: Every woman's quest for wisdom and beauty.* Berkeley, CA: Conari Press.

Klaiber, E. L. (2001). *Hormones and the mind. A woman's guide to enhancing mood, memory, and sexual vitality.* New York: HarperCollins Publisher.

Moore, S. L., Metcalf, B., & Schow, E. (2000). Aging and meaning in life: Examining the concept. *Geriatric Nursing, 21*(1), 27–29.

Mortimer, J. E. (2002). Hormone replacement therapy and beyond. *Geriatrics, 57*(6), 25–32.

Mount Sinai School of Medicine. (1999). Postmenopausal? See your gynecologist anyway! *Focus on Healthy Aging, 2*(11), 1, 6.

Northrup, C. (2001). *The wisdom of menopause. Creating physical and emotional health and healing during the change.* New York: Bantam Books.

Van Wynen, E. A. (2001). Key to successful aging: Learning-style patterns of older adults. *Journal of Gerontological Nursing, 27*(9), 6–15.

Wallace, M. (2001). Sexuality (Try this). *Journal of Gerontological Nursing, 27*(2), 10–11.

Warga, C. (1999). *Menopause and the Mind.* New York: The Free Press.

Writing Group for the Women's Health Initiative Investigators. (2002). Risks and benefits of estrogen plus progestin in healthy postmenopausal women. *Journal of the American Medical Association, 288,* 321–333.

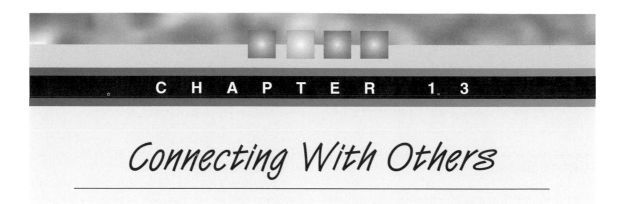

Connecting With Others

■ **Learning Objectives**

After reading this chapter, you should be able to:

- list communication obstacles resulting from hearing and visual impairments

- describe variables that affect socialization in late life

- list the effects of aging on sexual function

- describe factors that can contribute to sexual dysfunction

- list factors that facilitate connections with others

In the 1960s, Yale psychologist Stanley Milgram stirred excitment by suggesting that all humans were connected by "six degrees of separation" (Milgram, 1983). This was based on his experiment in which he had a group of midwesterners forward a letter to someone they did not know using their network of friends as intermediaries. The friends were allowed to pass the letter to their friends until it reached the stranger who originally was the targeted recipient. Milgram discovered that the letter had to pass through five friends, on average, to reach the intended party; therefore, he concluded that we live in a small world in which people are separated by only six connections. Milgram's work has since inspired a play and interesting entertainment as people attempted to test his theory.

Although a closer examination of Milgram's research disclosed flaws that showed that actually people are not as closely connected as proposed, the reality is that there is a profound interconnectedness among people. The ease of travel, widespread use of the Internet, and availability of affordable long-distance telephone calls have connected people from far corners of the world with extraordinary speed and ease. As active participants in a highly communicative society, the elderly connect with others—formally and informally, directly and indirectly, and casually and intimately. Assisting older adults in maintaining healthy connections is an important aspect of gerontological nursing.

Communication

The axiom that people are social beings is true for the elderly. Through social interaction, people share joys and burdens, derive feelings of normalcy, validate perceptions, and maintain a link with reality. The ability to communicate is an essential ingredient for social interaction, but because of a variety of intrinsic and extrinsic factors, older persons may face unique obstacles in their attempts to interact with others.

IMPACT OF HEARING IMPAIRMENT

Presbycusis (the age-related sensorineural hearing loss) may cause speech to be inaudible or distorted, as can impacted cerumen, which is a common problem in the elderly. Older people may be self-conscious of this limitation and avoid situations in which they must interact. In turn, others may avoid them because of this difficulty. Telephone conversations can be affected by this problem, limiting social contact even further for the individual who may be socially isolated for other reasons.

Approximately 10% of the elderly have some difficulty hearing telephone conversations. Corrective measures for hearing problems should be explored. The first step to managing or correcting hearing problems is to assess the underlying problem through professional evaluation, including an audiometric examination.

> ✔ **Point to Ponder**
>
> *Cellular phones have widespread use. In what ways do you believe these have facilitated and impaired communication?*

Hearing aids can benefit persons with some hearing disorders, but they may not solve all hearing problems. An audiometric evaluation can determine if the specific hearing problem can be improved by using a hearing aid. A hearing aid should never be purchased without being specifically prescribed. Sometimes elderly persons will attempt to improve hearing by purchasing an aid through a private party or a mail-order catalog, which often results in disappointment and a waste of money from an already limited budget. Nurses should educate the public about the realities of hearing aid use.

Even when a hearing aid is appropriate, problems can arise with its use. Inability to adjust to the presence of the aid and the distortion of sound caused by the amplification of environmental noise, along with speech sounds, may make the patient reject its use. New hearing aid users need support during the adjustment phase and should be advised to wear the aid for progressively longer periods each day until comfort is gained and to avoid its use in noisy environments, such as airports, train stations, and stadiums. The aid must be checked regularly to ensure that the earpiece is not blocked with cerumen and that the battery is working. This appliance may easily correct a hearing problem and reintroduce the older individual to a socially active life.

If a hearing aid cannot correct the problem, efforts should be made to speak clearly and distinctly, in a low frequency but at an audible level, when facing the individual. Shouting should be avoided because it raises the high-frequency sounds that older persons already have difficulty hearing, causing even greater hearing problems. Cupping the hands over the less deficient ear and talking directly into the ear may be helpful. Using gestures and pictures and pointing to items when talking about them can assist in communication. Chapter 30 discusses other considerations for communicating with hearing-impaired people.

> 🔑 **KEY CONCEPT**
> Shouting raises the frequency of the voice, thereby reducing what the older ear can hear.

The nurse should examine an older adult's ears frequently for cerumen accumulation. Cerumen removal can be aided by gentle irrigation with warm water or a hydrogen peroxide and water solution; commercial preparations also are available. It is wise for older persons to have assistance when irrigating ears because dizziness often occurs during the procedure. Even allowing water to run in the ears during showers or shampoos can aid in loosening cerumen. Cotton-tipped applicators should not be used for cerumen removal, because they can push the cerumen back into the ear canal and cause an impaction.

 KEY CONCEPT
Ear irrigations can help to remove cerumen accumulations; however, care must be taken to protect the older person from the potential dizziness associated with this procedure.

It is beneficial for nurses to provide health education about the effects of environmental noise on hearing and general health. Nurses also should take an active role in advocating legislation to control noise pollution and the enforcement of that legislation.

IMPACT OF VISUAL IMPAIRMENT

The ability to see is equally important in communication. Most elderly people require some form of corrective lenses, and approximately half of all individuals who are identified as legally blind each year are 65 years of age or older. Visual limitations can make communication problematic because facial expressions and gestures, which are as important as the words themselves, may be missed or misinterpreted. Lip reading to compensate for hearing deficits may be difficult, and written correspondence may be limited because independent reading and writing become almost impossible tasks. Remaining aware of current events through newspapers and socialization through playing cards and other games may be hampered.

For visual deficits, one of the first assistive measures is a thorough eye examination, including tonometry, by an ophthalmologist. The importance of an annual eye examination, not only to detect vision changes and needs for alterations in corrective lenses but also for early discovery of problems, such as cataracts, glaucoma, and other disease processes, must be stressed. The financial ability of the individual to afford an eye examination and glasses must be evaluated because health insurance seldom covers this important service; community resources or the negotiation of special payment plans may help the elderly to acquire the necessary aid.

To compensate for visual limitations, one should face the individual and exaggerate gestures and facial expressions when speaking. To compensate for poor peripheral vision, which is common in older people, one should approach these individuals from the front rather than the side where their vision is limited and ensure that seating allows for full sight of persons or objects with which they are interacting. Ample lighting is important and should be provided by several soft indirect lights rather than a single, bright, glaring source. Interaction can be promoted by using large-print games and playing cards, telephone dials with enlarged numbers that glow in the dark, and cassette recorders. Books and magazines with large print and recordings of current events and popular literature can provide a source of recreation and a means of keeping informed.

 KEY CONCEPT
To compensate for poor peripheral vision, approach the older person from the front rather than from the side.

Social Interaction and Nursing Intervention

Because of declining physical function, the older person may have less energy to invest in social interaction. Urinary frequency and incontinence make people reluctant to engage in social activities, as do stiff, painful joints and other discomforts. Changes in appearance may alter the individual's self-concept and interfere with the motivation for and quality of social interaction. Although many of these problems cannot be eliminated, nursing intervention can help to reduce the limitations they cause. Education of younger adults regarding the normal aging process can enhance their sensitivity and patience and help them understand the socialization handicaps that elderly persons face, perhaps thereby also helping them learn how to minimize and manage these limitations as they grow older. Assuring the elderly that their problems are shared by many others and that some of their limitations are a natural part of aging may help them feel "normal" and thus promote social interaction (Fig. 13-1).

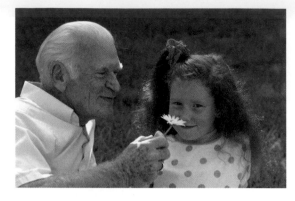

FIGURE 13·1

Social interaction can be beneficial to all age groups.

Using common sense in nursing care will facilitate social activity. The nurse can review and perhaps readjust the person's schedule to conserve energy and maximize opportunities for socialization. Medication administration should be planned so that during periods of social activity analgesics will provide relief, tranquilizers will not sedate, diuretics will not reach their peak, and laxatives will not begin working. Likewise, fluid intake and bathroom visits before activities begin should be planned to reduce the fear or actual occurrence of incontinence; activities for the elderly should include frequent break periods for bathroom visits. The control of these minor obstacles can often facilitate social interaction.

Given the capacity to interact socially and manage their problems independently, the elderly must then confront social factors over which they have no control. Their circles of friends and relatives may become smaller through deaths, and a limited budget may necessitate giving food and shelter priority over social functions. A youth-oriented, fast-paced society may not provide an atmosphere that is conducive to active social involvement. If segments of society disengage from the elderly, the ability to socially interact is lessened. Fortunately, as described in Chapter 40, families become a strong source of socialization for the elderly. Nurses need to promote social activity among the elderly, including helping persons of all ages see the attributes of the unique human being housed within the aged body (see the Nursing Diagnosis Highlight at the end of this chapter).

> **KEY CONCEPT**
> Nurses play an important advocacy role by helping younger persons see the individuality and attributes of older persons.

Sex and the Elderly

For many years, sex was a major conversational taboo in the United States. Discussion and education concerning this natural, normal process were discouraged and avoided in most circles. Literature on the subject was minimal and usually secured under lock and key. An interest in sex was considered sinful and highly improper. Although there was an awareness that sexual intercourse had more than a procreative function, the other benefits of this activity were seldom openly shared; sexual expression outside of wedlock was viewed as disgraceful and indecent. The reluctance to accept and intelligently confront human sexuality led to the propagation of numerous myths, the persistence of ignorance and prejudice, and the relegation of sex to a vulgar status.

Fortunately, attitudes have changed over the years, and sexuality has come to be increasingly understood and accepted as natural and pleasurable. Education has helped erase the mysteries of sex for both adults and children, and magazines and books on the topic flourish. Sex courses, workshops, and counselors throughout the country are helping people gain greater insight about and enjoyment of sex. Not only has the stigma attached to premarital sex been greatly reduced, but also increasing numbers of unmarried couples are living together with society's acceptance. To a large degree, sex is now viewed as a natural, good, and beautiful shared experience.

> ✔ **Point to Ponder**
> *How comfortable are you acknowledging that your older relatives could be sexually active?*

Natural, good, and beautiful—seldom are these terms used to describe the sexual experiences of aged individuals. When the topic of sex and the aged is confronted, much ignorance and prejudice concerning sex reappear. Education about the sexuality of old age is minimal; literature abounds on the sexuality of all individuals in society except the elderly. Any signs of interest in sex or open discussions of sex by older persons are discouraged and often labeled as lecherous. The same criteria that make a man a "playboy" at 30 years of age make him a "dirty old man" at 70 years of age. Unmarried young and middle-aged adults who engage in pleasurable sexual experiences are accepted, but widowed grandparents seeking the same enjoyment are often viewed with disbelief and ridicule. Myths run rampant. How many times do we hear that women lose all desire for sex after menopause, that older men cannot achieve an erection, and that older people are not interested in sex? Respect for the elderly as vital, sexual beings is minimized by the lack of privacy afforded them, by the lack of credence given to their sexuality, and by the lack of acceptance, respect, and dignity granted to their continued sexual expression. The myths, ignorance, and vulgar status previously associated with sex in general have been conferred on the sexuality of the aged. Such misconceptions and prejudices are an injustice to persons of all ages. They reinforce any fears and aversion the young have to growing old. They impose conformity on the aged, which requires that they either forfeit warm and meaningful sexual experiences or suffer feelings of guilt and abnormality. Nurses can play a significant role in educating and counseling about sexuality and the aged; they can encourage attitude changes by their own examples.

> 🔑 **KEY CONCEPT**
> Often, society conveys the same attitudes regarding sex and the elderly as it has in the past concerning sex in general.

Sexual Intercourse

With the exception of the outstanding work by Kinsey (1948) and Masters and Johnson (1966), there has been minimal exploration into the realities of sex in old age until recently. Several possible factors have contributed to this lack of research and information. First, the acceptance and expansion of sexology has been relatively recent. Second, impropriety was formerly associated with open discussions of sex. Furthermore, there is a misconception on the part of many professionals, the aged, and the general public that the aged are neither interested in nor capable of sex. Finally, practitioners lack experience in and do not have an inclination toward discussing sex with any age group. Even today, medical and nursing assessments frequently do not reflect inquiry into sexual history and activity.

Nurses should be aware of recent interest and research in the area of sex in old age and communicate these research findings to colleagues and clients to promote a more realistic understanding of the aged's sexuality. Research has disproved the belief that older persons are not interested in or capable of engaging in sex; elders can and do enjoy the pleasures of sexual foreplay and intercourse. Because the general pattern of sexual behavior is basically consistent throughout life, individuals who were disinterested in sex and had infrequent intercourse throughout their lifetime will not usually develop a sudden insatiable desire for sex in old age. On the other hand, a couple who has maintained an interest in sex and continued regular coitus throughout their adult life will most likely not forfeit this activity at any particular age. Homosexuality, masturbation, a desire for a variety of sexual partners, and other sexual patterns also continue into old age. Sexual styles, interests, and expression must be placed in the perspective of the individual's total life experience.

> 🔑 **KEY CONCEPT**
> Sexuality and sexual interest in late life reflect lifelong patterns.

Despite the physical ability to maintain a sexually active state in old age, various factors threaten the elderly person's ability to remain sexually active (Nursing Diagnosis Table 13-1). Although clinical data are minimal and additional research is necessary, some general statements can be made about sex and the older person.

- There is a decrease in sexual responsiveness and a reduction in the frequency of orgasm (Greenberg, 2001; Masters & Johnson, 1981).
- Older men are slower to erect, mount, and ejaculate.
- Older women may experience dyspareunia (painful intercourse) as a result of less lubrication, decreased distensibility, and thinning of the vaginal walls.

Nursing Diagnosis

ND **TABLE 13-1** ● *Aging and Risks to Sexuality*

Causes or Contributing Factors	Nursing Diagnosis
Wrinkling and sagging of tissues; age spots; graying and loss of hair; arthritic joints; loss of muscle tone; high prevalence of tooth loss; increased incidence of disabling disease	Disturbed Body Image and Sexual Dysfunction related to altered appearance
Increased physical stimulation required to achieve erection and lubricate vagina	Sexual Dysfunction related to inadequate preparation for intercourse
Increased prevalence of chronic disabling	Sexual Dysfunction related to discomfort, diseases, preoccupation with health, or positional restrictions
Higher ratio of women to men in advanced years	Sexual Dysfunction related to unavailability of a sexual partner
Ageism	Sexual Dysfunction related to belief that sex in old age is inappropriate

• Many older women gain a new interest in sex, possibly because they no longer have to fear an unwanted pregnancy or because they have more time and privacy with their children grown and gone.

Although individual differences occur in the intensity and duration of sexual response in older people, regular sexual expression for both sexes is important in promoting sexual capacity and maintaining sexual function. With good health and the availability of a partner, sexual activity can continue well into the seventh decade and beyond.

The work of Masters and Johnson (1966) provided the first major insight into the sexual responses of older persons. Table 13-1 summarizes their findings.

Sexual Dysfunction

Various physical, emotional, and social variables threaten the elderly person's ability to remain sexually active (Table 13-2). A comprehensive nursing assessment should include a sexual history, which can reveal these problems. Display 13-1 offers sample questions that can be incorporated into the assessment to identify issues pertaining to sexual function. Sensitive attention to the maintenance of sexual function and identity is significant in promoting wellness and normality.

KEY CONCEPT
The unavailability of a partner, ageism, changes in body image, boredom, misconceptions, physical conditions, medications, and cognitive impairments are among the factors that can interfere with sexual function in later life.

UNAVAILABILITY OF A PARTNER

A practical interference with sexual function in later life is the lack of a partner, particularly for older women. By 65 years of age, there are only 7 men to every 10 women; by 85 years of age, the ratio becomes 1:5. Furthermore, there is a tendency for men to marry women who are younger than themselves; one third of men older than 65 years of age have wives younger than 65 years of age; therefore, most older men are married, and most older women are widowed.

Even when an older person has a spouse or partner, that person may be too infirm to remain sexually active and, in some cases, may be institutionalized.

PSYCHOLOGICAL BARRIERS

The elderly are not immune to the attitudes around them. As they hear comments about the inappropriateness of older people engaging in sex and watch television shows that portray sex among the elderly in a

TABLE 13-1 ● *Human Sexual Response Cycle and the Elderly*

Phase	Older Women	Older Men
Excitement: results from stimulation from any source	Same clitoral response and nipple erection as younger women; sex flush (vasocongestive skin response) occurs less frequently; less muscle tension elevation in response to sexual stimuli; unlike in younger women, labia majora does not separate, flatten, and elevate; reduced reactions of labia minora; less secretory activity of Bartholin's gland; less vaginal lubrication and wall expansion	Takes two to three times longer for erection to be achieved; less firm erection; increased difficulty regaining erection if lost; less sex flush
Plateau: sexual tensions intensified; if they reach an extreme, orgasm will be achieved; if tension level drops, resolution phase will be entered	Reduced intensity; less degree of engorgement of areolae; decreased vasocongestion of labia; less uterine elevation	Slower; full erection may not occur until just prior to ejaculation; less intense muscle tension; delayed and diminished testicular elevation
Orgasm: lasts a few seconds; sexual stimuli released; although entire body is involved to varying degrees, primarily concentrated in genitalia	Same vaginal contractions as younger woman but of decreased intensity and duration; similar slight degree of involuntary distention of external urinary meatus	Similar response as younger man only slower; during ejaculation, more of a seepage of semen rather than a forceful emission; orgasm may not occur with every intercourse, especially if it is frequent
Resolution: sexual tensions subside	Nipple erection can continue for hours; urinary symptoms may be present	Longer duration; rapid penile detumescence

condescending or ridiculing manner, they may feel foolish or unnatural in having sexual desires and activity. If they happen to have sexual partners who are disinterested in sex and negatively label their advances, the problem is intensified. As the impact of others' reactions is internalized, they may have a reluctance or inability to engage in sexual activity, and this function may be forfeited unnecessarily. Nurses can advocate for the elderly by educating persons of all ages in the realities and importance of sexual function in later life and ensuring that nursing care does not reinforce negative attitudes about sex.

It is not unusual for older men occasionally to have difficulty achieving an erection; erections also may be easily lost if there is an interruption (eg, a ringing telephone or a partner who leaves the bed to use the bathroom). These factors may lead older men to believe that they are losing their sexual capabilities. A cycle of problems can then be triggered, whereby an episode of impotence causes anxiety over the potential loss of sexual function permanently, and this anxiety inter-

feres with the ability to become erect, which heightens anxiety. Aging persons need realistic explanations—preferably before the situation arises—that occasional impotence is neither unusual nor an indication that one is "too old for sex." Open discussions and reassurance are beneficial. The partner needs to be included in this process and made aware of the importance of patience and sensitivity in helping the man deal with this problem. The couple should be encouraged to continue their efforts and, if erection is occasionally a problem, compensate with other forms of sexual gratification. Of course, chronic impotence can indicate a variety of disorders and deserves a thorough evaluation.

Body image and self-concept affect sexual activity. In a society in which beauty is youthful, older persons may believe that their wrinkles, gray hair, and sagging torsos make them physically unappealing. This can be particularly difficult for single elderly people who must deal with baring their bodies to new partners. The fear of being unattractive and rejected may cause

TABLE 13-2 ● *Physical Conditions Interfering with Sexual Function*

Condition	Problem Created	Intervention
Men		
Prostatitis	Discomfort, interference with ejaculation	Treat infection; prostatic massage
"Open" type prostatectomy	Disturbed function of internal sphincter, causing impotency	Penile prosthesis
Peyronie's disease	Painful, dorsal bending of penis from fibrous scarring associated with inflammatory process	Local injections of corticosteroids Surgery
Infections of genitalia	Pain, inhibition of erection, scarring that narrows urethral outlet	Treat infection Surgical dilation of narrow outlet
Arteriosclerosis	Testicular cellular function disturbed, leading to decline in male sex hormone	Testosterone therapy
Parkinsonism	Decrease in sexual interest secondary to loss of potency	Levodopa therapy
Cord compression from arthritic changes	Impotency	Surgery may not restore potency if reflex arc is permanently broken Penile prosthesis
Women		
Decreased level of estrogen	Excessive vaginal dryness	Local estrogens
Virginity	Thick or large hymen	Surgery Dilation
Infection of genitalia	Discomfort, itching	Treat infection and underlying cause (poor hygiene, hyperglycemia)
Prolapsed uterus	Pain, difficulty with penile penetration	Pessary Surgery
Cystocele	Discomfort, dribbling urine	Surgery
Both Sexes		
Cardiovascular, respiratory disease	Shortness of breath, coughing, discomfort, fear of heart attack or death during sex, decreased libido	Counseling on realistic restrictions necessary Instruction in alternative positions to avoid strain Advise to avoid large meals for several hours before, relax, plan medications for peak effectiveness during sex
Arthritis	Limited movement	Instruction on alternative positions
Diabetes mellitus	Local genital infection	Treat infection
	Failure of erection due to inhibition of parasympathetic nervous system	Penile prosthesis
	Absence of or difficulty achieving orgasm	Instruction in alternative positions and
	Delayed and decreased vaginal lubrication	forms of sexual expression
Stroke	Decreased libido	Counseling
	Fear	Instruction in alternative positions
Alcoholism	Decreased potency	Counseling and treatment for alcoholism
	Delayed orgasm (women)	

older adults to avoid encountering such situations and assume a sexually inactive role.

For single older people, developing a sexual relationship can be difficult. Older women were social-

ized during a period when sex was considered appropriate only in wedlock and, to some persons, only for the purpose of procreation. The thought of seeking sexual gratification with a partner to whom one is not

---

DISPLAY 13-1

Assessment of Sexual Health

Begin this component of the assessment by explaining that you're going to ask questions pertaining to his or her sex life to identify problems that could be improved and to learn about possible existing conditions that could be revealed through sexual problems. Ask the elder if he or she has your permission to ask these questions:

Are you sexually active?

If the answer if *no,* ask for reasons (eg, no partner, not enough energy, erectile dysfunction). Based on the reason, inquire about the elder's interest in changing the situation to become sexually active and recommend plans accordingly (eg, offer location of senior centers, evaluate possible causes of low energy, refer to sexual dysfunction clinic).

If the answer is *yes,* proceed with the following questions:

- How frequently do you have sex? Is this a satisfying frequency to you? If not, how would you change the frequency of sex?
- Do you have sex with a single or multiple partners? Male or female partner?
- If you have sex with new partners, do you use a condom?
- Do you obtain pleasure from sex? If not, why not?
- Do you or your partner(s) ever been treated for a sexually transmitted disease? If yes, for what disease and when?
- Do you or your partner(s) have risk factors for HIV/AIDS, such as a history of blood transfusions, IV drug use, sex with prostitutes?
- *Male:* Are you able to get an erection when you want to engage in sex? Do you have orgasms and ejaculate when you have sex? If not, describe what happens. Do you have any sores on your penis or discharge?
- *Female:* Is sex comfortable for you? If not, describe. Do you have orgasms? Do you have any vaginal discharge or bleeding?
- Is your partner satisfied with your sex life? If not, why not?
- Have you ever been or are you currently being sexually abused? Raped? If yes, describe.
- *If health conditions or disabilities are present, ask* How has this condition affected your ability to enjoy sex?
- What concerns do you have regarding your sex life?
- Do you have any questions about your sexual function that you'd like me to answer?

---

married creates anxiety and guilt in many older women. The older man, who was socialized in the aggressor role, may not have had to practice his courtship skills for years if he has been monogamous for a long period, and he may feel insecure in his ability to seduce a partner or find one who understands his individual preferences. He, too, may be emotionally uncomfortable in establishing a sexual relationship. Financial considerations can affect sexual activity also when the single elder has concern that commitment to a relationship and marriage could reduce social security income or create problems in sharing assets. The hurdle of building new sexual re-lationships can be so great that many older people may find it easier to repress their sexual needs.

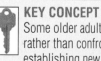 **KEY CONCEPT**
Some older adults may repress sexual needs rather than confront the stresses associated with establishing new sexual relationships.

Married elderly also may experience problems with sex. Not all marriages enjoy fulfilling sex. Some women conceded to sex because it was a "wife's duty," yet they never achieved satisfaction from this intimate experience. Some spouses may have become bored with the same partner or form of sex. Perhaps physical changes or an inattention to appearance causes dissatisfaction with the partner. Love and caring may have been lost from the marriage. Sexual interest may be diminished if one is the caregiver for a partner or if a disability causes the partner to be perceived as sexually undesirable. Elderly couples experience sexual problems for many of the same reasons that younger couples do.

Misconceptions are often responsible for creating obstacles to a fulfilling sex life in old age and can include the following:

- erections are not possible after prostatectomy
- penile penetration can be harmful to a woman after a hysterectomy
- menopause eliminates sexual desire
- sex is bad for a heart condition
- after a hip fracture, intercourse can refracture the bone
- sexual ability and interest are lost with age

Straightforward explanations and public education can help correct these misconceptions, as can realistic descriptions of how illness, surgery, and drugs do and do not affect sexual function.

PHYSICAL BARRIERS

A variety of physical conditions, many of which respond to treatment (see Table 13-2), can affect sexual function in later life. Thorough evaluation is crucial in determining a realistic approach to aiding the elderly with these problems. Interventions of value to younger people also can benefit the elderly, including medications, penile prostheses, lubricants, surgery, and sex counseling. Nurses should communicate their understanding of the importance of sexual functioning to the elderly and a willingness to assist them in preserving sexual capabilities.

ERECTILE DYSFUNCTION

Erectile dysfunction, which is commonly referred to as impotence, is a condition characterized by the inability of a man to attain and maintain an erection of the penis sufficient to allow him to engage in sexual intercourse. An estimated 10 to 20 million American men are believed to suffer from erectile dysfunction and the prevalence increases with age, affecting as many as 25% of men at age 65 years (Kubin, Wagner, & Fugl-Meyer, 2003). Erectile dysfunction can have multiple causes, including atherosclerosis, diabetes, hypertension, multiple sclerosis, thyroid dysfunction, alcoholism, renal failure, structure abnormalities (eg, Peyronie's disease), medications, and psychological factors. Obviously, with the range and complexity of potential causes, a thorough physical examination is essential. (Even if the older man is not interested in being sexually active, he should be encouraged to have this dysfunction evaluated to identify underlying conditions that warrant medical attention.)

In 1998, a major breakthrough occurred in the treatment of erectile dysfunction with the Food and Drug Administration approval of sildenafil citrate, better known by its brand name of Viagra. Within its first year on the market, nearly 4 million prescriptions were written for Viagra, demonstrating the scope of erectile dysfunction and the desire of men to correct this problem. **(For more information about how Viagra works, visit the Connection website.)** There are other options to treat erectile dysfunction, such as alprostadil (a drug that is injected into the penis to increase blood flow), vacuum pumps, and penile implants. Men need to discuss with their physicians the options that are best for them.

DRUGS

Frequently, medications prescribed to the elderly affect potency, libido, orgasm, and ejaculation. Some of these drugs include the following:

- anticholinergics
- benztropine
- clonidine
- cytoxic agents
- digoxin
- diphenhydramine
- guanethidine
- haloperidol
- phenothiazines
- reserpine
- sedatives
- thiazide diuretics
- tranquilizers
- trihexyphenidyl
- tricyclic antidepressants

It is important to prepare older people for the potential changes in sexual function that drugs can produce. Imagine what it does to a patient with newly diagnosed hypertension when he experiences drug-related impotency and begins to feel anxious about the sudden changes in both health and sexual function. Drugs should be reviewed when new sexual dysfunction occurs and, whenever possible, nondrug treatment modalities should be used to manage health problems.

COGNITIVE IMPAIRMENT

The sexual behavior of individuals with dementia tends to be more difficult for those around them than for the affected persons. Inappropriate behavior, such as undressing and masturbating in public areas and grabbing and making sexual comments to strangers, can occur. The spouse may be accused of being a stranger improperly trying to share the bed, and care procedures (eg, baths, and catheterization) may be confused as sexual advances. Sometimes touching and statements such as "How's my sweetheart?" or "Are you going to give me a big hug?" can be misinterpreted as invitations to become sexually intimate. Family members and caregivers need to understand that this is a normal feature of the illness. Rather than become upset or embarrassed, they need to learn to respond simply, for example, by taking the individual to a private area when masturbating or stating "I'm not a stranger, I'm Mary, your wife."

> **KEY CONCEPT**
> Unintentionally, caregivers can make comments to the cognitively impaired person that can be misinterpreted as flirtatious and trigger inappropriate sexual behaviors.

> ✔ **Point to Ponder**
> *What measures do you use to sustain old friendships and develop new ones?*

Facilitating Connections

Relationships are the essence of connections; unfortunately, relationships can be more challenging to create and sustain in late life. The circle of friends and family gradually diminishes with each passing year; health and economic limitations decrease one's participation in social activities; and preoccupation with health conditions of self and significant others narrows one's sphere of interests. The risks resulting in a shrinking of the elderly's social world are real and often significant; however, nurses can offer interventions that can minimize and compensate for them. Display 13-2 offers suggestions for helping older adults to maintain satisfying, healthy connections.

DISPLAY 13-2

Strategies to Facilitate Connections

- *Assist patients in evaluating current relationships.* Guide them in examining relationship patterns that are effective and those that could be improved. Discuss impact of relationships on health and quality of life.
- *Guide patients in becoming aware of their behaviors and responses that impact relationships.* Help them to gain insight into roles and dynamics and impact of responses.
- *Teach strategies that promote effective expression of inner feelings.* Offer suggestions and role plays that support feeling-based communication, such as making statements that reflect how they feel rather than impersonal generalities (eg, "I feel angry when you make my decisions for me"). Help patients to respect others' expressions of feelings.

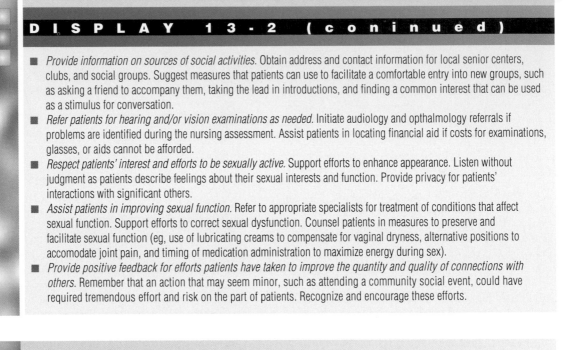

DISPLAY 13-2 (coninued)

■ *Provide information on sources of social activities.* Obtain address and contact information for local senior centers, clubs, and social groups. Suggest measures that patients can use to facilitate a comfortable entry into new groups, such as asking a friend to accompany them, taking the lead in introductions, and finding a common interest that can be used as a stimulus for conversation.

■ *Refer patients for hearing and/or vision examinations as needed.* Initiate audiology and opthalmology referrals if problems are identified during the nursing assessment. Assist patients in locating financial aid if costs for examinations, glasses, or aids cannot be afforded.

■ *Respect patients' interest and efforts to be sexually active.* Support efforts to enhance appearance. Listen without judgment as patients describe feelings about their sexual interests and function. Provide privacy for patients' interactions with significant others.

■ *Assist patients in improving sexual function.* Refer to appropriate specialists for treatment of conditions that affect sexual function. Support efforts to correct sexual dysfunction. Counsel patients in measures to preserve and facilitate sexual function (eg, use of lubricating creams to compensate for vaginal dryness, alternative positions to accomodate joint pain, and timing of medication administration to maximize energy during sex).

■ *Provide positive feedback for efforts patients have taken to improve the quantity and quality of connections with others.* Remember that an action that may seem minor, such as attending a community social event, could have required tremendous effort and risk on the part of patients. Recognize and encourage these efforts.

Critical Thinking Exercises

1. Describe features of public places (eg, malls, restaurants, and waiting rooms) that could interfere with communication with elderly individuals.
2. List the age-related changes that occur for men and women in the following sexual phases: excitement, plateau, orgasm, and resolution.
3. List at least six factors that can interfere with sexual function in late life.
4. What attitudes and actions of health care providers can have a negative effect on the sexuality of older adults? What can have a positive effect?

Web Connect

Learn more about erectile dysfunction by visiting the National Kidney and Urologic Disease Information Clearinghouse at www.niddk.nih.gov/health/urolog/pubs/impotnce/impotnce.htm.

● **Resources**

American Association of Sex Educators, Counselors, and Therapists
P.O. Box 238
Mount Vernon, IA 52314
www.aasect.org

Pride Senior Network
1756 Broadway
Suite 11H
New York, NY 10019
(212) 757-3203
www.pridesenior.org

Sexuality Information and Education Council of the United States
130 West 42nd Street
Suite 350
New York, NY 10036
(212) 819-9770
www.siecus.org

●References

Greenberg, S. A. (2001). Sexual health. In M. B. Mezey. *The encyclopedia of elder care. The comprehensive resource on geriatric and social care* (pp. 589–592). New York: Springer Publishing Company,

Kinsey, A. (1948). *Sexual behavior in the human male.* Philadelphia: Saunders.

Kubin, M., Wagner, G., Fugl-Meyer, A. R. (2003). Epidemiology of erectile dysfunction. *International Journal of Impotency Research, 15*(1), 63–71.

Masters, W., & Johnson, V. (1966). *Human sexual response.* Boston: Little Brown.

Masters, W., & Johnson, V. (1981). Sex and the aging process. *Journal of the American Geriatrics Society, 9,* 385.

Milgram, S. (1983). *Obedience to authority: An experimental view.* New York: Harper/Collins.

●Recommended Readings

Alford-Cooper, F. (1998). *For keeps: Marriages that last a lifetime.* Armonk, NY: Sharpe.

Barba, B. E., Tesh, A. S., & Courts, N. F. (2002). Promoting thriving in nursing homes: The Eden alternative. *Journal of Gerontological Nursing, 28*(3), 7–13.

Bauer, M. (1999). Their only privacy is between their sheets: Privacy and sexuality of elderly nursing home residents. *Journal of Gerontological Nursing, 25*(8), 37–41.

Berardicci, A., & Lenacher, C. A. (1998). Osteoporosis in perimenopausal women: Current perspectives. *American Journal for Nurse Practitioners, 2*(9), 9–14.

Berrin, S. (1997). *A heart of wisdom: Making the Jewish journey from midlife through the elder years.* Woodstock, VT: Jewish Lights Publishers.

Bitzan, J. E. (1998). Emotional bondedness and subjective well-being between nursing home roommates. *Journal of Gerontological Nursing, 24*(9), 8–15.

Bidikov, I., & Meier, D. E. (1997). Clinical decision-making with the woman after menopause. *Geriatrics, 52*(3), 28–35.

Borysenko, J. (1998). *A woman's book of life: The biology, psychology, and spirituality of the feminine life cycle.* New York: Riverhead Books.

Brumberg, E. (1997). *Ageless: What every woman needs to know to look and feel great.* New York: HarperCollins.

Carbone, D. J., & Seftel, A. D. (2002). Erectile dysfunction. *Geriatrics, 57*(9), 18–24

Cary, C. (1998). *A foxy old woman's guide to living with friends.* Freedom, CA: Crossing Press.

Conway, J. (1997). *Men in midlife crisis.* Colorado Springs, CO: Chariot Victor Publishers.

Cumming, D. C., & Cumming, C. E. (1998). Hormone replacement therapy: Part I: Should your patient do with—or without—it? *Consultant, 38,* 2417–2420, 2425–2427, 2431.

Cumming, D. C., & Cumming, C. E. (1998). Hormone replacement therapy: Part II: Should your patient do without it? *Consultant, 38,* 2435—2438, 2441–2442.

Dean, A. (1997). *Growing older, growing better: Daily meditations for celebrating aging.* Carlsbad, CA: Hay House.

Disch, R., & Dobrof, R. (1998). *Dignity and old age.* Binghamton, NY: Haworth Press.

Eli Lilly and Company. (1997). *Beyond menopause: Taking charge of your health.* Indianapolis, IN: Author.

Gershick, Z. Z. (1998). *Gay old girls.* Los Angeles: Alyson Publications.

Hendrix, C. C., & Sakauye, K. M. (2001). Teaching elderly individuals on computer use. *Journal of Gerontological Nursing, 27,* 47–53.

Hertz, J.E. and Anschutz, C.A. (2002). Relationships among perceived enactment of autonomy, self-care, and holistic health in community-dwelling older adults. *Journal of Holistic Nursing, 20,* 166–186.

Hicks, T. J. (2000). What is your life like now? Loneliness and elderly individuals residing in nursing homes. *Journal of Gerontological Nursing, 26*(8), 15–19.

Hill, J., Bird, B., & Thorpe, R. (2003). Effects of rheumatoid arthritis on sexual activity and relationships. *Rheumatology, 42*(2), 280–286.

Hillman, J. (1999). *The force of character and the lasting life.* New York: Random House.

Jarow, J. P., Kloner, R. A., & Holmes, A. M. (1998). *Viagra: How the miracle drug happened and what it can do for you* (pp. 8–9). New York: M. Evans.

Kaiger-Walker, K. (1997). *Positive aging: Every woman's quest for wisdom and beauty.* Berkeley, CA: Conari Press.

Kaiser, F. E. (2002). Disorders of sexual function. *Clinical Geriatrics, 10*(3), 38–46.

Kaiser, F. E. (1996). Sexuality in the elderly. *Urologic Clinics of North America, 23,* 99–109.

Kamel, H. K. (2001). Sexuality in aging: Focus on institutionalized elderly. *Annals of Long-Term Care, 9*(5), 64–72.

Klingman, L. (1999). Assessing the male genitalia. *American Journal of Nursing, 99*(7), 47–50.

Klingman, L. (1999). Assessing the female reproductive system. *American Journal of Nursing, 99*(8), 37–42.

Lee, G. (1997). *On the way to over the hill: A guide to aging gracefully.* Seattle, WA: Educare Press.

Mount Sinai School of Medicine. (1999). Postmenopausal? See your gynecologist anyway! *Focus on Healthy Aging, 2*(11), 1, 6.

Puentes, W. J. (2000). Using social reminiscence to teach therapeutic communication skills. *Geriatric Nursing, 21*(6), 311–317.

Redburn, D. E. (Ed.). (1998). *Social gerontology.* New York: Auburn House.

Rice, R. (1999). A little art in home care: Poetry and storytelling for the soul. *Geriatric Nursing, 20*(3), 165–166.

Smith, C. A., Neal, M., Penrod, J., Ryder, J., Dye, M., et al. Patterns of telephone use among nursing home residents. *Journal of Gerontological Nursing, 27*(5), 35–41.

Tremethick, M. J. (2001). Alone in a crowd: A study of social networks in home health and assisted living. *Journal of Gerontological Nursing, 27*(5), 42–47.

Voda, A. M. (1997). *Menopause, me and you: The sound of women pausing.* New York: Harrington Park Press.

Wallace, M. (2001). Sexuality: Try this. *Journal of Gerontological Nursing, 27*(2), 10–11.

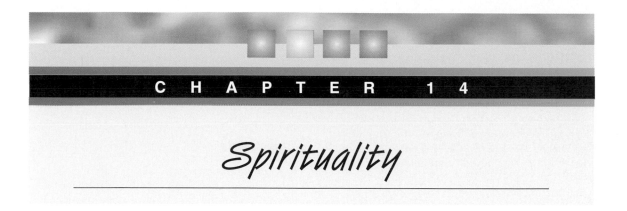

Spirituality

■ Learning Objectives

After reading this chapter, you should be able to:

- Describe basic spiritual needs
- List questions that could be used for spiritual assessment
- Discuss measures to support spiritual needs

*M*ost people are comforted with the knowledge that they have a connection with a power that is greater than themselves. A positive, harmonious relationship with God or other higher power (the Divine) helps individuals to feel unified with other people, nature, and the environment. It offers them love and a sense of having value, despite their imperfections or errors. Joy, hope, peace, and purpose are derived when people transcend beyond themselves. Suffering and hardship can have meaning and be faced with added strength.

Spirituality is the essence of our being that transcends and connects us to the Divine and other living organisms. It involves relationships and feelings. Spirituality differs from religion, which consists of human-created structures, rituals, symbolism, and rules for relating to the Divine. Religion is a significant expression of spirituality, but highly spiritual individuals may not identify with a specific religion.

KEY CONCEPT
Spirituality and religion are not synonymous.

Spiritual Needs

All humans have spiritual needs, regardless of whether or not they realize or acknowledge them. Some of these needs become particularly relevant in late life when the high prevalence of chronic illness and reality of death are evident; they can include love, purpose, hope, dignity, forgiveness, gratitude, transcendence, and faith.

LOVE

Love is probably the most important spiritual need of all. People need to feel that they are cared about and can offer caring feelings. Spiritual love is not a quid pro quo in which it is offered to obtain something. Rather, it is unconditional—offered unselfishly, completely. People need to feel loved regardless of their physical or mental condition, social position, material possessions, or productivity. In the Judeo-Christian tradition, this type of love is exemplified by the type God has for people.

MEANING AND PURPOSE

The final developmental task of aging that Erikson described (see Chap. 2) claims that the end result of healthy psychological aging is for the elder to achieve a sense of integrity. This integrity, or wholeness, is supported by the belief that life experiences—both good and bad—make sense and have served a purpose. Some individuals' faith may cause them to believe that suffering and sorrow have eternal purposes or allow God to be glorified. With this perspective, nothing is in vain and one's significance in the world is better understood.

HOPE

Hope is the expectation for something in the future. For some people, hope consists of the anticipation that opportunities for new adventures, pleasures, and relationships will unfold with each tomorrow. For others, hope propels them to face the future in the presence of pain and suffering, because they believe relief and eternal reward are possible.

DIGNITY

In Western society, self-worth often is judged by one's appearance, function, and productivity. Yet, every human being has intrinsic worth. When elders lack the attributes that command dignity for most of secular society, they can derive a sense of value and worth through their connection with God or higher power.

FORGIVENESS

It is human nature to err and sin. Carrying the burden of the wrongs committed by or to them is significantly stressful and can have a detrimental effect on their health. Furthermore, being unforgiving can rob people of the love and fulfillment derived through relationships. It is healing for people to forgive and accept forgiveness. For the elderly, forgiveness can facilitate the important process of putting things in order and achieving closure to unfinished business.

GRATITUDE

The abundance that is so prevalent in Western society sometimes causes much to be taken for granted. Rather than appreciate that they needn't go hungry or homeless, people complain that they haven't dined at certain restaurants or that their home lacks a pool. They focus on having large thighs rather than giving thanks that they are able to walk. Instead of being appreciative that their children are healthy, they are distressed that they are not the parents of an honor roll student. It is easy to fall into the trap of focusing on the negatives. However, an attitude of thankfulness nourishes the spirit and strengthens the ability to cope with any situation. At a time when losses may be many, elders may benefit from a guided review of the positive aspects of their lives. The life review process is a good approach to use in this effort (see Chap. 11).

TRANSCENDENCE

People need to feel that there is a reality beyond themselves, that they are connected to a greater power that surpasses logical thinking, and that they have a source to draw on that empowers them to achieve that which they cannot achieve independently. Transcendence affords people life beyond material existence and equips them to make sense of the difficult circumstances they face (Fig. 14-1).

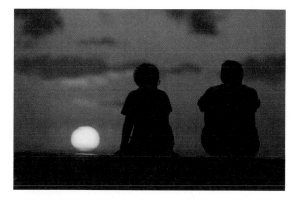

FIGURE 14-1

Transcendence helps people make sense of the difficult circumstances they face.

EXPRESSION OF FAITH

Religious beliefs and practices are encompassed in faith. These can include prayer, worship, scripture reading, rituals (eg, fasting on certain days or wearing special articles of clothing), and celebration of specific holy days. Disruption in the ability to express one's faith because of illness or disability can lead to spiritual distress. Likewise, spiritual distress can arise during illness from a person feeling resentful that God has seemingly abandoned him, guilty that the illness may be a means of punishment for sin, or regretful that he lacks a strong faith to support him through the situation.

> ✔ **Point to Ponder**
> *Which spiritual need is most difficult for you to fulfill? Why?*

Assessing Spiritual Needs

Asking about spiritual matters as part of the initial and ongoing assessment fosters holistic care. Although various clinical settings will have assessment tools preferred for use, elements of a spiritual assessment should address faith beliefs and practices, affiliation with faith community, and extent to which spiritual needs (eg, love, meaning, purpose, hope,

dignity, forgiveness, gratitude, transcendence, and expression of faith) are satisfied. The response to spiritual/religious preference on routine admission forms can give some indication of the patient's spirituality and provide a lead for a discussion of other issues pertaining to spirituality. Visible cues, such as the wearing of a religious article or presence of religious symbols, Bible, Koran, and inspirational books, can provide insights useful in spiritual assessment. A keen ear to comments (eg, "All I can do now is pray" or "I can't understand why God would allow this to happen") offers clues about spiritual needs. Depression, a flat affect, crying, and other observable signs can be a red flag for spiritual distress. Also, specific questions can explore spiritual needs. Display 14-1 outlines questions that could be used to assess a patient's spirituality.

Supporting Spiritual Needs

Evidence suggests that strong spiritual beliefs facilitate health and healing; therefore, it is therapeutically beneficial to support patients' spirituality and assist them in fulfilling spiritual needs. **(Visit the Connection website to learn about specific research findings.)** There are a variety of interventions nurses can use to assist patients, such as:

Identifying needs. Observations and responses to spiritual assessment questions can highlight specific spiritual needs and signs of spiritual distress (see Nursing Diagnosis Highlight). Strategies to address specific needs should be planned.

Being available. The closeness and trust that they feel toward nurses facilitate patients sharing deep feelings with nurses more than with other members of the health care team. Nurses need to honor this trust and be available for patients to express their feelings. This means being not only physically available but also fully present with patients when in their presence without being distracted or having thoughts on other activities. There may be times when nurses may not know how to respond to spiritual needs or hear expressions of beliefs that differ from their own; in these situations, attentive listening and encouraging communication remain important.

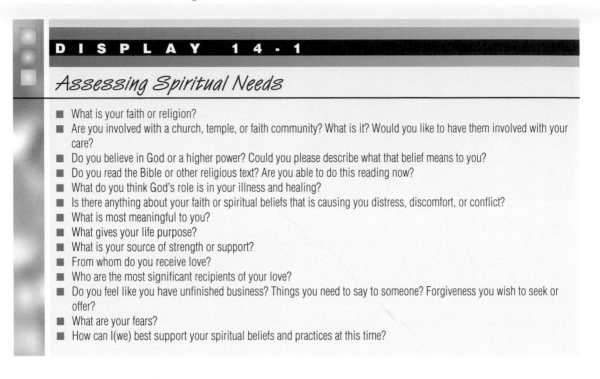

DISPLAY 14-1

Assessing Spiritual Needs

- What is your faith or religion?
- Are you involved with a church, temple, or faith community? What is it? Would you like to have them involved with your care?
- Do you believe in God or a higher power? Could you please describe what that belief means to you?
- Do you read the Bible or other religious text? Are you able to do this reading now?
- What do you think God's role is in your illness and healing?
- Is there anything about your faith or spiritual beliefs that is causing you distress, discomfort, or conflict?
- What is most meaningful to you?
- What gives your life purpose?
- What is your source of strength or support?
- From whom do you receive love?
- Who are the most significant recipients of your love?
- Do you feel like you have unfinished business? Things you need to say to someone? Forgiveness you wish to seek or offer?
- What are your fears?
- How can I(we) best support your spiritual beliefs and practices at this time?

Honoring beliefs and practices. A good spiritual assessment should reveal specific beliefs and practices that may need to be facilitated. These can include special diets, refusal to participate in certain care activities on one's Sabbath, wearing of specific articles of clothing, and prayer at specific times of the day (see Display 14-2).

✔ Point to Ponder

How much time do you build into your typical week for private time or solitude?

Providing opportunities for solitude. Solitude can be an important aspect of the expression of spirituality. Uninterrupted time allows personal communication with one's God or other higher power. One can offer prayers, reflect, meditate, and listen for answers from the divine source (Display 14-3). Periods of solitude must be respected and protected. **(Visit the Connection website for more information about Solitude.)**

 KEY CONCEPT
Choosing solitude differs from being socially isolated.

Promoting hope. Hope is important to human beings. When people believe in the future and that something positive is possible, they are likely to commit to goals and actions. For elders, especially those with serious health conditions or disabilities, maintaining hope can be challenging. The risk of feeling hopeless and depressed is real. Hopelessness can interfere with self-care and healing and drain energies that are needed to face life's challenges. Promoting hope begins with establishing a trusting relationship with the patient so that there will be comfort in expressing feelings openly. A careful assessment can assist in identifying factors that contribute to hopelessness, such as strained family relationships, unrelieved pain, and growing financial problems; interventions should be planned

D I S P L A Y   1 4 - 2

Religious Beliefs and Practices Relevant to Gerontological Nursing Practice

Protestant

■ *Assemblies of God (Pentecostal):* Encourage abstinence from tobacco, alcohol, and illegal drugs; believe in divine healing through prayer and laying on of hands; communion provided by clergy; believe in Jesus Christ as Savior

■ *Baptist:* Encourage abstinence from alcohol; communion provided by clergy; Scripture reading important as Bible viewed as word of God; believe in Jesus Christ as Savior (more than two dozen different groups in United States)

■ *Christian Church (Disciples of Christ):* Communion part of regular Sunday worship, provided by clergy; clergy and church elders can provide spiritual support; believe in Jesus Christ as Savior

■ *Church of the Brethren:* Clergy provides anointing of sick for physical healing and spiritual well-being; communion provided by clergy

■ *Church of the Nazarene:* Abstinence from tobacco and alcohol; believe in divine healing but accept medical treatment; communion provided by clergy

■ *Episcopal (Anglican):* Fasting not required, although some Episcopalians may abstain from meat on Fridays; communion provided by clergy; anointing of sick may be offered although not required; believe in Jesus Christ as Savior

■ *Lutheran:* Communion provided by clergy; anointing of sick by clergy; provide service of Commendation of the Dying; believe in Jesus Christ as Savior (10 different branches)

■ *Mennonite:* Abstain from alcohol; prayer has important role during crisis or illness, as well as anointing with oil; may oppose medications; women may desire to wear head covering during hospitalization; simple and plain lifestyle and dress style; communion provided twice a year with foot washing part of ceremony (12 different groups)

■ *Methodist:* Communion provided by clergy; anointing of sick; praying and reading Bible important during illness; organ donation encouraged; believe in Jesus Christ as Savior (more than 20 different groups)

■ *Presbyterian:* Communion provided by clergy; clergy or elders can provide prayer for the dying; believe in Jesus Christ as Savior (10 different groups)

■ *Quaker (Friends):* Believe God is personal and real, and that any believer can achieve communion with Jesus Christ without use of clergy or church rituals; no special death ceremony because of belief that present life is part of God's kingdom; abstain from alcohol; may oppose use of medications

■ *Salvation Army:* Follow Bible as foundation for faith; Scripture reading important; no special ceremonies; offers social welfare programs and centers; open to medical treatment; officer of local Army can be called for visitation and assistance

■ *Seventh-Day Adventist:* Healthy lifestyle practices are promoted as the body is seen as a temple of the Holy Spirit; alcohol, tobacco, coffee, tea, and recreational drugs are prohibited; pork and shellfish are avoided by most, and many are vegetarians; Sabbath is observed on Saturday; treatment may be opposed on Sabbath; communion provided by clergy; Bible reading important

Roman Catholic

Believe in Pope as head of the church on earth; express faith mainly in formulated creeds, such as Apostle's Creed; fasting during Lent and on Fridays optional, although older Catholics may adhere to practice; priest provides communion, Sacrament of the Sick, and hears confession; rosary beads, medals, statues, and other religious objects important

(Continued)

DISPLAY 14-2 (Continued)

Eastern Orthodox

Includes Greek, Serbian, Russian, and other orthodox churches; believe Holy Spirit proceeds from Father (rather than Father and Son), therefore, reject authority of Pope; fast from meat and dairy products on Wednesdays and Fridays during Lent and on other holy days; follow different calendar for religious celebrations; fast during Lent and before communion; holy unction administered to sick but not necessarily as last rites; last rites must be provided by ordained priest

Other Christian Religions

- *Christian Science:* Religion based on use of faith for healing; may decline drugs, psychotherapy, hypnotism, vaccination, and some treatments; use Christian Science nurses and other practitioners and may desire that they be active participants in care
- *Jehovah's Witnesses:* Discourage use of alcohol and tobacco; blood transfusions not accepted although alternative methods can be used
- *Mormons (Church of Jesus Christ of Latter Day Saints):* No professional clergy; communion and anointing of sick/laying on of hands can be provided by member of church priesthood; abstain from alcohol; discourage use of caffeine, alcohol, and other substances that are considered unhealthy and harmful; a sacred undergarment may be worn at all times that is only removed in absolute emergencies; prayer and reading sacred writings important; may oppose some medical treatments and use divine healing through laying on of hands
- *Unitarian:* Highly liberal branch of Christianity; belief in God as single being rather than doctrine of the Trinity; believe individuals are responsible for their own health state; advocate donation of body organs

Judaism

Believe in one universal God and that Jews were specially chosen to receive God's laws; observe Sabbath from sundown Friday to nightfall Saturday; three branches:

- *Orthodox (observant):* Strictly adhere to traditions of Judaism; believe in divinely inspired five Books of Moses (Torah); follow Kosher diet (not mixing of milk and meat at a meal, no pork or shellfish, no consumption of meat not slaughtered in accordance with Jewish law, use of separate cooking utensils for meat and milk products); strict restrictions during Sabbath (no riding in car, smoking, turning lights on/off, handling money, using telephone or television; medical treatments may be postponed until after Sabbath); men do not shave with razor but may use scissors or electric razor so that blade does not come in contact with skin, men wear skullcaps at all times; beard is considered sign of piety; Orthodox man will not touch any woman other than those in his family; married women cover hair; family and friends visit and may remain with dying person; witness needs to be present when person prays for health so that if death occurs family will be protected by God; after death body should not be left alone and only Orthodox person should touch or wash body; if death occurs on Sabbath, Orthodox persons cannot handle corpse but nursing staff can care for body wearing gloves; body must be buried within 24 hours; autopsy not allowed; any removed body parts must be returned for burial with the remaining body as they believe all parts of the body need to be returned to earth; prayer and quiet time important
- *Conservative:* Follow same basic laws as Orthodox; may only cover heads during worship and prayer; some may approve of autopsy
- *Reform:* Less stringent adherence to laws; do not strictly follow Kosher diet; do not wear skullcaps; attend temples on Fridays for worship but do not follow restrictions during Sabbath; men can touch women

(Continued)

D I S P L A Y   1 4 - 2   (C o n t i n u e d)

Islam (Muslim)

Second largest monotheistic (belief in one God) religion; founded by prophet Mohammed who was a human messenger or prophet used by God to communicate His word; Koran is scripture; Koran cannot be touched by anyone ritually unclean and nothing should be placed on Koran; may pray five times a day facing Mecca; privacy during prayer important; abstain from pork and alcohol; all permissible meat must be blessed and killed in special way; cleanliness important; at prayer time, washing is required, even by the sick; accept medical practices if these do not violate religious practices; women are very modest and not allowed to sign consent or make decisions without husband; may wear a *taviz* (black string with words of Koran attached); family or any practicing Muslim can pray with dying person; most Muslims prefer family to wash and prepare body of deceased (if necessary, nurses can care for deceased body wearing gloves); autopsy prohibited except when legally mandated; organ donation not allowed

Hinduism

Considered world's oldest religion; religion of most of India's residents; no scriptures, fixed doctrine, or common worship; belief in karma (every person born into position based on deeds of previous life) and reincarnation; illness may be viewed as sin from past life; mostly vegetarian; abstain from alcohol and tobacco

Buddhism

Offshoot of Hinduism with most followers in Japan, Thailand, and Myanmar; believe enlightenment found in individual meditation rather than communal worship; follow moral code known as Eightfold Path that leads to nirvana (form of liberation and enlightenment); vegetarian; abstain from alcohol and tobacco; may oppose medications and refuse treatments on holy days; private, uninterrupted time for meditation important

---

D I S P L A Y   1 4 - 3

Meditation

Solitude provides an opportunity for meditation, an activity that calms the mind and assists on focusing thoughts to the present. It can take the form of:

- *concentrative meditation*—attention is focused on breathing, a sound, or an image; this calms and promotes mental clarity and acuity
- *mindfulness meditation*—attention is paid to sensations being experienced, such as sounds or thoughts; this promotes a calm, nonreactive mental state
- *transcendental meditation*—introduced by Maharishi Mahesh Yogi, this form involves guiding the body to a level of profound relaxation while the mind becomes more alert;

Meditation has many health benefits, including stress reduction, stimulation of immune function, and pain control. Older adults may benefit from the improved self-esteem and higher levels of mental function that are allegedly achieved.

to address specific factors. Other beneficial actions include:

- assisting the patient in developing realistic short-term goals and acknowledging the achievement of goals
- guiding the patient in life review to highlight past successes in meeting life challenges that can be linked to current situations
- helping the patient to find pleasure and enjoyment in current life activities
- encouraging a relaxing, uplifting environment (eg, flowers, fresh air, sunlight, pleasant scents, pets, stimulating colors)
- facilitating the patient's spiritual practices; referring to clergy as needed
- assisting the patient in participating in religious services
- developing affirmations for the patient to use and recommending they be repeated daily
- suggesting that the patient maintain a personal journal to promote self-understanding and personal growth
- using music therapeutically; consulting with music therapist for selections that promote optimism and hope
- referring to a support group
- using humor therapeutically; conveying hope and optimism

> **KEY CONCEPT**
> Some people's faith can enable them to be comforted in believing that their current challenges serve a positive purpose for God.

Assisting in discovering meaning in challenging situations. Patients may question the purpose of the difficulties they face or believe that God has abandoned them. Persons of faith may want to discuss their perspective on how their current situation fits into a larger plan. An open, non-judgmental attitude when encouraging the expression of feelings can prove useful.

Arranging for religious needs to be met. Patients may have a desire for communion, confession, and other religious sacraments. Contact clergy as needed. Assist patients in wearing or displaying religious articles and ensure the safe care of these articles during nursing activities.

Praying with and for. People of faith have long understood the value of prayer and now growing research evidence supports the positive relationship between prayer and health and healing. One needn't be an ordained clergy to hold a patient's hand and offer a prayer. Prayers can be specific, for example, that the medication just administered will relieve the pain soon. The use of flowery or "religious" vocabulary is less important than having a heart to ask a higher power to intervene on the patient's behalf. Intercessory prayers can be offered for patients. Nurses who are not comfortable offering prayers themselves can ask coworkers to pray with and for their patients who so desire.

> ✔ **Point to Ponder**
> *What would it mean to you to have someone pray for your needs or struggles?*

People are spiritual beings; therefore, spiritual care must be an integral component of comprehensive, holistic care. Realizing their connection to something greater than themselves—other people, nature, the universe, and the Divine—empowers elders to rise above their physical, intellectual, emotional, and social challenges and discover the peace and harmony that facilitates healing and well-being. Self-worth and hope can be achieved, thereby imprinting the last segment of life with integrity and joy.

Web Connect

Visit www.beliefnet.com to get facts and updates on a range of religious and spiritual issues.

NURSING DIAGNOSIS HIGHLIGHT

SPIRITUAL DISTRESS

Overview

Spiritual distress is a state in which one's relationship to God or other higher power is disrupted or at risk of being disrupted and/or spiritual needs cannot be fulfilled. Illness or declining health of self or significant others, losses, awareness of mortality, and conflicts between beliefs and medical treatments are factors that could promote spiritual distress. Signs of spiritual distress could include anger, anxiety, complaints, crying, cynicism, depression, guilt, hopelessness, isolation, low self-esteem, powerlessness, refusal to make plans, sarcasm, suicidal thoughts or plans, and physical symptoms (fatigue, poor appetite, sleep disturbances, sighing). The person may question his or her faith and beliefs.

Causative or Contributing factors

Serious illness, losses, added burdens, inability to engage in religious practices, association of current health problems with past sinful behavior or lack or faith

Goal

The patient maintains religious practices to maximum degree possible; discusses issues pertaining to spiritual distress; develops support systems to promote spiritual well-being.

Interventions

- Assist patient in identifying factors contributing to spiritual distress.
- Support patient's religious practices: learn about patient's religious practices and implications for care; provide Bible, religious articles, and inspirational music; respect periods of solitude; respect and assist with practice of rituals; read scripture or arrange for volunteer to do so
- Pray with or for patient if this does not violate the patient's or your own faith
- Provide patient with privacy and time for prayer, meditation, and solitude
- Refer to clergy, native healer, support group, or other resources
- Contact patient's church or temple for visitation and follow-up (cg, via parish nurse); link patient with community health ministry if patient desires
- Respect patient's desire not to be visited by clergy or participate in religious activities
- Do not challenge patient's religious beliefs or attempt to change them

Critical Thinking Exercises

1. Why may spirituality become increasingly important to people as they age?
2. Describe the ways in which spiritual needs can be difficult for older adults to fulfill.
3. Consider the older adult who is a patient in a hospital or a resident of a long-term care facility. What opportunities exist for that person to have periods of solitude? What could be done to facilitate periods of solitude?
4. What questions could you ask an older adult to assess his or her spiritual beliefs and needs?
5. How can the mystery inherent in life events foster spirituality?

●Recommended Readings

Autry, J. A. (2002). *The spirit of retirement.Creating a life of meaning and personal growth.* New York: Prima Press.

Barnum, B. S. (2003). *Spirituality in nursing.* (2nd ed.). New York: Springer Publishing Company.

Berrin, S. (1997). *A heart of wisdom: Making the Jewish journey from midlife through the elder years.* Woodstock, VT: Jewish Lights Publishers.

Bitzan, J. E. (1998). Emotional bondedness and subjective well-being between nursing home roommates. *Journal of Gerontological Nursing, 24*(9), 8–15.

Conway, J. (1997). *Men in midlife crisis.* Colorado Springs, CO: Chariot Victor Publications.

Dean, A. (1997). *Growing older, growing better: Daily meditations for celebrating aging.* Carlsbad, CA: Hay House.

Disch, R., & Dobrof, R. (1998). *Dignity and old age.* Binghamton, NY: Haworth Press.

Dossey, L. (1997). *Prayer is good medicine.* New York: HarperCollins.

Hicks, T. J. (1999). Spirituality and the elderly: Nursing implications with nursing home residents. *Geriatric Nursing, 20*(3), 144–146.

Hillman, J. (1999). *The force of character and the lasting life.* New York: Random House.

Kimble, M. A., McFadden, S. H., Ellor, J. W., & Seeber, J. J. (Eds.). (1995). *Aging, spirituality, and religion.* Minneapolis: Fortress Press.

Kirkland, K. H., & McIlveen, H. (1999). *Full circle: Spiritual therapy for the elderly.* Binghamton, NY: Haworth Press.

Koenig, H. G. (1994). *Aging and God. Spiritual pathways to mental health in midlife and later years.* New York: Haworth Pastoral Press.

Koenig, H. G. (2002) *Purpose and power in retirement.* New York: Templeton Foundation.

Larson, D. B., Sawyers, J. P., & McCullough, M. E. (Eds.) (1998). *Scientific research on spirituality and health: A consensus report.* Rockville, MD: National Institute for Healthcare Research.

Leder, D. (1997). *Spiritual passages: Embracing life's sacred journey.* New York: Jeremy P. Tarcher/Putnam.

Lowry, L. E., & Conco, D. (2002). Exploring the meaing of spirituality with aging adults in Appalachia. *Journal for Holistic Nursing, 20*(4), 388–402.

Matthews, D. A., & Larson, D. B. (1995). *The faith factor: An annotated bibliography of clinical research on spiritual subjects* (Vol. III). Rockville, MD: National Institute for Health Care Research.

Myss, C. (1996). *Anatomy of the spirit.* New York: Three Rivers Press.

Pargament, K. I. (1997). *The psychology of religion and coping.* New York: Guilford Press.

Shelly, J. A., & Miller, A. B. (1999). *Called to care. A Christian theology of nursing.* Downers Grove, IL: InterVarsity Press.

Redburn, D. E. (Ed.). (1998). *Social gerontology.* New York: Auburn House.

Rice, R. (1999). A little art in home care: Poetry and storytelling for the soul. *Geriatric Nursing, 20*(3), 165–166.

Rybarczyk, B., & Bellg, A. (1997). *Listening to life stories.* New York: Springer.

Schweitzer, R., Norberg, M., & Larson, L. (2002). The parish nurse coordinator: A bridge to spiritual health care leadership for the future. *Journal of Holistic Nursing, 20,* 212–231.

Stanley, C. (1997). *The blessings of brokenness.* Grand Rapids, MI: Zondervan Publishing House.

Thomas, E. L., & Eisenhandler, S. A. (1999). *Religion, belief, and spirituality in late life.* New York: Springer.

VandeCreek, L. (1998). *Scientific and pastoral perspectives on intercessory prayer.* New York: Harrington Park Press.

Wallace, S. (2000). Rx RN: A spiritual approach to aging. *Alternative and Complementary therapies, 6*(1), 47–48.

Weaver, A. J., Flannelly, L. T., & Flannelly, K. J. (2001). Review of research on religious and spiritual variables in two primary gerontological nursing journals: 1991 to 1997. *Journal of Gerontological Nursing, 27*(9), 47–54.

Weaver, A. J., & Koenig, H. G. (1998). *Reflections on aging and spiritual growth.* Nashville, TN: Abingdon Press.

Wicks, R. J. (1997). *After 50: Spiritually embracing your own wisdom years.* New York: Paulist Press.

Wilt, D. L., & Smucker, C. J. (2001). *Nursing the spirit.* Washington, DC: American Nurses Publishing.

Wimberly, A. S. (1997). *Honoring African American elders: A ministry in the soul community.* San Francisco: Jossey-Bass.

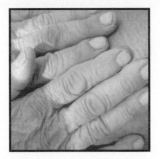

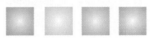

Facilitating Physiological Balance

Respiration and Circulation

■ Learning Objectives

After reading this chapter, you should be able to:

- list factors that can alter tissue perfusion
- describe nursing measures that could improve circulation
- describe measures to reduce the risk of respiratory infection and other respiratory complications

The exchange of carbon dioxide with oxygen in the lungs (ie, respiration) and in all blood-carrying vessels throughout the body (ie, circula-tion) is essential to life. These acts, of which we are seldom conscious in daily life, can become major foci of attention in later years because of the impact of age-related changes (Nursing Diagnosis Table 15-1). It is crucial that actions be planned to prevent and address some of the potential nursing problems related to ventilation and circulation.

Tissue Health

Good tissue health depends on adequate tissue perfusion (ie, circulation to and from a body part). To ensure good tissue perfusion, arterial blood pressure must be maintained within a normal range. Factors that can alter tissue perfusion include:

- cardiovascular disease: arteriosclerotic heart disease, hypertension, congestive heart failure, varicosities
- other diseases: diabetes mellitus, cancer, renal failure
- blood dyscrasias: anemia, thrombus, transfusion reactions
- hypotension: arising from anaphylactic shock, hypovolemia, hypoglycemia, hyperglycemia, orthostatic hypotension
- medication side effects: antihypertensives, vasodilators, diuretics, antipsychotics
- other conditions: edema, inflammation, prolonged immobility, hypothermia, malnutrition

The adequacy of tissue circulation should be assessed in older adults by reviewing the individual's health history, evaluating vital signs, inspecting the tissues, and noting signs or symptoms. Display 15-1 lists indications of ineffective tissue perfusion.

ND *Nursing Diagnosis*

TABLE 15-1 ● Aging and Risks to Adequate Respiration and Circulation

Causes or Contributing Factors	Nursing Diagnosis
Respiration	
Reduced elastic recoil of lungs during expiration	Impaired Gas Exchange
	Ineffective Breathing Pattern
Increase in residual capacity	Ineffective Breathing Pattern
Decrease in vital capacity	Risk for Infection
Decrease in maximum breathing capacity	Ineffective Airway Clearance
Hyperinflation of lung apices and underinflation of lung bases	Impaired Gas Exchange
Reduced number and elasticity of alveoli	Activity Intolerance due to decreased respiratory efficiency
Calcification of tracheal and laryngeal cartilage	Ineffective Airway Clearance
Reduced ciliary activity	Risk for Infection
Increased diameter of bronchioles and alveolar ducts	
Loss of skeletal muscle strength in thorax and diaphragm	
Increased rigidity of thoracic muscles and ribs	
Increased diameter of anteroposterior chest	
Less efficient cough response	
Circulation	
Decreased elasticity of blood vessels	Ineffective Tissue Perfusion
Increased resistance of peripheral vessels	
Decreased coronary blood flow	
Less efficient cardiac oxygen usage	Activity Intolerance
Reduced proportion of oxygen extracted from arterial blood by tissues	Ineffective Tissue Perfusion
	Impaired Gas Exchange
Reduced cardiovascular responsiveness to adrenergic stimulation	Ineffective Tissue Perfusion
	Activity Intolerance

DISPLAY 15-1

Indications of Ineffective Tissue Perfusion

Hypotension	Pallor, coolness of skin
Tachycardia, decreased pulse quality	Cyanosis
Claudication	Decreased urinary output
Edema	Delirium (altered cognition and level of consciousness)
Loss of hair on extremities	
Tissue necrosis, stasis ulcers	Restlessness
Dyspnea, increased respirations	Memory disturbance

Because the elderly possess age-related changes and a high prevalence of health conditions that heighten their risk of altered tissue perfusion, gerontological nurses should promote interventions that improve tissue circulation to:

* ensure that blood pressure is maintained within an acceptable range (usually under 140 mm Hg systolic and 90 mm Hg diastolic)
* prevent and eliminate sources of pressure on the body
* remind or assist patients to change positions frequently
* prevent pooling of blood in the extremities
* encourage physical activity
* prevent hypothermia, maintain body warmth (particularly of the extremities)
* massage the body unless contraindicated (eg, in the presence of deep vein thrombosis and pressure ulcer)
* monitor drugs for the side effect of hypotension
* educate to reduce risks (eg, avoiding excess alcohol ingestion, cigarette smoking, obesity, inactivity)
* periodically evaluate physical and mental health to identify signs and symptoms of altered tissue perfusion.

> **KEY CONCEPT**
> In addition to traditional aerobic, strengthening, and balance exercises, yoga and t'ai chi are good ways to enhance circulation and respiration.

Tips on the prevention of pressure ulcers can be found in Chapter 31, which offers guidance in keeping skin healthy and intact. An often overlooked measure to promote tissue circulation is the maintenance of an adequate blood pressure level. Hypotension can reduce cerebral circulation and subsequently decrease the amount of oxygenation of that tissue; this is an important consideration for the elderly taking antihypertensive drugs.

Effective Breathing

To ensure adequate ventilation, respiratory infection must be prevented. In addition to the precautions any adult would take, older persons need to be particularly attentive to obtaining influenza and pneumonia vaccines and avoiding exposure to individuals who have respiratory infections. The susceptibility of older people to drafts necessitates that indirect room ventilation be used—fibrosis, which is common in the elderly, can be aggravated by chilling and drafts. The elderly should be advised to seek medical attention promptly if any sign of a respiratory infection develops. Frequently, older people do not experience the chest pain associated with pneumonia to the same degree younger adults do, and their normally lower body temperature can cause an atypical appearance of fever (ie, at lower levels than would occur for younger persons). Thus, by the time symptoms are visible to others, pneumonia can be in an advanced stage. The elderly should be taught to report changes in the character of sputum, which could be associated with certain disease processes. For example, the sputum is tenacious, translucent, and grayish white with chronic obstructive pulmonary disease; it is purulent and foul smelling with a lung abscess or bronchiectasis; and it is red and frothy with pulmonary edema and left-sided heart failure.

Approximately 80% of the elderly population have some degree of chronic obstructive pulmonary disease; people with this disorder tend to retain a higher amount of carbon dioxide in their lungs. Nurses should teach deep-breathing exercises to all older persons and encourage that they be done regularly (Fig. 15-1). To aid in making these exercises a daily routine, they can be linked to other routines, for example, before meals or every time the person sits down to watch the news. Yoga is another practice that can aid respiration and circulation.

> **KEY CONCEPT**
> To help make respiratory exercises a daily routine, combine them with other routines.

Carbon dioxide retention increases the risk of developing the serious complication of carbon dioxide narcosis during the administration of oxygen therapy. Oxygen should be used prudently with the elderly; blood gases should be monitored and the patient should be observed for symptoms of carbon dioxide narcosis. These include confusion, muscle twitching,

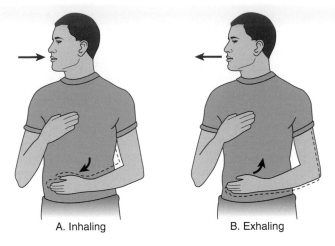

A. Inhaling   B. Exhaling

FIGURE 15-1

Breathing exercises should emphasize forced expiration. (**A**) With one hand on the stomach (below the ribs) and the other over the middle anterior chest, the patient should inhale to the count of one. The hand over the stomach should move outwardly as the diaphragm and stomach move downward; the hand over the chest should not move. (**B**) Expire air to the count of three. The hand over the stomach should be pulled closer to the body as the diaphragm and stomach move upward; the hand over the chest should not move.

visual defects, profuse perspiration, hypotension, progressive degrees of circulatory failure, and cerebral depression, which may be displayed as increased sleeping or a deep comatose state.

> ✔ **Point to Ponder**
>
> *Take a few minutes to do deep-breathing exercises with your eyes closed. What effects did this have on your body, mind, and spirit? How could these exercises benefit you if you did them several times throughout the day?*

Although it may appear to be a relatively minor consideration, hair in the nostrils becomes thicker with age and may readily accumulate a greater amount of dust and dirt particles during inspiration. Unless these particles are removed and the nasal passage is kept patent, there may be an interference with the normal inspiration of air. Blowing the nose and mild manipulation with a tissue may adequately rid the nostrils of these particles. When particles are difficult to remove, a cotton-tipped applicator moistened with warm water or saline solution may help loosen them. Caution should be taken not to insert the cotton-tipped applicator too far into the nose because trauma can easily result. Any nasal obstruction not easily removed should be brought to a physician's attention. Some considerations for promoting effective breathing can be found in the Nursing Diagnosis Highlight.

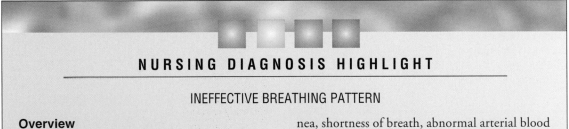

NURSING DIAGNOSIS HIGHLIGHT

INEFFECTIVE BREATHING PATTERN

Overview

In late life there is a high prevalence of conditions that limit the ability to adequately inflate the lungs or rid them of sufficient amounts of carbon dioxide. Signs such as confusion, dyspnea, shortness of breath, abnormal arterial blood gases, cyanosis, pursed-lip breathing, retraction of respiratory muscles during breathing, and shallow respirations could be associated with this diagnosis.

Causative or contributing factors

Weakness, fatigue, pain, paralysis, immobility, altered mental status, respiratory or musculoskeletal disease

Goal

The patient displays an effective breathing pattern, is free from signs of ineffective breathing, and possesses normal arterial blood gases.

Interventions

- Instruct patient in breathing exercises (Fig. 15-1).
- Control symptoms (eg, pain) that could threaten effective respirations.
- Raise head of bed at least 30° when patient is lying down, unless contraindicated.
- Instruct patient to turn, cough, and deep breathe at least once every 2 hours.
- Monitor rate, depth, and rhythm of respirations; coloring; coughing pattern; blood gases; and mental status.

Critical Thinking Exercises

1. What are some practical hints that can be given to older adults to improve circulation?
2. What is the rationale for the coordination of stomach movements with inhalation and expiration? For the 1:3 ratio of inspiration to expirations?
3. Describe the advantages of educating older adults to detect their own symptoms of health problems.

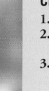 *Web Connect*

Search "Breathing Exercises" on the Internet. Visit some of the sites listed and compare the different types of breathing exercises described.

● **Recommended Readings**

Barker, W. H., Borisute, H., & Cox, C. (1998). A study of the impact of influenza on the functional status of frail older people. *Archives of Internal Medicine, 158,* 645–650.

Blazer, D. G., Landerman, L. R., Hays, J. C., Grady, T. A., Havlik, R., & Corti, M. C. (2001). Blood pressure and mortality risk in older people: Comparison between African Americans and whites. *Journal of the American Geriatrics Society, 49*(3), 375–381.

Chen, K. M., & Snyder, M. (1999). A research-based use of tai chi/movement therapy as a nursing intervention. *Journal of Holistic Nursing, 17*(3), 267–278.

Garcia-Palmieri, M. (2001). Cardiovascular disease prevention in the elderly. *Clinical Geriatrics, 9*(13), 69–77.

Lai, J. S., et al. (1995). Two-year trends in cardiorespiratory function among older tai chi chuan practitioners and sedentary subjects. *Journal of the American Geriatrics Society, 43*(9), 1222–1227.

McBride, S., Graydon, J., Sidani, S., & Hall, L. (1999). The therapeutic use of music for dyspnea and anxiety in patients with COPD who live at home. *Journal of Holistic Nursing, 17*(3), 227–228.

Monahan, K. (1999). A joint effort to affect lives: The COPD wellness program. *Geriatric Nursing, 20*(5), 200–202.

Narsavage, G. L. Cardiovascular health for older adults. *Journal of Gerontological Nursing, 26*(5), 5–6.

Regan, S. F., & Fowler, C. (2002). Influenza: Past, present, and future. *Journal of Gerontological Nursing, 28*(11), 30–37.

Robinson, A. W., & Sloan, H. L. (2000). Heart health and older women. *Journal of Gerontological Nursing, 26*(5), 38–45.

Rosenberg, H., & Resnick, B. (2003). Exercise intervention in patients with chronic obstructive pulmonary disease. *Geriatric Nursing, 24*(2), 90–98.

Sheahan, S. L., & Musialowski, R. (2001). Clinical implications of respiratory system changes in aging. *Journal of Gerontological Nursing, 27*(5), 26–34.

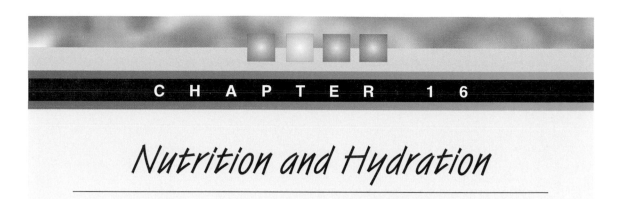

Nutrition and Hydration

■ Learning Objectives

After reading this chapter, you should be
able to:

- list age-related factors that affect
  dietary requirements in late life
- list the special nutritional needs of
  aging women
- identify causative factors and signs of
  dehydration
- describe oral health problems that
  could influence nutritional status and
  recommended oral hygiene for older
  adults
- identify risks associated with the use of
  nutritional supplements
- outline threats to good nutrition in late
  life and ways to minimize them

*T*he impact of nutrition on health and functional capacity is profound. The ability to defend the body against disease, maintain anatomic and structural normality, think clearly, and possess the energy and desire to engage in social activity is influenced by one's nutritional status. Numerous age-related changes, which are often subtle and gradual, can progressively jeopardize the ability of the elderly to maintain good nutritional status; these changes demand special nursing attention (Nursing Diagnosis Table 16-1).

Nutritional Needs of Elders

Although the body's needs for basic nutrients are consistent throughout life, the required amount of specific nutrients may vary. One of the most signifi-

ND *Nursing Diagnosis*
TABLE 16-1 ● *Aging and Risks to Nutritional Status*

Causes or Contributing Factors	Nursing Diagnosis
Teeth have various degrees of erosion; abrasions of crown and root structure; high prevalence of tooth loss	Imbalanced Nutrition: Less Than Body Requirements related to limited ability to chew foods
	Pain related to poor condition of teeth
Reduction in saliva to approximately one-third the volume of earlier years	Imbalanced Nutrition: Less Than Body Requirements related to less efficient mixing of foods
Inefficient digestion of starch due to decreased salivary ptyalin	Imbalanced Nutrition: Less Than Body Requirements related to reduced breakdown of starches
Atrophy of epithelial covering in oral mucosa	Impaired Oral Mucous Membrane
Increased taste threshold; approximately one-third the number of functioning taste buds per papilla of earlier years	Disturbed Sensory Perception: gustatory
	Imbalanced Nutrition: More Than Body Requirements related to excessive intake of salts and sweets to compensate for taste alterations
Decreased thirst sensations; reduced hunger contractions	Imbalanced Nutrition: Less Than Body Requirements related to reduced ability to sense hunger sensations
	Deficient Fluid Volume related to decreased thirst
Weaker gag reflex; decreased esophageal peristalsis; relaxation of lower esophageal sphincter; reduced stomach motility	Risk for Injury from aspiration
	Imbalanced Nutrition: Less Than Body Requirements related to self-imposed restrictions to avoid discomfort
Less hydrochloric acid, pepsin, and pancreatic acid produced	Imbalanced Nutrition: Less Than Body Requirements related to ineffective breakdown of food
Lower fat tolerance	Pain related to indigestion
Decreased colonic peristalsis: reduced sensation for signal to defecate	Imbalanced Nutrition: Less Than Body Requirements related to reduced appetite and self-imposed restrictions related to constipation
Less efficient cholesterol stabilization and absorption	Risk for Infection related to risk of gallstone formation
Increased fat content of pancreas; decreased pancreatic enzymes	Imbalanced Nutrition: Less Than Body Requirements related to problems in normal digestion

cant differences in nutrient requirements among people of different ages involves caloric intake. Several factors contribute to the elderly's reduced need for calories:

- The older body has less body mass and a relative increase in adipose tissue. Adipose tissue metabolizes more slowly than lean tissue and does not burn calories as quickly.
- Basal metabolic rate declines 2% for each decade of life, which contributes to weight increasing with the same caloric intake as consumed in younger years.
- The activity level for most older adults is usually lower than it was during their younger years.

Although the nutritional needs of older adults are best determined on an individual basis, some generalizations can be made (Fig. 16-1). Quantity and quality of caloric intake must be monitored. One useful way to determine resting caloric needs that considers age, among other factors, is the Harris-Benedict equation, also called the Resting Energy Expenditure:

Males
$$66 + [13.7 \times weight~(kg)] + [5 \times height~(cm)] - [6.8 \times age] = kcal/day$$

Females
$$655 + [9.7 \times weight~(kg)] + [1.8 \times height~(cm)] - [4.7 \times age] = kcal/day$$

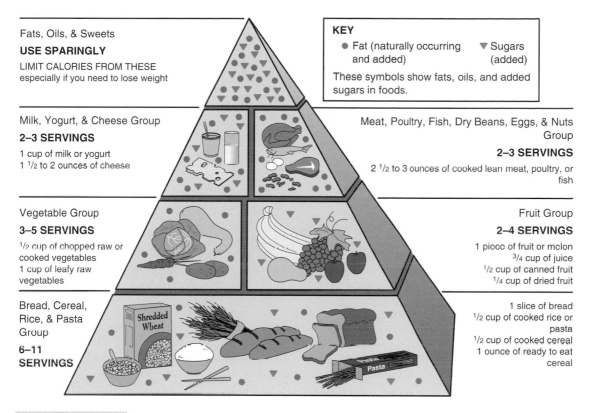

Fats, Oils, & Sweets
USE SPARINGLY
LIMIT CALORIES FROM THESE
especially if you need to lose weight

KEY
● Fat (naturally occurring and added)   ▼ Sugars (added)
These symbols show fats, oils, and added sugars in foods.

Milk, Yogurt, & Cheese Group
2–3 SERVINGS
1 cup of milk or yogurt
1 ½ to 2 ounces of cheese

Meat, Poultry, Fish, Dry Beans, Eggs, & Nuts Group
2–3 SERVINGS
2 ½ to 3 ounces of cooked lean meat, poultry, or fish

Vegetable Group
3–5 SERVINGS
½ cup of chopped raw or cooked vegetables
1 cup of leafy raw vegetables

Fruit Group
2–4 SERVINGS
1 piece of fruit or melon
¾ cup of juice
½ cup of canned fruit
¼ cup of dried fruit

Bread, Cereal, Rice, & Pasta Group
6–11 SERVINGS

Shredded Wheat

Pasta

1 slice of bread
½ cup of cooked rice or pasta
½ cup of cooked cereal
1 ounce of ready to eat cereal

FIGURE 16-1

The Food Guide Pyramid (serving sizes depicted in boxes).

The diet of the elderly should contain high-quality calories (Fig. 16-2). Carbohydrates provide important sources of energy and fiber. Soluble fibers help to lower serum cholesterol and improve glucose tolerance in diabetics; oats and pectin contain soluble fibers. Insoluble fibers promote good bowel activity and can be found in grains and many vegetables and fruits. Limiting dietary fat intake to less than 30% of total calories consumed is a good practice for older adults. The decreased ability of the older person to maintain a regular blood glucose level emphasizes the need for a reduced carbohydrate intake. A high-carbohydrate diet can stimulate an abnormally high release of insulin in the elderly. This can cause hypoglycemia, which can first present in the elderly as a confused state. At least 1 g protein per kilogram of body weight is necessary to renew body protein

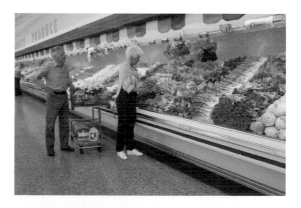

FIGURE 16-2

Although they usually need to ingest fewer calories than younger persons, older adults' diets must include a high quality of nutrients.

and protoplasm and to maintain enzyme systems. If 15% of daily caloric intake is derived from protein, protein requirements should be met. Several protein supplements are available commercially and may be useful additives to the older person's diet. Although the ability to absorb calcium decreases with age, calcium is still required in the diet to maintain a healthy musculoskeletal system, as well as to promote the proper functioning of the body's blood-clotting mechanisms.

It is recommended that older adults eat at least five servings of fruits and vegetables daily. Unfortunately, only about one third of the elderly consume the recommended amounts (Walker, 2003). It might be useful for the nurse to discuss the importance of consuming adequate fruits and vegetables and suggestions on the variety of ways that they can be consumed (eg, smoothies or mixed in yogurt or gelatin).

The use of calcium supplements may benefit older persons but first should be discussed with the physician to ensure that other medical problems do not contraindicate them. In addition, caution is needed to ensure that excess calcium consumption does not occur—a possibility with the increasing number of calcium-fortified products available. Patients should be advised to check labels and total the amount of calcium they're getting from various sources. Excess calcium consumption (ie, in excess of 2000 mg/day) can lead to such problems as kidney stones. If calcium supplements are used, it is best that no more than 500 mg are taken at any one time because larger amounts are not absorbed as well. Consideration also must be given to the food with which calcium supplements are taken, because wheat bran, soybeans, and other legumes can interfere with the calcium absorption. A good intake of vitamin D and magnesium facilitates calcium absorption.

Each person will have a unique caloric need based on individual body size, metabolism, health status, and activity level. Because caloric requirements and intake are often reduced in later life, the ingested calories need to be of higher quality to ensure an adequate intake of other nutrients. Table 16-1 lists the recommended daily allowances (RDAs) for older adults.

Researchers at Tufts University have offered a modification to the U.S. Department of Agriculture's Food Guide Pyramid to more accurately reflect the dietary needs of persons over age 70 (Davis, Britten, & Myers, 2001; Tufts University, 1999). They have added a base layer to the pyramid for water, advising

TABLE 16-1 ● *Recommended Dietary Allowances for People over 50 Years of Age*

	Men	Women
Protein (g)	56	44
Vitamin A (mg)	1000	800
Vitamin D (μg)	15	15
Vitamin E (IU)	12	12
Vitamin C (mg)	90	75
Thiamin (mg)	1.2	1
Riboflavin (mg)	1.4	1.2
Niacin (mg)	16	14
Vitamin B6 (mg)	1.7	1.5
Folate (mg)	400	400
Vitamin B12 (mg)	3	3
Calcium (mg)	1200	1200
Phosphorus (mg)	700	700
Magnesium (mg)	420	320
Iron (mg)	10	10
Zinc (mg)	12	12
Iodine (μg)	150	150
Potassium (gm)	2	2
Selenium (μg)	55	55

(Recommended dietary needs of mature Americans. National Dairy Council Digest, www.nationaldairycouncil.org/lvl04/nutrilib/digest/dairydigest_694.htm, 2003).

that older adults drink at least 8 glasses of fluids daily. A flag has been added to the top to represent the need for dietary supplements, particularly calcium, vitamin D, and vitamin B_{12}, which have decreased absorption with age. To ensure sufficient essential nutrients in light of reduced calorie intake, "nutrient-dense" choices in each food category are outlined, emphasizing whole grains, varied colored fruits and vegetables, low-fat dairy products, and lean meats, fish, and poultry. This modified Food Guide Pyramid for people over age 70 has merit and may affect changes in future models of the Food Guide Pyramid.

✔ **Point to Ponder**

How do you see your diet affecting your body, mind, and spirit and vice versa? Are there patterns that need to be changed, and, if so, how?

Special Needs of Women

Heart disease, cancer, and osteoporosis are among the nutrition-related conditions to which older women are susceptible. Attention to dietary requirements and reduction of diet-related risks can reduce some of these problems.

From 64 to 74 years of age, the rate of heart disease among women equals that of men. The reduction of fat intake to 30% kilocalories or less (70 g in an 1800-calorie diet) can be beneficial in reducing the risk of heart disease in older women. Research is attempting to disclose the role of low fat intake and reduced risk of breast cancer, which could support another benefit to limiting fat intake. Alcohol consumption also has a role in breast cancer; the daily intake of 40 g or more of alcohol has been linked to an increased risk of breast cancer (40 g of alcohol equals 30 oz of beer or 3 oz of 100 proof whiskey). Thus, reducing alcohol intake is advisable.

Nearly all women are affected by some degree of osteoporosis by the time they reach their seventh decade of life. The risk of bone loss is increased by estrogen reduction, obesity, inactivity, smoking, and the excessive consumption of caffeine and alcohol. The risk of fracture from brittle bones and the complications that follow warrant consideration to prevent bone loss by controlling risks. Postmenopausal women should have a daily calcium intake of at least 1000 mg.

A wide range of physical, mental, and socioeconomic factors affect nutritional status in later life. Because these factors can change, regular nutritional assessment is necessary. Effective nutritional assessment involves collaboration among physician, nurse, nutritionist, and social worker. Display 16-1 describes the basic components of the nutritional assessment.

KEY CONCEPT
Nutritional status is affected by a variety of physical, psychological, and socioeconomic factors.

Hydration

With age, intracellular fluid is lost, resulting in decreased total body fluids. Whereas water comprises approximately 60% of body weight in younger adults, it constitutes 50% or less of body weight in older adults. This reduces the margin of safety for any fluid loss; a reduced fluid intake or increased loss that would be only a minor problem in younger persons could be life-threatening to the elderly. Special measures must be taken to ensure a minimum fluid intake of 1500 mL daily. The elderly should be evaluated for factors that can cause them to consume less fluid, such as:

- age-related reductions in thirst sensations
- fear of incontinence (physical condition and lack of toileting opportunities)
- lack of accessible fluids
- inability to obtain or drink fluids independently
- lack of motivation
- altered mood or cognition
- nausea, vomiting, gastrointestinal distress

When such factors are present or there is any suspicion regarding the adequacy of fluid intake, fluid intake and output should be recorded and monitored. (See the Nursing Diagnosis Highlight at the end of the chapter.)

Fluid restriction not only predisposes the elderly to infection, constipation, and decreased bladder distensibility, but it also can lead to serious fluid and electrolyte imbalances. Dehydration, a life-threatening condition to older persons because of their already reduced amount of body fluid, is demonstrated by dry, inelastic skin; dry, brown tongue; sunken cheeks; concentrated urine; blood urea value elevated above 60 mg/dL; and, in some cases, confusion. At the other extreme, the elderly are also more sensitive to overhydration caused by decreased cardiovascular and renal function. Overhydration is a consideration if intravenous fluids are needed therapeutically.

KEY CONCEPT
The age-related decline in body fluids reduces the margin of safety when insufficient fluid is consumed or extra fluid is lost.

Oral Health

Painless, intact gums and teeth will promote the ingestion of a wider variety of food. The ability to meet nutritional requirements in old age is influenced by

DISPLAY 16-1

Components of the Nutritional Assessment

History

■ Review health history and medical record for evidence of diagnoses or conditions that can alter the purchase, preparation, ingestion, digestion, absorption, or excretion of foods.

■ Review medications for those that can affect appetite and nutritional state.

■ Patient's description of diet, meal pattern, food preferences, and restrictions.

■ Diary of all food intake for a week.

Physical Examination

Inspect hair. Hair loss or brittleness can be associated with malnutrition

Inspect skin. Note persistent "goose bumps" (vitamin-B6 deficiency), pallor (anemia), purpura (vitamin-C deficiency), brownish pigmentation (niacin deficiency), red scaly areas in folds around eyes and between nose and corner of mouth (riboflavin deficiency), dermatitis (zinc deficiency), fungus infections (hyperglycemia).

Test skin turgor. Skin turgor, although poor in many older adults, tends to be best in the areas over the forehead and sternum; therefore, these are preferred areas to test.

Note muscle tone, strength, and movement. Muscle weakness can be associated with vitamin and mineral deficiencies.

Inspect eyes. Ask about changes in vision, night vision problems (vitamin-A deficiency). Note the patient's percentile rank

Inspect oral cavity. Note dryness (dehydration), lesions, condition of tongue, breath odor, condition of teeth or dentures.

Ask about signs and symptoms: sore tongue, indigestion, diarrhea, constipation, food distaste, weakness, muscle cramps, burning sensations, dizziness, drowsiness, bone pain, sore joints, recurrent boils, dyspnea, dysphagia, anorexia, appetite changes.

Observe person drinking or eating for difficulties.

Biochemical Evaluation

Obtain blood sample for screening of total iron binding capacity, transferrin saturation, protein, albumin, hemoglobin, hematocrit, electrolytes, vitamins, prothrombin time.

Obtain urine sample for screening of specific gravity.

Cognition and Mood

Test cognitive function.

Note alterations in mood, behavior, cognition, level of consciousness. Be alert to signs of depression (can be associated with deficiencies of vitamin B6, magnesium, or niacin).

Ask about changes in mood or cognition.

Anthropometric Measurement

Measure and ask about changes in height and weight. Use age-adjusted weight chart for evaluating weight. Note weight losses of 5% within the past 1 month and 10% with the past 6 months.

Determine triceps skinfold measurement (TSM). To do so, grasp a fold of skin and subcutaneous fat halfway between the shoulder and elbow and measure with a caliper. Note the patient's percentile rank.

Measure the midarm circumference (MC) with a tape measure (using centimeters) and use this to calculate midarm muscle circumference (MMC) with formula:

MMC in cm = MAC in cm − (0.314 × TSM in mm)

The standard MMC is 25.3 for men and 23.2 for women. MMC below 90% of the standard is considered undernutrition; below 60% is considered protein-calorie malnutrition.

basic dental care throughout one's lifetime. Poor dental care, environmental influences, inappropriate nutrition, and changes in gingival tissue commonly contribute to severe tooth loss in older persons. After the third decade of life, periodontal disease becomes the first cause of tooth loss; by 70 years of age, most people have lost all their teeth. Growing numbers of aging adults are preserving their teeth as they grow older; however, without attention to the prevention of periodontal disease, they, too, could face their senior years without their natural teeth. In addition to teaching methods to prevent periodontal disease, nurses must ensure that older adults and their caregivers understand the signs of this condition so that they can seek help in a timely manner. Signs of periodontal disease include:

- bleeding gums, particularly when teeth are brushed
- red, swollen, painful gums
- pus at gumline when pressure is exerted
- chronic bad breath
- loosening of teeth from gumline

Obviously, a lifetime of poor dental care cannot be reversed. Geriatric dental problems need to be prevented early in a person's life. Although the specialty of geriatric dentistry has grown, many persons do not have access to this service or the financial means to avail themselves of this care.

Through education, nurses should make the public aware of the importance of good, regular dental care and oral hygiene at all ages, as well as informing them that aging alone does not necessitate the loss of teeth. The use of a toothbrush is more effective than swabs or other soft devices in improving gingival tissues and removing soft debris from the teeth. However, care should be taken not to traumatize the tissues because they are more sensitive, fragile, and prone to irritation in the elderly. Loose teeth should be extracted to prevent them from being aspirated and causing a lung abscess.

Many older adults believe that having dentures eliminates the need for dental care. Nurses must correct this misconception and encourage continued dental care for the individual with dentures. Lesions, infections, and other diseases can be detected by the dentist and corrected to prevent serious complications from developing. Changes in tissue structure may have affected the fit of the dental appliances and require readjustment. Poorly fitting dentures need not always be replaced; sometimes they can be lined to ensure a proper fit. This should be made known to the elderly, who may resist correction because of concern for the expense involved. Most important, dental appliances should be used and not kept in a pocket or dresser drawer! Wearing dental appliances allows proper chewing, encouraging the elderly to introduce a wider variety of foods into their diets.

Nutritional Supplements

Today, approximately half of all adults take nutritional supplements on a daily basis. Vitamin and mineral requirements for the elderly are undetermined and, presently, the RDAs for the general adult population are applicable to the older age group. Although not a panacea, nutritional supplements can compensate for inadequate intake of nutrients and deficiencies resulting from diseases and medication effects. Niacin, riboflavin, thiamine, and vitamins B_6, C, and D are the most common nutrients found to be deficient in elders. However, caution is needed because vitamins, minerals, and herbs, particularly in high doses, can produce adverse effects (Displays 16-2 and 16-3) and interact with many medications (Display 16-4). The nursing assessment should include a review of the type and amount of nutritional supplements used. Older adults should be encouraged to avoid excess intake of supplements and to review the use of nutritional supplements with their health care providers.

KEY CONCEPT
Dental problems can affect virtually every system of the body; therefore, they must be identified and corrected promptly.

KEY CONCEPT
Vitamin, mineral, and herbal supplements can be beneficial, but caution is needed to avoid adverse consequences from their misuse.

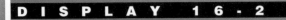

D I S P L A Y 1 6 - 2

Risks Associated With Excess Intake of Selected Vitamins and Minerals

High doses of:	Can cause:
Vitamin D	calcium deposits in kidneys and arteries
Vitamin K	blood clots
Folic acid	masking of vitamin B_{12} deficiency (a cause of dementia)
Calcium	renal calculi; impairment of ability to absorb other minerals
Potassium	cardiac arrest

Threats to Good Nutrition

INDIGESTION AND FOOD INTOLERANCE

Indigestion and food intolerance are common among the elderly because of decreased stomach motility, less gastric secretion, and a slower gastric emptying time. Older persons frequently attempt to manage these problems by using antacids or limiting food intake—both potentially predispose them to other risks. Other means for managing these problems should be explored. For example, one can eat several small meals rather than three large ones. This not only provides a smaller amount of food to be digested at one time but also helps to maintain a more stable blood glucose level throughout the day. Also, one can avoid or limit fried foods. It is easier to digest broiled, boiled, or baked food. Third, one can identify and eliminate specific foods from the diet to which an intolerance exists. Often, the elderly need help identifying prob-

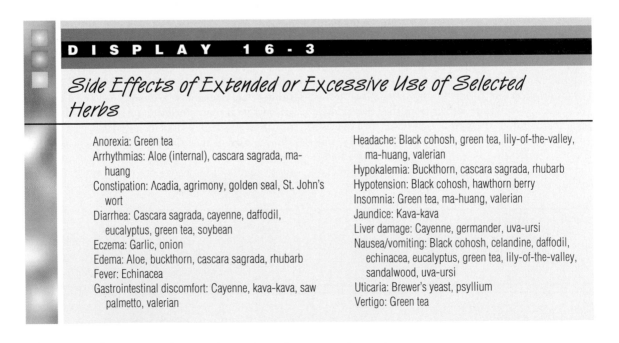

D I S P L A Y 1 6 - 3

Side Effects of Extended or Excessive Use of Selected Herbs

Anorexia: Green tea
Arrhythmias: Aloe (internal), cascara sagrada, ma-huang
Constipation: Acadia, agrimony, golden seal, St. John's wort
Diarrhea: Cascara sagrada, cayenne, daffodil, eucalyptus, green tea, soybean
Eczema: Garlic, onion
Edema: Aloe, buckthorn, cascara sagrada, rhubarb
Fever: Echinacea
Gastrointestinal discomfort: Cayenne, kava-kava, saw palmetto, valerian

Headache: Black cohosh, green tea, lily-of-the-valley, ma-huang, valerian
Hypokalemia: Buckthorn, cascara sagrada, rhubarb
Hypotension: Black cohosh, hawthorn berry
Insomnia: Green tea, ma-huang, valerian
Jaundice: Kava-kava
Liver damage: Cayenne, germander, uva-ursi
Nausea/vomiting: Black cohosh, celandine, daffodil, echinacea, eucalyptus, green tea, lily-of-the-valley, sandalwood, uva-ursi
Uticaria: Brewer's yeast, psyllium
Vertigo: Green tea

DISPLAY 16-4

Herb-Drug Interactions

Herb	Combined with	Can cause
Aloe Barbadensis	Cardiac glycosides	Increased effects of drug
	Corticosteroids	Increased potassium loss
	Thiazide diuretics	Increased potassium loss
Cascara sagrada	Thiazide diuretics	Increased potassium loss
Feverfew	Salicylates	Increased antithrombotic effect
	Warfarin sodium	Increased antithrombotic effect
Ginkgo biloba	Antithrombotic drugs	Increased antithrombotic effect
Kava-kava	CNS depressants	Increased sedation
White willow	Salicylates	Increased antithrombotic effect

lem foods, particularly if they have included those foods in their diets throughout their entire lives. Fourth, one can sit in a high Fowler position while eating and for 30 minutes after meals. Sitting upright increases the size of the abdominal and thoracic cavities, provides more room for the stomach, and facilitates swallowing and digestion. Finally, one should ensure adequate fluid intake and activity to assist the motility of food through the digestive tract.

KEY CONCEPT

Self-imposed dietary restrictions and misuse of antacids to manage indigestion can create a new set of problems for older adults.

DYSPHAGIA

The incidence of dysphagia increases with age and can take several forms, such as difficulty moving food from the mouth to the esophagus *(transfer dysphagia),* down the esophagus *(transport dysphagia),* or from the esophagus into the stomach *(delivery dysphagia).* Neurological conditions, such as a stroke, can cause dysphagia, although most cases result from gastroesophageal reflux disease.

A careful assessment that identifies specific swallowing problems is useful in planning the best interventions for the person experiencing dysphagia. Factors to consider include: onset, types of foods that present the most problem (solids or liquids), if it occurs consistently or periodically, and other symptoms and related complications (eg, aspiration or weight loss). A referral to a speech pathologist is beneficial in evaluating the problem and developing a care plan that is best suited for the individual. Often, thickened liquids or mechanically altered foods may prove beneficial. Although specific interventions will be used to address an individual's needs, some general measures prove useful for all persons with dysphagia, such as having the person sit upright whenever food or fluid is being consumed, allowing sufficient time for eating, assuring there is no residual food in the mouth before feeding additional food, placing small portions in the mouth, discouraging the person from talking while eating, keeping a suction machine readily available, and monitoring intake, output, and weight. Tilting the head to a side and placing food on a particular part of the tongue may be recommended, as may correction of an underlying problem, such as obesity or removal of a structural obstruction.

CONSTIPATION

Constipation is a common problem among the elderly because of slower peristalsis, inactivity, side effects of drugs, and a tendency toward less bulk and fluid in the diet. If food intake is reduced to relieve discomfort, nutritional status can be threatened. Laxatives, another relief measure, can result in diarrhea, leading to dehydration; if oil-based laxatives are used, fat-soluble vitamins (eg, A, D, K, and E) can be drained from the body, leading to vitamin deficiencies.

Constipation must be recognized as a frequent problem for the elderly, and preventive measures should be encouraged. Plenty of fluids, fruits, vegetables, and activity are advisable, as is regular and adequate time allowance for a bowel movement. Activity promotes peristalsis and should be encouraged. Fiber is important but must be used with care. Excessive fiber intake can cause bowel obstruction, diarrhea, or the formation of bezoars, which are dense masses of seeds, skins, and other fiber-containing components of plants that form in the stomach (Steinberg and Eitan, 2003). The lower gastric acidity contributes to bezoar development, which is demonstrated by nausea, vomiting, fullness, abdominal pain, and diarrhea. Senna is an effective natural laxative that can be consumed in tablet or tea form. Often, individuals are aware that certain foods (eg, bananas, prunes, carrots, or oatmeal) facilitate bowel elimination; these should be incorporated into the diet on a regular basis. Laxatives should be considered only after other measures have proved unsuccessful and, when necessary, should be used with great care.

MALNUTRITION

Because malnutrition is a potential and serious threat to the elderly, it should be closely monitored. The factors contributing to this problem include decreased taste and smell sensations, reduced mastication capability, slower peristalsis, decreased hunger contractions, reduced gastric acid secretion, and less absorption of nutrients because of reduced intestinal blood flow and a decrease in cells of the intestinal absorbing surface. The effects of medications can contribute to malnutrition (Display 16-5), reinforcing the significance of using nonpharmacologic means to address health conditions when possible. Socioeconomic factors contributing to malnutrition also must be considered, along with lifelong eating patterns (eg, history of skipping breakfast or high consumption of "junk foods").

The appearance of the elderly can be misleading and delay the detection of a malnourished state. Some of the clinical signs of malnutrition include:

- weight loss greater than 5% in the past month or 10% in the past 6 months
- weight 10% below or 20% above ideal range
- serum albumin level lower than 3.5 g/100 mL
- hemoglobin level below 12 g/dL
- hematocrit value below 35%

Of course, other problems can indicate malnutrition, such as delirium, depression, visual disturbances, dermatitis, hair loss, pallor, delayed wound healing, lethargy, and fatigue. It is crucial that keen assessment skills be used to recognize early malnourishment in the elderly and that good nutritional practices be encouraged to prevent its occurrence.

Often, it is a minor service link that can enhance an older adult's nutritional status. In addressing the nutritional needs of elders, the nurse must consider a wide range of services, including Food Stamps, Meals on Wheels, shopping and meal preparation assistance through volunteer organizations, home health aides for feeding assistance, congregate eating programs, and nutritional and psychological counseling.

Cultural variables affecting nutrition must also be considered. Ethnic and religious factors can influence food selection and preparation and eating patterns and practices. In some cultures, specific foods are seen as having healing benefit. For example, Asian Americans who believe that health is a balance of yin and yang may select certain hot or cold foods to restore balance. An understanding of unique cultural factors affecting dietary practices is essential to individualized care.

Critical Thinking Exercises

1. List the various physical, mental, and socioeconomic requisites for good nutritional intake.
2. What topics could be included in an oral health education program for older adults?
3. How have the media and advertisements influenced the use of dietary supplements? What can nurses do to assist older adults in separating fact from myth regarding the claims made by manufacturers and distributors of dietary supplements?
4. Describe factors that can negatively influence dietary intake in a nursing home, a hospital, and at home.
5. Describe the components of a comprehensive nutritional assessment.

D I S P L A Y   1 6 - 5

Nutritional Risks Associated With Selected Medications

Anemia
   Colchicine
   Indomethacin
   Methyldopa
   Nitrofurantoin
   Nonsteroidal antiinflammatory drugs
   Oxyphenbutazone
   Phenylbutazone
   Sulfonamides
Anorexia
   Aminosalicylic acid
   Cardiac glycosides
   CNS stimulants
   Propranolol
   Pyrazinamide
Constipation
   Aluminum hydroxide
   Calcium carbonate
   Cimetidine
   Codeine
   Narcotics
   Nonsteroidal antiinflammatory drugs
   Sedatives-hypnotics
Diarrhea
   Ampicillin
   Ascorbic acid
   Cardiac glycosides
   Cimetidine
   Laxatives
   Magnesium-based preparations
   Neomycin
   Nonsteroidal antiinflammatory drugs
   Penicillins
   Tetracyclines
Fluid and electrolyte disturbances
   Corticosteroids
   Diuretics
   Estrogens
   Laxatives
   Prednisone
Gastrointestinal upset
   Aspirin

   Colchicine
   Corticosteroids
   Erythromycin
   Estradiol
   Estrogens
   Fenoprofen
   Ibuprofen
   Indomethacin
   Naproxin
   Nonsteroidal antiinflammatory drugs
   Oxyphenbutazone
   Phenylbutazone
   Probenecid
   Tetracycline
   Tolmetin
Nausea/vomiting
   Allopurinol
   Antibiotics
   Anticancer drugs
   Anticholinesterases
   Anticonvulsants
   Antidysrhythmics
   Antihistamines
   Antihypertensives
   Cardiac glycosides
   Chloral hydrate
   Codeine
   Colchicine
   Diuretics
   Ibuprofen
   Levodopa
   Naproxen
   Narcotics
   Nonsteroidal antiinflammatory drugs
   Potassium
   Probenecid
   Propranolol
   Reserpine
   Tamoxifen
   Thiamine
   Tolmetin
   Vasodilators

NURSING DIAGNOSIS HIGHLIGHT

DEFICIENT FLUID VOLUME

Overview

Deficient fluid volume refers to a state of dehydration in which intracelluar, extracellular, or vascular fluid is less than that required by the body. This condition can be indicated by increased output, reduced intake, concentrated urine, weight loss, hypotension, increased pulse, poorer skin turgor, dry skin and mucous membranes, increased body temperature, weakness, and elevated serum creatinine, blood urea nitrogen, and hematocrit.

Causative or contributing factors

Vomiting, diarrhea, polyuria, excessive drainage, profuse perspiration, increased metabolic rate, insufficient intake due to physical or mental limitation, inaccessible fluids, medications (e.g., diuretics, laxatives, sedatives).

Goal

The patient possesses an intake and output balance within 200 ml and has cause of problem identified and corrected.

Interventions

- Perform a comprehensive assessment to identify underlying cause of fluid volume deficit; obtain treatment for underlying cause as appropriate.
- Maintain a strict record of intake and output.
- Closely monitor vital signs, urine specific gravity, skin turgor, mental status.
- Monitor patient's weight daily until problem corrected.
- Encourage fluids, at least 1500 ml during a 24-hour period unless contraindicated; offer foods that are high in fluid content (eg, gelatin, sherbets, soup); keep fluids easily accessible.
- Consult with physician regarding need for intravenous fluid replacement; if prescribed, monitor carefully because of high risk of overhydration in elderly persons.
- Assist with or provide good oral hygiene.
- Identify persons at high-risk for dehydration and closely monitor their intake and output.

Web Connect

Explore the warnings and safety information pertaining to nutritional supplements on the U.S. Food and Drug Administration's website at www.cfsan.fda.gov/~dms/ds-warn.html.

● Resources

American Dietetic Association
216 West Jackson Boulevard
Suite 800
Chicago, IL 60606
(800) 366-1655
www.eatright.org

American Vegan Society
501 Old Harding Highway
Malaga, NJ 08328
(856) 694-2887
www.social.com/health/nhic/data/hr0100/hr01

Food and Nutrition Information Center
National Agriculture Library Building
Room 304

Beltsville, MD 20705
(301) 504-6409
www.nal.usda.gov/fnic.html

National Oral Health Information Clearinghouse
1 NOHIC Way
Bethesda, MD 20892
(301) 402-7364
www.aerie.com/nohicweb/special.html

Overeaters Anonymous
World Services Office
P.O. Box 92870
Los Angeles, CA 90009
(213) 936-4206
www.overeaters.org

● **References**

Davis, C. A., Britten, P., & Myers, E. F. (2001) Past, present, and future of the Food Guide Pyramid. *Journal of the American Dietetic Association, 101*(8), 881–885.

Steinberg, J. M., & Eitan, A. (2003). Prickly pear fruit bezoar presenting as rectal perforation in an elderly patient. *International Journal of Colorectal Disease, 18*(4), 5–7.

Tufts University. (1999). New food guide pyramid specifically for people 70 and older. *Tufts University Health and Nutrition Letter, 17*(2), 8.

Walker, S. N. (2003). Bigger is not always better. *Journal of Gerontological Nursing, 29*(5), 3.

● **Recommended Readings**

Amella, E. J. (1998). Assessment and management of eating and feeding difficulties for older people: A NICHE protocol. *Geriatric Nursing, 19,* 269–275.

Bartlett, S. (1998). *Geriatric nutrition handbook.* New York: Chapman & Hall.

Burckhardt, P., & Dawson-Hughes, B. (1998). *Nutritional aspects of osteoporosis.* New York: Springer.

de Castro, J. M., & Stroebele, N. (2002). Food intake in the real world: Implications for nutrition and aging. *Clinical Geriatric Medicine, 18*(4), 685–697.

Drewnowski, A., & Warren-Mears, V. A. (2001) Does aging change nutrition requirements? *Journal of Nutrition and Healthy Aging, 5*(2), 70–74.

Dror, Y. (2003). Dietary fiber intake for the elderly. *Nutrition, 19*(4), 388–389.

Gasper, P. M. (1999). Water intake of nursing home residents. *Journal of Gerontological Nursing, 25*(4), 23–29.

Johns Hopkins Medical Institutions. (1999, May). The truth about diet and cancer. *Health After 50, 11*(3), 1–2.

Kennedy, K. L. (2001). Documenting nutritional status and its impact. *Annals of Long-Term Care, 9*(12), 35–38.

McDonald, A., & Hildebrandt, L. (2003). Comparison of formulaic equations to determine energy expenditure in the critically ill patient. *Nutrition, 19*(3), 233–239.

Resnick, B. (2001). Weight loss and failure to thrive: Evaluating and motivating older adults toward recovery. *Annals of Long-Term Care, 9*(7), 21–31.

Robinson, S. B., & Rosher, R. B. (2002). Can a beverage cart help improve hydration? *Geriatric Nursing, 23*(4), 208–211.

Schlenker, E. D. (1998). *Nutrition in aging* (3rd ed.). Boston: McGraw-Hill/WCB.

Shanley, C., & O'Loughlin, G. (2000). Dysphagia among nursing home residents: An assessment and management protocol. *Journal of Gerontological Nursing, 26*(8), 35–48.

Sharkey, J. R., Giuliani, C., Haines, P. S., Branch, L. G., Busby-Whitehead, J., & Zohoori, N. (2003). Summary measure of dietary musculoskeletal nutrient (calcium, vitamin D, magnesium, and phosphorus) intakes is associated with lower-extremity physical performance in homebound elderly men and women. *American Journal of Clinical Nutrition, 77*(4), 847–856.

Wahlqvist, M. L. (2002) Malnutrition in the aged: The dietary assessment. *Public Health and Nutrition. 5*(6A), 911–913.

Yen, P. K. (1999). The supplement dilemma. *Geriatric Nursing, 20,* 167–168.

Yen, P. K. (2003). Maintaining cognitive function with diet. *Geriatric Nursing, 24*(1), 62–63.

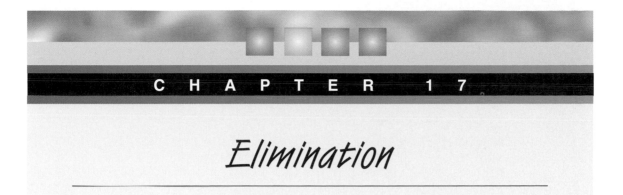

CHAPTER 17

Elimination

■ *Learning Objectives*

After reading this chapter, you should be able to:

- describe age-related changes that affect bladder and bowel elimination

- list nursing measures to promote voiding

- describe nursing interventions to prevent and correct constipation

- list common signs of fecal impaction

- discuss unique aspects of skin care in older adults

- discuss the effects of fasting

*T*o maintain a healthy state, the body must rid itself of waste material, and that eliminated material must be properly disposed. Excretory processes are seldom given considerable thought; they are automatic and natural. With age, however, these processes are less efficient and demand more conscious thought and assistance to be performed satisfactorily (Nursing Diagnosis Table 17-1).

Bladder Elimination

Age-related changes in the urinary tract may cause various elimination problems. One of the greatest annoyances is urinary frequency caused by hypertrophy of the bladder muscle and thickening of the bladder, which decreases bladder ability to expand and reduces storage capacity. This factor should be kept in mind when individuals who are unable to ambulate independently are placed in wheelchairs; they will not be able to sit all day without needing to void, and unnecessary incontinence may result if toileting assistance is not provided. Trips and activities should be planned to allow bathroom breaks at frequent intervals. Older people not only find more frequent voiding necessary during the day, but they also find that night frequency may be a bothersome problem. Often, kidney circulation improves when a recumbent position is assumed, and voiding may be required a few hours after the individual lies down and at other times during the night. Age-related changes in cortical control of micturition also contribute to nocturia; this problem, along with incontinence, can be noted in persons with dementia or other conditions affecting the cerebral cortex.

ND *Nursing Diagnosis*
TABLE 17-1 ● *Aging and Risks to Normal Excretion of Wastes*

Causes or Contributing Factors	Nursing Diagnosis
Loss of nephrons; approximately 50% decrease in glomerular filtration rate	Ineffective Health Maintenance related to ineffective filtration of drugs, wastes from blood
Decreased resorption of glucose from filtrate; less concentration of urine	Ineffective Health Maintenance related to unreliable urine specimen findings on which to identify health deviations
Weaker bladder muscles; decreased bladder capacity; slower micturition reflex; prostate enlargement	Impaired Urinary Elimination: Urgency, Frequency, Nocturia related to age-related changes
Decreased colonic peristalsis; duller neural impulses for signal to defecate	Constipation related to age-related changes
Weaker respiratory muscles; inefficient cough response	Risk for Infection related to ineffective breathing patterns, causing reduced ability to expel material

With the increased threshold for light perception of the elderly making night vision difficult, nocturia could predispose them to accidents and thus threaten their safety. Night-lights should be used to improve visibility during trips to the bathroom, and any clutter or environmental hazards that could cause a fall should be removed. Reducing fluids immediately before bedtime may help, although they should not be significantly restricted. If multiple episodes of nocturia occur, medical evaluation may be warranted to ensure that no urinary tract problem is present. The elderly and their caregivers should be advised that long-acting diuretics, such as the thiazides, even when administered in the morning, can cause nocturia.

Inefficient neurologic control of bladder emptying and weaker bladder muscles can promote the retention of large volumes of urine. In women, the most common cause of urinary retention is a fecal impaction; prostatic hypertrophy, present to some degree in most older men, is the primary cause in men. Symptoms of retention include:

- urinary frequency
- straining
- dribbling
- palpable bladder
- feeling that the bladder has not been emptied

Retention can predispose older individuals to the development of a urinary tract infection. Good fluid intake and efforts to enhance voiding should be emphasized, including:

- voiding in upright position
- massaging bladder area
- rocking back and forth
- running water
- soaking hands in warm water

The filtration efficiency of the kidneys decreases with age, which is an important factor in the elimination of drugs. The nurse should observe the patient for signs of adverse drug reactions resulting from an accumulation of toxic levels of medications. Higher blood urea nitrogen levels may occur due to reduced renal function, causing lethargy, confusion, headache, drowsiness, and other symptoms. Decreased tubular function may cause problems in the concentration of urine; the maximum specific gravity at 80 years of age is 1.024, whereas at younger ages it is 1.032. Reduced ability to concentrate and dilute urine in response to water or sodium excess or depletion occurs. Decreased reabsorption from the filtrate makes a proteinuria of 1.0 usually of no diagnostic significance in the elderly. An increase in the renal threshold for glucose is a serious concern, because the elderly can be hyperglycemic without evidence of glycosuria. False-negative results in diabetic urine testing can occur for this reason.

KEY CONCEPT
Changes in the renal threshold for glucose can cause older adults to be hyperglycemic without having any evidence of glycosuria.

The inability to control the elimination of urine (ie, incontinence) is not a normal occurrence with advanced age, although age-related changes increase the risk for this problem. Incontinence reflects a physical or mental disorder and demands a thorough evaluation. Some stress incontinence may be present, particularly in women who have had multiple pregnancies or in persons who postpone voiding after they sense the urge. More information on incontinence can be found in Chapter 28.

Bowel Elimination

CONSTIPATION

Bowel function is often a major concern of the elderly, many of whom were raised with the belief that anything other than a single daily bowel movement is abnormal. Slower peristalsis, inactivity, reduced food and fluid intake, drugs, and the ingestion of less bulk food are responsible for the high incidence of constipation in the elderly (see the Nursing Diagnosis Highlight at the end of this chapter). Decreased sensory perception may cause the signal for bowel elimination to go unnoticed, which can promote constipation. There also is a tendency toward incomplete emptying of the bowel with one bowel movement; 30 to 45 minutes after the initial movement, the remainder of the bowel movement may need to occur and, if not heeded, problems may develop.

Laxative abuse as a reaction to real or anticipated constipation is a concern. These drugs are not benign substances, as many people believe, and their habitual use should be discouraged. The problems associated with chronic laxative use include:

- Dehydration—diarrhea can occur and deplete fluids rapidly.
- Electrolyte imbalances—the high amounts of sodium and other substances in laxative preparations can alter blood levels of electrolytes.
- Digestion disturbances—magnesium-based preparations can reduce the already lowered amount of gastric acid.
- Vitamin depletion—fat-soluble vitamins A, D, K, and E can dissolve in oil-based laxatives and be excreted.

Education is important to help the elderly and their caregivers learn natural means of bowel elimination, including good fluid intake, a diet rich in fruits and vegetables, activity, and the establishment of a regular time for bowel elimination (Fig. 17-1). Dietary fiber intake of 20 to 35 grams/day is advisable; however, if fiber intake has been low, the amount should be gradually increased to prevent gas, bloating, diarrhea, and other symptoms. If a person dislikes eating high-fiber foods, these foods can be added to other foods (eg, adding wheat bran to ground beef or muffins) to mask the taste. Plenty of fluid intake should accompany increased fiber intake. Because of the tendency for incomplete emptying of the bowel at one time, opportunity should be provided for full emptying and for repeated attempts at subsequent elimination. Sometimes, an older person's request to be taken to the bathroom or to have a bedpan for bowel elimination shortly after a movement occurred is viewed as an unnecessary demand and ignored; it is then wondered why fecal incontinence results. It is useful for older adults to attempt a bowel movement following breakfast, because the morning activity and ingestion of food and fluid following a period of rest stimulate peristalsis. Suppositories occasionally may be necessary to stimulate elimination and should be administered 30 minutes before bowel elimination is desired. Fecal softeners are commonly prescribed to promote elimination in older persons. Itching and discomfort around the rectum may result from poor

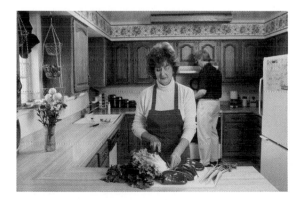

FIGURE 17-1

A diet rich in fruits and vegetables can be beneficial in maintaining a regular bowel elimination pattern.

hygienic practices, hemorrhoids, or dryness caused by reduced secretions of the mucous membrane. Scratching and dryness can irritate the tissue and lead to skin breaks and infection. Regular, thorough cleansing with mild soap and water, followed by the application of a small amount of a lubricant, can minimize this problem. Coarse toilet tissue always should be avoided.

> **KEY CONCEPT**
> Constipation can be prevented by the inclusion of herbs in the diet that have a laxative effect, such as aloe, dandelion root, cascara sagrada, senna, and rhubarb.

FLATULENCE

Flatulence, which is common in the elderly, is caused by constipation, irregular bowel movements, certain foods (eg, the high-fiber foods promoted for increased dietary intake in recent years), and poor neuromuscular control of the anal sphincter. Achieving a regular bowel pattern and avoiding flatus-producing foods may relieve this problem, as may the administration of specific medications intended for this purpose. Sitting upright after meals is helpful in allowing gas to rise to the fundus of the stomach and be expelled.

Discomfort associated with the inability to expel flatus can occur occasionally. Increased activity can provide relief, as may a knee-chest position, if possible. A flatus bag consisting of a rectal tube with an attached plastic bag that prevents the entrance of air into the rectum can be beneficial (Fig. 17-2).

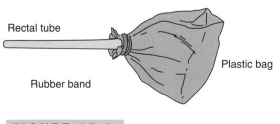

Rectal tube

Plastic bag

Rubber band

FIGURE 17-2

A flatus bag can be made by attaching a plastic bag to a rectal tube.

FECAL IMPACTION

Prevention of constipation aids in avoiding fecal impaction. Observation of the frequency and character of bowel movements may aid in detecting the development of an impaction; a defecation record is essential for older people in a hospital or nursing home. Indications of a fecal impaction include:

- distended rectum
- abdominal and rectal discomfort
- oozing of fecal material around the impaction; often mistaken as diarrhea
- palpable, hard fecal mass
- fever

Fecal impactions should be corrected promptly and carefully. Sometimes an oil retention enema will soften the impaction and facilitate its passage. If this initial procedure is not effective, it may be essential to break up the impaction with a lubricated gloved finger. Inserting 60 mL hydrogen peroxide before the digital attempt at removal sometimes will assist in breaking the impaction. This procedure should be done only after having consulted with the physician and confirming that no lower gastrointestinal disorders exist (eg, tumors).

Excretion Through the Skin

The cleansing process of waste excretion through the skin is different in advanced age because of age-related changes. Perspiration and oil production are decreased, making less frequent bathing necessary. Reduced hydration and vascularity of the dermis make the skin less elastic and more delicate. Consequently, dryness, itching, and breakage of the skin can result from too much bathing. Unless some problem warrants a different pattern, complete bathing is not required more than every third or fourth day. Daily partial sponge baths to the face, axillae, and perineum should be sufficient to prevent odor and irritation. Neutral or superfatted soaps and bath oils should be used for bathing, followed by the application of skin softeners and moisturizers. Tub baths not only are effective for good cleansing but also enhance circulation and provide an opportunity to exercise stiff joints. Showers also may be enjoyed by the elderly; the use of shower chairs, shower lifts, hand-controlled shower heads, and other appliances can assist with this activity. The individual's unique bathing habits, schedule, and preferences should be appreciated and respected, as should the right to privacy and protection from exposure during bathing activities. To reduce the risk of burns, the temperature of the bath water should range from 100° to 105°F.

KEY CONCEPT
Excess bathing can result in dryness, itching, and breakage of fragile older skin.

Elimination of Toxins via Fasting

As Americans increasingly use complementary and alternative therapies for wellness and healing, fasting is growing in popularity. Many people seek enhanced physical, emotional, and spiritual health through the elimination of toxins via fasting.

KEY CONCEPT
Properly done, fasting can eliminate toxins and energize the body.

People view a fast differently. For some it means the ingestion of nothing but water; for others, juices and fruits may be included. Fasting can last anywhere from a day to several weeks. This emphasizes the important of asking people for a detailed description when they say they fast as a health practice.

For someone without health conditions that would otherwise prohibit fasting, there usually is no problem with a 2-day fast consisting of only water intake or a 5-day fast in which only water and juices are ingested. Prolonged fasts or fasts in the presence of health conditions need to be conducted under supervision. Fasting is contraindicated in persons with diabetes, eating disorders, malnutrition, cancer, infectious diseases, renal disease, ulcerative colitis, and bronchial asthma.

Fasting stimulates a cleansing and removal of toxins within the body, which can cause some physical effects, including coated tongue, unpleasant taste, halitosis, increased body odor, skin dryness, fatigue, dizziness, insomnia, nausea, aching joints, and reduced pulse and blood pressure. In some persons, cardiac arrhythmias may occur. A weight loss of several pounds is common.

Drastic modifications in activity level are not required for short-term fasts, although it is best to avoid strenuous exercise. Additional rest periods should be built into the days when fasting occurs.

Good personal hygiene is important during fasting. Because toxins will be eliminated through the skin, frequent bathing is useful, including gently scrubbing the skin with a soft brush. Frequent oral hygiene is essential as well. (Rinsing the mouth with lemon juice can reduce tongue coating and unpleasant tastes.)

There is some belief that the elimination of toxins and other beneficial effects of fasting can be accomplished in a gentler way with cleansing diets (Davis, 2003). An example of a cleansing diet that could be used for one to several days is as follows:

- morning: noncaffeinated herbal tea without sweetener, fresh fruit
- midmorning: at least one full glass of water or noncaffeinated herbal tea
- lunch: steamed vegetables or vegetables cooked in clear broth, grain product, one full glass of water or noncaffeinated herbal tea
- midafternoon: unsweetened fruit or vegetable juice, one full glass of water or noncaffeinated herbal tea
- supper: clear broth vegetable soup or salad, one full glass of water or noncaffeinated herbal tea
- evening: fresh fruit, one full glass of water or noncaffeinated herbal tea

This low-fat, high-fiber vegetarian diet provides a continuous cleansing effect without the stress of a fast.

> **✔ Point to Ponder**
> *What benefit could an occasional day of fasting and respite from responsibilities have on you? How could you build this into your life?*

Nurses need to be aware that the effects of fasting in persons of advanced age are not fully understood. However, with complementary and alternative therapies increasingly being practiced among aging baby boomers, gerontological nurses can expect to encounter growing numbers of elders who fast. Careful assessment of the impact of this practice in light of existing conditions and general health needs is crucial.

NURSING DIAGNOSIS HIGHLIGHT

CONSTIPATION

Overview

Constipation is a condition in which there is an infrequent passage of dry, hard stools. Some of the findings consistent with constipation include decreased frequency of bowel movements (as compared to patient's normal pattern); straining to have bowel movement; hard, dry stools; abdominal distention and discomfort; palpable mass and sense of pressure or fullness in rectum; poor appetite; backache, headache; reduced activity level; and request for or use of laxatives or enemas.

Causative or contributing factors

Age-related decrease in peristalsis, inactivity, immobility, hemorrhoidal pain, poor dietary intake of fiber and fluids, dehydration, surgery, dependency on laxatives or enemas, side effects of medications (eg, antacids, calcium, anticholinergics, barium, iron, narcotics)

Goal

The patient establishes a regular pattern of bowel elimination and passes a stool of normal consistency without straining or experiencing discomfort.

Interventions

- Establish and maintain record of frequency and characteristics of bowel movements.
- Ensure patient consumes at least 1300 mL fluids daily (unless contraindicated).
- Review dietary pattern with patient and educate as needed regarding the inclusion of high-fiber foods in diet; monitor dietary intake.
- Assist patient in developing a program to increase activity level as appropriate.
- Assist patient in developing a regular schedule for toileting; provide toileting assistance as needed; ensure privacy is provided during toileting; if bedpan must be used, be sure patient is in upright position, unless contraindicated, and made comfortable.
- Consider use of herbs with laxative effects, such as aloe, dandelion root, cascara sagrada, senna, and rhubarb.
- Consult with physician regarding use of vitamin C supplements several times daily until stool is soft (not to exceed 5000 mg/d).
- Administer laxatives, as prescribed; avoid long-term use of laxatives unless patient's condition warrants otherwise.
- Monitor for fecal impaction.
- Assess patient's use of laxatives and enemas; if dependency on laxatives or enemas for bowel elimination exists, educate patient about hazards associated with this dependency and develop a plan to gradually taper usage of laxative or enema (abrupt discontinuation is contraindicated).
- Educate patient as to nonpharmacologic means to stimulate bowel movement.

Critical Thinking Exercises

1. What age-related changes affect bladder and bowel elimination?
2. In planning activities for a group of senior citizens, what type of schedule would be most appropriate to their unique elimination patterns?
3. What natural measures for bowel elimination could you recommend to older adults?
4. List the safety risks and complications that older adults are subjected to as a result of age-related changes in elimination patterns.

Web Connect

Review content for teaching bladder control for women at the National Kidney and Urologic Diseases Information Clearinghouse, www.niddk.nih.gov/health/urolog/uibcw/bcw/bcw.htm.

● Reference

Davis, J. L. (2003). Detox diets: Cleansing the body. *WebMD*. Retrieved May 25, 2003, from http://content. health.msn.com/content/article/11/1671_52826.htm.

● Recommended Readings

Abyad, A., & Mourad, F. (1996). Constipation: Common-sense care of the older patient. *Geriatrics, 51*(12), 28–36.

Bradway, C., Hernly, S., & the NICHE Faculty. (1996). Urinary incontinence in older adults admitted to acute care. *Geriatric Nursing, 19*, 98–101.

Luft, J., & Vriheas-Nichols, A. A. (1998). Identifying the risk factors for developing incontinence: Can we modify individual risk? *Geriatric Nursing, 19*, 66–70.

Mueller, C., & Cain, H. (2002). Comprehensive management of urinary incontinence through quality improvement efforts. *Geriatric Nursing, 23*(2), 82–97.

Penn, C., Lekan-Rutledge, D., Joers, A. M., Stolley, J. M., & Amhof, N. V. (1996). Assessment of urinary incontinence. *Journal of Gerontological Nursing, 22*(1), 8–19.

Specht, J. K. P., Lyons, S. S., & Mass, M. L. (2002). Patterns and treatments of urinary incontinence on special care units. *Journal of Gerontological Nursing, 28*(5), 13–21.

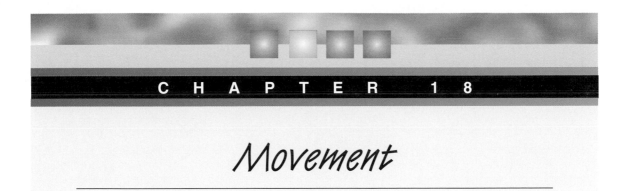

Movement

■ Learning Objectives

After reading this chapter, you should be able to:

- list the benefits of activity
- discuss the challenges elders may face in maintaining an active state
- describe the adjustments that may need to be made in exercise programs in late life
- list actions that could benefit an elder who has impaired mobility

A variety of physical, psychological, and social benefits are gained through regular activity. Physical activity aids respiratory, circulatory, digestive, excretory, and musculoskeletal functions. The physiological effects of exercise enhance mental acuity and mood. The act of engaging in exercise and the health benefits achieved by being physically fit promote socialization. Multiple health problems, such as atherosclerosis, obesity, joint immobility, pneumonia, constipation, pressure ulcers, depression, and insomnia, can be avoided when an active state is maintained. However, as Nursing Diagnosis Table 18-1 describes, the effects of the aging process challenge the older person's ability to remain active and demand special attention by gerontological nurses.

Physical Activity

Maintaining a physically active state is an increasingly difficult task not only for the elderly but also for many younger adults. Fewer occupations require hard physical labor, and those that do often use technological innovations to perform the more strenuous tasks. Television viewing and spectator sports are popular forms of recreation. Automobiles, taxicabs, and buses provide transportation to destinations once conveniently reached by walking. Elevators and escalators minimize stair climbing. Modern appliances

ND *Nursing Diagnosis*
TABLE 18-1 ● *Aging and Risks to Maintaining an Active State*

Causes or Contributing Factors	Nursing Diagnosis
Decreased cardiac output	Activity Intolerance related to less efficient management of stress
Reduced breathing capacity and efficiency	Activity Intolerance related to shortness of breath
Delayed oxygen diffusion	Ineffective Tissue Perfusion related to delayed oxygen diffusion
Decrease in muscle mass, strength, and movements	Activity Intolerance related to muscle weakness and fatigue
Demineralization of bone; deterioration of cartilage, surface of joints	Impaired Physical Mobility related to decreased range of motion
High risk for injury related to brittleness of bones	Pain related to stiff joints
Poorer vision and hearing	Impaired Social Interactions related to sensory deficit
Social isolation related to sensory deficit	Impaired Verbal Communication related to sensory deficit
Wrinkling of skin; thinning, loss, and change in hair color	Disturbance in Self-Concept related to age-related changes to appearance
Lower basal metabolic rate	Impaired Physical Mobility related to slower functions
	Risk for Injury and infection related to decreased bodily functions during resting/sleeping states
Higher prevalence of chronic, disabling disease	Activity Intolerance related to chronic disease
	Impaired Physical Mobility related to chronic disease
	Pain related to chronic disease
	Social Isolation related to chronic disease
Reduced income	Deficient Diversional Activity related to fewer funds available for leisure pursuits
	Chronic Low Self-Esteem related to decreased income
	Social Isolation related to fewer funds available for transportation, entertainment, leisure pursuits

have considerably eased the physical energy expended in household chores. Youth are spending considerable amounts of time sitting in front of computer screens and playing video games. Growing numbers of Americans find that it is challenging to find the time for jogging or trips to the gym.

Educating and encouraging persons of all ages to exercise regularly is an important way that gerontological nurses can influence the health of today's and future generations of elders. All exercise programs should address:

• *Cardiovascular endurance.* The ability of the heart, lungs, and blood vessels to deliver oxygen to all body cells is enhanced by aerobic training. Aerobic exercises include walking, jogging, cycling, swimming, rowing, tennis, and aerobic dancing. For

cardiac endurance, these exercises must be performed long enough to require a continuous supply of oxygen, which puts a demand on the cardiopulmonary system to reach at least 55% of its maximum heart rate (Display 18-1). Ideally, the heart rate should fall within the target heart rate range during exercise. Depending on the exercise, these should be done for at least 20 minutes, at least 3 days a week. Adjustments to desirable target heart rate range may need to be made for persons with heart conditions or who are taking certain medications, reinforcing the importance of consultation with a physician before initiating an exercise program.

• *Flexibility.* The ability to freely move muscles and joints through their range of motion is another part of physical fitness. Gentle stretching exercises help

DISPLAY 18 - 1

Calculating Maximum and Target Heart Rates

Maximum heart rate = 220 − age
Target heart rate = maximum heart rate × 75%
Target heart rate range = 65% to 80% of maximum heart rate

(Commercial heart rate monitors, available at sports supplies stores, can provide feedback on heart rate during exercise without the inconvenience of having to stop to palpate the pulse.)

maintain flexibility of joints and muscles; stretching exercises for about 5–10 minutes before and after other exercises can reduce muscle soreness. Major muscle groups should be stretched at least twice weekly.

* *Strength training.* Strength and endurance are enhanced by exercises that challenge muscles. Key elements of strength training are resistance and progression. Resistance is achieved by lifting weights and the use of weight machines; isometric exercises or the use of one's own body weight through calisthenics, such as push-ups and pull-ups, are good means of strength training, too. Progression involves increasing the workload on the muscles, such as by lifting heavier weights. The recommendation for most adults is to exercise a muscle through a set of 8–12 repetitions at least twice weekly.

Every health assessment should include a review of the quality and quantity of exercise. Nurses should address identified exercise deficits by reviewing desirable exercise goals and strategies. Helping people to develop good exercise habits today promotes a healthier senior population in the future.

Because many real obstacles get in the way of being physically active in later life, special efforts are demanded by the elderly and those caring for them to compensate for this problem. A crucial basic measure is to educate the public, especially caregivers, about the importance of physical activity for older adults (eg, lowering blood pressure, maintaining muscle strength, preventing falls, aiding lymphatic circulation, sharpening mental acuity, elevating mood, and improving digestion and elimination). Sometimes families believe they are assisting their older relatives by "doing for" and allowing them to be sedentary. Often, assisting with household responsibilities not only enhances good functioning of the body's systems but also promotes a sense of worth by providing an opportunity for productivity. Although physical activity may be more uncomfortable or demanding than inactivity, future health problems and disability may be spared by its regular practice. Creativity in suggesting pastimes that can stimulate movement may be a key to increasing opportunities for activity. For instance, encouraging membership in a senior citizen's club can motivate many types of activity because the individual will have a reason to perform the following tasks, among others:

* get out of bed
* prepare and eat breakfast
* bathe
* dress
* comb hair
* travel to the club
* negotiate a new environment
* interact with others
* participate in activities
* travel home
* undress

Those caring for older people can enhance motivation by demonstrating a sincere interest in their activities, for example, asking how they spent their day, admiring crafts they made, or listening to the details of a trip. Recognizing housekeeping efforts, using their handmade gifts, and commenting on a well-groomed appearance are small but meaningful ways to reinforce the older person's efforts to be active.

The fitness craze continues in our society, and the elderly are not untouched by this movement. Regular physical activity can delay or prevent some of the age-related losses in cardiovascular function and improve maximal oxygen uptake. Resting systolic and diastolic blood pressure can decline with regular exercise. Physical activity can increase muscle strength and flexibility and slow the rate of bone loss.

Exercise can improve body tone, circulation, appetite, digestion, elimination, respiration, immunity, sleep, and self-concept. Opportunities for socialization and recreation can be enhanced through participation in exercise programs (Fig. 18-1). Growing numbers of older adults understand the benefits of and are engaging in exercise programs.

> **KEY CONCEPT**
> In addition to improving physical fitness, exercise programs can offer opportunities for socialization and recreation.

Although exercise is highly beneficial to the elderly, it can create problems if adjustments are not made for their advanced age. Display 18-2 describes some of the guidelines that can assist older adults to obtain maximum benefit from exercise programs.

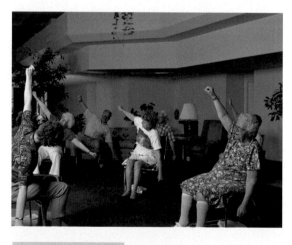

FIGURE 18-1

Planned activities can offer opportunities for socialization and exercise.

Exercise programs are best followed if they match the individual's interests and needs. Some people dislike playing organized sports but enjoy dancing, so helping them to find church and community groups that regularly sponsor evenings of dancing may do more to promote exercise than describing all the benefits of joining a tennis or bowling team. Likewise, people who may not be able or willing to workout at a gym may be open to lifting weights or jogging on a minitrampoline in their homes. A range of options should be considered, such as brisk walking, swimming, yoga, and aerobic exercises (Fig. 18-2). In addition, people can take advantage of opportunities to enhance physical activity during daily routines, such as climbing stairs instead of taking an elevator, parking the car farther away from the designation to increase walking, taking the dog on a longer route during regular walks, and doing one's own yardwork and housecleaning.

Special Adjustments for the Elderly

Consideration must be given to the impact of aging on the ability to exercise. The reduced stroke volume experienced with age usually is adequate during mild exercise, although it is unable to increase in response to more strenuous exercise as compared to younger hearts. This causes the heart rate to accelerate to supply adequate circulation to the tissues. Not only does an increased resistance to blood flow result in a higher systolic blood pressure during rest, but also systolic pressures can rise above 200 mm Hg during exercise. Reduced vital capacity and increased residual capacity limit air movement, causing the respiratory muscles to work harder and the respiratory rate to increase. The decline in the number and size of muscle fibers and subsequent reduction in muscle mass decreases body strength; grip strength endurance declines. Connective tissue changes reduce the flexibility of joints and muscles. The proportionate increase in body fat in older bodies causes heat to dissipate less effectively, making older persons more susceptible to heat stroke if they exercise in hot temperatures. The 10% to 15% decline in total body fluid that is experienced by late life means that older persons can dehydrate more easily from perspiration during exercise. These factors emphasize the importance of assessing older adults before they start an ex-

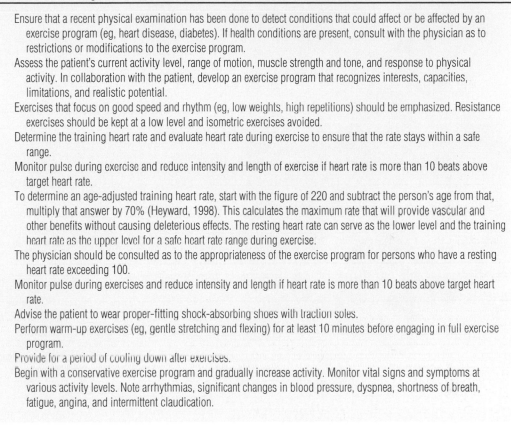

DISPLAY 18-2

Exercise Program Guidelines for Older Adults

Ensure that a recent physical examination has been done to detect conditions that could affect or be affected by an exercise program (eg, heart disease, diabetes). If health conditions are present, consult with the physician as to restrictions or modifications to the exercise program.

Assess the patient's current activity level, range of motion, muscle strength and tone, and response to physical activity. In collaboration with the patient, develop an exercise program that recognizes interests, capacities, limitations, and realistic potential.

Exercises that focus on good speed and rhythm (eg, low weights, high repetitions) should be emphasized. Resistance exercises should be kept at a low level and isometric exercises avoided.

Determine the training heart rate and evaluate heart rate during exercise to ensure that the rate stays within a safe range.

Monitor pulse during exercise and reduce intensity and length of exercise if heart rate is more than 10 beats above target heart rate.

To determine an age-adjusted training heart rate, start with the figure of 220 and subtract the person's age from that, multiply that answer by 70% (Heyward, 1998). This calculates the maximum rate that will provide vascular and other benefits without causing deleterious effects. The resting heart rate can serve as the lower level and the training heart rate as the upper level for a safe heart rate range during exercise.

The physician should be consulted as to the appropriateness of the exercise program for persons who have a resting heart rate exceeding 100.

Monitor pulse during exercises and reduce intensity and length if heart rate is more than 10 beats above target heart rate.

Advise the patient to wear proper-fitting shock-absorbing shoes with traction soles.

Perform warm-up exercises (eg, gentle stretching and flexing) for at least 10 minutes before engaging in full exercise program.

Provide for a period of cooling down after exercises.

Begin with a conservative exercise program and gradually increase activity. Monitor vital signs and symptoms at various activity levels. Note arrhythmias, significant changes in blood pressure, dyspnea, shortness of breath, fatigue, angina, and intermittent claudication.

ercise program and monitoring their status during physical activity.

> **✔ Point to Ponder**
>
> *Do you have regular exercise built into your life? If not, what factors prevent this?*

Some older individuals may be unable to participate in formal exercise programs. For these persons, it can be beneficial to build less aggressive exercises into their daily activities and promote maximum activity during routine care activities. For example:

- Suggest that the patient do foot, leg, shoulder, and arm circling while watching television.
- Instruct the patient to do deep-breathing and limb exercises in the period between awakening and rising from bed.
- Encourage the patient to wash dishes or light laundry by hand to exercise the fingers with the benefit of warm water.
- When greeting a patient in the hall, ask the person to raise both arms as high as possible and wave.

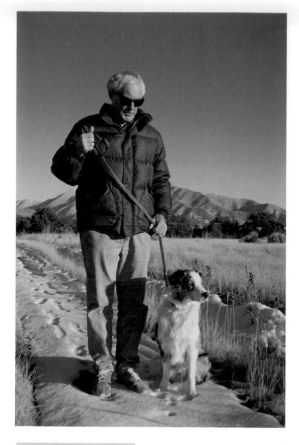

FIGURE 18-2

Walking the dog promotes outdoor exercise.

- When giving a medication, ask the patient to bend each extremity several times.
- During bathing activities, ask the patient to flex and extend all body parts.

Figure 18-3 depicts several exercises that can easily be incorporated into the older adult's daily activities.

KEY CONCEPT

Persons unable to participate in an aggressive exercise program can stretch and exaggerate movements during routine activities to promote joint mobility and circulation.

It is advisable to pace exercises throughout the day and avoid fatigue from exercising because of potential muscle pain and cramping. Morning stretching exercises loosen stiff joints and muscles, which encourages activity, whereas bedtime exercises promote relaxation and encourage sleep. If an older person is not accustomed to a great deal of physical activity, introduce exercises gradually and increase them according to individual progress. Some tachycardia normally may occur during the exercises and continue for as long as several hours thereafter in the elderly. Longer periods must be allowed for the older person to perform exercises, and rest periods should follow activity. Warm water and warm washcloths or towels wrapped around the joints may ease joint motion and facilitate exercising.

The thinner, weaker, and more brittle bones of the elderly heighten the risk for fractures. Exercises that stress an immobilized joint, strenuous sports, and running and jumping exercises must be avoided to prevent trauma. Older adults with cardiac or respiratory problems should seek advice from their physician about the amount and type of exercise best suited for their unique capacities and limitations.

At times, older persons may need partial or complete assistance with exercises. The nurse or other caregivers will find it useful to remember the following points:

- Exercise all body joints through their normal range of motion at least three times daily.
- Support the joint and distal limb during the exercise.
- Do not force the joint past the point of resistance.

Chapter 37 reviews some of the assistive devices that can help the elderly be active.

Increasing numbers of older adults are using exercises that were once limited to the complementary and alternative therapy arena. T'ai chi and yoga are examples of such practices. These practices seem to have many beneficial uses among the elderly. After the first major study was published that showed that t'ai chi exercises helped to reduce falls in the elderly by 25% (Province et al., 1995), several other studies have demonstrated that in addition to improving flexibility and balance, t'ai chi is beneficial in promoting positive mood in the elderly (McCann, 2003; Ross, Bohannon, Davis, & Gurchiek, 1999). **(Visit the Connection website to learn more about yoga and t'ai chi.)**

Exercise to Do While in Bed

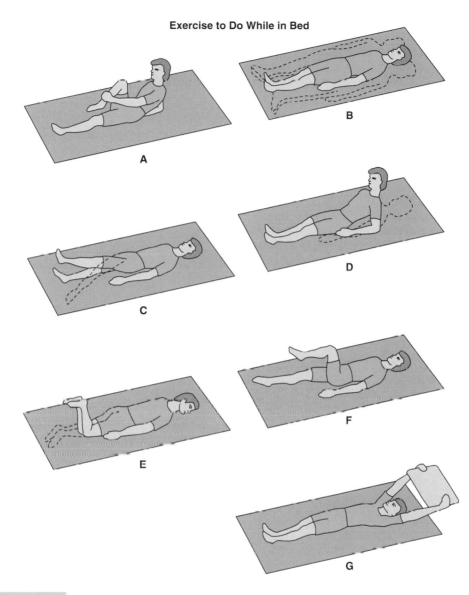

FIGURE 18-3

Exercises to do while in bed: (**A**) Flexing the knee with the opposite hand holding the foot for assistance. (**B**) Rolling from side to side. (**C**) Scissorlike crossing of the legs. (**D**) Raising the chest. (**E**) Flexing the knees while lying on the abdomen. (**F**) Bicycling. (**G**) Lifting a pillow over the head with the arms straight. Exercises to do while sitting: (**A**) Circling motion of the shoulder joint with the arm at the side. (**B**) Circling the arms. (**C**) Rotating the head. (**D**) Flexing and extending the neck. (**E**) Pushing up in a chair with the use of the arms. (**F**) Kicking the legs while sitting. (**G**) Rolling the foot on a can.

All exercises can be built into regular activities. Exercises to do anytime: (**A**) Rolling a pencil on a hard surface. (**B**) Flexing the fingers around a pencil. (**C**) Exaggerating chewing motions. (**D**) Rubbing the back with a towel. (**E**) Tightening the rectoperineal muscles. (**F**) Holding the stomach in to tighten the abdominal muscles.

(*continued*)

Exercises to Do While Sitting

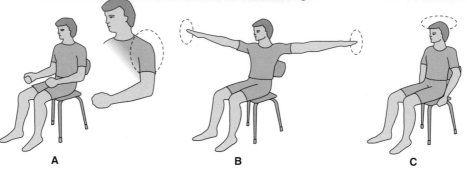
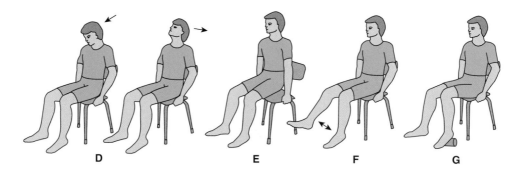

Exercises to Do Anytime

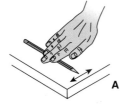

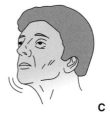

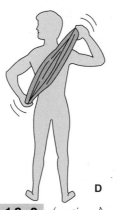
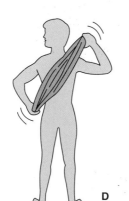
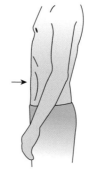

FIGURE 18-3 (continued)

Mind-Body Connection

Cognitive and emotional states can influence physical activity. Depressed individuals may be poorly motivated to engage in exercise or lack the energy to be physically active. Persons with Alzheimer's disease and other cognitive impairments may lack the memory, judgment, or coordination to safely exercise. On the other hand, inactive states lead to the ill effects of immobility (eg, poor circulation, fatigue, reduced release of endorphins) that can affect the mind. Promotion of physical activity, therefore, can have positive effects on mood and cognition. Patients with mood or cognitive disorders should be helped in the development and implementation of an exercise program appropriate for their capabilities and needs. Activities must be planned according to the unique interests of the individual and could include arts, crafts, travel, classes, gardening, auto repair, dancing, listening to music, people watching, and collecting. Pets are frequently a source of interest, activity, and companionship for the elderly. Old age can also be the time for the development of new hobbies and interests.

> **KEY CONCEPT**
> Mental stimulation is as vital to an individual's well-being as physical activity.

Therapeutic recreation is structured leisure with a specific goal in mind, for example, working with clay to exercise fingers, painting to express feelings, and cooking classes to restore or maintain roles. Specialists in recreation, music, art, or dance therapy can provide valuable assistance in matching activities to the unique needs, interests, and capacities of older persons.

With any activity, adequate time and patience are necessary. Slower passage of impulses through the nervous system, sensory deficits, and the vast storehouse of information being triggered and sorted in response to psychological stimuli are just a few of the factors that interfere with rapid reactions in older people.

Hazards of Inactivity

Maintaining an active state can be challenging for the elderly. Age-related changes in muscle strength and endurance, reduced opportunities for activity, and fatigue, pain, dizziness, dyspnea, and other symptoms associated with health problems prevalent in later life can reduce activity levels.

As listed in Display 18-3, the deconditioning effects of inactivity are significant to older adults, so every effort must be made to maximize the activity level of the elderly. Learning about patients' interests can assist nurses in identifying activities that will be familiar and enjoyable. Patients should be made aware of local resources that can promote activity, such as senior centers, exercise classes, educational and recreational programs at local schools or colleges, volunteer opportunities, and local clubs. In addition, activity can be promoted by arranging transportation for the elderly to and from activities. For homebound elderly, special services offered by libraries, vision associations, Pets on Wheels, social service organizations, faith communities, and other agencies can provide resources and companionship that promote activity. Refer to the listing of resources at the end of Chapter 10 for agencies that address specific needs. The featured Nursing Diagnosis Highlight describes additional interventions for promoting mobility.

> **KEY CONCEPT**
> Inactivity can result in deconditioning in which multiple organ systems deteriorate.

Gerontological nurses can make a difference by identifying patients at high risk for developing this complication, implementing interventions to prevent it, and implementing a reconditioning program for persons with chronic deconditioning.

Self-Fulfilling Prophecy

An older adult's unique capacities and limitations will dictate the appropriate activities for that individual. Individual differences, preferences, and abilities must be considered and appreciated. Stereotyping the elderly by assuming they all enjoy exactly the same activities violates the underlying nursing principle of individualized care and severely limits the opportunities available for older persons. If it is assumed that elderly persons are normally inactive, disinterested in exercise, and unable to participate in physical activity,

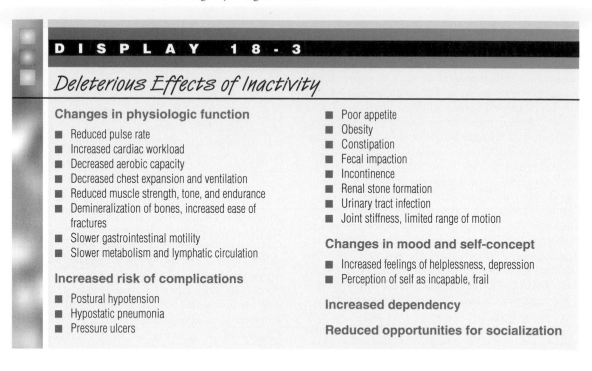

DISPLAY 18-3

Deleterious Effects of Inactivity

Changes in physiologic function

- Reduced pulse rate
- Increased cardiac workload
- Decreased aerobic capacity
- Decreased chest expansion and ventilation
- Reduced muscle strength, tone, and endurance
- Demineralization of bones, increased ease of fractures
- Slower gastrointestinal motility
- Slower metabolism and lymphatic circulation

Increased risk of complications

- Postural hypotension
- Hypostatic pneumonia
- Pressure ulcers

- Poor appetite
- Obesity
- Constipation
- Fecal impaction
- Incontinence
- Renal stone formation
- Urinary tract infection
- Joint stiffness, limited range of motion

Changes in mood and self-concept

- Increased feelings of helplessness, depression
- Perception of self as incapable, frail

Increased dependency

Reduced opportunities for socialization

and if they are treated as though they are, they most likely will fulfill these expectations. On the other hand, if they are expected to keep active and interested in the world around them, they have a better probability of remaining capable, independent, and physically and mentally functional.

KEY CONCEPT
Older adults are more likely to keep active and involved in the world around them if society conveys this as a normal expectation.

NURSING DIAGNOSIS HIGHLIGHT

IMPAIRED PHYSICAL MOBILITY

Overview

Impaired physical mobility is a state in which movement is limited. Some degree of mobility limitation will be observed, ranging from the use of special equipment for movement to total dependency on others for movement. Other signs associated with this diagnosis could include decreased muscle strength or control, restricted range of motion, impaired coordination, altered gait, decreased level of consciousness, pain, paralysis, and imposed restrictions on movement.

Causative or contributing factors

Arthritis, malnutrition, neuromuscular disease, sensory deficits, edema, missing limb, cardiovascular disease, pulmonary disease, obesity, side effects of medications, altered mood or cognition

Goal

The patient will increase mobility to optimal level. The patient will be free from complications associated with impaired mobility.

Interventions

- Assess muscle strength and tone, active and passive range of motion, and mental status. Review history for conditions that can limit mobility or require alteration in level of mobility. Consult with physician as to restrictions on mobility and any necessary modifications for exercises.
- Develop an individualized exercise program, which could include passive or active range-of-motion exercises, structured exercise classes, walking programs.
- Assist patient in maintaining good body alignment and hourly position changes.
- Promote a good nutritional status. Consult with nutritionists as needed.
- If necessary, refer for canes, walkers, wheelchairs, braces, traction devices, and other aids to increase mobility. Provide related health teaching as needed.
- Collaborate with physical therapist, occupational therapist, recreational therapist, and other health team members to develop a program to increase the patient's mobility.
- Encourage family and significant others to assist in efforts to increase the patient's mobility.
- Provide diversional activities based on the patient's interests and level of function.
- Observe for complications associated with immobility and seek prompt correction. Instruct patient in recognition of complications.

- Ensure that a recent physical examination has been done to detect conditions that could affect or be affected by an exercise program (eg, heart disease, diabetes). If health conditions are present, consult with the physician as to restrictions or modifications to the exercise program.
- Assess the patient's current activity level, range of motion, muscle strength and tone, and response to physical activity. In collaboration with the patient, develop an exercise program that recognizes interests, capacities, limitations, and realistic potential.
- Exercises that focus on good speed and rhythm (eg, low weights, high repetitions) should be emphasized.
- Resistance exercises should be kept at a low level and isometric exercises avoided.
- Determine the training heart rate and evaluate heart rate during exercise to ensure that the rate stays within a safe range. The physician should be consulted as to the appropriateness of the exercise program for persons who have a resting heart rate exceeding 100.
- Advise the patient to wear proper-fitting shock-absorbing shoes with traction soles.
- Perform warm-up exercises (eg, gentle stretching and flexing) for at least 10 minutes before engaging in full exercise program.
- Provide for a period of cooling down after exercises.
- Begin with a conservative exercise program and gradually increase activity. Monitor vital signs and symptoms at various activity levels. Note arrhythmias, significant changes in blood pressure, dyspnea, shortness of breath, fatigue, angina, and intermittent claudication.

Critical Thinking Exercises

1. What obstacles do older adults face when trying to maintain an active state? What aspects of society at large discourage physical activity in the elderly?
2. Outline the contents of an exercise education program for a group of healthy senior citizens.
3. List special problems the following older individuals may experience in achieving adequate exercise: a resident of a long-term care facility who has dementia, a depressed widow who lives alone in the community, and a man who must seek re-employment after retiring.
4. Describe how a nurse's attitude toward the elderly can affect their participation in activities.

Web Connect

Watch video clips of t'ai chi movements at www.taichiwebsite.com/videoclips.html, and see examples of yoga movements at www.yogabasics.com/, www.hathayogalesson.com/, and www.poweryoga.net/yoga-postures.html.

●Resources

Information on t'ai chi and yoga exercises can be obtained by contacting the following groups:

International Association of Yoga Therapists
109 Hillside Avenue
Mill Valley, CA 94941
(415) 383-4587
www.iayt.org

Iyengar Yoga
2404 27th Avenue
San Francisco, CA 94116
(415) 753-0909
www.iyoga.com

Tai Chi Network
(603)227-9185
www.taichinetwork.org

Tai Chi Tao Center
433 South Boulevard
Oak Park, IL 60302
(708) 386-0266
www.taichitaocenter.com

●References

Allsen, P. E., Harrison, J. M., & Vance, B. (1997). *Fitness for life.* New York: McGraw-Hill.

Heyward, V. H. (1998). *Advanced fitness assessment & exercise prescription.* Champaign, IL: Human Kinetics.

Province, M. A., et al. (1995). The effects of exercise on falls in elderly patients. *Journal of the American Medical Association, 273*(17), 1341–1347.

Ross, M. C., Bohannon, A. S., Davis, D. C., & Gurchiek, D. A. (1999). The effects of a short-term exercise program on movement, pain, and mood in the elderly. *Journal of Holistic Nursing, 17*(2), 139–147.

●Recommended Readings

Alexander, N. B., Galecki, A. T., Grenier, M. L., Nyquist, L. V., Hofmeyer, M. R., et al. (2001) *Journal of the American Geriatrics Society, 49*(11), 1418–1427.

Allison, M. J., & Keller, C. (2000). Physical activity maintenance in elders with cardiac problems. *Geriatric Nursing, 21*(4), 200–203.

Brach, J. S., Berthold, R., Craik, R., VanSwearingen, J. M., & Newman, A. B. (2001). *Journal of the American Geriatrics Society, 49*(12), 1646–1650.

Chen, K. M., & Snyder, M. (1999). A research-based use of t'ai chi/movement therapy as a nursing intervention. *Journal of Holistic Nursing, 17*(3), 267–279.

Cooper, K. M., Bilbrew, D., Dubbert, P. M., Kerr, K., & Kirchner, K. (2001). Health barriers to walking for exercise in elderly primary care. *Geriatric Nursing, 22*(5), 259–262.

Corbett, B. (1998). *More than a game: A new focus on senior activity services.* State College, PA: Venture Publishing.

Cotton, R. T., & Ekeroth, C. J. (1998). *Exercise for older adults: ACE's guide for fitness professionals.* Champaign, IL: American Council on Exercise.

Gielen, S., Schuler, G., & Hambrecht, R. (2001). Benefits of exercise training for patients with chronic heart failure. *Clinical Geriatrics, 9*(4), 32–45.

Golczewski, J. A. (1998). *Aging: Strategies for maintaining good health and extending life.* Jefferson, NC: McFarland & Co.

Hagberg, J. M., Zmuda, J. M., McCole, S. D., Rodgers, K. S., Ferrell, R. E., et al. (2001). Moderate physical activity is associated with higher bone mineral density in postmenopausal women. *Journal of the American Geriatrics Society, 49*(11), 1411–1417.

Jitramontree, N., Tang, J. H., & Titler, M. G. (2001). Evidence-based protocol: Exercise promotion— encouraging older adults to walk. *Journal of Gerontological Nursing, 27*(10), 7–18.

Judge, J. O. (2001). Physical activity. *Clinical Geriatrics, 9*(13), 17–18.

Judge. J. O. (2001). Promoting physical activity in assisted living and long-term care facilities. *Annals of Long-Term Care, 9*(10), 29–37.

Katzel, L. I., Sorkin, J. D., & Fleg, J. L. (2001). *Journal of the American Geriatrics Society, 49*(12), 1657–1664.

Kelly, M. (1995). Consequences of visual impairment on leisure activities of the elderly. *Geriatric Nursing, 16*(6), 273–275.

Konradi, D. B., & Anglin, L. T. (2003). Walking for exercise self-efficacy appraisal process: Use of a focus group methodology. *Journal of Gerontological Nursing, 29*(5): 29–37.

Lai, J. S., Lan, C., Wong, M. K., & Teng, S. H. (1995). Two year trends in cardiorespiratory function among older t'ai chi chuan practitioners and sedentary subjects. *Journal of the American Geriatrics Society, 43*(9), 1222–1227.

Lord, S. R., Lloyd, D. G., Nirui, M., Raymond, J., Williams, P., & Stewart, R. A. (1995). The effect of a 12-month exercise trial on balance, strength, and falls in older women. *American Geriatrics Society, 43*(9), 1198–1206.

Resnick, B. (2000). Functional performance and exercise of older adults in long-term care settings. *Journal of Gerontological Nursing, 26*(3), 7–16.

Rosenberg, H., & Resnick, B. (2003). Exercise intervention in patients with chronic obstructive pulmonary disease. *Geriatric Nursing, 24*(2), 90–98.

Roth, S. M., Ivey, F. M., Martel, G. F., Lenner, J. T., Hurlbut, D. E., et al. (2001) *Journal of the American Geriatrics Society, 49*(11), 1428–1433.

Shephard, R. J. (1997). *Aging, physical activity, and health.* Champaign, IL: Human Kinetics.

Skelton, D. A., et al. (1995). Effects of resistance training on strength, power, and selected functional abilities of women aged 75 and older. *Journal of the American Geriatrics Society, 43*(10), 1081–1087.

Vincent, K., & Braith, R. (2002). Resistance exercise and bone turnover in elderly men and women. *Medicine and Science in Sports and Exercise, 34*(1), 17–23.

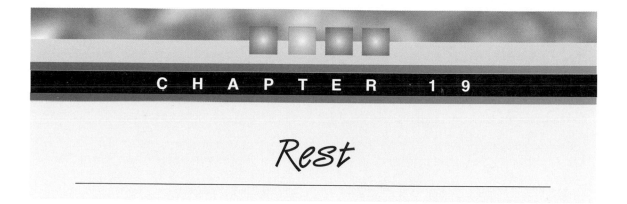

CHAPTER 19

Rest

■ Learning Objectives

After reading this chapter, you should be able to:

• list differences between younger and older adults in sleep stages

• describe nonpharmacological means to induce sleep

• describe health conditions that could cause altered sleep patterns

• discuss schedules of activity and rest that could benefit elders

• list nonpharmacological measures for pain control

• list the body's reaction to stress

• describe approaches to reduce stress

All human beings must retreat from activity and stimulation to renew their reserves. Several periods of relaxation throughout the day and a block of sleep help promote a healthy pattern of rest. However, conditions experienced in later years can interfere with the ability to achieve adequate sleep and rest (Nursing Diagnosis Table 19-1). Astute assessment is necessary to ensure that sleep and rest requirements are fulfilled and to identify obstacles for which intervention is warranted.

Sleep

When we consider that nearly one third of our lifetime is spent sleeping and resting, the significance of these activities is profound. Sleep often is a mirror into our state of health and well-being in that we may be restless and unable to obtain sufficient sleep in the

229

ND *Nursing Diagnosis*

TABLE 19-1 ● *Aging and Risks to the Ability to Achieve Rest*

Causes or Contributing Factors	Nursing Diagnosis
Increased awakening during sleep; sleep stages III and IV less prominent	Disturbed Sleep Pattern related to less prominent sleep stages
Increased incidence of nocturia	Disturbed Sleep Pattern related to nocturia
Altered perception of night environment, resulting from visual and hearing deficits	Anxiety and Fear related to difficulty in falling asleep
Increased incidence of muscle cramps during resting states	Pain related to muscle cramps

presence of pain, stress, or impaired bodily functions. It also is a factor in creating our level of health and well-being due to the risks to physical and mental health associated with an inadequate quality or quantity of sleep.

With age there are changes in the *circadian rhythm*—the body's natural day-night cycle. Over the years, many people begin to feel sleepy at an earlier hour and, consequently, achieve their full night's sleep requirements. The quantity of sleep doesn't change, but the hours in which it occurs may. This can prove frustrating for elders who find themselves nodding off during evening activities and wide awake in the early morning hours when everyone else is asleep. Adjusting schedules to accomodate the altered biorhythms could prove useful. Increasing natural light also is useful in pushing the circadian rhythm toward a later hour of sleep.

Although the normal aging process has minimal effect on the quantity of sleep, the same does not hold true for the quality of sleep. Older people sleep less soundly, shift in and out of stage I sleep to a greater degree than younger adults, and have a decline in stage IV sleep to the point that it is absent in many older adults (Display 19-1).

Environmental factors play a significant part in sleep disturbances. Beginning in midlife, people become more sensitive to noise while they are sleeping and are awakened by noises that may not cause a reaction in younger adults. Likewise, elders are more likely than the young to be awakened by having lights turned on and having changes in room temperature. It is important to consider these factors when caring for older adults in institutional settings. If the sleeping area is noisey, a *white-light generator* that produces

soothing sounds that mask other noises could prove useful. Some people find that leaving a radio on achieves the same purpose.

> **KEY CONCEPT**
> Nurses need to be aware that older adults can be easily awakened by noise and lighting associated with caregiving and other staff activities during the night.

Some older people initially may be disoriented and confused when they waken in a dark room; this, combined with visual deficiencies and postural hypotension, may predispose them to falls. A night-light in the bedroom is helpful, and, if possible, bathroom lighting should be on throughout the night. Clutter and furniture should not obstruct the path from the bedroom to the bathroom. It may be beneficial to provide a urinal, bedpan, or commode in the bedroom if the bathroom is on a different floor of the home.

The attachment of side rails to the bed may be a beneficial protective measure for the older person at home. This prevents falls from bed, assists with movement, and provides a means of orientation to place. It is important that individuals feel confident that they can remove these rails to get out of bed or that someone will be readily available to help them do so when necessary. Falls resulting from attempts to climb over the side rails may be prevented by prompt caregiver response to calls for assistance.

Vision and hearing limitations of the elderly produce difficulties for care providers who need to communicate necessary questions, warnings, or di-

DISPLAY 19-1

Stages of Sleep and Late Life Differences

Stage	Characteristics	Late Life Differences
I	Begins nodding off Can be easily awakened If undisturbed, will reach next stage in a few minutes	More time spent in this stage, most likely due to frequent awakening; increased number of arousals and shifts into non-REM sleep
II	Deeper stage of relaxation reached Some eye movement noted through closed lids Can be easily awakened	No significant change
III	Early phase of deep sleep Reduced temperature and heart rate Muscles relaxed More difficult to be awakened	No significant change
IV	Deep sleep and relaxation All body functions reduced Considerable stimulation needed to be awakened Insufficient amount of this stage of sleep can cause emotional dysfunction	May disappear completely in extreme old age
REM	Rapid eye movement (REM) occurs Increased vital signs (sometimes irregular) Will enter REM sleep approximately once every 90 minutes of stage IV sleep	Decreased due to reduced amount of sleep time in general

Certain drugs can decrease REM sleep, including alcohol, barbiturates, and phenothiazine derivatives. Insufficient REM sleep can cause emotional dysfunction, including psychosis.

rections during the night. Whispering to avoid awakening other sleeping individuals may be missed by the older person who has a reduced ability to hear or whose hearing aid is removed, and lip reading is difficult in dimly lit bedrooms. Focusing a flashlight on the lips of the speaker can help the individual read lips, and cupping the hands over the ear and speaking directly into it can aid hearing. A stethoscope also can be used to amplify conversation by placing the earpieces into the individual's ear and speaking into the bell portion. It is a good idea to explain these procedures during the day so that the patient will understand your actions during the night.

KEY CONCEPT
Conversation with a hearing-impaired individual during the night can be facilitated by placing the earpieces of a stethoscope into the impaired person's ears and speaking into the bell or diaphragm.

The elderly often have difficulty falling asleep. Unfortunately, frequently the first means used to encourage sleep is the administration of a sedative. Sedatives must be used with the utmost care. Barbiturates are general depressants, especially to the central nervous system, and they can significantly depress some vital body functions, lowering basal metabolic rate more than it already is and decreasing blood pressure, mental activity, and peristalsis to the extent that other problems may develop. These serious effects, combined with a greater susceptibility to adverse reactions, warrant that barbiturates be used with extreme caution. Nonbarbiturate sedatives also create problems and should be used only when absolutely necessary. Because of the prolonged half-life of medications in the elderly, the effects of sedatives may exist into the daytime and result in confusion and sluggishness. Sometimes these symptoms are treated with medications, further complicating the situation. Occasionally, sleeping medications will reverse the normal sleep rhythm. All sedatives may decrease body movements during sleep and predispose the older person to the many complications of reduced mobility.

> **Point to Ponder**
>
> *What are your unique sleep and rest requirements, and how well do you meet them? What do you notice about your physical and emotional states when you have had inadequate sleep and rest?*

Alternatives to sedatives should be used to induce sleep whenever possible. The activity schedule of the elderly should first be evaluated. If they have been inactive in a bed or wheelchair all day, most likely they will not be sleepy at bedtime. Including more stimulation and activity during the day may be a solution. Exposure to sunlight during the day can also facilitate sleep. Furthermore, the amount of time allotted for sleep must be evaluated. One should not expect the older person who goes to bed at 8 PM to be able to sleep until 8 AM the following day. A warm bath at bedtime can promote muscle relaxation and encourage sleep, as can a back rub, a comfortable position, a protein and carbohydrate snack (foods high in carbohydrates tend to raise the level of serotonin in the brain which could have a sedating effect), and the alleviation of pain or discomfort. A quiet environment at a temperature preferred by the individual should be provided. Flannel sheets and electric blankets can promote comfort and relaxation; electric blankets should be used to preheat the bed and should be

turned off when the individual enters the bed to reduce the health hazards associated with electromagnetic fields. Eliminating caffeine and alcohol is advisable if sleep disorders are present. Elders may need to be educated about the caffeine content of food and beverages (Display 19-2).

Medications being taken that could interfere with sleep should be identified and reviewed with the physician; examples of such medications include Benadryl capsules, Nicoderm Nicotine Transdermal System, Prozac, Theo-X Extended-Release tablets, and Xanax.

Valerian root tea or herbal tincture consumed 45 minutes before bedtime can also facilitate sleep. The supplement melatonin (a synthetic form of the hormone that is naturally stimulated by darkness) has gained popularity for improving the quality of sleep in adults of all ages by correcting imbalances in the body's circadian rhythm. It is advisable not to use melatonin with light therapy because melatonin photosensitizes the retina, thereby working in opposition to light; they can be used in combination if the light is used at a different time of day from the administration of the melatonin (Kohl, 1999). Also, it is contraindicated in persons who are using immunosuppressants or who have an autoimmune disease (Lippincott Williams & Wilkins, 2002).

> **KEY CONCEPT**
>
> Regular exercise, exposure to sunlight during the day, and noncaffeinated herbal teas at bedtime are three measures to help elders fall asleep naturally.

Sleep Disturbances

Changes in sleep patterns may indicate signs of other problems in the elderly (see Nursing Diagnosis Highlight at the end of the chapter). Although early morning rising is not unusual for the elderly, a sudden change to earlier awakening or insomnia may be symptomatic of an emotional disturbance or alcohol abuse. Sleep disturbances also may arise from cardiac or respiratory problems, which produce difficulties, such as orthopnea and pain related to poor peripheral circulation. Restlessness and confusion during the

DISPLAY 19-2

Caffeine as a Contributor to Poor Sleep

It is important to assess caffeine consumption in individuals who offer complaints related to sleeping. The effects of a cup of a caffeinated beverage begin to be felt in about 15–20 minutes and can last approximately 4 hours. However, some people may feel the effects of caffeine for 10 or more hours. So, an after-dinner cup of coffee can interfere with ability to achieve satisfying sleep. It is important for people to understand the amount of caffeine they are consuming. For example, these are the milligrams of caffeine in an 8-ounce serving of the following beverages:

Cappuccino	120
Coffee	85–110
Tea, brewed	40–60
Shasta cola	45
Pepsi ONE	37
Mountain Dew	34
Diet Coke	31
Sunkist Orange soda	28
Iced tea	25
Diet Pepsi	24
Coca Cola	23
Snapple iced tea	21
Decaf espresso	10

Medications also need to be checked for their caffeine content. Examples of the milligrams of caffeine in a single tablet of popular medications include:

NoDoz Maximum Strength	200
Aqua Ban	100
Excedrin Maximum Strength	65
Anacin	13

Source: National Sleep Foundation (2002).

night may indicate an adverse reaction to a sedative. Nocturnal frequency may be a clue to the presence of diabetes. It is important that the quality and quantity of sleep be assessed.

Approximately half of the adult population complains of sleep disorders, with the major complaint being insomnia. It can be difficult to get a fair estimate of the problem because insomnia can have various meanings. People may report that they have insomnia because they awaken at 5 AM, have difficulty falling asleep, do not sleep soundly, or travel to the bathroom several times during the night. This rein-forces the importance of recognizing insomnia as a symptom and thoroughly assessing for factors that contribute to disrupted sleep. Insomnia can be a short-term problem associated with a changed environment, illness, added stress, or anxiety. Chronic insomnia (ie, insomnia lasting 3 or more weeks) can be related to physical or mental illnesses, substance abuse, or medications. Sedatives may be unnecessary if the underlying cause of insomnia can be addressed.

Jerking leg movements during sleep, known as nocturnal myoclonus, can cause awakenings during the night. This condition is characterized by at least five leg jerks or movements per hour during sleep. It is estimated that more than one third of all older adults experience this problem; therefore, its potential role in causing reported insomnia needs to be evaluated. Noctural myoclonus is associated with the use of tricyclic antidepressants and chronic renal failure.

Sleep apnea is a significant disorder in which at least five episodes of cessation of breathing occur per hour of sleep. It is characterized by snoring and sudden awakening and gasping for air. The prevalence is two times greater in men than women.

This disorder can be caused by a defect in the central nervous system that affects the diaphragm (central sleep apnea), a blockage in the upper airway that interferes with normal air flow (obstructive sleep apnea), or a combination of both (mixed). Snoring usually accompanies the obstructive type. The interruption of sleep can result in daytime fatigue and sleepiness; nurses should assess for sleep apnea when these symptoms are present.

Sleep disorder clinics and other resources can assist in evaluating the disorder and determining the best treatment plan, which could consist of:

- weight reduction
- continuous positive pressurized air
- surgery to remove obstructions or realign bite

Sleeping in a supine position should be avoided because it allows the tongue to fall back and block the airway. Alcohol and other drugs with depressant effects can aggravate the problem by decreasing respiratory drive and relaxing throat muscles. Patients need to be cautioned about driving and using machinery if daytime drowsiness is present.

Health conditions, particularly chronic diseases, can interfere with sleep by producing symptoms such as nocturia, incontinence, pain, orthopnea, apnea, muscle cramps, and tremors. Cardiovascular conditions that produce nocturnal cardiac ischemia can interfere with sleep due to the dyspnia and transient angina that occurs. Fluctuating blood glucose levels can interfere with the sleep of persons who have diabetes. Gastric pain can awaken persons with gastroesophageal reflux disease (GERD). Chronic obstructive pulmonary disease (COPD) and other respiratory conditions can disrupt sleep with coughing and dyspnea. Musculoskeletal conditions can cause pain. People with dementia have minimal stage II and rapid eye movement (REM) sleep, no stage IV sleep,

and frequent arousals from sleep. Depression and other emotional disturbances can alter sleep. Likewise, medications used to treat those conditions can alter sleep; examples of drugs that can interrupt sleep include anticholinergics, antidepressants, antihypertensives (centrally acting ones), benzodiazepines, β-blockers, diuretics, levodopa, steroids, theophylline, and thyroid preparations. Hypnotics interfere with REM and deep sleep stages and can cause daytime drowsiness (due to their extended half-lives in the elderly), thereby creating difficulties in falling asleep for the patient.

Activity and Rest

Satisfying, regular activity promotes rest and relaxation (Fig. 19-1). Greater amounts of rest are required by older people and should be interspersed with periods of activity throughout the day. On awakening, the elderly should spend several minutes resting in bed and stretching their muscles, followed by several more minutes of sitting on the side of the bed before rising to a standing position. This will reduce morning stiffness of the muscles and prevent dizziness and falls resulting from postural hypotension. Many older adults focus all their activity in the early part of the day so that they will have the evening free. For instance, the early morning hours may be used for household cleaning, marketing, club meetings, gardening, cooking, and laundering; the evening hours may then be spent watching television, reading, or sewing. This pattern may be an outgrowth of decades of employment, whereby one worked during the day and relaxed in the evening. Older people need insight into the advantages of pacing activities throughout the entire day and providing ample periods for rest and naps between activities. The nurse may find it useful to review the older person's daily activities hour by hour and assist in developing patterns that more equally distribute activity and rest throughout the day.

Pain Control

The presence of pain can threaten the ability of elders to obtain adequate rest and sleep. Although the results of studies regarding the effects of aging on pain

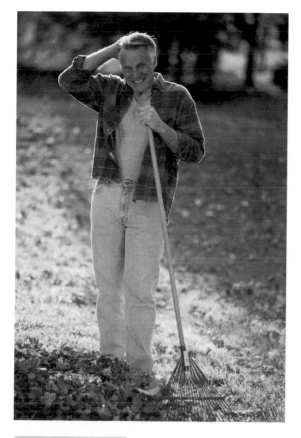

FIGURE 19-1

Daytime activity promotes night sleep.

sensitivity are inconclusive, the prevalence of chronic pain-causing conditions, such as osteoarthritis and postherpetic neuralgia, is high among the elderly. Not only can pain interfere with sleep, but it can also reduce activity levels, depress mood, and result in other factors that can affect sleep and rest patterns.

Identifying the cause of pain is the essential first step to controlling it. Undiagnosed medical conditions can be the source of the problem, but so can psychological factors, poor positioning, and adverse drug reactions. A comprehensive assessment is crucial. Consideration should be given to factors that precipitate, aggravate, and relieve pain. Patients can be assisted in self-evaluating pain with the use of rating scales that use numbers or diagrams to indicate severity of pain.

Because of the risks associated with drugs, non-pharmacologic measures to control pain should be attempted whenever possible. Among these measures are proper positioning, diversional activities, guided imagery, biofeedback, yoga, massage, therapeutic touch, acupuncture, and magnet therapy.

If nonpharmacologic means of pain relief are ineffective and drugs are necessary, it is advisable to begin with the weakest type and dosage of analgesic and gradually increase as necessary. Trials of nonopioids should be used before resorting to opioids. Adjuvant drugs (eg, tricyclic antidepressants, anticonvulsants, antihistamines, caffeine) can be useful in the control of nonmalignant pain or in combination with opioid drugs.

Narcotics should be used discriminately in older persons because of the high risk for delirium, falls, decreased respirations, and other side effects. Administering a nonnarcotic analgesic with the narcotic could decrease the amount of narcotic that is needed. Analgesics should be administered regularly to maintain a constant blood level; fear of addiction should not be a factor in appropriately using analgesics to assist patients in achieving relief.

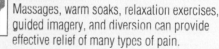

KEY CONCEPT
Massages, warm soaks, relaxation exercises, guided imagery, and diversion can provide effective relief of many types of pain.

Stress Management

Stress is a normal part of life. Most individuals confront a variety of physical and emotional stressors daily; temperature changes, pollutants, viruses, injury, interpersonal conflicts, time pressures, fear, bad news, and unpleasant or difficult tasks are some examples of stressors.

Many real or perceived threats to our physical, emotional, and social well-being and balance can create stress. Demands and activity levels are not necessarily correlated with stress; a busy schedule or numerous responsibilities to juggle may be less stressful than a boring, monotonous existence.

Regardless of the source of the stress, the body reacts in a similar manner in that the sympathetic nervous system is stimulated. This causes stimulation of the pituitary gland; the release of adrenocorticotropic hormone (ACTH) and an increase in the body's adrenaline supply. The following series of changes also occur:

- mental alertness increases
- fingers, hands, and toes become cold as more blood goes to the body's muscles
- glycogen converts to glucose
- heart rate and respirations increase
- pupils dilate
- hearing becomes more acute
- blood-clotting activity increases
- sexual interest and drive are reduced, menstrual irregularities occur, testosterone level is lowered
- ability to concentrate decreases, causing more errors and irrational decisions
- anxiety, fear, or a sense that "something isn't right" occurs

Life is a series of stress and recovery episodes that produce no harmful effects. However, chronic stress without recovery can produce serious consequences, including heart disease, hypertension, cerebrovascular accident, cancer, ulcers, skin eruptions, complications of existing illnesses, and a variety of social and emotional problems.

> **KEY CONCEPT**
> Unrelieved chronic stress can lead to heart disease, hypertension, cerebrovascular accident, ulcers, and other health disorders.

It is important, therefore, to prevent chronic stress from developing. The key to stress control is not avoiding stress but managing it by learning compensatory measures. Some of these measures are outlined as follows.

Respond to stress in a healthy manner. Good nutrition, rest, exercise, and other sound health practices strengthen the body's ability to confront stress. When in a stressful situation, adherence to these principles continues to be important. It is beneficial to learn to remain calm when faced with stress; reacting in an unhealthy manner worsens the situation.

Manage lifestyle. Little in the lives of most people would bring the world to a halt if not completed at a certain time or in a specific manner. Things should be put in perspective; for example, what difference will it really make if the clothes are not washed today or if one is 10 minutes late? Whenever possible, anticipate the consequences of a situation so that the stress of an unpredictable situation can be reduced.

Relax. Be it a good book, swimming, weaving, travel, music, or woodcarving, find something in which to get absorbed so that there is some respite from life's demands. Yoga, meditation, qigong, guided imagery, and relaxation exercises can be effective. Also, herbs can be of benefit, including chamomile and lavender to promote relaxation, and American ginseng to protect the body from the ill effects of stress.

Pray. People of faith look to a higher power with whom they can share and understand life's burdens. The "unloading" of one's problems during prayer also can be a rest-inducing activity in that it clears the mind of the day's stresses. Furthermore, the repeated words or rituals associated with prayer can offer the same therapeutic benefits as meditation and relaxation exercises.

> ✔ **Point to Ponder**
> *What are the three major stresses in your life? What are you doing to minimize their negative effects? What more could you be doing to control stress in your life?*

NURSING DIAGNOSIS HIGHLIGHT

DISTURBED SLEEP PATTERN

Overview

A sleep pattern disturbance exists when the quantity or quality of sleep causes disruption to daily function. This disturbance can be displayed by problems falling or staying asleep, night-time sleep of less than 4 hours, daytime drowsiness, frequent yawning, lack of energy or motivation to engage in activities, dark circles under eyes, weakness, and disturbances in mood or cognition.

Causative or contributing factors

Age-related decrease in stage IV sleep, nocturia, muscle cramps, orthopnea, dyspnea, angina, poor peripheral circulation, cough, incontinence, diarrhea, insufficient activity or exercise, immobility, pain, new environment, depression, confusion, anxiety, medications (eg, antidepressants, antihypertensives, tranquilizers), noise, interruptions, high caffeine consumption

Goals

The patient will:

- obtain 5 to 8 hours of sleep daily
- be free from symptoms and signs associated with sleep pattern disturbance.

Interventions

- Assess sleep pattern. Ask the patient about number, length and quality of naps; activity pattern; bedtime; quality of sleep; awakening time; symptoms and interruptions of sleep. Attempt to identify and correct factors associated with sleep disturbance.

- Increase daytime activity; limit naps, reduce caffeine.
- Consult with physician regarding eliminating medications that are known to disrupt sleep.
- Maintain bedroom temperature between 70°F (21°C) and 75°F (24°C); control interruptions; provide a night-light.
- Assist patient with toileting at bedtime. Be aware that renal circulation improves when one lies down; therefore, the patient may need to toilet shortly after going to bed.
- Use measures that are known to stimulate sleep, such as soft music, television, drinking warm milk.
- Offer back rubs, evening care, and other comfort measures to relax the patient and induce sleep.
- Instruct patient in measures to improve sleep.
- If sedatives are necessary, use those that are least disruptive to sleep cycle and monitor 24-hour effects from the drug.
- Reduce the potential for injury by having bed in lowest position, using side rails, providing night-light, adjusting lighting so that patient does not have to travel from dark bedroom to bright bathroom, encouraging patient to ask for assistance with transferring and ambulating as needed.
- Record or have patient record sleep pattern (eg, time to bed, time when asleep, times awakened during the night, signs and symptoms during sleep, rising time, self-assessment of restfulness).

Critical Thinking Exercises

1. What nonpharmacologic measures can be incorporated into an older adult's lifestyle to facilitate sleep?
2. What stresses do the elderly face that are different from those encountered by other age groups?

Web Connect

Review the MedLine Plus discussion of sleep disorders at www.nlm.nih.gov/medlineplus/ency/article/000800.htm; search the Web for a sleep disorder clinic in your community.

● Resources

Additional information about sleep apnea can be obtained by contacting:

American Sleep Apnea Association
1424 K Street NW
Suite 302
Washington, DC 20005
(202) 293-3650
www.sleepapnea.org

National Sleep Foundation
1522 K Street NW
Suite 500
Washington, DC 20005
(202) 347-3471
www.sleepfoundation.org

Information on pain management can be obtained by contacting:

American Academy of Pain Management
3600 Sisk Road
Suite 2D
Modesto, CA 95356
(209) 545-2920
www.aapainmanage.org/index.html

American Chronic Pain Association
P.O. Box 850
Rocklin, CA 95677
(916) 632-0922
www.theacpa.org

● References

Kohl, M. (1999). Treating insomnia: Helping your patients get enough sleep. *Alternative and Complementary Therapies, 5,* 130–135.

Lippincott Williams & Wilkins. (2002). *Nurse's handbook of complementary and alternative therapies* (2nd ed., pp. 331–332). Philadelphia: Author.

National Sleep Foundation. (2002). Caffeine calculator. [On-line]. Available: www.sleepfoundation.org.

● Recommended Readings

Ancoli-Israel, S. (1997). Sleep problems in older adults: Putting myths to bed. *Geriatrics, 52*(1), 20–30.

Beck-Little, R., & Weinrich, S. P. (1998). Assessment and management of sleep disorders in the elderly. *Journal of Gerontological Nursing, 24*(2), 21–29.

Chasens, E. R. (2003). Nocturia: A problem that disrupts sleep and predicts obstructive sleep apnea. *Geriatric Nursing, 24*(2), 76–81.

Cricco, M., & Simonsick, E. M. (2001). The impact of insomnia on cognitive functioning of older adults. *Journal of the American Geriatrics Society, 49*(9), 1185–1189.

Davis, S. (1996). Why we must sleep. *American Health, 15*(3), 76–79.

Floyd, J. A. (1995). Another look at napping in older adults. *Geriatric Nursing, 16,* 136–138.

Foley, D., Monjan, A., Masaki, K., Ross, W., Havlik, R., White, L., & Launer, L., (2001). Daytime sleepiness is associated with 3-year incident of dementia and cognitive decline in older Japanese-American men. *Journal of the American Geriatrics Society, 49,* 1628–1632.

Foreman, M. D., & Wykle, M. (1995). Nursing standard of practice protocol: Sleep disturbances in elderly patients. *Geriatric Nursing, 16,* 238–243.

Galloway, S., & Turner, L. (1999). Pain assessment in older adults who are cognitively impaired. *Journal of Gerontological Nursing, 25*(7), 34–39.

Herrera, C. O. (1995). Sleep disorders. In W. B. Abrams, R. Berkow (Eds.), *The Merck manual of geriatrics* (p. 128). Rahway, NJ: Merck Sharp & Dohme Research Laboratories.

Johns Hopkins Medical Institutions. (1999, August). Sleep problems. *Health After 50,* 4.

Richards, K. C., Sullivan, S. C., Phillips, R. L., Beck, C. K., & Overton-McCoy, A. L. (2001). Effect of individualized activities on the sleep of nursing home residents who are cognitively impaired: A pilot study. *Journal of Gerontological Nursing, 27*(9), 30–37.

O'Rourke, D. J., Klaasen, K. S., & Sloan, J. A. (2001). Redesigning nighttime care for personal care residents. *Journal of Gerontological Nursing, 27*(7), 30–37.

Sandberg, O., Franklin, K. A., Bucht, G., & Gustafson, Y. (2001). Sleep apnea, delirium, depressed mood, cognition, and ADL ability after stroke. *Journal of the American Geriatrics Society, 49,* 391–397.

Swanson, J. (1999). *Sleep disorders sourcebook.* Detroit: Omnigraphics.

Tabloski, P. A., Cooke, K. M., & Thomas, E. B. (1998). A procedure for withdrawal of sleep medication in elderly women who have been long-term users. *Journal of Gerontological Nursing, 24*(9), 20–28.

Yantis, M. A. (1999). Identifying depression as a symptom of sleep apnea. *Journal of Psychosocial Nursing, 37*(10), 28–34.

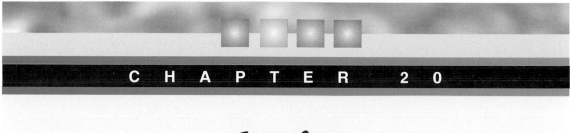

Comfort

■ Chapter Outline

Comfort
  Meaning varies among individuals
  Increased incidence of factors threatening
    comfort with age
Pain—a complex phenomenon
  Defined by patient's perception
Types of pain
  Nociceptive
  Neuropathic
Pain management
  Begins with qualitative and quantitative
    assessment
  Impact of aging on pain unclear
  Cultural factors
  Special challenges with cognitively
    impaired
An integrative approach to pain
    management
  Use of complementary and alternative
    therapies
  Impact of diet on pain
Medication
  Safe use
Comforting
  Comforting strategies
  Continuous process of assuring
    comfort

■ Learning Objectives

After reading this chapter you should be able to:

- describe the characteristics and scope of pain
- list the types of pain
- describe the components of a comprehensive pain assessment
- outline major complementary and alternative therapies useful in pain management
- identify levels of analgesics used for various types of pain
- describe comforting strategies

Comfort

Comfort is a relative term. To some people it can mean sufficient control of pain to capture a few hours of rest; other individuals may view comfort as freedom from physical and mental stress; and still others may consider luxurious, pampered living synonymous with comfort. The word *comfort* is derived from the Latin word *confortare* that means to strengthen greatly. *Webster's Dictionary* offers definitions that include to relieve from distress, lessen misery, have freedom from pain and worry, calm, and inspire with hope. From a holistic perspective, comfort can be viewed as a sense of physical, emotional, social, and spiritual peace and well-being.

Comfort tends to be a state often taken for granted until it is threatened. People coast along without pain or distress, not giving much thought to the comfort they are experiencing. But then something happens—unrelenting gastric pain develops, joints ache while doing routine tasks, a suspicious lump is found in a breast—and the comfort cart is upset. Unfortunately, with advancing age, the incidence of factors that can threaten comfort increases.

Pain—A Complex Phenomenon

Pain is the greatest threat to comfort. The definition of pain, accepted for decades, as being "an unpleasant sensory and emotional experience associated with actual or potential tissue damage" (American Pain Society, 1999) is now being expanded by a broader understanding of pain that relies on and accepts the patient's perception and report (St. Marie, 2002). A Gallup survey of the general adult population revealed that more than 4 of 10 people report experiencing pain on a daily basis, with a majority (89%) saying that they experience pain each month (PR Newswire, 2000). This same survey showed that persons over age 65 are more likely to experience pain than younger adults, with 75% of the elderly suffering weekly pain compared to 66% of persons aged 18–34, and that these elders suffer moderate to severe pain twice as long as younger persons.

It may be difficult to determine the accuracy of the prevalence of pain in the elderly. On one hand, elders may underreport pain because they don't want to be viewed as complainers, lack the funds to seek treatment, or erroneously believe that pain is a normal part of being old. On the other hand, pain could be overreported by some elders who see reporting this symptom as an effective means to get the attention of family members and health care professionals. These possibilities reinforce the importance of exploring pain during every assessment and reviewing the relationship of other factors (physical, emotional, socioeconomic, and spiritual) to this symptom.

KEY CONCEPT
The complex phenomenon of pain is a stressor to physical, emotional, and spiritual well-being.

Types of Pain

Pain is classified according to its pathophysiological mechanism. *Nociceptive pain* arises from mechanical, thermal, or chemical noxious stimuli to the A delta and C afferent nociceptors. These nociceptors are found in fasciae, muscles, joints, and other deep structures, and their activation causes a transduction of painful stimuli along the primary afferent fiber of the dorsal horn of the spinal column. Neurotransmitters (eg, somatostatin, cholecystokinin, and substance P) carry the pain signal through secondary neurons to the brain where the signal is interpreted. Common forms of nociceptive pain are:

- Somatic pain: characteristic of pain in the bone and soft tissue masses. This pain is well localized and described as throbbing or aching.
- Visceral pain: associated with disorders that can cause generalized or referred pain. The pain is described as deep and aching.

Neuropathic pain is another major category and is associated with diabetic neuropathies, postherpetic neuralgias, and other insults to the nervous system. The pain is sharp, stabbing, tingling, or burning, with a sudden onset of high intensity. It can last a few seconds or linger for a longer period.

Point To Ponder
Reflect on the worse pain you have experienced. How did that affect your activities, relationships, and outlook?

Pain Management

Unrelieved pain can lead to many complications for the elderly. For example, if movement causes pain, the person may limit mobility and, consequently, develop pressure ulcers, pneumonia, and constipation.

The individual experiencing pain may have a poor appetite or lack the motivation to properly eat and drink; malnutrition and dehydration can result. The experience of chronic or unrelenting pain can cause a person to become depressed, hopeless, and spiritually distressed. To provide adequate relief from pain and reduce the risk of complications, effective pain management is essential.

Effective pain management begins with qualitative and quantitative assessment of this symptom. Inquiries into the presence of pain are an essential component of every assessment. Patients who indicate that they experience pain should be asked to describe it through the use of questions similar to those shown in Display 20-1. Questions that facilitate descriptive rather than yes-or-no answers offer better insights into the pain experience. If medications are used for pain management, ask specific questions about the type, dosage, frequency, and effectiveness. The more detailed the pain history, the better the likelihood of developing an effective pain management plan.

Physical examination offers additional insights into patients' pain. Areas described as having pain during the interview should be examined for discoloration, swelling, trigger points, and other signs. Sensitivity to touch and restricted movement to the area should be noted, along with body language indicative of pain (eg, grimacing, favoring a side, or rubbing an area).

Ongoing assessment is essential to determine the status of the pain and effectiveness of interventions.

The role of aging on pain perception is unclear. Studies examining the effects of aging on pain sensitivity vary according to the type of pain. There seems to be some evidence that there is a reduced sensitivity for thermal pain with advancing age (Gagliese & Katz, 2003). Research on aging and mechanical pain threshold has been minimal, although the limited studies that have been done indicate a decrease in mechanical pain sensitivity in the elderly (Meliala, Gibson, & Helme, 1999). Studies have not revealed an age effect for electrical pain thresholds. Furthermore, an understanding of the effects of aging on the experience of pain is complicated by the chronic diseases that are common in late life. For example, it could be that it isn't a reduced pain sensitivity but a decreased transmission of signals associated with diseased tissues. There remains much to be learned about the relationship of aging and pain perception.

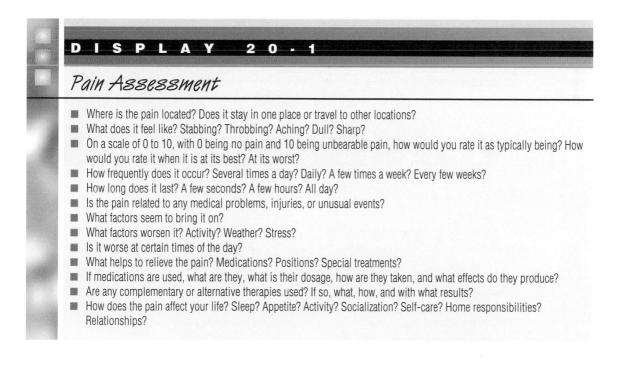

DISPLAY 20-1

Pain Assessment

- Where is the pain located? Does it stay in one place or travel to other locations?
- What does it feel like? Stabbing? Throbbing? Aching? Dull? Sharp?
- On a scale of 0 to 10, with 0 being no pain and 10 being unbearable pain, how would you rate it as typically being? How would you rate it when it is at its best? At its worst?
- How frequently does it occur? Several times a day? Daily? A few times a week? Every few weeks?
- How long does it last? A few seconds? A few hours? All day?
- Is the pain related to any medical problems, injuries, or unusual events?
- What factors seem to bring it on?
- What factors worsen it? Activity? Weather? Stress?
- Is it worse at certain times of the day?
- What helps to relieve the pain? Medications? Positions? Special treatments?
- If medications are used, what are they, what is their dosage, how are they taken, and what effects do they produce?
- Are any complementary or alternative therapies used? If so, what, how, and with what results?
- How does the pain affect your life? Sleep? Appetite? Activity? Socialization? Self-care? Home responsibilities? Relationships?

> **KEY CONCEPT**
> Research is inconclusive concerning the role of aging on pain perception and tolerance; therefore, every patient's unique pain experience must be assessed and understood.

Patients with cognitive impairments present special challenges to pain assessment. These individuals may not have the ability to interpret or report their symptoms; therefore, a greater burden falls on the nurse to adequately identify and assess pain. Display 20-2 offers signs that could indicate pain in persons who are cognitively impaired. That patients with cognitive impairments do not offer specific complaints does not mean they are free from pain. When patients' unique manifestations of pain are identified, these should be well documented in the health record for future reference in assessment.

Cultural factors also must be considered during the pain assessment. In some cultures, people may be socialized to tolerate pain without expression, whereas in other groups, dramatic expression of pain may be the norm. Likewise, some men may have been raised with the belief that "real men don't admit to pain" and not acknowledge the severity of their discomfort. These factors support that the nurse must be thorough and astute when assessing pain.

A variety of pain assessment instruments provide standardized methods for objectively evaluating pain such as:

- *Numeric rating scale:* This commonly used tool asks the patient to rate pain on a scale from 1 to 10, with 1 representing minimal pain and 10 the worst pain imaginable. The scale can be difficult for elders who have trouble thinking in abstract terms and has been found unreliable in persons who are cognitively impaired (Ferrell, Ferrell, & Rivera, 1995).
- *Visual analog scale.* This simple although effective pain assessment tool uses a horizontal line with "no pain" on the left end and "pain as bad as it can possibly be" on the right end (Carr, Jacox, & Chapman, 1992). The patient indicates where his or her pain falls on the scale. A modified version of this tool uses faces, with 0 being a smile and 6 being a crying grimace.
- *McGill Pain Questionnaire.* This popular and widely used tool contains 78 words categorized into 20 groups, a drawing of the body, and a Present Pain Intensity (PPI) scale (Melzack & Katz, 1992). This tool is effective for use with persons who are either cognitively normal or impaired (Ferrell, Ferrell, & Rivera, 1995). Its length and reliance on reading or hearing the items can pose problems with some individuals.

Barriers to using standardized tools must be considered. Patients need to be given clear instructions and an opportunity to practice its use. Using the same tool consistently facilitates the collection of data that is comparable and meaningful.

The fact that patients have not complained about pain doesn't guarantee its absence in their lives. Only

---

DISPLAY 20-2

Signs That Could Indicate Pain in Persons With Cognitive Impairments

Grimacing	Splinting or guarding body part
Crying, moaning	Agitation
Increased vital signs	Poorer function
Perspiration	Change in sleep pattern
Increased pacing, wandering	Change in appetite or intake
Aggressive behaviors	Decreased socialization
Hitting, banging on objects	

about half of pain sufferers sought medical attention for their pain, with nearly two thirds seeing a doctor only when the pain was absolutely unbearable (PR Newswire, 2000). The reality that many people attempt to live with pain reinforces the importance of nurses inquiring about this symptom with routine assessments.

An Integrative Approach to Pain Management

Nurses can be influential in guiding the development of a pain management plan that is individualized and comprehensive. Before implementing symptomatic treatment, underlying causes for the pain need to be identified and corrected as possible. Goals set the foundation for the interventions planned and need to be realistic, specific, and achievable, such as:

- reduce pain level from 9 to ≤ 5 within the next 5 days
- obtain at least 5 hours of sleep without interruptions from pain
- independently bathe and dress without restrictions from pain within the next week

> **KEY CONCEPT**
> In addition to medical problems, poor positioning or posture, inactivity, emotional issues, and adverse drug reactions could be at the root of new or worsened pain. Improving these underlying factors is the first step in pain management.

Although medications have a significant role in pain management, they should not be the only approach used. Increasingly, therapies that once were considered "alternative" or "unorthodox" are being used as complementary approaches to pain management as part of effective integrative care. Using this vision for added options to address pain, possible interventions that could be used in a comprehensive pain management program include :

- Acupressure: use of pressure over points along meridians (what in Traditional Chinese Medicine are believed to be invisible channels of energy {*qi*} running through the body) to unblock energy flow and restore or promote the balance of *qi*
- Acupuncture: placement of needles under the skin at acupoints along meridians to unblock energy flow and restore or promote the balance of *qi*
- Aromatherapy: branch of herbal medicine that uses scents from the essential oils of plants to create physiological and emotional effects (eg, use of lavender, geranium, rose, and sandalwood scents to calm)
- Biofeedback: process of teaching people to bring specific bodily functions under voluntary control
- Chiropractic: use of manipulation or adjustment of the spine and joints to correct misalignments that can be causing dysfunction and pain
- Electrical stimulation: use of electrical currents administered to the skin and muscles via electrodes placed on the painful part of the body
- Exercises: gentle stretching, range of motion exercises
- Guided imagery: suggesting images that can create specific reactions in body
- Heat and cold therapies: use of hot or cold pads, packs, dips (eg, paraffin), baths, massage, or environments (eg, sauna)
- Herbal medicine: use of plants for therapeutic benefit (Display 20-3)
- Homeopathic remedies: use of dilute forms of biological material (plant, animal, or mineral) that produce symptoms similar to that caused by the disease or condition
- Hypnosis: guiding person into trancelike state in which increased receptivity to suggestion is possible
- Massage: manipulation of soft tissue by using rubbing, kneading, rolling, pressing, slapping, and tapping movements (called *bodywork* when combined with deep tissue manipulation, movement awareness, and energy balancing)
- Meditation: using deep relaxation to calm the body and mind and focus on the present
- Naturopathy: use of proper nutrition, pure water, fresh air, exercise, rest, and other natural means
- Osteopathy: branch of physical medicine that uses physical therapy, joint manipulation, and postural correction
- Prayer: petition to God or Divine through direct or intercessory praying
- Progressive relaxation: series of exercises that help body achieve a state of deep relaxation
- Supplements: use of specific nutritional products (eg, B-complex vitamins to enhance function of

DISPLAY 20-3

Herbs Used for Pain Management

Capsaicin/Capsicum (Chili Pepper Oil): used topically for joint and nerve pain; relief provided within a few days

Devil's Claw: effective for inflammatory-related pain; taken orally in dried or extract form; can take several weeks to work

Feverfew: beneficial for prevention of migraines; used orally; best to take in capsule or extract form because plant leaves can be highly irritating to the mouth

Ginger: reduces inflammation and nausea

Kava: sedative effects relieve anxiety and muscle tension; avoid long-term use with liver conditions

St. John's wort: effective for mild to moderate depression

Tumeric: useful with inflammatory conditions

Valerian: relaxes muscles; has a mild sedative effect

White Willow: relieves inflammation and general pain

Because many herbs can interact with medications, it is advisable to consult with a herb-knowledgeable professional before suggesting the use of any herb

nervous system; bromelain, fish oil, ginger, tumeric, and devil's claw to reduce inflammation; topical capsaicin to block pain signal; feverfew and vitamin B_2 to reduce migraines)

- Yoga: discipline that combines breathing exercises, meditation, and specific postures (asanas) to aid in achieving sense of balance and health

✔ Point to Ponder

What methods do you use, other than medications, to manage pain? What facilitates and limits your use of complementary and alternative pain management approaches?

Nurses need to be knowledgeable about the uses and contraindications of various therapies to be able to offer guidance to patients. Also, nurses should be familiar with the licensing requirements for various complementary and alternative practitioners and assist patients in locating qualified therapists. Education and counseling are important to ensure patients make informed choices about their therapists.

Diet can influence inflammation and its pain, particularly arthritic pain that is common in the older population. Arachidonic acid is a primary precursor in the synthesis of omega-6 to proinflammatory eicosanoids. Therefore, eliminating foods that contain arachidonic acid or that are converted into arachidonic acid can be beneficial to persons who suffer from inflammatory conditions. Foods to consider avoiding include animal products, high-fat dairy products, egg yolks, beef fat, safflower, corn, sunflower, soybean, and peanut oils. White flour, sugars, and "junk foods" also are believed to contribute to inflammation. On the other hand, foods rich in omega-3 fatty acids can reduce inflammation; these include cold-water fish (eg, salmon, tuna, sardines, mackerel, and halibut) and their oils, flaxseed and flaxseed oil, canola oils, walnuts, pumpkin seeds, and omega-3 enhanced eggs. Antioxidants offer protection against inflammation, and chief among them are flavonoids. Flavonoids inhibit enzymes that synthesize eicosanoids, thereby interfering with the inflammatory process. Sources of flavonoids include red, purple, and blue fruits, such as berries and their juices; black or green tea; red wine; chocolate; and cocoa. Fresh pineapple also is considered helpful in reducing inflammation. The herbs garlic, ginger, and tumeric (the main ingredient in curry powder) also are believed to have anti-inflammatory effects.

> **KEY CONCEPT**
> A deficiency of B-complex vitamins can contribute to pain caused by damaged or misfiring nerves. Consuming green leafy vegetables can provide B-complex vitamins, along with chemicals that enhance serotonin.

Medication

Medication use in older adults is a complicated process because of the high number of drugs this age group consumes and unique pharmacokinetics and pharmacodynamics (see Chapter 35). The risk for side effects and adverse reactions is higher than in younger age groups, yet this should not deter analgesic use in the elderly. Rather, analgesics need to be used appropriately and monitored closely.

Acetaminophen is the most commonly used drug for mild to moderate pain relief in the elderly, followed by nonsteroidal anti-inflammatory drugs (NSAIDs), with ibuprofen the most used of this drug group. Before advancing to an opioid analgesic, a different NSAID should be tried. For moderate to severe pain, opioids of choice include codeine, oxycodone, and hydrocodone; these are available in combination with nonopioids to offer enhance benefits from the additive effect. Morphine and fentanyl patches are used for severe pain.

Propoxyphene is contraindicated for the elderly, because it does not offer any added benefits but has the potential for central nervous system (CNS) and cardiac toxicity. Pentazocine is another drug that should not be used by older persons because of its high risk for causing delirium, seizures, and cardiac and CNS toxicity.

Nurses should closely observe responses to medications to determine if the drug and its schedule of administration are appropriate. Around-the-clock dosing or the use of sustained-release drugs is useful in the management of continuous pain. If at all possible, medications should be administered on a schedule to prevent pain, rather than treat it after it develops.

Regular reevaluation of patients' response to medications is essential. Medications may change in their effectiveness over time, necessitating a change in the prescription. Also, side effects and adverse reactions can develop with drugs that have been used for a long time without incident.

Comforting

Heavy assignments, fast-paced schedules, and pressures to complete tasks are common experiences for nurses in today's health care system. In the midst of all the *doing* that is demanded, the significance of *being* with patients can be minimized. However, comforting and healing occur through the time spent being with patients.

> **KEY CONCEPT**
> Healing is not synonymous with cure. Rather, it implies living in harmony and peace with a health condition.

Granted, the quantity of time nurses have available to spend with patients is limited, but the quality of that time is significant to comforting and healing. Quality time with patients that fosters comforting is reflected by:

- *giving the patient undivided attention regardless of the length of the interaction.* One method for achieving this is to pause before coming in contact with the patient, take a deep breath, and mentally affirm that you are going to focus on the patient during the time you are together. Sometimes it is helpful to visualize a basket that you are leaving the burdens and tasks of the day in as you enter the patient's room or home.
- *listening attentively.* Encourage the patient to speak and through body language and feedback, demonstrate interest. Feeling that he or she is not heard adds to the patient's discomfort.
- *explaining.* Describe procedures, changes, and progress. Don't assume that a routine procedure is understood by the patient.
- *touching.* Gently rubbing the patient's shoulders, massaging the feet, or holding a hand offers a caring, comforting connection.
- *perceiving.* Pick up signs that could indicate distress, such as sighing, tear-filled eyes, and flat affect. Validate your observations and inquire about their cause (eg, "Mrs. Haines, you seem a little distracted today. Is there something you'd like to talk about?"). As tempting as it may be to ignore a problem that isn't verbalized, this would not be a healing approach.

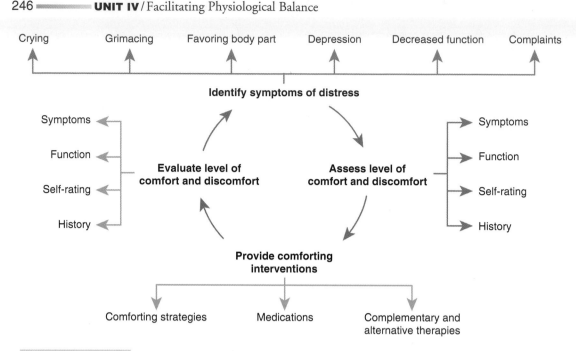

FIGURE 20-1

Pain and comforting cycle.

Point to Ponder

Have you ever been tempted to ignore a problem that you suspect but that the person hasn't verbalized? What were your motives for doing this?

Assuring patients' comfort is a dynamic process (Fig. 20-1) that requires reevaluation and readjustment as needs and status change. It requires sensitivity by nurses to patients' cues of distress and a commitment to alleviate suffering. It affords an opportunity for nurses to demonstrate the healing art of their profession.

NURSING DIAGNOSIS HIGHLIGHT

CHRONIC PAIN

Overview

Chronic pain is a state in which the uncomfortable sensation of pain is not time limited and must be managed on a long-term basis.

Causative or contributing factors

Arthritis, shingles, terminal cancer, phantom limb, depression, ineffectiveness of analgesic

Goal

The patient will experience a reduction in or elimination of pain and safely use effective pain-relief measures

Interventions

- Perform a comprehensive assessment to assist in identifying the underlying cause and nature of pain. Review pain-relief measures used and their effectiveness.
- If patient currently is not using one, instruct in the use of a scale for self-assessment of pain.
- Teach patient and/or caregivers pain control measures such as guided imagery, self-hypnosis, biofeedback, yoga

- Discuss benefits of acupuncture, chiropractic, homeopathy, herbs, and other complementary therapies with health care providers and refer accordingly
- Assure analgesics are used properly
- Control environmental stimuli that may affect pain (eg, loud noise, bright lights, and extreme temperatures)
- Use music therapeutically for relaxation
- Refer to resources for pain management, such as the American Pain Society and National Chronic Pain Outreach Association.
- Monitor level of pain and continued effectiveness of pain-relief measures

Critical Thinking Exercises

1. How does society reinforce symptomatic treatment of pain rather than correction of the underlying problem?
2. Develop an integrative care plan for the management of an elder who experiences chronic arthritis pain.
3. Why could prayer offer relief to someone who is suffering physically and emotionally?
4. Describe possible reasons for reimbursement to be provided for medical procedures for pain relief rather than for comforting strategies that nurses could provide.

 Web Connect

Select a type of pain (eg, back pain, angina pain, or wrist pain), and search the range of sites devoted to that specific pain.

● Resources

American Academy of Pain Management
3600 Sisk Road
Suite 2D
Modesto, CA 95356
(209) 545-2920
www.aapainmanage.org

American Pain Society
4700 W. Lake Avenue
Glenview, IL 60025

(847) 375-4715
www.ampainsoc.org

Pain Links
Extensive listing of foundations, societies, and literature related to pain management
www.painlinks.org

National Chronic Pain Outreach Association
P.O. Box 274
Millboro, VA 24460
(540) 862-9437
www.medhelp.org/amshc/amshc504.htm

● References

American Pain Society. (1999). *Principles of analgesic use in the treatment of acute pain and cancer pain* (4th ed.) Glenview, IL: American Pain Society.

Carr, D. B., Jacox, A. X., & Chapman, B. (1992). *Acute pain management: Operative or medical procedures or trauma. Clinical practice guideline.* (Report No. 92-0032). Rockville, MD: U.S. Department of Health and Human Services, Public Health Agency, Agency for Health Care Policy and Research.

Ferrell, B. A., Ferrell, B. R., & Rivera, L. (1995). Pain in cognitively impaired nursing home patients. *Journal of Pain and Symptom Management, 10*, 591–598.

Gagliese, L., & Katz, J. (2003) Age differences in postoperative pain are scale dependent: A comparison of measures of pain intensity and quality in younger and older surgical patients. *Pain, 103*(1), 11–20.

Meliala, A., Gibson, S. J., & Helme, R. D. (1999). The effect of stimulation site on detection and pain thresholds in young and older adults. *Abstracts: IXth World Congress on Pain.* Seattle: IASP Press, p. 559.

Melzack, R., & Katz, J. (1992). The McGill Pain Questionnaire: Appraisal and current status. In D. Turk and R. Melzack (Eds.), *Handbook on Pain Assessment* (pp. 152–168). New York: Guilford.

PR Newswire. (2000, April 6). Four of 10 Americans suffer pain daily, Gallup survey shows. Atlanta: *PR Newswire Issue.*

St. Marie, B. (2002). *Core curriculum for pain management nursing.* Philadelphia: W.B. Saunders.

● Recommended Readings

Chinall, J. T., & Tait, R. C. (2001). Pain assessment in cognitively impaired and unimpaired older adults: A comparison of four scales. *Pain, 92*(1), 173–186.

Coyle, N., & Layman-Goldstein, M. (2001). Pain assessment and management in palliative care. In M. L. Matzo and D. W. Sherman (Eds.), *Palliative care nursing: Quality care to the end of life.* New York: Springer, p. 362–486.

Dahl, J. L., Joranson, D. E., & Stein, W. (2001). Pain management standards: Their role in improving the quality of care. *Annals of Long-Term Care (Special Issue), 9*(8), 25–30.

Dillard, J. N. (2002). *Chronic pain solution: Your personal path to pain relief.* New York: Bantam Books.

Epps, C. D. (2001). Recognizing pain in the institutionalized elder with dementia. *Geriatric Nursing, 22*(2), 71–79.

Feldt, K. S., & Finch, M. (2002). Older adults with hip fractures: Treatment of pain following hospitalization. *Journal of Gerontological Nursing, 28*(8), 27–35.

Hawk, C. (2002). An evidenced-based look at chiropractic: Tailoring treatment for older adults. *Journal of Gerontological Nursing, 28*(4), 6–14.

Herr, K. A. (2001). Assessment and measurement of pain in older adults. *Clinical Geriatric Medicine, 17*(3), 457–478.

Kolcaba, K., & Steiner, R. (2000). Empirical evidence for the nature of holistic comfort. *Journal of Holistic Nursing, 18*(1), 46–62.

Herr, K. (2002). Chronic pain: Challenges and assessment strategies. *Journal of Gerontological Nursing, 28*(1), 20–27.

Herr, K. A. (2002). Pain assessment in cognitively impaired older adults. *American Journal of Nursing, 102*(12), 65–67.

Horgas, A. L. & Dunn, K. (2001). Pain in nursing home residents: Comparison of residents' self-report and nursing assistants perceptions. *Journal of Gerontological Nursing, 27*(3), 44–53.

The management of persistent pain in older persons. (2002). *Journal of the American Geriatrics Society. Special Supplement, 50*(6), 205–224.

Morse, J. M. (2000). On comfort and comforting. *American Journal of Nursing, 100*(9), 34–37.

Otis, J. A. D., & McGeeney, B. Managing pain in the elderly. *Clinical Geriatrics, 9*(5), 82–88.

Panke, J. T. (2002). Difficulties in managing pain at the end of life. *American Journal of Nursing, 102*(7), 26–33.

Ray, A. (2002). Pain perception. *Clinical Geriatrics, 10*(3), 38–46.

Smith, D. W., Arnstein, P., Rosa, K. C., & Wells-Federman, C. (2002). Effects of integrating Therapeutic Touch into a cognitive behavioral pain treatment program: Report of a pilot clinical trial. *Journal of Holistic Nursing, 20*, 367–387.

Tsai, P. F., & Tak, S. (2003). Disease-specific pain measures for osteoarthritis of the knee or hip. *Geriatric Nursing, 24*, 106–109.

Wallace, M. (2001). Pain in older adults. *Annals of Long-Term Care, 9*(7), 50–58.

Wynne, C. F., Ling, S. M., & Remsburg, R. (2000). Comparison of pain assessment instruments in cognitively intact and cognitively impaired nursing home residents. *Geriatric Nursing, 21*(1), 20–23.

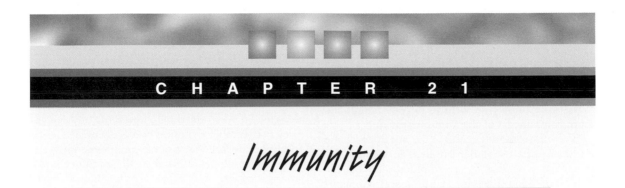

CHAPTER 21

Immunity

■ *Learning Objectives*

After reading this chapter, you should be able to:

- list major changes in immunologic function as the result of aging

- discuss natural approaches to boosting immunologic health

- describe the risks associated with overuse and misuse of antibiotics

*O*lder adults experience infectious diseases that usually are more severe than those of younger adults. *Immune senescence,* an age-related decline in the immune system's function, increases the body's susceptibility to infections and diminishes the strength of the immune response. The high prevalence of chronic conditions in late life enables infectious agents to easily invade, and the high rate of hos-

pitalization and institutionalization increases the exposure to pathogens. Strengthening the immune system and protecting against factors that promote infection are essential to gerontological nursing care.

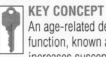

KEY CONCEPT
An age-related decline in the immune system's function, known as immune senescence, increases susceptibility to infections.

The Immune System in Late Life

Our bodies are exposed to many bacteria over the course of the average day, yet we do not develop infectious diseases from each exposure. Our ability to protect ourselves is the result of the effectiveness of the immune system; simply put, this system works in the following manner:

An antigen (invading bacteria) enters the body
↓
A macrophage attacks the antigen and retains some of the antigen's protein on its surface
↓
The macrophage carries the protein markers to lymphoid tissue where T lymphocytes interpret them as foreign
↓
Antibodies attack the antigens

Once the body has been exposed to an antigen, it stores information about the antigen in its memory

249

system to use in the future for protection of the body. (This is the principle on which vaccination works.) When functioning optimally, this system offers resistance to infection that enables health to be maintained. **(Visit the Connection website to learn about the main components of the immune system.)**

There are some differences in the way in which the immune system responds in late life. The thymus gland progressively declines in size with age, although the number of T and B cells in circulation does not significantly decrease; however, there is an increased number of immature T cells in the thymus and blood. T-cell function declines, resulting in a reduced response to foreign antigens because of decreases in cell-mediated immunity and humoral immunity. There is a deficiency of cell-mediated immunity. The inability of many older adults to raise a delayed cutaneous hypersensitivity response (eg, with a tuberculin test) is related to this. The total concentration of immunoglobulins in the blood is not significantly altered with age, although there are changes in the serum distribution of IgA and IgG, which increase, and IgM and IgD, which decrease. A reduced antibody response to pneumococcus, influenza, and tetanus vaccines is noted (although these are recommended for older people). The skin loses macrophages (Langerhans cells), and when this is combined with reduced thickness and circulation to the skin, local defenses against infections are weakened.

KEY CONCEPT

The inability of many older adults to raise a delayed cutaneous hypersensitivity response can alter the results of skin tests.

Promoting Immunologic Health

To compensate for the elderly's compromised immune function and high prevalence of health conditions that increases the risk for infections, health practices that stimulate immunity are essential nursing interventions in gerontolotical care. Some interventions that could prove useful are discussed in the following sections.

DIET

In addition to maintaining a good nutritional state, older people can be encouraged to include foods in their diet that positively affect immunity; some of these include milk, yogurt, nonfat cottage cheese, eggs, fresh fruits and vegetables, nuts, garlic, onion, sprouts, pure honey, and unsulfured molasses. A daily multivitamin and mineral supplement is also helpful; specific nutrients that have immune-boosting effects are listed in Display 21-1. Intake of refined carbohydrates, saturated and polyunsaturated fats, caffeine, and alcohol should be limited.

Fasting, the abstinence of solid foods for 1 to 2 days, is becoming increasingly popular as a means to promote health and healing. The effects of fasting on the immune system include (Chaitow, 1998; Muller, 2001):

- increased macrophage activity, immunoglobulin levels, and neutrophil antibacterial activity
- improvement of cell-mediated immunity, ability of monocytes to kill bacteria, and natural killer cell activity
- reductions in free radicals and antioxidant damage

DISPLAY 21-1

Nutrients With Immune-Boosting Effects

Protein	Magnesium
Vitamins A, E, B_1, B_2, B_6, B_{12}, C	Manganese
Folic acid	Selenium
Pantothenic acid	Zinc
Iron	

For most persons, a day or two without food is safe; however, an assessment of health status is essential before beginning a fast because some health conditions and medication needs can be altered. Also, it is essential that good fluid intake be maintained during a fast (see Chap. 17 for more discussion of fasting).

> ☑ **Point to Ponder**
>
> *In what types of practices do you engage that boost your immune system and offer you protection from infection? What can you do to improve on this?*

EXERCISE

Any type of regular physical activity can enhance immune function. Exercises such as yoga and t'ai chi are low impact and have a positive effect on immunity. There are exercises that can benefit persons with various levels of physical function, and nurses should assist patients in developing a regular exercise program that is tailored to their unique needs (see Chap. 18 for more information on physical activity and exercise).

IMMUNIZATION

General immunizations that are recommended for elders, unless contraindicated, include:

* pneumococcal polysaccharide vaccine: once in a lifetime unless vaccinated before age 65
* influenza vaccine: annually
* tetanus and diphtheria toxoids: every 10 years

If there is significant risk of exposure and immunity does not exist as a result of having the disease or being vaccinated, older adults should be immunized against:

* measles, mumps, and rubella: once
* varicella: once

There are special circumstances that demand immunization against hepatitis:

* hepatitis A: for individuals who are IV drug users, engage in homosexual sexual activity, or who reside or travel in areas with high rates of infection
* hepatitis B: for persons who are IV drug users, engage in homosexual sexual activity, receive hemodialysis, or have received blood transfusions

STRESS MANAGEMENT

The thymus, spleen, and lymph nodes are involved in the stress response; therefore, stress can affect the function of the immune system. Some stress-related diseases, including arthritis, depression, hypertension, and diabetes mellitus, cause a rise in serum cortisol, a powerful immunosuppressant. Elevated cortisol levels can lead to a breakdown in lymphoid tissue, inhibition of the production of natural killer cells, increases in T-suppressor cells, and reductions in the levels of T-helper cells and virus-fighting interferon. Some stress reduction measures that nurses can encourage elders to use include progressive relaxation, meditation, prayer, yoga, imagery, exercise, diversional activity, and substitution of caffeine and "junk" foods with juices and nutritious snacks (Fig. 21-1).

MIND–BODY CONNECTION

The ability of our psychological state to affect physical health is recognized; in fact, the specialty of psychoneuroimmunology has emerged in recognition that thoughts and emotions affect the immune system. Studies have identified traits consistent with strong immune systems to include the following (Cohen, 2002; Cohen & Miller 2001):

* assertiveness
* faith in God or a higher power
* ability to trust and offer unconditional love
* willingness to be open and confide in others

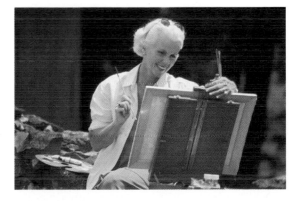

FIGURE 21-1

Managing stress and developing an optimistic attitude can promote good immunologic health.

- purposeful activity
- control over one's life
- acceptance of stress as a challenge rather than a threat
- altruism
- development and exercise of multiple facets of personality

> ✔ **Point to Ponder**
>
> *Do your psychological traits positively support your immunity?*

Nursing interventions that assist elders with the developmental tasks of aging (see Chap. 2) and their connection to others (see Chap. 13) are useful in promoting an immune-enhancing psychological state.

In addition to releasing endorphins and increasing the body's oxygenation and heart rate, laughter and humor can stimulate immunologic function. Nurses can use therapeutic humor by sharing jokes, providing comedy videos or audiotaped comedy programs, and finding laughter and levity among the occurrences in the average day.

CAREFUL USE OF ANTIBIOTICS

More than 133 million courses of antibiotics are prescribed annually to community-based persons and 190 million daily doses of antibiotics are administered in hospitals in the United States (Centers for Disease Con-

trol and Prevention, 2003). Serious consequences have resulted from the overuse and misuse of antibiotics. Some strains of bacteria are resistant to penicillin and ampicillin, and many are resistant to all antibiotics except highly potent and toxic form. Furthermore, antibiotics can produce side effects and adverse reactions that can cause serious consequences (Display 21-2). A trend has been noted in long-term care facilities in which multiple antibiotic-resistant *Klebsiella* and *Escherichia coli* are being observed, attributable to the use of broad-spectrum oral antibiotics and poor infection control techniques (Wiener, Quinn, Bradford, et al., 1999).

> 🔑 **KEY CONCEPT**
> The overuse and misuse of antibiotics have resulted in many strains of bacteria becoming resistant to antibiotics.

Nurses play a significant role in promoting safety in antibiotic use. Some suggestions include:

- assist patients in health promotion efforts to increase their resistance to infections
- adhere to strict infection control practices
- use alternatives to antibiotics whenever possible (Display 21-3)
- educate consumers about the realities and risks of antibiotics
- advise patients not to save and use antibiotics for future illnesses

DISPLAY 21-2

Adverse Effects of Antibiotics

Antibiotic	Effect
Cephalosporin, penicillin, fluoroquinolones, macrolides, erythromycin	Nausea, gastrointestinal upset
Vancomycin, cotrimoxazole	Kidney toxicity
Isoniazid, penicillin, cephalosporin, erythromycin, cotrimoxazole	Liver toxicity
Penicillin-like antibiotics	Neutropenia
Nalidixic acid, methronidazole	Convulsions
Aminoglycosides	Hearing impairments
Tetracyclines	Photophobia
Penicillin	Muscle inflammation

D I S P L A Y 2 1 - 3

Alternatives to Antibiotics

Some herbs have gained popularity for their effectiveness in preventing and treating infections. *Echinacea,* long used by Native Americans, has been shown to increase the number and activity of white blood cells, promote phagocytosis, and stimulate the reproduction of T-helper cells and cytokines (Libster, 2002). Because echinacea can activate autoimmune aggressions and other overreactive immune responses, it is contraindicated in persons with AIDS, multiple sclerosis, or tuberculosis. *Garlic* is known for its antibiotic, antifungal, and antiviral properties. *Siberian ginseng* is a general tonic that can boost the immune system.

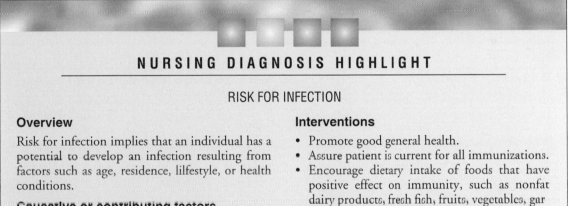

NURSING DIAGNOSIS HIGHLIGHT

RISK FOR INFECTION

Overview

Risk for infection implies that an individual has a potential to develop an infection resulting from factors such as age, residence, lifestyle, or health conditions.

Causative or contributing factors

Age-related decline in immune system's function, high prevalence of chronic conditions, high rate of hospitalization and institutionalization, and age-related changes to body systems (eg, enlarged prostate, weaker bladder muscles, increased residual capacity of lungs, increased fragility of skin).

Goal

The patient will be free from infection.

Interventions

- Promote good general health.
- Assure patient is current for all immunizations.
- Encourage dietary intake of foods that have positive effect on immunity, such as nonfat dairy products, fresh fish, fruits, vegetables, garlic, grains, pure honey, unsulfured molasses.
- Assist patient in maintaining skin integrity.
- Instruct in stress management techniques.
- Encourage and assist with regular exercise.
- Counsel patient against overuse of antibiotics. Consider use of immune-boosting herbs, such as echinacea, garlic, ginseng, and goldenseal.
- Instruct patient in infection control measures and early recognition of infection.
- Assure all caregivers adhere to strict infection prevention and control measures.

Critical Thinking Exercises

1. What major points would you discuss if you were presenting a health education class at a senior citizen center on the topic of "Boosting Your Immunity?"
2. What are the differences between your generation and that of your grandparents in regard to lifestyle and environmental factors that could influence immunity to infection and disease?
3. What factors have contributed to the overuse of antibiotics? How were these factors related to society's attitude and priorities?
4. How did conventional medical care in the United States contribute to antibiotic overuse? What can be done to change this?

Web Connect

To learn about the growing field of psychoneuroimmunology and opportunities to participate in research, visit the Norman Cousins Center for Psychoneuroimmunology at www.prototype.neuropsychiatricinstitute.org/center/cousins/ed_psychneuroim.

● References

Centers for Disease Control and Prevention, (2003). *Promoting appropriate antibiotic use in the community.* Division of Bacterial and Mycotic Diseases Website. Retrieved May 25, 2003, from www.cdc.gov/drugresistance/community/.

Chaitow, L. (1998). *Antibiotic crisis: Antibiotic alternatives* (p. 141). London: Thorsons.

Cohen, S. (2002). Psychosocial stress, social networks, and susceptibility to infection. In H. G. Koenig & H. J. Cohen (Eds.). *The link between religion and health: Psychoneuroimmunology and the faith factor.* New York: Oxford University Press.

Cohen, S., & Miller, G. E. (2001). Stress, immunity, and susceptibility to upper respiratory infections. In R. Ader, D. Felten, & N. Cohen (Eds.). *Psychoneuroimmunology* (3rd ed.). New York: Academic Press.

Libster, M. (2002). *Delmar's integrative herb guide for nurses* (pp. 263–272). Florence, KY: Delmar/Thompson Learning.

Muller, H. (2001). Fasting followed by vegetarian diet in patients with rheumatoid arthritis: A systematic review. *Scandinavian Journal of Rheumatology, 30*(1),1–10.

Saputo, L., & Faass, N. (Eds.) (2002). *Boosting Immunity. Creating Wellness naturally.* Novato, CA: New World Library.

Spake, A. (1999, May 10). Losing the battle of the bugs. *U.S. News and World Report, 126*(18), pp. 52, 55.

Weiner, J., Quinn, J. P., Bradford, P. A., et al. (1999). Multiple antibiotic-resistant *Klebsiella* and *Escherichia coli* infections in nursing homes. *Journal of the American Medical Association, 281,* 517–523.

● Recommended Readings

Ader, R., Felten, D., & Cohen, N. (Eds.). (2001). *Psychoneuroimmunology* (3rd ed.). New York: Academic Press.

Cheraskin, E. (1999). Are antibiotics our best choice? *International Journal of Integrative Medicine, 1*(3), 36–38.

Fazzari, T. V. (1997). Stability of individual differences in cellular immune responses to acute psychological stress. *Advances: The Journal of Mind-Body Health, 13*(3), 36–37.

Gallucci, B. B. (1997). Neuroendocrine and immunological responses of women to stress. *Advances: The Journal of Mind-Body Health, 13*(3), 36.

Golczewski, J. A. (1998). *Aging: Strategies for maintaining good health and extending life.* Jefferson, NC: McFarland.

Jacelon, C. S. (1999). Preventing cascade iatrogenesis in hospitalized elders: An important role for nurses. *Journal of Gerontological Nursing, 25*(1), 27–30.

Kaufman, D. L. (1997). *Injuries and illness in the elderly.* St. Louis: Mosby.

Meydani, S. N., Meydani, M., Blumberg, J. B., et al. (1997). Vitamin E supplementation and in vivo immune response in healthy elderly subjects. *Journal of the American Medical Association, 277,* 1380–1386.

Moldawer, N., & Carr, E. (2000). The promise of recombinant interleukin-2. *American Journal of Nursing, 100*(5), 35–40.

Stern, E. (1997). Two cases of hepatitis C treated with herbs and supplements. *Journal of Alternative and Complementary Medicine: Research on Paradigm, Practice, and Policy, 3*(1), 77–82.

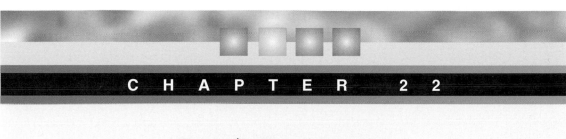

C H A P T E R   2 2

Risk Reduction

Preventing falls
Managing falls
Restraints
Safety aids
Measures to compensate for age-related
changes and health conditions

■ *Learning Objectives*

After reading this chapter, you should be
able to:

- describe the effects of aging on safety
- discuss the significance of the
  environment to physical and
  psychological health and well-being
- list the impact of age-related changes
  on the function and safety of the
  environment
- describe adjustments that can be
  made to the environment to promote
  safety and function of older persons
- identify bathroom hazards and ways to
  minimize them
- discuss the effect of the environment
  on psychosocial health
- list measures to reduce the elderly's
  risks to safety and well-being
- discuss unique safety risks of
  individuals with functional impairments
- list factors that contribute to falls in the
  elderly
- describe safety aids that can be of
  benefit to the elderly

*T*hroughout life, human beings confront threats
to their lives and well-being, such as acts of nature, pollutants, communicable diseases, accidents, and crime. Normally, adults take preventive
action to avoid these hazards and, should they occur,
attempt to control them to minimize their impact.
Older persons face the same hazards as any adult, but

their risks are compounded by age-related factors that
reduce their capacity to protect themselves from and
increase their vulnerability to safety hazards. Gerontological nurses need to identify safety risks when assessing older adults and provide interventions to address existing and potential threats to safety, life, and
well-being.

> **KEY CONCEPT**
> Age-related changes can reduce the capacity of
> the elderly to protect themselves from injury and
> increase their vulnerability to safety hazards.

Aging and Risks to Safety

The injury rate for the elderly falls in the midrange for
all age groups (Table 22-1). Older women have a
higher rate of injuries than any adult female age
group, whereas the rate among men declines through
adult years. The death rate from accidents is lower
among the older population than among other adult
age groups (Table 22-2); accidents rank as the sixth
leading cause of death for the elderly.

Age-related changes, altered antigen–antibody response, and the high prevalence of chronic disease
cause older persons to be highly susceptible to infections. Pneumonia and influenza rank as the fourth
leading cause of death in this age group, and pneumonia is the leading cause of infection-related death.
Older adults have a threefold greater incidence of

TABLE 22-1 ● *Incidence of*
Injuries for Various Age Groups

Age (years)	Persons Injured (Rate per 1000 Population)
<12	110.8
12–21	167.5
22–44	132.4
45–64	109.5
65+	113.8

(From U.S. Department of Commerce. [2001] *Statistical abstract of
the United States* [121st ed.]. Washington, DC: Bureau of the Census.)

TABLE 22-2 ● *Deaths From Injuries by Gender and Age*

Age (years)	Total	Men	Women
1–4	1935	1155	780
5–14	3254	2086	1158
15–24	13,349	9887	3462
25–44	27,172	20,232	6940
45–64	18,286	12,971	5315
65 and older	32,975	16,176	16,799

(From U.S. Department of Commerce. [2001]. *Statistical abstract of the United States* [121st ed., p. 82]. Washington, DC: Bureau of the Census.)

nosocomial pneumonia as compared with younger age groups; the elderly experience gastroenteritis caused by *Salmonella* species more frequently than persons younger than 65 years of age; and urinary tract infections increase in prevalence with age. The elderly account for more than half of all reported cases of tetanus, endocarditis, cholelithiasis, and diverticulitis. Atypical symptomatology often results in delayed diagnosis of infection, contributing to the elderly's higher mortality rate from infections; for instance, older persons are more likely to die from appendicitis than younger persons.

Altered pharmacokinetics, self-administration problems, and the high volume of drugs consumed by older individuals can lead to considerable risks to safety. It is estimated that 5% to 30% of geriatric admissions to hospitals are associated with inappropriate drug administration.

Nursing Diagnosis Table 22-1 lists the various age-related factors that can pose risks to the safety and well being of older adults and potential nursing problems associated with these risks.

Impact of Environment

The environment is a statement by and to us, an expression of our unique selves. Whether it is filled with family heirlooms, accented by our handiwork, dramatic in design, or stark and simple, our environment expresses a great deal about our preferences, attitudes, lifestyles, and personalities. In turn, we perceive messages from environments, such as the

behavior expected, the degree to which we are welcome, and the consideration for our needs. Although it is seldom given conscious thought, the communication between us and our surroundings is dynamic and significant.

The environment can be considered in two parts, the microenvironment and the macroenvironment. The *microenvironment* refers to our immediate surroundings with which we closely interact (eg, furnishings, wall coverings, lighting, room temperature, and room sounds). The *macroenvironment* consists of the elements in the larger world that affect groups of people or even entire populations (eg, the weather, pollution, traffic, and natural resources). Although nurses should be concerned with improving the macroenvironment to benefit public health, the microenvironment, which can be more easily manipulated and from which more immediate benefits can be realized, is the focus of this discussion.

Ideally, the environment provides more than shelter; it should promote continued development, stimulation, and satisfaction to enhance our psychological well-being. This is particularly important for the elderly, many of whom spend considerable time in their homes or in a bedroom of an institution and have reduced interaction with the larger environment of their communities. To achieve the fullest satisfaction from their microenvironments, the elderly must have various levels of needs met within their surroundings. This can be exemplified by comparing environmental needs with the basic human needs postulated by Maslow (Table 22-3). Similar to Maslow's theory, it can be hypothesized that higher-level satisfaction from the environment cannot be achieved unless lower-level needs are fulfilled. This may explain why some elderly have the following priorities and problems:

- They do not think installing a free smoke detector is important when there are rodents in their apartment.
- They refuse to have their house painted because it will make them look too affluent in a high-crime neighborhood and be a target for burglary.
- They believe their home is no longer their own because a daughter-in-law has decided to redecorate it.
- They remain socially isolated rather than invite guests to a house perceived as shabby.
- They are unwilling to engage in creative arts and crafts if they are adjusting to a new and unfamiliar residence.

ND *Nursing Diagnosis*

TABLE 22-1 • *Aging and Risks to Safety*

Causes or Contributing Factors	Nursing Diagnosis
Decrease in intracellular fluid	Deficient Fluid Volume related to easier development of dehydration
Loss of subcutaneous tissue; less natural insulation; lower basal metabolic rate	Risk for Injury and Disturbed Thought Processes related to hypothermia
Decreased efficiency of heart	Activity Intolerance related to alterations (decrease) in cardiac output
Reduced strength and elasticity of respiratory muscles; decreased lung expansion; inefficient cough response; less ciliary activity	Risk for Infection related to reduced ability to expel accumulated or foreign matter from lungs
Reduced oxygen use under stress	Ineffective Tissue Perfusion related to changes in cardiovascular response to stress
Poor condition of teeth	Risk for Infection related to dental disease or aspirated tooth particles
Weak gag reflex	Risk for Infection related to aspiration
Altered taste sensation	Imbalanced Nutrition: More Than Body Requirements of salt or sweets related to taste deficit
Reduction in filtration of wastes by kidneys	Risk for Injury related to ineffective elimination of wastes from blood stream
Higher prevalence of urinary retention	Risk for Infection related to stasis of urine
More alkaline vaginal secretions	Risk for Infection related to inadequate acid environment to inhibit bacterial growth
Decreased muscle strength	Risk for Injury related to reduced muscle strength
Demineralization of bone	Risk for Injury and Impaired Physical Mobility related to increased tendency of bones to fracture
Delayed response and reaction time	Risk for Injury related to inability to respond in timely manner
Poor vision and hearing	Risk for Injury, Impaired Home Maintenance, and Disturbed Sensory Perception related to misperception of environment
Reduced lacrimal secretions	Risk for Injury and Risk for Infection related to decreased ability to protect cornea
Distorted depth perception	Risk for Injury related to decreased ability to judge changes in level of walking surface
Increased threshold for pain and touch	Risk for Injury, Risk for Infection, Disturbed Sensory Perception and Impaired Skin Integrity related to less ability to sense problems, such as pain and pressure
Less elasticity and more dryness and fragility of skin	Impaired Skin Integrity and Risk for Infection related to easier skin breakdown
Poor short-term memory	Risk for Injury and Noncompliance related to inability to recall medication administration, treatments
High prevalence of polypharmacy	Ineffective Management of Therapeutic Regimen and Risk for Injury related to combining drugs inappropriately, drug interactions, and side effects
Reduced income	Risk for Injury related to limited ability to afford protection of safe neighborhood, home repairs, adequate environmental temperature

TABLE 22-3 ● *Environmental Needs Based on Maslow's Hierarchy*

Basic Human Needs*	Environmental Needs
Self-actualization	A space that promotes the realization of all potential, inspiring objects, beautiful grounds, relaxation aids
Self-esteem	A home one can feel pride in having, elegant decor, status symbols
Trust	A niche in which one can feel confident, control over lifestyle, consistent layout/furnishings/temperature/lighting
Love	A place one derives pleasure from being, familiar and comfortable furniture, favorite objects, attractive
Security	A haven from external threats, ability to safeguard personal possessions, adequate lighting, locks, smoke detectors, alarms
Physiological needs	A shelter in which to live, adequate ventilation, room temperature about 75°F (24°C), functioning utilities and appliances, pest control

(*Data from Maslow, A.H. [1968]. *Toward a psychology of being*. New York: Van Nostrand Reinhold.)

Nurses must be realistic in their assessment of the environment to determine which levels of needs are being addressed and to plan measures to promote the fulfillment of higher level needs. **(Visit the Connection website to obtain an Environmental Assessment Tool. You will also find fhe most common nursing diagnosis related to this assessment,** *Impaired Home Maintenance Management.***)**

✔ **Point to Ponder**
What aspects of your home environment contribute to the fulfillment of the higher level needs based on Maslow's hierarchy?

Impact of Aging on Environmental Safety and Function

Previous chapters have described some of the changes experienced with aging. These, along with limitations imposed by highly prevalent chronic diseases, create special environmental problems for elderly people, such as those listed in Table 22-4.

Of course, specific disabilities accompany various diseases and create unique environmental problems, as is witnessed with a person who is cognitively impaired. Based on common limitations found among older people, most elderly need an environment that is safe, functional, comfortable, personal, and normalizing and that compensates for their limitations.

Lighting

Light has a more profound effect than simply illuminating an area for better visibility. For example, light affects the following:

- *Function.* An individual may be more mobile and participate in more activities in a brightly lit area, whereas a person in a dim room may be more sedate.
- *Orientation.* An individual may lose the perspective of time if in a room that is constantly lit or darkened for long periods, as witnessed by persons exposed to the bright lighting in intensive care units for several days who cannot determine if it is day or night. A person who awakens in a pitch-dark room may be disoriented for a few seconds.
- *Mood and behavior.* Blinking psychedelic lights cause a different reaction from candlelight. In restaurants, customers are quieter and eat more slowly with soft, low illumination levels than with harsh, high ones.

Several diffuse lighting sources rather than a few bright ones are best in areas used by the elderly. Fluorescent lights are the most bothersome because of eye strain and glare. The use of fluorescent lighting for economic reasons actually may not be cost effective; although less expensive to operate, they have higher maintenance costs. Sunlight can be filtered by sheer curtains. The environment should be assessed for glare, paying particular attention to light bouncing off shining floors and furniture. Observe the

TABLE 22-4 ● *Potential Environmental Impact of Various Physical Limitations*

Limitation	Potential Environmental Impact
Presbyopia	Decreased ability to focus and visualize near objects
Cornea less translucent, transmits less light	More external light needed to produce adequate image on retina
Decreased opacity of sclera, allows more light to enter eye	Colors more washed out, more contrast required
Yellowing of lens	Distorted color vision, particularly for browns, beiges, blues, greens, violets
Senile cataracts cloud lens	Glare more bothersome
Macular degeneration	Vision more difficult, more magnification needed
Senile miosis, pupil size decreased, less light reaches retina	Slower light-to-dark accommodation
Decreased visual field	Peripheral vision narrower
Presbycusis	Distortion of normal sounds
Dependency on hearing aid	Amplification of all environmental sounds
Reduced olfaction	Odors, smoke, gas leaks difficult to detect
Less discriminating touch sensation	Less stimulation from textures
Less body insulation, lower body temperature	More sensitivity to lower environmental temperatures
Slower nerve conduction	Slower response to stimuli, less ability to regain balance
Decreased muscle tone and strength	Increased difficulty rising from a seated position, fatigue easier, less elevation of toes during ambulation, shuffling gait
Stiff joints	Difficulty climbing stairs, manipulating knobs and handles
Urinary frequency, nocturia	Frequent need for easily accessible bathroom
Shortness of breath, easily fatigued	Stairs, long hallways difficult to negotiate
Poor short-term memory	Forget to lock doors, turn off appliances
High use of medications, causing hypotension, dizziness	Increased risk of falls

environment's lighting from a seated position, because insufficient lighting, shadows, glare, and other problems can appear differently from chair or bed level than from a standing position.

KEY CONCEPT
Evaluate lighting from both seated and standing positions, because insufficient lighting, shadows, and glare can appear differently from chair or bed level than from a standing position.

Night-lights help facilitate orientation during the night and provide visibility to locate light switches or lamps for nighttime mobility. A soft red light can be useful at night in the bedroom because it improves night vision.

Natural light helps to maintain body rhythms, which, in turn, influence body temperature, sleep cycles, hormone production, and other functions. Exposure to light during the normal 24-hour dark–light

cycle keeps the body's biologic functions regulated; when the sleep–wake cycle is interrupted, the body's internal rhythms can be disrupted. This factor warrants attention to lighting in hospital and nursing home settings, where areas may be lit around the clock to facilitate staff activities; darkening areas at night can assist in maintaining normal body rhythms. Along this line, institutionalized or homebound ill elderly may have limited opportunities to go outdoors and be exposed to natural sunlight. Consideration should be given to taking these individuals outdoors, when possible, and opening windows to allow natural sunlight to enter.

Temperature

It has been known from Galen's time in 160 AD that hot and cold temperatures affect human beings and their performance. Research has shown that a direct correlation exists between body temperature and performance (Coaching Science Abstracts, 2001); tactile sensitivity, vigilance performance, and psychomotor tasks become impaired in temperatures below 55°F (13°C).

Their normally lower body temperature and decreased amount of natural insulation make the elderly especially sensitive to lower temperatures; thus, maintaining adequate environmental temperature becomes significant. The recommended room temperature for an older person should not be lower than 75°F (24°C). The older the person is, the narrower the range of temperature tolerated without adverse reactions. Room temperatures less than 70°F (21°C) can lead to hypothermia in the elderly.

> **KEY CONCEPT**
> Older adults are sensitive to lower environmental temperatures because of their lower body temperature and decreased amount of natural insulation.

Although not as significant a problem as hypothermia, hyperthermia can also create difficulty for older persons, who are more susceptible to its ill effects than younger adults. Brain damage can result from temperatures exceeding 106°F (41°C). Even in geographic areas that do not experience excessively high temperatures, consideration must be given to the temperature of rooms or homes in which doors and windows are not opened and no air conditioning is present. Persons with diabetes or cerebral atherosclerosis are at high risk for becoming hyperthermic. Refer to Chapter 38 for a discussion of heatstroke.

Colors

There is much debate concerning the best environmental color scheme for older people. Colors such as red, yellow, and white can be stimulating and increase pulse, blood pressure, and appetite, whereas blue, brown, and earth tones can be relaxing. Orange can stimulate appetite, whereas violet has the opposite effect. Green is considered the master healer color and gives a sense of well-being. Black and gray can be depressing. Although certain colors are associated with certain effects, experiences with colors play a significant part in individual reactions to and meanings inferred from various colors. Because individual response can vary, it may be best to focus on the use of colors to enhance function and, whenever possible, on the personal preference of the room's resident. Contrasting colors are helpful in defining doors, stairs, and level changes within an area. When the desire is to not draw attention to an area (eg, a storage closet), walls should be a similar color or within the same color family. Certain colors may be used to define different areas; bedrooms may be blue and green, eating and activity areas orange and red, and lounge areas gray and beige.

Patterned wall and floor coverings can add appeal to the environment; however, wavy patterns and diagonal lines can cause a sensation of dizziness and could worsen the confusion of persons with cognitive impairments. Using a simple pattern or a mural on one wall of the room can be effective and pleasing.

Scents

Scents have been used for aesthetic and medicinal purposes from the earliest of times. Although the use of perfumes and colognes is hardly new, the therapeutic use of scents, aromatherapy (or phytomedicine), has become popular in the United States only recently. However, it is a commonly used extension of orthodox medicine in countries such as Germany and France.

Aromatherapy implies more than the smelling of pleasant fragrances. Instead, it is the therapeutic use of essential oils. Essential oils are highly volatile droplets made by plants that are stored in their veins, glands, or sacs; when they are released (by crushing or breaking open the plant), the aroma is released along with them. When the chemicals within the essential oils are inhaled, they are carried to the olfactory bulb, stimulating nerve impulses that travel to the limbic system of the brain for processing. An organ called the amygdala is housed in the limbic system and stores memories associated with different scents. In some cases, the memories can be dormant for many years.

Essential oils also can be absorbed through the skin through baths, compresses, or rubbing or massaging them onto the skin surface. Like topical medications, these oils are absorbed and produce physiologic effects. **(Visit the Connection website to learn about therapeutic uses of scents and related precautions.)**

Floor Coverings

Most people believe that carpeting represents warmth, comfort, and a homelike atmosphere and that it is an effective sound absorber. There even has been speculation that the use of carpeting in institutional settings can reduce the number of fractures associated with falls. However, carpeting does create problems, which include the following:

- *Static electricity and cling.* Many older persons have a shuffling gait and incomplete toe lift during ambulation; uncomfortable static electricity can be produced, and the clinging of slippers and shoe soles to the carpeting could cause falls.
- *Difficult wheelchair mobility.* The more plush the carpet, the more difficult it becomes to roll wheels on its surface.
- *Cleaning.* Spills are more difficult to clean on a carpeted surface; even with washable surfaces, discoloration can result.
- *Odors.* Cigarette smoke and other odors can cling to carpeting, creating unpleasant odors. Urine, vomitus, and other substances demand special deodorizing efforts that may not prove effective.
- *Pests.* The undersurface of carpeting provides a wonderful environment in which cockroaches, moths, and other pests can reside.

To derive some of the benefits of carpeting, consideration may be given to carpeting some of the wall surface rather than the floor. This can provide a noise buffer, textural variation, and a decor with fewer housekeeping and maintenance problems than floor carpeting.

KEY CONCEPT

Carpeting a portion of the wall can provide a buffer for noise and offer a variation in room decor.

Scattered and area rugs provide an ideal source for falls and should not be used. Tiled floor covering should be laid on a wood foundation rather than directly on a cement surface for better insulation and cushion. Bold designs can cause dizziness and confusion in ambulation; a single solid color is preferable. A nonglare surface is essential for the elderly. Floor treatments that create a nonslip surface are particularly useful in bathrooms, kitchens, and areas leading from outside doors.

Furniture

Furnishings should be appealing, functional, and comfortable. A firm chair with arm rests provides support and assistance in rising from or lowering into the seat; low, sinking cushions are difficult for older people to use. Chairs should also be of an appropriate height to allow the individual's feet to rest flat on the floor with no pressure behind the knees. Rockers provide relaxation and some exercise to older people. Love seats are preferable to larger sofas because no one risks being seated in the center without arm rests for assistance.

Upholstery for all furniture should be easy to clean; thus, leather and vinyl coverings are more useful than cloth. Upholstery should be fire resistant, with a firm surface without buttons or seams in areas that come in contact with the body. Rather than the back, seat, and arm rest being one connecting unit, open space where these sections meet allows for ventilation and easier cleaning. Recliners can promote relaxation and provide a means for leg elevation, but they should not require strenuous effort to change positions.

Tables, bookcases, and other furniture should be sturdy and able to withstand weight from persons leaning for support. If table lamps are used, one should consider bolting them to the table surface so they are not knocked over in an attempt to locate them in the dark. Foot stools, candlestick tables, plant stands, and other small pieces of furniture would be best placed in low-traveled areas, if they must be present at all.

Drawers should be checked for ease of use. Sanding and waxing the corners and slides can facilitate their movement. In hanging mirrors, the height and function of the user must be considered; obviously, persons confined to wheelchairs will need a lower level than their ambulatory counterparts.

Individuals with cognitive impairments need a particularly simple environment. Furniture should look like furniture and not pieces of sculpture. The use of furniture should be clear. Placement of a commode chair next to a sitting chair can be confusing and result in the improper use of both.

Sensory Stimulation

By making thoughtful choices and capitalizing on the objects and activities of daily life, much can be done to create an environment that is pleasing and stimulating to the senses. Some suggestions are:

- textured wall surfaces
- soft blankets and spreads
- differently shaped and textured objects to hold (eg, a round sheepskin-covered throw pillow and a square tweed-covered one)
- murals, pictures, sculptures, and wall hangings
- plants and freshly cut flowers
- coffee brewing, food cooking, perfumes, and oils
- birds to listen to and animals to pet
- soft music

Different areas in the person's living space can be created for different sensory experiences. The appetite of nursing home residents could be much improved if, within their own dining area, they could smell the aroma of their coffee brewing or bread toasting rather than just having the finished product placed on a tray before them.

For bedbound persons or those with limited opportunity for sensory stimulation, special efforts are necessary. In addition to the suggestions given, one could regularly change the wall hangings in their rooms. Many libraries and museums will loan artwork free of charge. Collaboration with a local school can yield unique art for the older person and meaningful art projects for the students. One could also use a "sensory stimulation box" that contains objects of different textures, shapes, colors, and fragrances for an activity.

Noise Control

Sound produces a variety of physiologic and emotional effects. Many of the sounds we take for granted—television, traffic noise, conversation from an adjoining room, appliance motors, leaking faucets, and paging systems—can create difficulties for the older person. Many elderly already experience some hearing limitation as a result of presbycusis and need to be especially attentive to compensate for this deficit.

Environmental sounds compete with the sounds that the elderly want or need to hear, such as a telephone conversation or the evening news, resulting in poor hearing and frustration. Unwanted, unharmonic, or chronic noise can be a stressor and cause physical and emotional symptoms.

Ideally, noise control begins with the design of the building. Careful landscaping and walls can buffer outdoor noise. Acoustical ceilings, drapes, and carpeting—also useful on walls—are helpful, as is attention to appliance and equipment maintenance. Radios and televisions should not be playing when no one is listening; if one person needs a louder volume, earphones for that individual can prevent others from being exposed to high volumes. In institutional settings, individual pocket pagers are less disruptive than intercoms and paging systems. (**Visit the Connection website to learn more about sound.**)

Bathroom Hazards

Many accidental injuries occur in the bathroom and can be avoided with common sense and inexpensive measures. Particular attention should be paid to the following aspects.

Lighting. A small light should be on in the bathroom at all times. Because urinary frequency and nocturia are the norm, the elderly use the bathroom often and can benefit from the increased visibility. This is especially helpful if the switch is located inside the bathroom, so that the individual does not have to enter a dark area and then search for a switch.

Floor surface. Towels, hair dryers, and other items should not be left on the bathroom floor, and throw rugs should not be used. For older people, falls are dangerous under any circumstance, but with the high likelihood of falling and striking one's head on the hard surface of a tub or toilet, the potential seriousness of the fall increases. Leaks should be corrected to avoid creating slippery floors, which is another cause of falls.

Faucets. Lever-shaped faucet handles are easier to use than round ones or those that must have pressure exerted on them. Older people can risk falling or burning themselves by releasing too much hot water as they struggle to turn a faucet handle. This problem supports the need to control hot water temperature centrally. Color coding the faucet handles makes differentiation of hot and cold easier than small letters alone.

> **🗝 KEY CONCEPT**
> Lever-shaped faucet handles are easier than round ones for older adults to use.

Tubs and shower stalls. Nonslip surfaces are essential for tubs and shower floors. Grab bars on the wall and safety rails attached to the side of the tub offer support during transfers and a source of stabilization when bathing (Fig. 22-1). A shower or bath seat offers a place to sit when showering and, for tub bathers, a resting point when lifting to transfer out of the tub. Because a drop in blood pressure may follow bathing, it may be beneficial to have a seat alongside the tub to enable the bather to rest when drying.

Toilets. Grab bars or support frames aid in the difficult task of sitting down and rising from a toilet seat. Because the low height of toilet seats makes them difficult for many elderly to use, a raised seat attachment could prove useful.

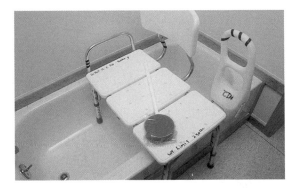

FIGURE 22-1

Safety features in this shower include grab bars, safety rails, shower seat, and transfer seat. (Craven, R.F., & Hirnle, C.J. [2003]. *Fundamentals of nursing: Human health and function* (4th ed., p. 665). Philadelphia: Lippincott Williams & Wilkins)

Electrical appliances. The use of electric heaters, hair dryers, and radios in the bathroom produces a considerable safety risk. Even healthy, agile persons can accidentally slip and pull an electric appliance into the tub with them.

Medical supply stores and health care equipment suppliers offer a variety of devices that can make the bathroom and other living areas safer and more functional. Sometimes less expensive replicas can be homemade and be equally effective. It is much wiser to invest in and use these assistive devices to prevent an injury than to wait until an injury occurs.

Psychosocial Considerations

Objects form only a partial picture of the environment. The human elements make the picture complete. Feelings and behavior influence and are influenced by the individual's surroundings.

From the homeless woman who claims the same department store alcove as her resting place each night to the nursing home resident who forbids anyone to open her bedside stand, most people want a space to define as their own. This territoriality is natural and common; many of us would become uncomfortable with a visitor to our office sifting through the papers on our desk, a house guest looking through our closets, or a stranger snuggling close to us on a subway when the rest of the seats are empty. The annoyance we feel at having someone looking into our window, peering over a privacy fence into our yard, playing music loudly enough to be heard in our home, or staring at us demonstrates that our personal space and privacy can be invaded without direct physical contact.

> **🗝 KEY CONCEPT**
> From the homeless woman who claims the same department store alcove each night to the nursing home resident who forbids anyone from opening her bedside stand, most people desire their own defined space.

To the dependent, ill, elderly person, privacy and personal space are no less important, but they are more difficult to achieve. In an institutional setting, staff and other patients may make uninvited contact with a person's territory and self at any time, ranging from the confused resident who wanders into others' rooms to staff members who lift blankets to check if the bed is dry. Even in the home, well-intentioned relatives may not think twice about discarding or moving personal possessions in the name of house-keeping or entering a bathroom unannounced just to ensure that all is well. The more dependent and ill individuals are, the more personal space and privacy may be invaded. Unfortunately, for these individuals who have experienced multiple losses and a shrinking social world, the regulation of privacy and personal space may be one of the few controls they can exercise. It is important that this be realized and respected by caregivers through several basic measures:

- Define a specific area and possessions that are the individual's (eg, this side of the room; this room in the house; this chair, bed, or closet).
- Provide privacy areas for periods of solitude. If a private room is not available, arrange furniture to achieve maximum privacy (eg, beds on different sides of the room facing different directions, use of bookshelves and plants as room dividers).
- Request permission to enter personal space. Imagine an invisible circle of about 5 to 10 feet around the person and ask before coming into it: "May I sit your new roommate next to you?" "Is it all right to come in?" "May I clean the inside of your closet?"
- Allow maximum control over one's space.

> **KEY CONCEPT**
> Regulation of personal space and privacy may be among the few existing controls that can be exercised by persons who have experienced multiple losses and a shrinking social world.

Components of the environment can facilitate or discourage mental and social activity. Clocks, calendars, and newspapers promote orientation and knowledge of current events. Easily accessible books and magazines challenge the mind and expand horizons. Games and hobbies can offer stimulation and an alternative to watching television. The placement of chairs in clusters or in busy but not heavily trafficked areas is conducive to interaction and involvement with a larger world.

Although fewer than 5% of the elderly reside in nursing homes, approximately 25% of older persons will spend some time in such a facility during their last years of life. Nursing homes are not reflections of normal homelike environments; adjustment to them can be difficult. Familiar surroundings are replaced with new and strange sights, sounds, odors, and people. Cues that triggered memory and function are gone, and new ones must be mastered at a time when reserves are low. Relatives and neighbors who gave love and understanding are replaced with people who know only that person before them now and who have many tasks to be done. The individual who is experiencing this may have a variety of reactions, such as:

- depression over the loss of health, personal possessions, and independence
- regression because of the inability to manage the stress at hand
- humiliation by having to request basic necessities and minor desires, such as toileting, a cup of tea, or a cigarette
- anger at the loss of control and freedom

Nursing homes cannot offer the same satisfaction as the person's own home, but the institutional environment can be enhanced through the following:

- an attractive decor
- inclusion of the individual's personal possessions
- respect for privacy and personal territory
- recognition of the individuality of the resident
- allowance of maximum control over activities and decision making
- environmental modifications to compensate for deficits

The human environment will be more important to the nursing home resident than the physical surroundings. Superior interior decoration and lovely color schemes mean little when respect, individuality, and sensitivity are absent.

Reducing Risks

Good preventive practices form the foundation for safety. In addition to the usual practices that would promote safety for persons of any age, additional measures must be promoted for older adults. These measures not only aid in avoiding injury and illness but also can increase self-care capacity in older adults. These considerations include the following.

SUFFICIENT FLUID INTAKE

Adequate fluid intake can be difficult for the elderly, particularly if they are depressed, demented, or physically incapable of maintaining good fluid and food intake. Thirst perception declines with age, causing older persons to be less aware of their fluid needs. Sometimes a self-imposed fluid restriction is a means of managing urinary frequency; in other situations the mental capacity to respond to the thirst sensation may be lacking. The result is insufficient fluid intake, which causes the body's already reduced tissue fluid reserves to be tapped. Unless contraindicated, the elderly should ingest at least 1300 mL of fluid each day. Many sources other than plain water can provide this requirement, including soft drinks, coffee, juices, Jello, ices, and fresh citrus fruits.

ADEQUATE NUTRITION

Poor oral health, gastrointestinal symptoms, altered cognition, depression, and dependency on others for food can lead to poor food intake. Even healthy elderly people may have difficulty ingesting a proper diet because of factors such as limited funds, problems in shopping for food, and lack of motivation to prepare healthy meals. The fatigue, weakness, dizziness, and other symptoms associated with a poor nutritional status can predispose the elderly to accidents and illness. An appropriate quality and quantity of food intake can increase the body's resistance to such problems (see Chap. 16 for specific information about nutritional needs).

VISION AIDS

Most people older than 40 years of age require corrective lenses, so it is no surprise that most elderly will use eyeglasses. The visual capacity of the elderly can change frequently enough that regular evaluation of vision and the effectiveness of prescribed lenses is warranted. Annual eye examinations are helpful not only in ensuring the appropriateness of corrective lenses but also in detecting, in a timely fashion, the many eye disorders that increase in prevalence with age.

HEARING AIDS

The ability to hear directions and warnings is basic to safety. Audiometric evaluation should be obtained for persons with hearing impairments to determine possible corrective measures and the benefit of hearing aids. Older persons should be advised not to purchase a hearing aid without an evaluation and prescription for their specific needs.

STABLE BODY TEMPERATURE

Temperature fluctuations can be hazardous to older individuals. The normal body temperature of many elderly persons is lower than that found in younger persons (eg, temperatures as low as 97°F [36°C] can be a normal finding in the elderly). Temperature elevation indicating a health problem can be missed if one is not aware of the person's baseline norm. For instance, a 99°F (37°C) temperature may not be alarming to the caregiver; however, if it is 2° above the individual's norm, an infection may be present and, if undiscovered, can lead to complications. In addition to having an undetected, untreated, underlying problem, an unrecognized temperature elevation places an added burden on the heart. For every 1°F elevation, the heart rate increases approximately 10 beats/min—a stress that older hearts do not tolerate well. At the other extreme, hypothermia develops more easily in older people and can cause serious complications and death.

INFECTION PREVENTION

In late life, the antigen–antibody reaction is altered because of immunologic changes, such as atrophy of the thymus gland and reticuloendothelial system and decreased immunoglobulin production. The elderly have decreased ability to produce antibodies in response to antigens. Furthermore, changes within various body systems can promote infections. Because the risk of developing infections is considerably greater in the elderly person than the younger adult, avoiding situations that contribute to infection is necessary. Contact with persons who have known or suspected infections should be avoided, as should crowds (eg, in shopping malls, classrooms, movie theaters) during flu season.

Vaccines should be kept up to date. The Centers for Disease Control and Prevention recommends that persons aged over 65 years, nursing home residents, and persons who have close contact with either of these groups be vaccinated against influenza annually. Pneumococcal vaccines, administered once in a lifetime, and tetanus vaccines every 10 years should also be current. In addition to avoiding external sources of infection, the elderly must be careful to ensure they do not create situations that predispose them to infection, such as immobility, malnutrition, and poor hygiene. Of course, good infection control practices are a must for preventing iatrogenic infections in elderly persons who receive services from health care providers.

Some evidence suggests that the herbs echinacea, goldenseal, and garlic can help prevent infection and that ginseng can assist with infection prevention by protecting the body from the ill effects of stress.

KEY CONCEPT

Vaccinations for older adults should include pneumococcal vaccination once in a lifetime, influenza vaccination annually, and tetanus and diphtheria vaccinations every 10 years. Other vaccines may be administered under special conditions. (See Chap. 21 for additional discussion of infections.)

SENSIBLE CLOTHING

Shoes that are too large, offer poor support, or have high heels can lead to falls, as can loose hosiery and robes or slacks that drag on the floor. Garters and tight-fitting shoes or garments can obstruct circulation. Hats and scarves can decrease the visual field. Clothing that is practical, properly fitting, and conducive to activity is advisable.

CAUTIOUS MEDICATION USE

The high number of drugs consumed by the elderly and the differences in the pharmacokinetics in the aged can lead to serious adverse effects. Drugs should be prescribed only when necessary and after nonpharmacologic measures of treatment have proved ineffective. The elderly and their caregivers should be taught the proper use, side effects, and interactions of all drugs they are taking, and be advised in the discreet use of over-the-counter drugs. (See Chap. 35 for more information on drugs.)

CRIME AVOIDANCE

The elderly are particularly vulnerable to criminals who view them as ready targets. Older people should use caution in negotiating contracts and seek the advice of family members or professionals as needed. Likewise, discretion should be used in traveling alone or at night and in opening doors to strangers.

SAFE DRIVING

It is estimated that the elderly drive an estimated 84 billion miles annually. Although when examined as a group, drivers over age 60 have lower accident rates than persons under age 30, accident rates begin to skyrocket after age 75. After age 85, older drivers are involved in four times the number of accidents on a mile-per-mile basis as persons aged 50 to 59, and when they are involved in accidents, they are 15 times more likely to die as drivers in their 40s (Carr, 2000; Straight & Jackson, 1999). Nurses should assist older drivers in identifying risks to safe driving (eg, poor vision, use of medications that reduce alertness, slower reflexes) and encourage them to evaluate their continued ability to drive safely. Rather than cease driving altogether, some older adults may find it useful to restrict their driving to daylight hours, noncongested areas, and good weather. Local chapters of the Automobile Association of America and senior citizen groups can be contacted for safe driving classes that could be offered to older adults. If such programs do not exist in the community, the gerontological nurse could stimulate interest and assist in developing them as a means of advocating for the safety of older drivers.

✔ Point to Ponder

Many people take calculated risks, such as exceeding the speed limit, practicing unsafe sex, abusing drugs, and failing to perform regular breast self-examinations. What risks do you take and why do you do so? What can you do to change this behavior?

Early Detection

The early identification and correction of health problems helps minimize risks to safety. Regular professional assessment is important; however, self-evaluation by the elderly can be equally beneficial because they will recognize changes or abnormalities in themselves that signal problems. It could be useful for older people to be taught how to perform the following measures:

- take their own temperature and pulse (do not assume that everyone knows the right way to use and read a thermometer or palpate a pulse)
- listen to their own lungs with a stethoscope (they may not be able to diagnose the sounds they hear, but they will be able to recognize a new or changed sound)
- observe changes in their own sputum, urine, and feces that could indicate problems
- identify the effectiveness, side effects, and adverse reactions of their medications
- recognize symptoms that should warrant professional evaluation

> **KEY CONCEPT**
> Changes, problems, and difficulties the elderly mention should be investigated, because they can be indicators of serious conditions.

Confusion, disorientation, poor judgment, and decreased memory handicap the elderly's ability to protect themselves from hazards to their health and well-being. When these symptoms occur, they are not to be taken lightly or accepted as normal. Often, the root of the problem can be a reversible disorder, such as hypotension, hypoglycemia, or infection. A competent evaluation is crucial to selecting the appropriate treatment modality and correcting the problem before complications occur. A review of the individual's behaviors and function can pinpoint potential safety risks. Examples of situations to note include:

- a person who smokes in bed
- an incontinent individual
- an individual who uses a walker inappropriately

- a person who is dizzy from a new medication
- an automobile driver with poor vision
- a frail individual who cashes Social Security checks in a high-crime area
- an active pet that is constantly underfoot

By observing and asking about routine activities, responsibilities, and typical tasks performed, these situations can be identified. Steps to correct potential problems should be taken before an incident occurs.

Risks Associated With Functional Impairment

A particularly high risk to safety exists when persons are functionally impaired, as exemplified by victims of Alzheimer's disease, for instance. These individuals may not understand the significance of symptoms, may lack the capability to avoid hazards, and may be unable to communicate needs and problems to others. Examples of impairments that could heighten safety risks include significant memory deficits, disorientation, dementia, delirium, depression, deafness, low vision, aphasia, and paralysis.

When such conditions exist, an assessment should be made to determine how activities of daily living (eg, food preparation, telephone use, medication administration, laundry, and housekeeping) are affected. Interventions are then planned to address specific problems and can include:

- referring the individual to occupational therapists, audiologists, ophthalmologists, psychiatrists, and other specialists for evaluation of the existing condition and prescription of appropriate treatment
- providing assistive devices and mobility aids and instruction in their use
- helping the person to prepare and label drugs for unit dose administration; develop a triggering and recording system for drug administration
- arranging for telephone reassurance, home health aid, home-delivered meals, housekeeper, emergency alarm system, or other community resources to assist the impaired person
- instructing and supporting family caregivers as they supervise and care for the impaired individual
- modifying the individual's environment to reduce hazards and promote function

Falls

One of the significant concerns about safety in later life relates to the incidence of falls. Studies have indicated that one third of persons age 75 years and older experience a fall each year and half of these experience multiple falls (Centers for Disease Control and Prevention [CDC], 2001). The consequences of falls are serious; 20% of the hospital and 40% of the nursing home admissions of older adults are related to falls (Sterling, O'Connor, & Bonadies, 2001). Even if no physical injury occurs, fall victims may develop a fear of falling again (ie, postfall syndrome) and reduce their activities as a result; this can lead to unnecessary dependency, loss of function, decreased socialization, and a poor quality of life.

Many factors contribute to the high incidence of falls in older adults.

* *Age-related changes:* reduced visual capacity; problems differentiating shades of the same color, particularly blues, greens, and violets; cataracts; poor vision at night and in dimly lit areas; less foot and toe lift during stepping; altered center of gravity leading to balance being lost more easily; slower responses; urinary frequency
* *Improper use of mobility aids:* using canes, walkers, wheelchairs without being prescribed, properly fitted, or instructed in safe use; not using brakes during transfers
* *Medications:* particularly those that can cause dizziness, drowsiness, orthostatic hypotension, and incontinence, such as antihypertensives, sedatives, antipsychotics, diuretics
* *Unsafe clothing:* poor-fitting shoes and socks, long robes or pants legs
* *Disease-related symptoms:* orthostatic hypotension, incontinence, reduced cerebral blood flow, edema, dizziness, weakness, fatigue, brittle bones, paralysis, ataxia, mood disturbances, confusion
* *Environmental hazards:* wet surfaces, waxed floors, objects on floor, poor lighting
* *Caregiver-related factors:* improper use of restraints, delays in responding to requests, unsafe practices, poor supervision of problem behaviors

A history of falls can predict an individual's risk of future falls; therefore, persons who have experienced a fall or even a minor stumble should be carefully assessed to identify factors that may increase their risk of this problem (Display 22-1). Interventions should be planned accordingly.

Health care facilities can find it beneficial to have an active program to prevent falls that incorporates some of the interventions described in the Nursing Diagnosis Highlight. Regular, careful inspection of the environment and prompt correction of environmental hazards (eg, leaks, cracks in walkways, and broken bed rails) are essential (Display 22-2). An evaluation of risk of falling should be incorporated into the assessment of each older client (see Nursing Diagnosis Highlight: *Risk for Injury*). Staff should orient older clients to new environments and reinforce safe practices, such as using bed rails, braking wheelchairs and stretchers during transfers, and promptly cleaning spills.

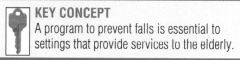

KEY CONCEPT
A program to prevent falls is essential to settings that provide services to the elderly.

Some falls will occur despite the best preventive measures. The fall victim should be assessed and kept immobile until a full examination for injury is done. Skin breaks or discoloration, swelling, bleeding, asymmetry of extremities, lengthening of a limb, and pain are among the findings to note. Medical examination and x-rays are warranted for even the slightest suspicion of a fracture or other serious injury. Fractures often are not readily apparent immediately after the fall; it may be only when the person attempts to resume normal activity that the injured bone becomes misaligned. Also, areas other than the direct point of impact may be injured in the fall; for instance, a person may have fallen on the knee, but the force of the fall may have placed enough stress on the hip to fracture the femur. Careful examination and observation can aid in the prompt diagnosis of injury and introduction of appropriate treatment.

Restraints

Throughout most of the 20th century, restraints were widely used in health care settings under the belief that they would prevent falls, promote patients' com-

DISPLAY 22-1

Risk Factors for Falls

History of falls
Female age 75 and older
Newly admitted to hospital/nursing home
Unfamiliar environment
Impaired vision
Gait disturbance
Physical disability
Incontinence, nocturia
Delirium, dementia
Mood disturbance
Dizziness
Weakness
Fatigue
Ataxia
Paralysis
Edema
Postural hypotension
Use of cane, walker, wheelchair, crutch, or brace
Use of restraint
Presence of IV, indwelling catheter
Unstable cardiac condition

Neurologic disease
Parkinsonism
Transient ischemic attack
Cerebrovascular accident
Diabetes mellitus
Peripheral vascular disease
Orthopedic disease
Foot problems
Multiple diagnoses
Medications
   Antidepressants
   Antihypertensives
   Antipsychotics
   Diuretics
   Sedatives
   Tranquilizers
   Multiple medications
Highly polished floors
Inadequate environmental lighting
Absence of railings, grab bars
Poor environmental design

pliance with treatments, and aid in managing behavioral symptoms. This practice was generally unchallenged until the 1990s, when studies began to emerge suggesting that restraints contribute to serious injuries and worsen cognitive function (Capezuti, Strumpf, Evans, Grisso, & Maslin, 1998). Since then, the combination of research-based clinical evidence, clinicial enlightenment, advocacy groups' efforts, and changed standards and regulations concerning restraints have contributed to a significant reduction in restraint use (CDC, 2000).

Restraints consist of anything that restricts freedom of movement. They can consist of physical restraints, such as seat belts, vests, wrist ties, "geri-chairs," bilateral full-length side rails, and chemical restraints, which are drugs given solely for the purpose of discipline or staff convenience.

As can be imagined, applying physical restraints to an already agitated person increases his or her fear and

worsens behavioral symptoms. This hardly reflects caring, compassionate practice. In addition, restraints can lead to serious complications, including aspiration, circulatory obstruction, cardiac stress, skin tears and ulcers, anorexia, dehydration, constipation, incontinence, fractures, and dislocations.

✔ **Point to Ponder**

How do you think you would react if you entered a hospital or nursing home room in which your loved one was being cared and found that person struggling to be freed from applied restraints?

Evidence now exists supporting that the use of physical restraints can be significantly reduced without increasing staffing or injuries (Strumpf, Evans, & Bourbonniete, 2001), therefore, nonuse of physical and chemical restraints is a standard that gerontolog-

D I S P L A Y   2 2 - 2

Environmental Checklist

Standard	Yes	No	Comments
Smoke detector			
Telephone			
Fire extinguisher			
Vented heating system			
Minimal clutter			
Functioning refrigerator			
Proper food storage			
Adequately lighted hallways and stairways			
Handrails on stairs			
Floor surface even, easy to clean, requiring no wax, free of loose scatter rugs and deep-pile carpets			
Doorways unobstructed, painted a contrasting color from wall			
Bathtub or shower with nonslip surface, safety rails, no electrical outlets nearby			
Hot water temperature less than 110°F (43°C)			
Windows screened, easy to reach and open			
Ample number of safe electrical outlets, probably 3 feet higher than level of floor for easy reach, not overloaded			
Safe stove with burner control on front			
Shelves within easy reach, sturdy			
Faucet handles easy to operate, clearly marked hot and cold			
Proper storage of medications, absence of outdated prescriptions			
For wheelchair use			

- Doorways and hallways clear and wide enough for passage
- Ramps or elevator
- Bathroom layout to provide maneuvering
- Sinks, furniture low enough to reach

ical nurses should promote in all clinical settings. A thorough assessment is beneficial in identifying factors that contribute to agitation and other negative behaviors; these factors could include visual deficits, impaired hearing, unrelieved pain, delirium, dyspnea, excess sensory stimulation, and lack of familiarity with a new environment. Addressing the specific factor contributing to the behavior could calm the patient and eliminate the need for restraints. When behaviors cannot be modified, alternatives to restraints can be considered, such as:

- placing patient in a room near the nursing station in which close observation and frequent contact are facilitated
- one-to-one supervision and companionship (often, family members and volunteers can provide this)
- use of electronic devices that alert staff when the patient attempts to get out of bed or leaves a designated area
- repositioning, soothing communication, touch, and other comfort measures

• frequent reality orientation and reassurance
• diversional activities

Close observation and documentation of patients' responses to restraints and alternatives to restraints are essential.

Safety Aids

When a fall, infection, or other problem occurs, the elderly take longer to recover and risk significantly more complications; thus, the key word in safety is *prevention*. A variety of practical methods, most of which are inexpensive, promote safety and should be considered in the care of the elderly.

> **KEY CONCEPT**
> Prevention is important because older adults require more time to recover from injuries and suffer more complications.

To compensate for reduced peripheral vision, affected individuals should be approached from the front rather than from the back or side, and furniture and frequently used items should be arranged in full view. Altered depth perception may hamper the ability of the aged to detect changes in levels; this may be alleviated by providing good lighting, eliminating clutter on stairways, using contrasting colors on stairs, and providing signals to indicate when a change in level is being approached. The filtering of low-tone colors is an important consideration when decorating areas for the elderly; bright reds, oranges, and yellows and contrasting colors on doors and windows can be appealing and helpful. Difficulty in differentiating between low-tone colors should be considered if urine testing is being taught to older diabetics because these tests often require color differentiation. Cleaning solutions, medications, and other materials should be labeled in large letters to prevent accidents or errors.

Directions and warnings can be missed because of poor hearing. Explanations and directions for diagnostic tests, medication administration, or other therapeutic measures should be explained in written, as well as verbal, form. These individuals should live close to someone with adequate hearing, who can alert them when fire alarms or other warnings are sounded. Specially trained dogs for the hearing impaired, similar to seeing-eye dogs, may prove useful; local hearing and speech associations can provide information on this and other resources.

Other sensory deficits, although more subtle, can predispose the elderly to serious risks. A decreased sense of smell can cause warnings to be missed and scents of harmful versus harmless substances to be undifferentiated. Electric stoves can help prevent gas intoxication from the inability to detect a gas odor. The loss of taste receptors may cause the elderly to use excessive amounts of salt and sugar in their diets, which is a possible health hazard. Reduced tactile sensation to pressure from shoes, dentures, or unchanged positions can cause skin breakdown, and the inability to differentiate between temperatures can cause burns. Careful observation, education, and environmental modifications to compensate for specific deficits should be planned.

Slower response and reaction times may be safety hazards. Older pedestrians may misjudge their ability to cross streets as traffic lights change, and older drivers may not be able to react quickly enough to avoid accidents; if family members are not available to escort and transport these individuals, assistance may be obtained through local social service agencies. Slower movement and poor coordination subject the elderly to falls and other accidents; loose rugs, slippery floors, clutter, and poorly fitting slippers and shoes should be eliminated. Rubber mats and nonslip strips are essential in the bathtub, where fainting and falls often occur as a result of hypotension caused first from the warm temperature of the bath water, which dilates the peripheral vessels, and then again from the orthostatic effect of rising to a standing position. Using a stool in the tub and resting before rising are useful measures. Because poor judgment, denial, or lack of awareness of their limitations may prevent them from protecting themselves, older people should be advised not to take risks, such as climbing ladders or sitting on ledges to wash windows.

The environmental checklist may also be useful in reviewing the safety of the elderly person's home.

NURSING DIAGNOSIS HIGHLIGHT

RISK FOR INJURY

Overview

Many older persons are limited in their ability to protect themselves from hazards to their health and well-being. Indications that this diagnosis exists can be manifested through a history of frequent falls or accidents, the presence of an unsafe environment, adverse drug reactions, infections, frequent hospitalizations, and altered mood or cognition.

Causative or contributing factors

Age-related changes, health problems, weak or immobile state, sensory deficits, improperly fitted or used mobility aids, unsafe use of medications, unsafe environment, altered mood or cognitive function

Goal

The patient is free from injury.

Interventions

- Assess risk of injury to patient (eg, falls risk, activities of daily living and impaired activities of daily living function, mental status, gait, medication use, nutritional status, environment, knowledge of injury prevention practices).
- Identify patients at high risk for injury and plan measures to reduce their specific risks.
- Orient patients to new environments.
- Encourage patients to wear prescribed eyeglasses, hearing aids, and prosthetic devices.
- Ensure patients use canes, walkers, and wheelchairs properly and only when prescribed.
- Avoid the use of physical or chemical restraints unless assessed to be absolutely necessary; use proper procedures to ensure safety when they are used.
- Advise patients to change positions slowly, holding on to a stable object as they do.
- Keep floors free from litter and clutter.
- Provide good lighting in all areas used by patient.
- Store cleaning solutions and other poisonous substances in a safe area.
- Encourage patients to use hand rails and grab bars.
- Assist patients as needed with transfers.
- Review medications used for continued need, effectiveness, appropriateness of dosage; instruct patients in safe medication use.
- Be sure patients wear well-fitted, low-heeled shoes and robes and pants of an appropriate length.
- Promptly detect and obtain treatment for changes in physical or mental health status.
- Review home environment for safety risks and assist patient in obtaining assistance in eliminating risks (eg, low-cost home improvements, housekeeping aid, or senior housing).
- If safety risks are associated with insufficient finances (inability to purchase prescriptions, heating oil, or home repairs) refer patient to social service agency to explore possibility of obtaining assistance.

Critical Thinking Exercises

1. Explain how Maslow's theory of low-level needs having to be fulfilled before one can concentrate on the fulfillment of high-level needs relates to satisfaction from one's environment.
2. What lighting, color selection, and decorations would be most therapeutic for the following areas used by older persons?
   bedroom
   recreation room
   dining room
3. List at least six hazards for the elderly in the average bathroom.
4. What measures can be taken to humanize an institutional environment?
5. Describe the safety risks that could result from the following health problems: hypertension, arthritis, right-sided weakness, and Alzheimer's disease.
6. What changes could be made to the average home to make it user friendly and safe for older adults?
7. What content could be included in a program to educate older adults about actions they can take to avoid accidents and injuries?

 Web Connect

Obtain older consumers' safety publications at the U.S. Consumer Product Safety Commission site www.cpsc.gov/cpscpub/pubs/older.html.

● References

Capezuit, E., Strumpf, N., Evans, L. K., Grisso, J. A., & Maslin, G. (1998). The relationship between physical restraint removal and falls and injuries among nursing home residents. *Journal of Gerontology, 53A,* M47–M52.

Carr, D. B. (2000). The older adult driver. *American Family Physician, 50*(1),141–150.

Centers for Disease Control and Prevention. (2000). *Falls in nursing homes.* National Center for Injury Prevention and Control, Centers for Disease Control and Prevention (producer). Retrieved from www.cdc.gov/ncipc/factsheets/nursing.htm.

Centers for Disease Control and Prevention. (2001). Web-based Injury Statistics Query and Reporting System (WISQARS) [database online]. National Center for Injury Prevention and Control, Centers for Disease Control and Prevention (producer). Retrieved April 1, 2004, from www.cdc.gov/ncipc/wisqars.

Coaching Science Abstracts. (2001). Temperature and performance 2. *Coaching Science Abstracts, 7*(2).

Sterling, D. A., O'Connor, J. A., & Bonadies, J. (2001). Geriatric falls: injury severity is high and dispropor-

tionate to mechanism. *Journal of Trauma-Injury, Infection and Critical Care, 50*(1), 116–119.

Straight, A., & Jackson, A. M. (1999). *Older drivers.* Washington, DC: AARP.

Strumpf, N., Evans, L., & Bourbonniere, M. (2001). Restraints. In M. Mezey (Ed.), *The encyclopedia of elder care* (pp.567–569). New York: Springer.

● Recommended Readings

American Geriatrics Association. *Position Paper on Restraints.* Retrieved April 1, 2004, from www.americangeriatrics.org/positionpapers/restrain.html.

Capezuti, E., Talerico, K. A., Cochran, I., Becker, H., Strumpf, N., & Evans, L. (1999). Individualized interventions to prevent bed-related falls and reduce siderail use. *Journal of Gerontological Nursing, 25*(11), 26–34.

Dunn, K. S. (2001). The effect of physical restraints on fall rates in older adults who are institutionalized. *Journal of Gerontological Nursing, 27*(10), 40–48.

Eagle, D. J., Salama, S., Whitman, D., Evans, L. A., Ho, E., & Olde, J. (1999). Comparison of three instruments in predicting accidental falls in selected inpatients in a general teaching hospital. *Journal of Gerontological Nursing, 25*(7), 4–45.

Fick, D., & Foreman, M. (2000). Consequences of not recognizing delirium superimposed on dementia in hospitalized elderly individuals. *Journal of Gerontological Nursing, 26*(1), 30–35.

Frandzel, S. (1996). The sound of healing: The role of music. *Alternative and Complementary Therapies, 2*(4), 225–229.

Hammer, R. M. (1999). The lived experience of being at home: A phenomenological investigation. *Journal of Gerontological Nursing, 25*(11), 10–18.

Harrison, B., Booth, D., & Algase, D. (2001). Studying fall risk factors among nursing home residents who fell. *Journal of Gerontological Nursing, 27*(10), 26–34.

Hausdorff, J. M., Rios, D. A., & Edelber, H. K. (2001). Gait variability and fall risk in community-living older adults: a 1-year prospective study. *Archives of Physical Medicine and Rehabilitation, 82*(8), 1050–1056.

Honeycutt, P. H. (2002). Factors contributing to falls in elderly men living in the community. *Geriatric Nursing, 23*(5), 250–257.

Horan, M., & Little, R. A. (1998). *Injury in the aging.* New York. Cambridge University Press.

Hughes, F. M. (1995). Creating functional environments for elder care facilities. *Geriatric Nursing, 16*(4), 172–176.

Kaufman, D. L. (1997). *Injuries and illness in the elderly.* St. Louis: Mosby.

Kelly, M. (1995). Consequences of visual impairments on leisure activities of the elderly. *Geriatric Nursing, 16*(6), 273–279.

Lin, B. A., et al. (1995). Falls among older people: Relationship to medication use and orthostatic hypotension. *Journal of the American Geriatrics Society, 43*(10), 1141–1145.

Lord, S. R., & Dayhew, J. (2001). Visual risk factors for falls in older people. *Journal of the American Geriatrics Society 49*, 508–515.

Luulinen, H., et al. (1995). Incidence of injury-causing falls among older adults by place of residence: A population-based study. *Journal of the American Geriatrics Society, 43*(8), 871–876.

Manion, P. S., & Rantz, M. J. (1995). Relocation stress syndrome: A comprehensive plan for long-term care admissions. *Geriatric Nursing, 16*(3), 108–112.

Middleton, H., Keene, R. G., Johnson, C., Elkins, A. D., & Lee, A. E. (1999). Physical and pharmacologic restraints in long-term care facilities. *Journal of Gerontological Nursing, 25*(7), 26–33.

Morse, J. M. (1997). *Preventing patient falls.* Thousand Oaks, CA: Sage.

Neufeld, R. R., et al. (1995). Can physically restrained nursing-home residents be untied safely? Intervention and evaluation design. *Journal of the American Geriatrics Society, 43*(9), 1264–1268.

Patrick, L., & Blodgett, A. (2001). Selecting patients for falls-prevention protocols: An evidence-based approach on a geriatric rehabilitation unit. *Journal of Gerontological Nursing, 27*(10), 22–25.

Patrick, L., Leber, M., Scrim, C., Gendron, I., & Eisner-Parsche, P. (1999). Standardized assessment and intervention protocol for managing risk for falls on a geriatric rehabilitation unit. *Journal of Gerontological Nursing, 25*(4), 40–47.

Pynoos, J. (1996). *Home modification resource guide* (2nd ed.). Los Angeles: Andrus Gerontology Center, University of Southern California.

Rantz, M. J., & McShane, R. E. (1995). Nursing interventions for chronically confused nursing home residents. *Geriatric Nursing, 16*(1), 22–26.

Rice, R. (1999). Environmental threats in the home: Home care nursing perspectives. *Geriatric Nursing, 20*, 165–166.

Roylance, F. D. (1995, October 4). Eye tests for elderly help cut traffic fatalities. *Baltimore Sunpapers*, p. A3.

Savage, T., & Matheis-Kraft, C. (2001). Fall occurrence in a geriatric psychiatry setting before and after a fall prevention program. *Journal of Gerontological Nursing, 27*(10), 49–53.

Silliman, R. A. (1995). Injury prevention in Alzheimer's disease patients: True possibility or pipe dream? *Journal of the American Geriatrics Society, 43*(7), 831–833.

Smith, D. B. (1995). Staffing and managing special care units for Alzheimer's patients. *Geriatric Nursing, 16*(3), 124–127.

Stevens, M., Holman, C. D., & Bennett, N. (2001). Preventing falls in older people: Impact of an intervention to reduce environmental hazards in the home. *Journal of the American Geriatrics Society, 49*(11), 1442–1447.

Stevens, M., Holman, C. D., & Bennett, N. (2001). Preventing falls in older people: Outcome evaluation of a randomized controlled trial. *Journal of the American Geriatrics Society, 49*(11), 1448–1455.

Sullivan-Marx, E. M. (2002). Achieving restraint-free care of acutely confused older adults. *Journal of Gerontological Nursing, 27*(4), 56–61.

Talerico, K. A., & Capezuti, E. (2001). Myths and facts about side rails. *American Journal of Nursing, 101*(7), 43–48.

Tideiksaar, R. (1997). *Falling in old age: Prevention and management* (2nd ed.). New York: Springer.

Tideiksaar, R. (1998). *Falls in older persons: Prevention and management* (2nd ed.). Baltimore: Health Professions Press.

Tinetti, M. E., et al. (1995). Risk factors for serious injury during falls by older persons in the community. *Journal of the American Geriatrics Society, 43*(9), 1214–1221.

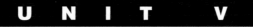

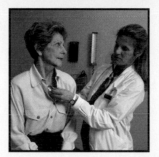

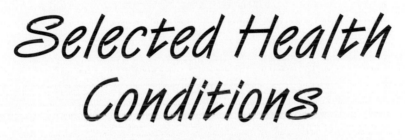

*Selected Health
Conditions*

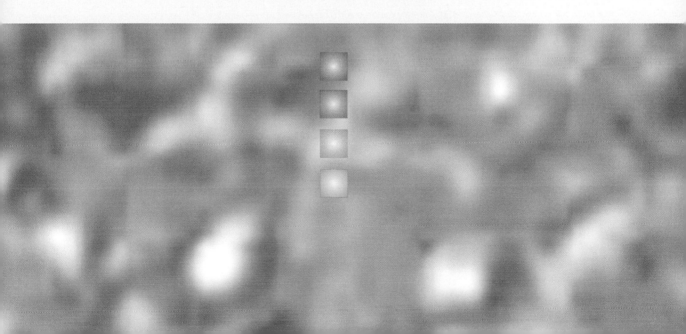

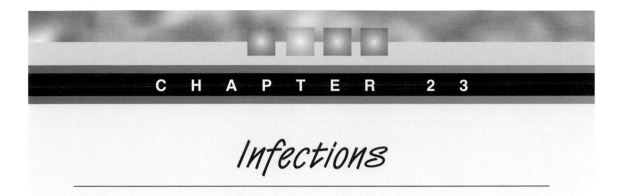

Infections

◼ Learning Objectives

After reading this chapter, you should be able to:

- describe unique features of the common infections of older adults

As described in Chapter 21, age-related changes in the immune system and the high prevalence of diseases in the older population heighten the risk for infections. Infections tend to have more profound effects in older adults, causing them significant consequences. Since the mid-1980s, the rates of hospitalization for septicemia among the elderly have more than doubled, with the primary sources being urinary tract infections, cystitis, pneu-monia, pressure ulcer, cellulitis, and renal infections (McBean & Rajamani, 2001). The elderly have a high rate of iatrogenic infections associated with their increased exposure to health care settings (ie, hospitalizations and nursing home residence). To compound matters, the elderly can have atypical presentations of infections (Display 23-1). Understanding the predisposing factors and related interventions to prevent the development of infections are basic to gerontological nursing practice.

Common Infections

URINARY TRACT INFECTIONS

Infections of the urinary tract are the most common infection of the aged, affecting as many as 1 in 10 elders annually (Foxman, 2002; Shortliffe & McCuc, 2002). Furthermore, urinary tract infections (UTIs) increase in prevalence with age. Although UTIs occur more frequently in women than men at younger ages, the gap between the sexes narrows in late life, which is attributable to reduced sexual intercourse in women and a higher incidence of bladder outlet obstruction secondary to benign prostatic hyperplasia in men. Organisms primarily responsible for UTIs are *Escherichia coli* in women and *Proteus* species in men. The presence of any foreign body in the urinary tract or anything that slows or obstructs the flow of urine (eg, immobilization, urethral strictures, neoplasms, or a clogged indwelling catheter) predisposes the individual to these infections. UTIs can result from poor hygienic practices, improper cleansing after bowel elimination, a predisposition created by low

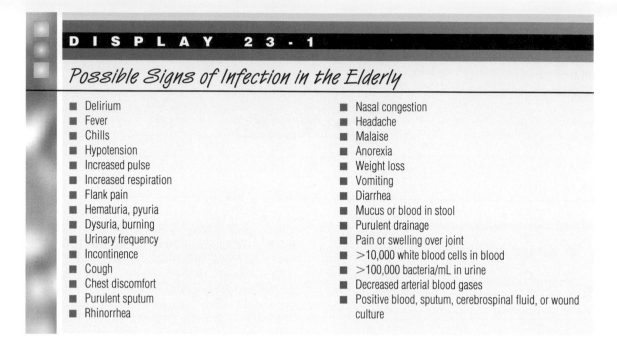

DISPLAY 23-1

Possible Signs of Infection in the Elderly

- Delirium
- Fever
- Chills
- Hypotension
- Increased pulse
- Increased respiration
- Flank pain
- Hematuria, pyuria
- Dysuria, burning
- Urinary frequency
- Incontinence
- Cough
- Chest discomfort
- Purulent sputum
- Rhinorrhea

- Nasal congestion
- Headache
- Malaise
- Anorexia
- Weight loss
- Vomiting
- Diarrhea
- Mucus or blood in stool
- Purulent drainage
- Pain or swelling over joint
- >10,000 white blood cells in blood
- >100,000 bacteria/mL in urine
- Decreased arterial blood gases
- Positive blood, sputum, cerebrospinal fluid, or wound culture

fluid intake and excessive fluid loss, and hormonal changes, which reduce the body's resistance. Persons in a debilitated state or who have neurogenic bladders, arteriosclerosis, or diabetes also have a high risk of developing UTIs.

> **KEY CONCEPT**
> Urinary tract infections can result from poor hygienic practices, prostate problems, catheterization, dehydration, diabetes, arteriosclerosis, neurogenic bladders, and general debilitated states.

The gerontological nurse should be alert to the signs and symptoms of this problem. Early indicators include burning, urgency, and fever. Some elders develop incontinence and delirium with UTIs. Awareness of the patient's normal body temperature helps the nurse recognize the presence of fever, for instance, 99°F (37°C) in a patient whose normal temperature is 96.8°F (35°C). Some urologists believe that many UTIs in older adults seem asymptomatic because of unawareness of elevations in normal temperature

from the baseline norm. The gerontological nurse can significantly facilitate diagnosis by informing the physician of temperature increases from the patient's normal level. Bacteriuria greater than 105 CFU/mL confirms the diagnosis of UTI. As a UTI progresses, retention, incontinence, and hematuria may occur.

Treatment aims to establish adequate urinary drainage and control the infection through antibiotic therapy. The nurse should carefully note the patient's fluid intake and output. Forcing fluids is advisable, provided that the patient's cardiac status does not contraindicate this action. Observation for new symptoms, bladder distention, skin irritation, and other unusual signs should continue as the patient recovers.

Severe UTIs leading to septicemia occur more frequently among older persons than the young, as do recurrent UTIs. Urosepsis (septicemia secondary to UTI) is a common complication of persons with indwelling catheters, emphasizing the importance of selective use of catheters.

Asymptomatic bacteriuria is a common finding in elders and usually is not treated, although it is important to assess underlying factors that could contribute to this condition.

Cranberry juice has long been promoted as a means to reduce UTIs; research now supports this belief. A study conducted at the Harvard Medical School demonstrated a reduction in the frequency of bacteria and white blood cells in the urine of women who regularly consumed cranberry juice (Goodine, 2002). The gerontological nurse may want to promote the daily inclusion of cranberry juice in the diet of older adults. (It may be best to use forms, such as capsules, that have no sugar added to avoid the high sugar content of some commercial brands; these capsules and other freeze-dried forms of cranberry juice are available at most health food stores.)

Prostatitis

Prostatitis is the most common UTI among older men. Although nonbacterial prostatitis is responsible for some cases, most infections are bacterial in origin. Acute bacterial prostatitis is characterized by the systemic symptoms of fever, chills, and malaise, whereas these symptoms are uncommon with chronic bacterial prostatitis. Both types will present urinary symptoms of frequency, nocturia, dysuria, and varying degrees of bladder obstruction secondary to an edematous, enlarged prostate, as well as lower back and perineal pain. A simple urinalysis usually can identify the pathogen responsible for acute bacterial prostatitis; with the chronic form, a special process may be used to collect a clean-catch urine sample, with prostatic secretions obtained by massaging the prostate during the procedure. Acute prostatitis usually responds well to antibiotic therapy; chronic prostatitis responds less well to antibiotics and is more difficult to treat.

> ### Point to Ponder
> *What self-care practices do you follow to strengthen your defenses against infection? In what ways could this be improved?*

PNEUMONIA

Pneumonia, especially bronchopneumonia, is common in the elderly and is one of the leading causes of death in this age group (Table 23-1). Several factors contribute to its high incidence:

TABLE 23-1 ● *Age and the Severity of Pneumonia*

	Death Rate/100,000
All ages	23.4
Ages 66–74 years	37.7
Ages 75–84	158
Ages 85+	748

(Source: National Vital Statistics Report. [2001]. *Deaths, percentage of total deaths, and death rates for 10 leading causes of death in selected age groups by race and sex,* Vol. 49, No. 11.)

- poor chest expansion and more shallow breathing due to age-related changes to the respiratory system
- high prevalence of respiratory diseases that promote mucus formation and bronchial obstruction
- lowered resistance to infection
- reduced sensitivity of pharyngeal reflexes that promotes aspiration of foreign material
- high incidence of conditions that cause reduced mobility and debilitation (Figure 23-1)
- greater likelihood for elders to be hospitalized or institutionalized and develop nosocomial pneumonia than younger persons

Pneumococcal pneumonia caused by *Streptococcus pneumoniae* is the most common type of pneumonia in the elderly. Other pneumonias are caused by gram-negative bacilli (*Klebsiella pneumoniae*), *Legionella pneumophila*, anaerobic bacteria, and influenza (*Haemophilus influenzae*).

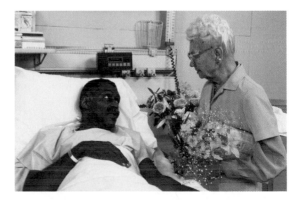

FIGURE 23-1

Immobile states increase the risk for pneumonia.

The signs and symptoms of pneumonia may be altered in older persons, and serious pneumonia may exist without symptoms being evident. Pleuritic pain, for instance, may not be as severe as that described by younger patients. Differences in body temperature may cause minimal or no fever. Symptoms may include a slight cough, fatigue, and rapid respiration. Confusion, restlessness, and behavioral changes may occur as a result of cerebral hypoxia. Nursing care for the older patient with pneumonia is similar to that used for the younger patient. Close observation for subtle changes is especially important. The aged patient can also develop the complication of paralytic ileus, which can be prevented by mobility.

> **KEY CONCEPT**
> Productive cough, fever, and chest pain may be atypical in older adults because of age-related changes and cause a delayed diagnosis of pneumonia.

Although their effectiveness continues to be debated, pneumococcal vaccines are recommended for persons over 65 years of age. The vaccine should not be administered during a febrile illness. Concurrent administration with influenza and some other vaccines is acceptable, providing that different injection sites are used. Common side effects are local redness, fever, myalgia, and malaise. Some individuals may experience arthritic flare-ups and, more rarely, paresthesias and other neuropathies. Despite the fact that the duration of protection from the vaccine is currently uncertain, the Centers for Disease Control and Prevention (CDC) recommend a single vaccination. Nurses should be sure to document the administration of the vaccine, along with the name of the manufacturer, lot number, and expiration date. The CDC also advised that if there is doubt whether the vaccine has already been given, it is best to administer the vaccine rather than risk pneumonia. The revaccination of elders with pneumococcal vaccines has been shown to cause local site reactions lasting several days but no life-threatening effects (Jackson et al., 2003).

INFLUENZA

Most deaths from influenza occur in the older population, emphasizing the seriousness of this infection to elders. Of the two subtypes of influenza, influenza A is the most frequent cause of serious illness and death in elders; influenza B is less severe, although it can produce serious problems for older adults. Age-related changes, including an impaired immune response to the virus, cause older persons to be highly susceptible to influenza. Typically, influenza causes fever (although not as high as in younger adults), myalgia, sore throat, and nonproductive cough. Once it attacks, influenza destroys ciliated epithelial cells of the respiratory tract and depresses mucociliary clearance. Secondary bacterial infections and other complications increase the risk of older adults dying as a result of influenza. Patients with chronic respiratory, cardiac, or metabolic disease are at particularly high risk of developing secondary bacteria pneumonia. Nonpulmonary complications can include myositis, pericarditis, Guillain-Barré syndrome, encephalitis, and a temporary loss of smell or taste.

Because influenza is acquired through inhalation of infected droplets, reducing contact with persons with known or suspected influenza is important. Prevention also can be achieved by annual influenza vaccination, which is recommended for persons over age 65 years. Although the elderly have lower antibody titers after vaccination than younger adults, vaccination can prevent severe complications associated with influenza, even if it does not prevent the disease itself. Approximately 2 weeks is needed for an antibody response to the vaccine; therefore, administration of the vaccine in October is recommended. Because the flu season can last through February, vaccinations for the elderly can be administered after October. Daily vitamin and mineral supplements with enhanced antioxidants have been shown to increase antibody titers in the elderly after influenza vaccines have been administered (Wouters-Wesseling et al., 2002), suggesting that the relatively safe practice of administering supplements be considered in gerontological care. Immunity gradually declines in the months following vaccination, which supports the need for annual revaccination. The vaccine is contraindicated in persons with febrile conditions and egg allergy and those with a history of Guillain-Barré syndrome. The blood level of carbamazepine, phenobarbital, phenytoin, theophylline, and warfarin can rise within 1 to 4 weeks after vaccination; therefore, patients using these drugs need to be closely monitored for toxic reactions. It is advisable for persons who work with older adults to be immunized.

KEY CONCEPT
Although the elderly have lower antibody titers than younger persons after vaccination, influenza vaccines can prevent severe complications associated with the disease, even if they do not prevent the disease itself.

TUBERCULOSIS

The incidence of tuberculosis has been increasing in the population as a whole since 1985, attributable, in part, to the acquired immunodeficiency syndrome (AIDS) epidemic, and a high incidence is found among persons residing in institutional settings. A reactivation of an earlier asymptomatic or improperly treated infection is more common than new infection in elders. Diagnosis may be delayed, either because the classic symptoms are not demonstrated or because symptoms resemble changes associated with many other geriatric conditions. For instance, anorexia, weight loss, and weakness may be the primary symptoms. Night sweats may not occur because of reduced diaphoresis with advanced age. Likewise, fever may not be detected because of alterations in body temperature in late life. These factors emphasize the importance of periodic evaluation for this disease.

Screening for tuberculosis should be performed for all patients entering a hospital or facility for geriatric care, and groups of older persons, such as senior citizen organizations, should be checked periodically. A two-step Mantoux test is recommended for elders because of the high incidence of false-negative results (ie, if the result is negative after the first test, the test should be repeated in 1 week, which could cause a conversion if the infection is present, owing to the booster phenomenon associated with a waned response).

KEY CONCEPT
Because of the risk of false-negative results, a two-step Mantoux test is recommended for tuberculosis screening in older adults.

Treatment follows the same principles as for any age group, basically consisting of rest, good nutrition, and medications. Some of the side effects of medications commonly prescribed for tuberculosis have special implications for older persons. Streptomycin can cause damage to the peripheral and central nervous systems, demonstrated through hearing limitations and disequilibrium, which create safety risks. Para-aminosalicylic acid can cause irritation to the gastrointestinal tract, anorexia, nausea, vomiting, and diarrhea, which can predispose elders to the risk of malnutrition. Changes in gastric secretions can cause these tablets to pass through the gastrointestinal system without being dissolved, thereby preventing a therapeutic benefit; stools should be examined for undissolved tablets. Isoniazid, although not as toxic as the other drugs mentioned, can have toxic effects on the peripheral and central nervous systems. The nurse must assess the patient regularly for the presence of adverse reactions to such medications.

A diagnosis of tuberculosis can be extremely difficult for some older persons to accept. Having lived through an era when people with tuberculosis were sent to sanitariums for long periods of time, older adults may be unaware of new approaches to treatment and fear institutionalization. Believing they could infect family and friends, they may avoid contact with others, promoting social isolation. It is possible that other people will fear contracting the disease and be reluctant to maintain social contact. Educating patients, their families, and friends is essential to clarify these misconceptions and promote a normal lifestyle. Patients should be taught their responsibilities in managing this disease. Medication is essential for the treatment of tuberculosis, and because the older person may have a problem remembering to take it, nurses should devise a system for helping the patient remember how to administer the medication. For example, medications and denture cream could be placed in the same box, so that during daily denture care, medications would be remembered. The patient, a family member, or a visiting nurse could fill seven envelopes with medications, labeling them for each day of the week, and devise a chart for recording when medication is taken. A family member or friend could call the patient daily to ask whether medication was taken. With prompt and proper therapy, the older person can recover from tuberculosis with minimal residual effects.

VAGINITIS

With advancing age, the vaginal epithelium thins, which is accompanied by a loss of tissue elasticity. Secretions become alkaline and of lesser quantity. The flora changes, affecting the natural protection that the vagina normally provides. These changes predispose the older woman to the common infection, senile vaginitis. Soreness, pruritus, burning, and a reddened vagina are symptoms, and the accompanying vaginal discharge is clear, brown, or white. As it progresses, vaginitis can cause bleeding and adhesions.

Local estrogens in suppository or cream form are usually effective in treating senile vaginitis. Nurses should ensure that patients understand the proper use of these topical medications and do not attempt to administer them orally. Boric acid, zinc, lysine, or gentian violet douches may also be prescribed. Some herbal medicine practitioners recommend a douche of antiseptic herbs, such as St. John's wort, goldenseal, echinacea, garlic, self-heal, and calendula. If the patient is to administer a douche at home, it is important to emphasize the need to measure the solution's temperature. Altered receptors for hot and cold temperatures and reduced pain sensation predispose the patient to burns from solutions excessively hot for fragile vaginal tissue. Good hygienic practices help treat and prevent vaginitis.

> **KEY CONCEPT**
> Older women should be advised to measure the temperature of douche solutions because altered receptors for temperatures and reduced pain sensations predispose them to burns.

Women can be advised to use a variety of natural approaches to the treatment of vaginitis. Vaginal infections have responded well to vitamins A, B complex, C, E, and β-carotene. An increased intake of acidophilus yogurt and garlic can help fight fungal infections, as can the avoidance of fermented foods and refined sugars.

HERPES ZOSTER

Herpes zoster, or shingles, is an acute viral infection usually caused in older adults by a reactivation of the latent varicella virus (the same virus that causes chickenpox) in the dorsal root ganglia. The weakening of immunity associated with aging is believed to contribute to the increased incidence of this problem with age; radiation, chemotherapy, or other factors that disturb immune mechanisms also can cause shingles.

The disease begins with pain and itching of the skin, followed in several days by the formation of vesicles. The eruption follows the path of a sensory nerve and can occur anywhere on the body, although the thoracic and abdominal areas are the most common sites. Treatment is symptomatic, consisting of analgesics, corticosteroids, and topical preparations to dry the lesions. Older adults are more likely than other age groups to experience postherpetic neuralgia. If herpes zoster is recurrent or if dissemination is widespread, the patient should be evaluated for the possibility of an underlying lymphoma or other immune deficiency.

> **KEY CONCEPT**
> Older adults are more likely than younger persons to experience postherpetic neuralgia.

SCABIES

Scabies is a highly contagious, pruritic skin eruption caused by a mite, the *Sarcoptes scabiei*. On contact, the female itch mite burrows under the skin and lays eggs. In 8 to 17 days, the larvae mature and travel to the skin surface to mate. After mating, the male dies on the skin surface while the female burrows back under the skin to lay eggs.

Intense pruritus, caused by an allergic reaction to the mites and their waste products, is characteristic of scabies. Pruritus worsens at night. On inspection, the skin appears excoriated. The rash typically is present in the interdigital webs, hands, wrists, elbows, abdominal folds, around the nipples, and on the genitalia, although older adults also can have a rash on the face, scalp, back, buttocks, and knees. Close examination of the rash can detect the burrow (a linear ridge with a vesicle on one end) where the mite is found. Without careful examination, the rash can be attributed to other dermatologic conditions, such as eczema; therefore, astute assessment is essential.

> **KEY CONCEPT**
> On inspection of the scabies rash, a burrow can be detected where the mite is located.

Diagnosis is made by scraping the lesions with a scalpel and having the material examined under a microscope for evidence of mites, eggs, or their wastes. A burrow ink test or application of mineral oil on the lesions can be done to enhance visualization of the burrows. Even with a negative finding on the scrapings, the patient may be treated if symptoms are consistent with scabies.

The case study in Display 23-2 describes the treatment and nursing care of patients with scabies.

HIV AND AIDS

Although HIV and AIDS are thought of as a younger person's disease, a little more than 10% of all cases occur in people over age 65—a number that has been consistent since the beginning of the AIDS epidemic (Centers for Disease Control and Prevention, 2003). Unfortunately, HIV and AIDS can be misdiagnosed due to the low index of suspicion in this age group. Health care professionals may not consider that older adults could be practicing unprotected sex (although without pregnancy to worry about, the probability of this is high) or be homosexual. Also, this infection can be overlooked due to the similarity of symptoms to common conditions in the elderly. For example, cognitive impairment may be attributed to Alzheimer's disease rather than HIV-related dementia.

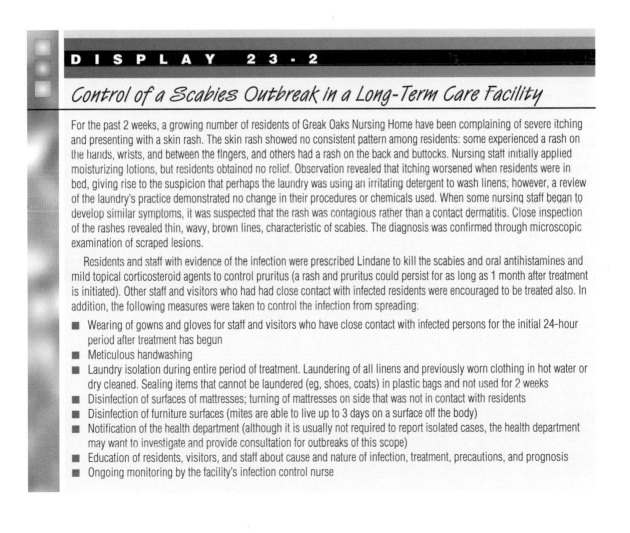

DISPLAY 23·2

Control of a Scabies Outbreak in a Long-Term Care Facility

For the past 2 weeks, a growing number of residents of Greak Oaks Nursing Home have been complaining of severe itching and presenting with a skin rash. The skin rash showed no consistent pattern among residents: some experienced a rash on the hands, wrists, and between the fingers, and others had a rash on the back and buttocks. Nursing staff initially applied moisturizing lotions, but residents obtained no relief. Observation revealed that itching worsened when residents were in bed, giving rise to the suspicion that perhaps the laundry was using an irritating detergent to wash linens; however, a review of the laundry's practice demonstrated no change in their procedures or chemicals used. When some nursing staff began to develop similar symptoms, it was suspected that the rash was contagious rather than a contact dermatitis. Close inspection of the rashes revealed thin, wavy, brown lines, characteristic of scabies. The diagnosis was confirmed through microscopic examination of scraped lesions.

Residents and staff with evidence of the infection were prescribed Lindane to kill the scabies and oral antihistamines and mild topical corticosteroid agents to control pruritus (a rash and pruritus could persist for as long as 1 month after treatment is initiated). Other staff and visitors who had had close contact with infected residents were encouraged to be treated also. In addition, the following measures were taken to control the infection from spreading:

- Wearing of gowns and gloves for staff and visitors who have close contact with infected persons for the initial 24-hour period after treatment has begun
- Meticulous handwashing
- Laundry isolation during entire period of treatment. Laundering of all linens and previously worn clothing in hot water or dry cleaned. Sealing items that cannot be laundered (eg, shoes, coats) in plastic bags and not used for 2 weeks
- Disinfection of surfaces of mattresses; turning of mattresses on side that was not in contact with residents
- Disinfection of furniture surfaces (mites are able to live up to 3 days on a surface off the body)
- Notification of the health department (although it is usually not required to report isolated cases, the health department may want to investigate and provide consultation for outbreaks of this scope)
- Education of residents, visitors, and staff about cause and nature of infection, treatment, precautions, and prognosis
- Ongoing monitoring by the facility's infection control nurse

KEY CONCEPT

Risk factors for HIV are the same for older people as younger adults and include vaginal or anal sex without using a condom; sharing needles or syringes; receiving transfusions, blood products, or organ transplants between 1978 and 1985; and getting tattoos or body piercings with a contaminated needle.

Point to Ponder

What values and attitudes do you hold that influence your feelings about people who have contracted HIV/AIDS in extramarital or homosexual relationships? How could this influence your care of these patients?

Initial symptoms appear within the first few weeks of being infected with the virus and resemble those of the flu, such as low-grade fever, headache, sore throat, fatigue, nausea, and a rash. These symptoms can last for several months, and then the infected person can be asymptomatic for several years. Blood will test positive for the HIV antibody about 2 months after the infection is contracted. Years after HIV has invaded the body, symptoms may appear again (Display 23-3). Infection with HIV needs to be considered when these symptoms are present. AIDS is diagnosed when people who are HIV positive develop decreased CD4+ lymphocyte count, an opportunistic infection (eg, pneumonia or septicemia), an opportunistic cancer (eg, Kaposi's sarcoma or invasive cervical cancer), wasting syndrome (loss of at least 10% of body weight), or dementia.

The high risk for infection of older adults is compounded when they have HIV/AIDS. Infection prevention measures need to be strictly adhered to, and signs of infection need to be identified early. Promotion of good nutrition can offer protection from infection and improve general health status. As these patients may become easily fatigued, mealtime assistance can spare their energy and facilitate good intake.

Emotional support is a crucial part of the care of any person with HIV/AIDS, and this may be even more significant for the elderly, particularly if their infection is associated with unprotected sex. Many people still feel uncomfortable with the notion of older adults being sexually active or engaging in homosexual relationships; therefore, older adults may have difficulty admitting their infection to close friends and family. In addition, the infected older adult may be rejected or treated with disdain by family and friends. A nonjudgmental attitude, listening ear, and emotional support are crucial components of the care of these patients.

D I S P L A Y   2 3 - 3

Symptoms That Can Develop Years After HIV Has Invaded the Body

Persistent fever	Herpes zoster
Drenching night sweats	Lymph node swelling
Headaches	Meningitis
Fatigue	Palsies
Chronic diarrhea	Pain
Thrush	Dementia
Persistent vaginitis	

ANTIBIOTIC-RESISTANT MICROORGANISMS

Methicillin-Resistant *Staphylococcus aureus* (MRSA)

A serious situation has evolved in recent years with the inability to control certain infections due to the resistance of pathogens to antibiotics. *Staphylococcus aureus*, a bacterium commonly found on the skin of healthy people, can enter the body and cause infections. The infections can range from minor (eg, boils or pimples) to quite serious (eg, pneumonia or septicemia). Until the introduction of penicillin, the fatality rate for bacteremia caused by *Staphylococcus aureus* was 90%, but the use of the antibiotic significantly improved survival. However, within a short period, a strain of *Staphylococcus aureus* grew that was resistant to penicillin. Methicillin was introduced in the 1960s as an effective new means of treating these infections, but in the 1980s, the pathogen grew resistant to this antibiotic and health care settings began to see epidemics of methicillin-resistant *Staphylococcus aureus* (MRSA) infections.

MRSA infection typically develops in hospitalized or institutionalized people who are elderly, are debilitated, or have an open wound or catheter that allows the bacteria to enter the body. It spreads through nasopharyngeal secretions and hands. For a time, vancomycin was effective against MRSA, but resistance to this antibiotic led to the need for new drugs. Linezolid (Zyvox) and the combination of quinupristin with dalfopristin (Synercid) have since offered treatment options.

Vancomycin-Resistant Enterococcus (VRE)

In the 1990s, strains of vancomycin-resistant *Enterococcus* (VRE) began to appear, which have now become a significant nosocomial infection. VRE infections tend to be resistant to most of the drugs previously used to treat such infections; furthermore, it is believed that genes present in VRE can be transferred to other gram-positive microorganisms, such as *Staphylococcus aureus*. Persons who are severely ill, debilitated, or immunosuppressed or who have had major surgical procedures, an indwelling urinary or central venous catheter, or antibiotic therapy are at risk for VRE infection. At present, Zyvox and Synercid are the only drugs effective against VRE.

It is important to promote immunologic health as part of infection prevention and control. Chapter 21 provides specific measures that can prove beneficial.

Critical Thinking Exercises

1. What would you include in a health education session to teaching elders about prevention, recognition, and care of influenza and pneumonia?
2. What are some of the reasons for HIV/AIDS not being identified in elders?
3. Describe potential implications for your community if the residents of a local senior citizen housing complex developed an acute respiratory infection that was resistant to all currently available antibiotics. What actions could be taken to protect the community?

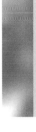

Web Connect

Find out about clinical trials, treatment options, and other facts about HIV/AIDS by visiting the website of the National Institute of Medicine's information page at http://sis.nlm.nih.gov/HIV.HIVMain.html.

● References

Centers for Disease Control and Prevention. (2003). *HIV/AIDS Surveillance Report: U.S. HIV and AIDS cases reported through December 1999 Year-End Edition Vol 11, No. 2* (Web Page). Retrieved January 15, 2003, from http://www.cdc.gov/hiv/stats/hasr1102.htm.

Foxman, B. (2002). Epidemiology of urinary tract infections: Incidence, morbidity, and economic costs. *American Journal of Medicine, 113*(Suppl 1A), 5S–13S.

Goodine, W. (2002). Regular drinking of cranberry-lingonberry juice concentrate reduced recurrent urinary tract infections in women. *Evidence Based Nursing, 5*(2), 43.

Jackson, L. A., Neuzil, K. M., Yu, O., Benson, P., Barlow, W. E., Adams, A. L., et al. (2003). Effectiveness of pneumococcal polysaccharide vaccine in older adults. *New England Journal of Medicine, 348*(18), 1747–1755.

McBean, M., and Rajamani, S. (2001). Septicemia rates double in the elderly. *Journal of Infectious Diseases, 183*(4), 596–603.

Shortliffe, L. M., and McCue, J. D. (2002). Urinary tract infection at the age extremes: Pediatrics and geriatrics. *American Journal of Medicine, 113*(Suppl 1A), 55S–66S.

Wouters-Wesseling, W., Rozendaal, M., Snijder, M., et al. (2002). Effect of a complete nutritional supplement on antibody response to influenza vaccine in elderly people. *Journals of Gerontology Series A: Biological Sciences and Medical Sciences, 57*(9), M563.

● Recommended Reading

Arden, N. H. (2001). Prevention and treatment of influenza in the long-term care facility. *Annals of Long-Term Care, 9*(12), 45–52.

Bockhold, K. M. (2000). Who's afraid of hepatitis C? *American Journal of Nursing, 100*(5), 26–32.

Cheraskin, E. (1999). Are antibiotics our best choice? *International Journal of Integrative Medicine, 1*(3), 36–38.

Cook, L. (1999). The value of lab values. *American Journal of Nursing, 99*(5), 66–68.

Cooper, J. W. (Ed.). (1996). *Antivirals in the elderly.* Binghamton, NY: Pharmaceutical Products Press.

Coyne, P. J., Lyne, M. E., & Watson, A. C. (2002). Symptom management in people with AIDS. *American Journal of Nursing, 102*(9), 48–64.

Fazzari, T. V. (1997). Stability of individual differences in cellular immune responses to acute psychological stress. *Advances: The Journal of Mind-Body Health, 13*(3), 36–37.

Gallucci, B. B. (1997). Neuroendocrine and immunological responses of women to stress. *Advances: The Journal of Mind-Body Health, 13*(3), 36.

Golczewski, J. A. (1998). *Aging: Strategies for maintaining good health and extending life.* Jefferson, NC: McFarland.

Jacelon, C. S. (1999). Preventing cascade iatrogenesis in hospitalized elders: An important role for nurses. *Journal of Gerontological Nursing, 25*(1), 27–30.

Kaufman, D. L. (1997). *Injuries and illness in the elderly.* St. Louis: Mosby.

Kirksey, K. M., Goodroad, B. K., Kemppainen, J. K., et al. (2002). Complementary therapy use in persons with HIV/AIDS. *Journal of Holistic Nursing, 20*(3), 250–263.

Lieberman, D., & Lieberman, D. (2001). Treating community-acquired pneumonia in the elderly. *Clinical Geriatrics, 9*(3), 66–74.

Mackenzie, D. L. (1999). When *E. coli* turns deadly. *RN, 62*(7), 28–32.

Maloney, C. (2002). Estrogen and recurrent UTI in postmenopausal women. *American Journal of Nursing, 102*(8), 44–60.

Metlay, J. P., Schultz, R., Li, Y. H., et al. (1997). Influence of age on symptoms at presentation in patients with community acquired pneumonia. *Archives of Internal Medicine, 157,* 1453–1459.

Meydani, S. N., Meydani, M., Blumberg, J. B., et al. (1997). Vitamin E supplementation and in vivo immune response in healthy elderly subjects. *Journal of the American Medical Association, 277,* 1380–1386.

Peters, P. H. (2001). Influenza and its impact on the elderly. *Clinical Geriatrics, 9*(2), 30–43.

Regan, S. F., & Fowler, C. (2002). Influenza: Past, present, and future. *Journal of Gerontological Nursing, 28*(11), 30–37.

Richards, C., Osterweil, D., & Stratton, C. W. (2001). From macrolides to ketolides: Meeting the antimicrobial needs in the current age of resistance. *Annals of Long-Term Care, 9*(8), 47–51.

Szirony, T. A. (1999). Infection with HIV in the elderly population. *Journal of Gerontological Nursing, 25*(10), 25–31.

Stern, E. (1997). Two cases of hepatitis C treated with herbs and supplements. *Journal of Alternative and Complementary Medicine: Research on Paradigm, Practice, and Policy, 3*(1), 77–82.

Trzcianowska, H., & Mortensen, E. (2001). HIV and AIDS: Separating fact from fiction. *American Journal of Nursing, 101*(6), 53–63.

Ungvarski, P. J. (2001). The past 20 years of AIDS. *American Journal of Nursing, 101*(6), 26–36.

Williams, A. B. (2001). Adherence to HIV regimens: Ten vital lessons. *American Journal of Nursing, 101*(6), 37–44.

Wisnivesky, J. P., Carnavali, F. C., & McGinn, T. G. (2001). Diagnosis and management of pulmonary tuberculosis in the elderly patient. *Clinical Geriatrics, 9*(8), 58–63.

Cardiovascular Conditions

■ Learning Objectives

After reading this chapter, you should be able to:

- list factors that promote cardiovascular health

- identify unique features of common cardiovascular diseases in the elderly

- describe nursing actions to assist patients with cardiovascular conditions

*I*mproved technology for early diagnosis and treatment and increased public awareness of the importance of proper nutrition, exercise, and smoking cessation have resulted in a decline in heart disease in the population as a whole. Future generations will experience fewer deaths and disabilities associated with cardiovascular diseases. Unfortunately, today's older population carries the insults of many years of inadequate preventive, diagnostic, and treatment practices and faces cardiovascular problems as the major cause of disability and death.

Facilitating Cardiovascular Health

The prevention of cardiovascular problems in all age groups is an important goal for all nurses to consider. By teaching the young and old to identify and lower risk factors related to cardiovascular disease, nurses promote optimum health and function. Important practices to reinforce include eating properly, getting adequate exercise, avoiding cigarette smoke, and managing stress.

PROPER NUTRITION

A diet that provides all daily requirements, maintains weight within an ideal range for height and age, and controls cholesterol intake is beneficial. Display 24-1 lists some general dietary guidelines for reducing the risk of cardiovascular disease. Some nutritional supplements can also help cardiovascular health (Display 24-2).

In recent years, Dr. Dean Ornish has promoted a diet that has been shown to be effective not only in preventing, but also in reversing, heart disease (Koertge et al., 2003; Ornish, 1996). The Reversal Diet for people who have cardiovascular disease consists of the following:

- less than 10% of calories from fat and very little of those from saturated fat
- high fiber intake
- exclusion of all oils and animal products, except nonfat milk and yogurt
- exclusion of caffeine and other stimulants
- allows, but does not encourage, less than 2 oz of alcohol per day
- no calorie restriction

Ornish's Prevention Diet is intended for persons with a cholesterol level less than 150 or a ratio of total cholesterol to high-density lipoprotein (HDL) cholesterol of less than 3 who have no cardiac disease and is similar to the Reversal Diet, with the exception that as much as 20% of calories can come from fat. (In addition to dietary modifications, Dr. Ornish's program advocates moderate exercise, increased intimacy, stress reduction, and other healthy practices.) In recent years, Ornish's diet has been criticized as being too restrictive of fats and contributing to the rise in obesity as people consume excess carbohydrates with the restricted fat intake. Despite the criticism and although many people find the restrictive diet proposed by Ornish to be difficult to follow on a long-term basis, any sustained dietary and lifestyle modifications that support the goals of reduced fats and stimulants, increased dietary fiber and exercise, and effective stress management certainly will move people in the right direction.

> **Point to Ponder**
> *Does your current diet increase your risk for cardiac disease? If so, what factors could present obstacles to you in changing your dietary pattern to one that is more vegetarian, and what could you do about overcoming these obstacles?*

D I S P L A Y 2 4 · 1

Dietary Guidelines for Reducing the Risk of Cardiovascular Disease

- Reduce the intake of fried foods, animal fats, and partially hydrogenated fats.
- Increase the intake of complex carbohydrates and fiber. Maintain caloric intake between ideal ranges.
- Use monounsaturated oils (eg, canola oil, cold-pressed olive oil) and omega-6 oils (eg, blackcurrant oil, evening primrose oil).
- Reduce intake of red meat, sugar, and highly processed foods.
- Consume alcoholic beverages in moderation

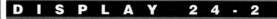

DISPLAY 24·2

Nutritional Supplements for Cardiovascular Health

Vitamin B6: effective in preventing the homocysteine-induced oxidation of cholesterol, which can aid in preventing heart attacks and strokes

Vitamin B12: can decrease homocysteine levels

Folic acid: essential for proper metabolism of homocysteine

Vitamin E: prevents abnormal blood clot formation, inhibits platelet aggregation, repairs lining cells of blood vessels

Vitamin C: helps prevent the formation of oxysterols, maintains integrity of arterial walls

Selenium: reduces platelet aggregation

Magnesium: aids in dilating arteries and facilitating circulation, may prevent calcification of vessels, lowers total cholesterol, raises high-density lipoprotein (HDL) cholesterol, inhibits platelet aggregation

Calcium: may decrease total cholesterol and inhibit platelet aggregation

Chromium: lowers total cholesterol and triglycerides (particularly when combined with niacin), raises HDL cholesterol

Potassium: can aid in reducing reliance on antihypertensives and diuretics

Fish oil: reduces deaths from coronary artery disease, lowers blood pressure

HYPERLIPIDEMIA

Hyperlipidemia is a significant risk factor in cardiovascular disease. In the past several decades, much has been learned about the significant reduction in cardiovascular and cerebrovascular incidents associated with the reduction of cholesterol levels in middle-aged persons. Although there is insufficient research to demonstrate the benefits in the elderly, reducing cholesterol intake is generally a positive practice. (For more discussion on hyperlipidemia, see Chapter 32.) Lifestyle modifications to lower cholesterol can also help people avoid the use of cholesterol medications, which, despite their benefits, can cause side effects, such as muscle pain, weakness, fatigue, erectile dysfunction, memory loss, and burning and tingling in the hands and feet.

ADEQUATE EXERCISE

Automobiles, elevators, modern appliances, and less physically exerting jobs lead to a more sedentary lifestyle than may be optimally healthy. Related to this may be the practice of being physically inactive during the week and then filling weekends with housecleaning, yard work, and sports activities. A sensible distribution of exercise throughout the week is advisable and is more beneficial to cardiovascular function than are periodic spurts of activity. The lack of physical exercise, known as physical deconditioning, can heighten many of the age-related functional declines that aging people can experience. On the other hand, a slower rate of decline and improved cardiovascular status has been found in middle-aged persons who exercised regularly. Persons who dislike scheduled exercise programs should be encouraged to maximize opportunities for exercise during their routine activities (eg, using stairs instead of an elevator, parking their car on the far end of the lot, or walking to the local newsstand to buy a newspaper instead of having it delivered).

CIGARETTE SMOKE AVOIDANCE

Although smokers are familiar with the health risks of cigarettes, breaking the habit is quite difficult, and, for this, people need more than to be *told* to stop. They require considerable support and assistance, which are often obtainable through smoking cessation programs. Acupuncture has proved helpful to some individuals for smoking cessation. Even if the patient has had repeated failures in attempting to quit, the next try could be successful and should be encouraged. In addition to avoiding cigarette smoking themselves, people should be instructed to limit their exposure to the cigarette smoke produced by others, which also can be detrimental.

STRESS MANAGEMENT

Stress is a normal part of all our lives. People should be taught to identify the stressors in their lives, their unique reactions to stress, and how they can more effectively manage stress. Relaxation exercises, yoga, meditation, and a variety of other stress-reducing activities can prove beneficial to nearly all persons.

Gerontological nurses understand that it is much easier and more useful to establish good health practices early in life than to change them or deal with their outcomes in old age. Furthermore, identifying cardiovascular problems early through astute assessment is critical (Display 24-3).

PROACTIVE INTERVENTIONS

Research continues to unfold that sheds light on routines that people can establish to promote healthy hearts. An aspirin a day can prove to be a good preventive measure, because low-dose aspirin has been shown to reduce the risk of heart attack (Yaes, 2003). A study of men who consumed alcohol at least 3 or 4 days per week showed a reduction in the risk of myocardial infarction, suggesting that moderate drinking could be beneficial (Mukamal et al., 2003). Of course, various nutritional supplements are suggested to have a role in cardiovascular health. Although additional insights are needed to fully understand the effects of these types of interventions, at this point it is reasonable to suggest that a daily low-dose aspirin, daily multivitamin supplement, and enjoyment of alcoholic beverages in moderation could be beneficial to adults of all ages in preventing cardiovascular disease.

> **KEY CONCEPT**
> Cardiovascular health in old age begins with positive health practices in younger years.

Cardiovascular Conditions

CONGESTIVE HEART FAILURE

The incidence of congestive heart failure (CHF) increases significantly with age and is a leading cause of hospitalization of elders. It is a potential complication in older patients with arteriosclerotic heart disease; the successful treatment of elders with myocardial infarction (MI) with thrombolytic agents contributes to the increasing incidence. Coronary artery disease is responsible for most cases of CHF, followed by hypertension; other conditions that can precipitate CHF in older adults include cor pulmonale, mitral stenosis, subacute bacterial endocarditis, hypothyroidism, anemia, vitamin deficiencies, bronchitis, pneumonia, and congenital heart disease. This problem is common in older adults because of age-related changes, such as reduced elasticity and lumen size of vessels and rises in blood pressure that interfere with the blood supply to the heart muscle. The decreased cardiac reserves limit the heart's ability to withstand effects of disease or injury.

Symptoms of this problem in older patients include dyspnea on exertion (the most common finding), confusion, insomnia, wandering during the night, agitation, depression, anorexia, nausea, weakness, shortness of breath, orthopnea, wheezing, weight gain, and bilateral ankle edema. On auscultation, moist crackles are heard. The detection of any of these symptoms should be promptly communicated to the physician.

History and physical examination assist in the confirmation of the diagnosis of CHF. The New York Heart Association has developed four categories of CHF that can be used in classifying the severity of the disease and guiding treatment (NYHA allows use of this classification system without permission):

- Class 1: Cardiac disease without physical limitation
- Class 2: Symptoms experienced with ordinary physical activity; slight limitations may be evident
- Class 3: Symptoms experienced with less than ordinary activities; physical activity significantly limited
- Class 4: Symptoms experienced with any activity and during rest; bedrest may be required

The management of CHF in elders is basically the same as in middle-aged adults, commonly consisting of bed rest, digitalis, diuretics, and a reduction in sodium intake. The patient may be allowed to sit in a chair next to the bed; usually, complete bed rest is discouraged to avoid the potential development of thrombosis and pulmonary congestion. The patient should be assisted into the chair, be adequately supported, and, while sitting, observed for signs of fatigue and dyspnea and changes in skin color and pulse.

Assessment of the Cardiovascular System

The early detection of cardiac problems can be difficult because of the atypical presentation of symptoms, the subtle nature of the progression of cardiac disease, and the ease with which cardiac symptoms can be mistakenly attributed to other health conditions (eg, indigestion, arthritis). Careful questioning and observation can yield valuable insight into problems that have recently developed or escaped recognition.

Clues to peripheral vascular disorders often can be detected through general contact with patients, who may comment that their feet always feel cold and numb, that they experience burning sensations in the calf, or that they become dizzy on rising. They may ambulate slowly, rub their legs, or kick off their shoes. Varicosities may be noted on the legs. Such observations can be used to introduce discussion of peripheral vascular problems.

General Observation

Assessment of the cardiovascular system can begin at the moment the nurse sees the patient by observing indicators of cardiovascular status. Such observations would note the following:

Generalized coloring: Pallor can accompany cardiovascular disorders.

Energy level: Fatigue and the amount of activity that can be tolerated should be noted.

Breathing pattern: Respirations can be observed while the patient ambulates, changes position, and speaks. Acute dyspnea warrants prompt medical attention because it can be a symptom of myocardial infarction in older adults.

Condition of nails: Inspection of the color, shape, thickness, curvature, and markings in nailbeds can give insight into problems. Blanching should be checked; circulatory insufficiency can delay the nails' return to pink after blanching. Advanced cardiac disease can cause clubbing of the nails.

Status of vessels: The vessels on the extremities, head, and neck should be inspected. Varicosities should be noted, as well as redness on the skin above a vessel.

Hair on extremities: Hair loss can accompany poor circulation.

Edema: Swelling of the ankles and fingers is often indicative of cardiovascular disorders.

Mental status: Inadequate cerebral circulation often manifests itself through confusion. Cognitive function and level of consciousness should be evaluated.

Interview

The interview should include a review of function, signs, and symptoms. Questions should be asked pertaining to the following:

Symptoms

Inquiry should be made into the presence of dizziness, light-headedness, edema, cold extremities, palpitations, blackouts, breathing difficulties, coughing, hemoptysis, chest pain or unusual sensations in chest, neck, back or jaws. It is helpful to use specific examples in questions: "Do you ever feel as though there is a vise pressing against your chest?" "Have you ever become sweaty and had trouble breathing while you felt that unusual sensation in your chest?" "Do you find that rings and shoes become tighter on you as the day goes on?" "Do you ever get the sensation of the room spinning when you rise from lying down?" When symptoms are reported, explore their frequency, duration, and management.

Some patients may be able to relate symptoms to vascular problems; however, others may be unaware that signs such as light-headedness, scaling skin, edema, or discoloration can be associated with peripheral vascular disorders; they must be asked specific questions. Information can be elicited through questions such as the following:

"Do your arms or legs ever become cold or numb?"
"Do dark spots or sores ever develop on your legs?"
"Do your legs get painful or swollen when you walk or stand?"

(Continued)

D I S P L A Y   2 4 - 3   (C o n t i n u e d)

"Do you ever have periods of feeling dizzy, lightheaded, or confused?"

"Does one leg ever look larger than the other?"

Family history of cardiac problems

Changes in function: the patient can be asked if changes in physical or mental function have been noticed using questions such as: "Do you have difficulty or have you noticed any changes in your ability to walk, work, or take care of yourself?" "Do you ever have periods in which your thinking doesn't seem clear?" "Have you had to restrict activities or change your lifestyle recently?"

Lifestyle practices

How often do you exercise and what type of exercises do you do?

What is your pattern of alcohol consumption?

What supplements (vitamin, herbal, homeopathic) are you using?

Do you do anything to promote health (e.g., take a daily aspirin, follow a special diet)?

Physical Examination

There should be an inspection of the patient from head to toe, noting areas of irritation or redness over a vessel, distended vessels, edema, and pallor. Blanching of the nailbeds gives information about circulation. An examination of the extremities should include palpitation of the pulses and temperature of the extremities and observation of hair distribution on the legs.

Assessment of apical and radial pulses is done and should normally reveal a pulse that ranges between 60 and 100 beats/min. Remember that older hearts take longer to recover from stress; thus, tachycardia may be detected as a result of a stress that occurred several hours earlier. If tachycardia is discovered in an elderly person, reassess in several hours.

Blood pressure assessment in three positions is important to determine the presence of postural hypotension; positional drops greater than 20 mm Hg are significant (Fig 24-1). Auscultation of the heart is done to detect thrills and bruits. Palpation of the point of maximal impulse can identify displacement, which can occur with problems such as left ventricular hypertrophy. Jugular venous pressure should be measured.

Pulses are palpated bilaterally for condition of the vessel wall, rate, rhythm, quality, contour, and equality at the following sites.

- Temporal pulse, the only palpable artery of the head, located anterior to the ear, overlying the temporal bone; normally appears tortuous
- Brachial pulse located in the groove between the biceps and triceps; usually palpated if arterial insufficiency is suspected
- Radial pulse branching from the brachial artery, the radial artery extends from the forearm to the wrist on the radial side and is palpated on the flexor surface of the wrist laterally
- Ulnar pulse also branching from the brachial artery, the ulnar artery extends from the forearm to the wrist on the ulnar side and is palpated on the flexor surface of the wrist medially; usually palpated if arterial insufficiency is suspected
- Femoral pulse, the femoral artery is palpated at the inguinal ligament midway between the anterosuperior iliac spine and the pubic tubercle
- Popliteal pulse located behind the knee, the popliteal artery is the continuation of the femoral artery; having the patient flex the knee during palpitation can aid in locating this pulse
- Posterior tibial pulse palpable behind and below the medial malleolus
- Dorsalis pedis pulse palpated at the groove between the first two tendons on the medial side of the dorsum of the foot; this and the posterior tibial pulse can be congenitally absent

Pulses are rated on a scale from 0 to 4:

0 = no pulse
1 = thready, easily obliterated pulse
2 = pulse difficult to palpate and easily obliterated
3 = normal pulse
4 = strong, bounding pulse, not obliterated with pressure.

(Continued)

Often, a stick figure is used to show the quality of pulses at different locations (Fig. 24–2). While the nurse assesses pulses, the vessels can be inspected for signs of phlebitis. Signs could include redness, tenderness, and edema over a vein. Sometimes, visible signs of inflammation may not be present, and the primary indication that phlebitis exists can be tenderness of the vessel detected through palpation. A positive Homans' sign (ie, pain when the affected leg is dorsiflexed) can accompany deep phlebitis of the leg. The legs should be inspected for discoloration, hair loss, edema, scaling skin, pallor, lesions, and tortuous-looking veins. Inspection of the nails can reveal thickness and dryness in the presence of cardiovascular disease. Skin temperature can be assessed by touching the skin surface in various areas.

Assure patient has had recent electrocardiogram and blood screening for cholesterol and CRP (Display 24-4).

Alterations in cerebral circulation can cause disruptions to cognitive function; therefore, a mental status evaluation can provide useful information about circulatory problems. During the assessment, actual and potential problems should be identified, and nursing diagnoses should be developed accordingly. Nursing Diagnosis Table 24-1 lists nursing diagnoses related to cardiovascular problems.

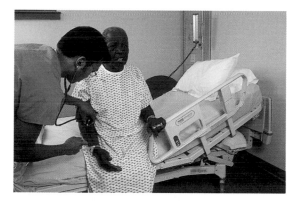

FIGURE 24-1

Assessing blood pressure in lying, sitting, and standing positions helps in identifying orthostatic hypotension. (Craven, R.F. & Hirnle, C.J. [2003]. *Fundamentals of nursing: Human health and function* [4th ed., p. 472]. Philadelphia: Lippincott Williams & Wilkins)

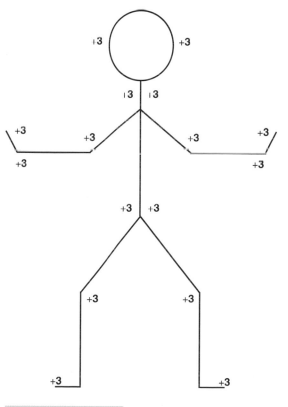

FIGURE 24-2

A stick figure may be used to describe the quality of the various pulses.

DISPLAY 24 - 4

Importance of C-Reactive Protein Screening

With the awareness that inflammation in the bloodstream can be a cause of heart attacks, the American Heart Association and the Centers for Disease Control and Prevention have recommended C-reactive protein (CRP) screening for persons at moderate risk of heart disease (Ridker, 2003). CRP is a marker of inflammation that is a stronger predictor of cardiovascular events than low-density lipoprotein (LDL) cholesterol. Two measures of CRP are suggested, with the lower value or the average being used to determine vascular risk. Because CRP levels are stable over long periods of time, are not affected by food intake, and demonstrate almost no circadian variation, there is no need to obtain fasting blood samples for CRP assessment. The cost of CRP testing is comparable to that of standard cholesterol screening and may be quite cost-effective in terms of avoiding serious complications and death.

Individuals with CRP levels > 3 mg/dL who have LDL cholesterol < 130 mg/dL are considered a high risk group and are advised to follow ATP III lifestyle interventions. People with an elevated CRP and LDL between 130–160 mg/dL are at elevated global risk and should be advised to adhere strictly to current ATP treatment guidelines. Those individuals with elevated CRP and LDL levels >160 mg/dL may need to be placed on medications and closely monitored for compliance to their treatment plan.

Significantly elevated levels of CRP could be related to other causes of systemic inflammation, such as lupus or endocarditis; additional diagnostic testing is warranted.

The nurse should be aware that the presence of edema and the poor nutrition of the tissues associated with this disease, along with the more fragile skin of the aged, all predispose the patient to a greater risk of skin breakdown. Regular skin care and frequent changes of positioning are essential. It must be recognized that this is a frightening, and often recurring, condition requiring a great deal of reassurance and emotional support.

Display 24-5 presents a care plan for the patient with CHF.

KEY CONCEPT

The risk of skin breakdown is high in persons with CHF because of the presence of edema and poor nutrition of the tissues.

PULMONARY EMBOLI

The incidence of pulmonary emboli is high in the elderly, but the detection and diagnosis of it in this age group are rare. Patients who are at high risk of developing this problem are those with a fractured hip, CHF, arrhythmias, and a history of thrombosis. Immobilization and malnourishment, which are frequent problems in the aged population, can contribute to pulmonary emboli. Symptoms that should be observed include confusion, apprehension, increasing dyspnea, slight temperature elevation, pneumonitis, and an elevated sedimentation rate. Older patients may not experience chest pain because of altered pain sensations, or their pain may be attributed to other existing problems. A lung scan or angiography may be done to confirm the diagnosis and establish the location, size, and extent of the problem. Treatment of pulmonary emboli in the elderly does not significantly differ from that used for the young.

CORONARY ARTERY DISEASE

Coronary artery disease is the popularly used phrase for ischemic heart disease. The prevalence of coronary artery disease increases with advanced age, so that some form of this disease exists in most persons 70 years of age or older.

ND *Nursing Diagnosis*

TABLE 24-1 ● *Nursing Diagnoses Related to Cardiovascular Problems*

Causes or Contributing Factors	Nursing Diagnosis
Insufficient oxygen transport, poor circulation, electrolyte imbalance, bed rest, pain, fatigue, effects of medications, fear of harming self	Activity Intolerance
Change in self-concept, fear of unknown procedures or diagnosis, hospitalization	Anxiety
Bed rest, medications, diet, stress, inactivity, insufficient fluids, pain, hospital environment	Constipation
Bradycardia, tachycardia, congestive heart failure, myocardial infarction, hypertension, cor pulmonale, stress, medications	Ineffective Tissue Perfusion
Vasospasm, occlusion, phlebitis, spasms, diagnostic tests, surgery, poor positioning, exertion	Acute Pain
Hospitalization, altered self-concept, helplessness	Ineffective Coping
Separation of patient from family, lack of knowledge	Compromised Family Coping
Hospitalization, forfeiture of activities, fear of impact	Deficient Diversional Activity
Patient's illness; financial, physical, and psychological burdens of illness; hospitalization; role changes	Interrupted Family Process
Change in function, disability, procedures, pain, lack of knowledge	Fear
Ascites, hypovolemia, anorexia	Deficient Fluid Volume
Decreased cardiac output, excess fluid intake, dependent venous pooling/stasis	Excess Fluid Volume
Change in body function or lifestyle, pain	Chronic Low Self-Esteem
Lack of knowedlge, loss of independence	Ineffective Health Maintenance
Disability, pain, fatigue	Impaired Home Maintenance
Impaired oxygen transport, invasive procedures, medications, immobility	Risk for Infection
Poor circulation, fatigue, immobility, pain, medications	Risk for Injury
Unfamiliar diagnostic tests, diagnosis, treatments, diet, ineffective coping, denial	Deficient Knowledge
Pain, fatigue, bed rest, edema, medications	Impaired Physical Mobility
Lack of knowledge or skill, prescribed plan in conflict with beliefs and practices, insufficient funds	Noncompliance
Anorexia, depression, stress, medications, nonacceptance of prescribed diet, anxiety	Imbalanced Nutrition: Less Than Body Requirements
Inability to participate in usual activities, lack of knowledge, hospitalization	Powerlessness
Immobility, pain, edema, fatigue	Self-Care Deficit
Change in body function, new diagnosis, hospitalization, immobility, pain	Disturbed Body Image
Metabolic changes, impaired oxygen transport, medications, immobility, pain, stress, hospital environment	Disturbed Sensory Perception

(continued)

ND *Nursing Diagnosis*

TABLE 24-1 ● *Nursing Diagnoses Related to Cardiovascular Problems* (continued)

Causes or Contributing Factors	Nursing Diagnosis
Pain, fatigue, fear, anxiety, depression, medications, hospitalization, lack of knowledge	Sexual Dysfunction
Edema, immobility, impaired oxygen transport	Impaired Skin Integrity
Impaired oxygen transport, immobility, hospitalization, pain, anxiety, inactivity, medications, depression	Disturbed Sleep Pattern
Metabolic or electrolyte imbalances, medications, anxiety, depression	Disturbed Thought Processes
Decreased cardiac output, myocardial infarction, angina, congestive heart failure, hypertension, vasoconstriction, hypotension, immobility, medications	Altered Tissue Perfusion
Diuretics, bed rest, hospital environment, anxiety	Impaired Urinary Elimination

Angina

A symptom of myocardial ischemia, the anginal syndrome presents in an atypical pattern, creating difficulty in detection. Pain may be diffuse and of a less severe nature than described by younger adults. The first indication of this problem may be a vague discomfort under the sternum, frequently after exertion or a large meal. The type of pain described and the relationship of the onset of pain to a meal may cause the patient and the health professional to attribute this discomfort to indigestion. As this condition progresses, the patient may experience precardial pain radiating down the left arm. Other symptoms can include coughing, syncope, sweating with exertion, and episodes of confusion.

The recurrence of anginal syndromes over many years can result in the formation of small areas of myocardial necrosis and fibrosis. Eventually, diffuse myocardial fibrosis occurs, leading to myocardial weakness and the potential risk of CHF.

Nitroglycerin has been effective in preventing and treating anginal attacks. Older persons are more likely to experience orthostatic hypotension with nitrates resulting from loss of vasomotor and baroreceptor reactivity. Because this drug may cause a drop in blood pressure, lower dosages may be indicated and the patient should be cautioned to sit or lie down after taking the tablet to prevent fainting episodes and falls. To prevent swallowing the tablet and thus blocking its absorption, patients should be reminded not to swallow their saliva for several minutes after sublingual administration. Long-acting nitrates are usually not prescribed for older adults. To prevent anginal syndromes, the patient should be taught and helped to avoid factors that may aggravate this problem, such as cold wind, emotional stress, strenuous activity, anemia, tachycardia, arrhythmias, and hyperthyroidism. Acupuncture has been shown to reduce the frequency and severity of angina attacks in some individuals and is a consideration. Because the pain associated with an MI may be similar to that of angina, patients should be instructed to notify the physician or nurse if pain is not relieved by nitroglycerin. Patients' charts should include factors that precipitate attacks, as well as the nature of the pain and its description by the patient, the method of management, and the usual number of nitroglycerin tablets used to alleviate the attack. Of course, education and support in reducing risk factors complement the plan of care.

KEY CONCEPT
Some anginal attacks can be prevented by avoiding factors such as cold wind, emotional stress, strenuous activity, anemia, and tachycardia.

DISPLAY 24-5

Sample Care Plan for the Patient With Congestive Heart Failure

Nursing Diagnosis

Activity Intolerance related to decreased cardiac output, pain, dyspnea, fatigue

Goal

The patient tolerates light-to-moderate activity without pain, dyspnea, or dysrhythmias

Actions

- Assess patient's ability to engage in activities of daily living; note presence of symptoms at various levels of activity.
- Schedule activities to avoid clustering of strenuous activities together (eg, shower, diagnostic test, physical therapy); plan rest periods before and after activities.
- Consult with physician to develop plan to gradually increase activity; monitor response and adjust activity accordingly.
- Administer oxygen as needed and prescribed; use nasal prongs rather than mask, because a mask tends to further increase anxiety and may not achieve an adequate seal against the patient's face. (Be aware that oxygen may be prescribed at lower levels or contraindicated for patients with chronic hypoxia.)
- Prevent and control pain; be alert to unique manifestations of pain in older adults (eg, altered mental status, apprehension, changes in functional capacity).
- Assess vital signs at rest and with activity. Note signs of decreased cardiac output (eg, drop in blood pressure, increased pulse).
- Monitor cardiac rhythm as ordered via electrocardiography or telemetry.
- Administer antidysrhythmic drugs as ordered; monitor response.
- Note alterations in mental status that could indicate cerebral hypoxia (eg, confusion, restlessness, decreased level of consciousness, agitation).

- Provide diversional activities to accommodate level of activity tolerance.

Expected Outcomes

The patient
- tolerates increasing levels of activity without pain or dyspnea
- maintains vital signs within normal range
- maintains normal mental status
- is free from dysrhythmias

Nursing Diagnosis

Impaired Skin Integrity related to edema and poor tissue nutrition

Goal

The patient is free from pressure ulcers and other impairments in skin integrity

Actions

- Assess amount of time patient can remain in position before signs of pressure are apparent; develop individualized turning and repositioning schedule.
- Use sheepskin, cushions, and other protective devices.
- Keep skin clean and dry.
- Ensure patient consumes adequate diet; consult with nutritionist for diet plan as needed.

Expected Outcome

- The patient maintains intact skin.

Nursing Diagnosis

Excess Fluid Volume related to ineffective pumping action of heart
Imbalanced Nutrition: Less Than Body Requirements related to decreased appetite, dyspnea, dietary restrictions, side effects of treatments

(Continued)

Goals

The patient
- maintains fluid and electrolyte balance
- ingests sufficient nutrients to meet body's metabolic needs without increasing cardiac workload

Actions

- Weigh patient daily (same time of day, same amount of clothing, same scale); record and report changes in weight that exceed 3 lb without relationship to dietary change.
- Inspect extremities, periorbital areas, and sacrum for edema; assess for jugular venous distension.
- Elevate and support extremities while patient sits.
- Apply antiembolism stockings or elastic wraps as ordered; remove for 10 minutes every 8 hours and inspect skin.
- Ensure patient complies with fluid and sodium restrictions as ordered; educate patient as necessary.
- Record and evaluate intake and output.
- Consult with dietitian regarding dietary restrictions and incorporating patient's preferences into diet.
- Administer diuretics as ordered; observe for signs of related fluid and electrolyte imbalances; educate patient as necessary.
- Monitor specific gravity and laboratory studies (eg, blood urea nitrogen, creatinine, electrolytes).
- Instruct patient to identify and report symptoms of worsening of condition (eg, swelling of ankles, loss of appetite, weight gain, shortness of breath).

Expected Outcomes

The patient
- demonstrates fluid and electrolyte balance
- complies with prescribed sodium and fluid restrictions
- demonstrates a reduction in weight or maintains weight within normal range
- demonstrates a reduction in or is free from edema

Nursing Diagnosis

Deficient Knowledge related to lifestyle modifications and caregiving needs associated with congestive heart failure

Goals

The patient
- describes care plan requirements and caregiving strategies
- demonstrates maximum self-care

Actions

- Assess learning needs.
- Consult with multidisciplinary team regarding recommendations pertaining to diet and fluid intake, activity, medications, exercise guidelines, and any precautions.
- Teach patient how to distribute rest and activity throughout the day to reduce workload of heart.
- Review symptoms that patient should identify and report, including weight gain of 3 or more pounds within a one to several days period of time, increased fatigue or weakness, dizziness, fainting or feeling faint, edema, shortness of breath, dyspnea with activities that were previously tolerated, cough, chest pain, abdominal pain or bloating, bleeding, bruising, or vomiting.
- Refer to community resources as needed (eg, support groups, healthy cooking classes).
- Supply with telephone numbers of physician, case manager, and other relevant contacts.

Expected Outcomes

The patient
- describes care plan and activities
- describes signs of complications that need to be reported to health care professional
- demonstrates self-care that adequately manages condition and reduces risk of complications

Myocardial Infarction

Myocardial infarction is frequently seen in older persons, especially in men with a history of hypertension and arteriosclerosis. The diagnosis of MI can be delayed or missed in older adults because of an atypical set of symptoms and the absence of pain. Symptoms include pain radiating to the left arm, the entire chest, the neck, and the abdomen; confusion; moist, pale skin; decreased blood pressure; syncope; cough; low-grade fever; and an elevated sedimentation rate. Output should be observed because partial or complete anuria may develop as this problem continues. Arrhythmias may occur, progressing to fibrillation and death, if untreated.

The trend in treating MI has been to reduce the amount of time in which the patient is limited to bed rest and to replace complete bed rest with allowing the patient to sit in an armchair next to the bed. The patient should be assisted into the chair with minimal exertion by him or her. Arms should be supported to avoid strain on the heart. Not only does this armchair treatment help to prevent many of the complications associated with immobility, but it also prevents pooling of the blood in the pulmonary vessels, thereby decreasing the work of the heart.

Early ambulation following an MI is encouraged. Typically, patients are allowed out of bed within a few days of an uncomplicated MI and are ambulating shortly thereafter. Getting out of bed early can be beneficial for the heart (using a bedpan puts more work on the heart than using a commode), maintains the body's condition, and assists in the prevention of complications associated with immobility.

Thrombolytic therapy is commonly used, and because older persons are more susceptible to cerebral and intestinal bleeding, close nursing observation for signs of bleeding is essential. Nurses should be alert to signs of developing pulmonary edema and CHF, potential complications for the geriatric patient with an MI. These and other observations, such as persistent dyspnea, cyanosis, decreasing blood pressure, rising temperature, and arrhythmias, reflect a problem in the patient's recovery and should be brought to the physician's attention promptly.

Fitness programs have shown to be beneficial for older persons with coronary artery disease in improving cardiac functional capacity, reducing ischemic episodes, decreasing the risk of complications, and promoting a sense of well-being and control over the disease. Walking, swimming, and bicycling are excellent rhythmic, aerobic means of exercise for older adults. Aggressive sports are not necessarily excluded but do present a greater challenge in controlling heart rate during the exercise. All exercise sessions should begin with a 5-minute warm-up and end with a 5- to 10-minute cool-down of low-intensity exercises. Nurses should advise patients to obtain a medical evaluation and exercise test before engaging in a fitness program. Usually, a target heart rate during the exercise is recommended, which is approximately 70% to 85% of the maximal heart rate.

> 🔑 **KEY CONCEPT**
> Fitness programs for older persons with coronary artery disease can improve cardiac functional capacity, reduce ischemic episodes, decrease the risk of complications, and promote a sense of well-being and control over the illness.

HYPERTENSION

The incidence of hypertension increases with advancing age and is the most prevalent cardiovascular disease of the elderly, making it a problem the gerontological nurse commonly encounters. Many elders have high blood pressure arising from the vasoconstriction associated with aging, which produces peripheral resistance. Hyperthyroidism, parkinsonism, Paget disease, anemia, and a thiamine deficiency can also be responsible for hypertension.

Individuals with a systolic pressure ≥ 140 and a diastolic > 90 are considered hypertensive, although treatment may not be initiated until the older person's blood pressure is equal to or greater than 180 mm Hg systolic and 90 mm Hg diastolic and the person is symptomatic. The nurse should carefully assess the patient's blood pressure by checking it several times with the person in standing, sitting, and prone positions. Anxiety, stress, or activity before the blood pressure check should be noted, because these factors may be responsible for a temporary elevation. The anxiety of being examined by a physician or of preparing for and experiencing a visit to a clinic frequently causes elevated blood pressure in a usually normotensive individual.

Awakening with a dull headache, impaired memory, disorientation, confusion, epistaxis, and a slow tremor may be symptoms of hypertension. The presence of these symptoms with an elevated blood pressure reading usually warrants treatment. Hypertensive older patients are advised to rest, reduce their sodium intake, and, if necessary, reduce their weight. Aggressive antihypertensive therapy is discouraged for older persons because of the risk of a sudden dangerous decrease in blood pressure. Nurses should observe for signs indicating blood pressure that is too low to meet the patient's demands, such as dizziness, confusion, syncope, restlessness, and drowsiness. An elevated blood urea nitrogen level may be present also. These signs should be observed for and communicated to the physician if they appear. In the management of the older hypertensive person, it is a challenge to achieve a blood pressure level high enough to provide optimum circulation yet low enough to prevent serious related complications.

Controversy still exists as to the proper treatment of hypertension in older patients; therefore, hypertensive elderly may receive a wide range of therapy, rather than antihypertensive drugs alone. Drugs that can be used to treat hypertension include diuretics, beta-blockers, calcium channel blockers, and angiotensin-converting enzyme (ACE) inhibitors. Because they have a higher risk for adverse reactions from antihypertensive drugs, older patients should be assisted in using nonpharmacologic measures to reduce blood pressure whenever possible. Biofeedback, yoga, meditation, and relaxation exercises have all proven effective in reducing blood pressure. In fact, the National Institutes of Health recommended meditation over prescription drugs for mild hypertension (Astin, Shapiro, Eisenberg, & Forys, 2003). Fish oil supplements can reduce blood pressure in hypertensive individuals. Some herbs have hypotensive effects, including garlic, hawthorn berries, rauwolfia, and periwinkle. On the other hand, herbs like ginseng and licorice can cause a rise in blood pressure when used regularly.

 KEY CONCEPT
Biofeedback, yoga, meditation, and relaxation exercises have been effective in reducing blood pressure.

HYPOTENSION

A decline in systolic blood pressure of 20 mm Hg or more after rising and standing for 1 minute is postural hypotension and a similar reduction within 1 hour of eating is postprandial hypotension. Various studies have shown that many elders experience problems related to postprandial and postural hypotension due to the increased intake of vasoactive medications and concomitant decrease in physiologic function, such as baroreceptor sensitivity (Frishman et al., 2003). This can be secondary to age-related changes, such as blunting of the baroreflex-mediated heart rate response to hypotensive and hypertensive stimuli and the presence of diseases that affect the heart. Postprandial hypotension also can be related to antihypertensive medications taken before eating and a high carbohydrate intake at meals (the effects of this can be prevented by drinking a caffeinated beverage after the meal). Hypotension can have serious consequences for elders, including a high risk for falls, stroke, syncope, and coronary complications.

ARRHYTHMIAS

Digitalis toxicity, hypokalemia, acute infections, hemorrhage, anginal syndrome, and coronary insufficiency are some of the many factors that cause an increasing incidence of arrhythmias with age. Of the causes mentioned, digitalis toxicity is the most common.

The basic principles of treatment for arrhythmias do not vary much for older adults. Tranquilizers, digitalis, and potassium supplements are part of the therapy prescribed. Patient education may be warranted to help the individual modify diet, smoking, drinking, and activity patterns. The nurse should be aware that digitalis toxicity can progress in the absence of clinical signs and with blood levels within a normal range, and that the effects can be evident even 2 weeks after the drug has been discontinued. This reinforces the importance of nursing assessment and monitoring to detect subtle changes and atypical symptoms. Older people have a higher mortality rate from cardiac arrest than other segments of the population, which emphasizes the necessity for close nursing observations and early problem detection to prevent this serious complication.

PERIPHERAL VASCULAR DISEASE

Arteriosclerosis

Arteriosclerosis is a common problem among older persons, especially those who have diabetes. Unlike atherosclerosis, which generally affects the large vessels coming from the heart, arteriosclerosis most often affects the smaller vessels farthest from the heart. Arteriography and radiography can be used to diagnose arteriosclerosis, and oscillometric testing can assess the arterial pulse at different levels. If surface temperature is evaluated as a diagnostic measure, the nurse should keep the patient in a warm, stable room temperature for at least 1 hour before testing. Treatment of arteriosclerosis includes bed rest, warmth, Buerger-Allen exercises (Fig. 24-3), and vasodilators. Occasionally, a permanent vasodilation effect is achieved by performing a sympathetic ganglionectomy.

Special Problems Associated With Diabetes

Persons with diabetes, who have a high risk of developing peripheral vascular problems and associated complications, commonly display the diabetes-associated neuropathies and infections that affect vessels throughout the entire body. Arterial insufficiency can present in several ways. Resting pain may occur as a re-

sult of intermittent claudication, arterial pulses may be difficult to find or totally absent, and skin discoloration, ulcerations, and gangrene may be present. Diagnostic measures, similar to those used to determine the degree of arterial insufficiency with other problems, include oscillometry, elevation-dependency tests, and palpation of pulses and skin temperatures at different sites. When surgery is possible, arteriography may be done to establish the exact size and location of the arterial lesion. The treatment selected will depend on the extent of the disease. Walking can promote collateral circulation and may constitute sufficient management if intermittent claudication is the sole problem. Analgesics can provide relief from resting pain.

Because many of today's elders may have witnessed severe disability and death among others with the disease they have known throughout their lives, they need to be assured that improved methods of medical and surgical management—perhaps not even developed at the time their parents and grandparents had diabetes—increase their chances for a full, independent life.

Aneurysms

In older adults, advanced arteriosclerosis is usually responsible for the development of aneurysms, although they may also result from infection, trauma,

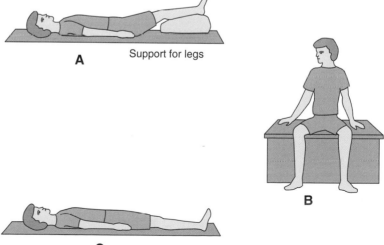

FIGURE 24-3

Buerger-Allen exercises. (**A**) The patient lies flat with legs elevated above the level of the heart until blanching occurs (about 2 minutes). (**B**) The patient lowers legs to fill the vessels and exercises feet until the legs are pink (about 5 minutes). (**C**) The patient lies flat for about 5 minutes before repeating the exercises. The entire procedure is done five times, or as tolerated by the patient, at three different times during the day. The nurse should assist the patient with position changes, because postural hypotension can occur. The patient's tolerance and the effectiveness of the procedure should be noted.

Support for legs

A

B

C

syphilis, and other factors. Some aneurysms can be seen by the naked eye and are able to be palpated as a pulsating mass; others can only be detected by radiography. A thrombosis can develop in the aneurysm, leading to an arterial occlusion or rupture of the aneurysm—the most serious complications associated with this problem.

Aneurysms of the abdominal aorta most frequently occur in older people. Patients with a history of arteriosclerotic lesions, angina pectoris, MI, and CHF more commonly develop aneurysms in this area. A pulsating mass, sometimes painful, in the umbilical region is an indication of an abdominal aortic aneurysm. Prompt correction is essential because, if not corrected, rupture can occur. Fewer complications and deaths result from surgical intervention before rupture. Among the complications that older adults can develop after surgery for this problem are hemorrhage, MI, cerebrovascular accident, and acute renal insufficiency. The nurse should observe closely for signs of postoperative complications.

> **KEY CONCEPT**
> Abdominal aortic aneurysms are a high risk in persons with a history of arteriosclerotic lesions, angina pectoris, MI, and CHF.

Aneurysms can develop in peripheral arteries, the most common sites being the femoral and popliteal arteries. Peripheral aneurysms can usually be palpated, thus establishing the diagnosis. The most serious complication associated with peripheral aneurysms is the formation of a thrombus, which can occlude the vessel and cause loss of the limb. As with abdominal aortic aneurysms, early treatment reduces the risk of complications and death. The lesion may be resected and the portion of the vessel removed replaced, commonly with a prosthetic material. For certain patients, a lumbar sympathectomy can be performed. The nurse should be aware that these patients can develop a thrombus postoperatively and should assist the patient in preventing this complication.

Varicose Veins

Varicosities, a common problem in old age, can be caused by lack of exercise, jobs entailing a great deal

of standing, and loss of vessel elasticity and strength associated with the aging process. Varicosities in all ages can be detected by the dilated, tortuous nature of the vein, especially the veins of the lower extremities. The person may experience dull pain and cramping of the legs, sometimes severe enough to interfere with sleep. Dizziness may occur as the patient rises from a lying position because blood is localized in the lower extremities and cerebral circulation is reduced. The effects of the varicosities make the skin more susceptible to trauma and infection, promoting the development of ulcerative lesions, especially in the obese or diabetic patient (Display 24-6).

> **KEY CONCEPT**
> Persons with varicose veins can experience dizziness when rising from a lying position because blood is localized in the lower extremities and cerebral circulation is reduced.

Treatment of varicose veins is aimed toward reducing venous stasis. The affected limb is elevated and rested to promote venous return. Exercise, particularly walking, also will enhance circulation. The nurse should make sure that elastic stockings and bandages are properly used and not constricting and that the patient is informed of the causes of venous status (eg, prolonged standing, crossing the legs, wearing constricting clothing) to prevent the development of complications and additional varicosities. Ligation and stripping of the veins require the same principles of nursing care used for other age groups undergoing this surgery.

Venous Thromboembolism

An increasing incidence of venous thromboembolism is found among older adults. Patients who have been restricted to bed rest or have had recent surgery or fractures of a lower extremity are high-risk candidates. Although the veins in the calf muscles are the most frequently seen sites of this problem, it also occurs in the inferior vena cava, iliofemoral segment, and various superficial veins. The symptoms and signs of venous thromboembolism depend on the vessel involved. The nurse should be alert for edema, warmth over the affected area, and pain in the sole of

D I S P L A Y 2 4 - 6

The Patient With a Leg Ulcer

Seventy-six-year-old Mrs. C, while participating in an activity at the adult day care center, is observed by the nurse to be rubbing her left ankle frequently and grimacing as she does. The nurse asks Mrs. C about the status of her ankle and learns that Mrs. C has been bothered with what she describes as an "annoying but not severe pain" for the past week. On inspecting Mrs. C's lower extremity the nurse sees a dime-sized ulcer on the medial aspect of Mrs. C's left ankle. The surrounding tissue is reddish purple and edematous. Peripheral pulses are present in both extremities, although stronger in the right extremity. Both of Mrs. C's legs possess severe varicosities.

Mrs. C is demonstrating classic signs of a venous ulcer (stasis ulcer). Venous ulcers are caused by chronic deep vein insufficiency or severe varicosities, as in Mrs. C's situation. Decreased circulation impairs the adequate exchange of oxygen and other nutrients which facilitates the development of an open necrotic lesion.

Mrs. C's symptoms are those that typically accompany venous ulcers. Arterial ulcers (ischemic ulcers) appear more necrotic because of oxygen being deprived to the tissue and are surrounded by pale or mottled skin; edema is uncommon and pain is more severe than that which occurs with venous ulcers.

The nurse's assessment actions were appropriate in asking about the history of symptoms and the characteristics of the pain, inspecting the ulcer and extremity, and palpating the pulse and edematous tissue.

Prompt referral to a physician can aid in preventing infection and getting the ulcer on the road to healing. Necrotic tissue must be debrided. Topical and systemic antibiotics may be prescribed to prevent infection.

An Unna boot (special type of impregnated gauze that hardens after application) may be applied to protect the area. Usually, the boot remains on the leg for 1 to 2 weeks, being changed more often if there is drainage.

Ulcers that do not heal or recur may require surgical intervention.

Patients with venous ulcers need to be taught to promote tissue perfusion and prevent complications (eg, infection, skin breakdown). Helpful measures to include in patient education are:

- Use gravity to promote circulation and reduce edema by elevating the lower extremity when sitting, and avoiding prolonged standing, sitting, and crossing the legs
- Prevent pressure on the ulcer by using an over-bed cradle to keep linens from touching the extremity
- Prevent constriction to circulation by avoiding tight socks or garters
- Control pain by using an analgesic; the use of the analgesic approximately 30 minutes prior to the dressing change can reduce some of the discomfort associated with the procedure
- Change the dressing as prescribed (if the patient is unable to perform the procedure independently, instruct a caregiver)
- Promote circulation by exercising (eg, walking, swimming, stationary bicycling, dorsiflexion of the feet)

the foot. Edema may be the primary indication of thromboembolism in the veins of the calf muscle, because discoloration and pain are often absent in aged persons with this problem. If the inferior vena cava is involved, bilateral swelling, aching and cyanosis of the lower extremities, engorgement of the superficial veins, and tenderness along the femoral veins will be present. Similar signs will appear with involvement of the iliofemoral segment, but only on the affected extremity.

The location of the thromboembolism will dictate the treatment used. Elastic stockings or bandages, rest, and elevation of the affected limb may promote venous return. Analgesics may be given to relieve any associated pain. Anticoagulants may be administered, and surgery may be performed as well. The nurse should help the patient to avoid situations that cause straining and to remain comfortable and well hydrated.

General Nursing Considerations

PREVENTION

The high incidence and potentially disabling effects of cardiovascular disease demand conscientious actions by gerontological nurses to incorporate preventive measures into their planning and caregiving. Education, counseling, coaching, and rehabilitative/restorative activities facilitate prevention on three levels:

- *Primary:* to prevent disease from developing in healthy elders.
- *Secondary:* to strengthen the abilities of persons who are diagnosed with disease to avoid complications and worsening of their conditions and achieve maximum health and function
- *Tertiary:* to maximize capabilities through rehabilitative and restorative efforts so that the disease doesn't create additional problems

The measures for facilitating cardiovascular health described at the beginning of this chapter are advantageous to incorporate into any health promotion plan for older adults.

KEEPING THE PATIENT INFORMED

Basic diagnostic and treatment measures for cardiovascular problems of the elderly will not differ greatly from those used with younger patients, and the same nursing measures can be applied. Because of sensory deficits, anxiety, poor memory, or illness, the older patient may not fully comprehend or remember the explanations given for diagnostic and treatment measures. Full explanations with reinforcement are essential. Patients and their families should have the opportunity to ask questions and to discuss their concerns openly. Often procedures that seem relatively minor to the nurse, such as frequent checks of vital signs, may be alarming to the unprepared patient and family.

PREVENTING COMPLICATIONS

The edema associated with many cardiovascular diseases may promote skin breakdown, especially in older people who typically have more fragile skin. Frequent changes of position are essential. The body should be supported in proper alignment, and dangling arms and legs off the side of a bed or chair should be avoided. A frequent check of clothing and protective devices can aid in detecting constriction due to increased edema. Protection, padding, and massage of pressure points are beneficial. If the patient is to be on a stretcher, an examining table, or an operating room table for a long time, protective padding can be placed on pressure points beforehand to provide comfort and prevent skin breakdown. When much edema is present, excessive activity should be avoided because it will increase the circulation of the fluid, with the toxic wastes it contains, and can subject the patient to profound intoxication. Weight and circumferences of extremities and the abdomen should be monitored to provide quantitative data regarding changes in the edematous state.

Accurate observation and documentation of fluid balance are especially important. Within any prescribed fluid restrictions, fluid intake should be encouraged to prevent dehydration and facilitate diuresis; water is effective for this. Fluid loss through any means should be measured; volume, color, odor, and specific gravity of urine should be noted. Intravenous fluids must be monitored carefully, particularly because excessive fluid infusion results in hypervolemia and can subject the elderly to the risk of CHF. Intravenous administration of glucose solution could stimulate the increased production of insulin, resulting in a hypoglycemic reaction if this solution is abruptly discontinued without an adequate substitute.

Vital signs must be checked regularly, with close attention to changes. A temperature elevation can reflect an infection or an MI. The body temperature for the elderly may be normally lower than for younger adults; it is important to record the patient's normal temperature when well to have a baseline for comparison. It is advisable to detect and correct temperature elevations promptly because a temperature elevation increases metabolism, thereby increasing the body's requirements for oxygen, and causes the heart to work harder. A decrease in temperature slows metabolism, causing less oxygen consumption and less carbon dioxide production and fewer respirations. A rise in blood pressure is associated with a reduced cardiac output, vasodilation, and lower blood volume. Hypotension can result in insufficient circulation to meet the body's needs; symptoms of confusion and dizziness could indicate insufficient cerebral circulation resulting from a reduced blood pressure. Pulse changes are significant. In addition to cardiac problems, tachycardia could indicate hypoxia caused by an obstructed airway. Bradycardia may be associated with digitalis toxicity.

Oxygen is frequently administered in the treatment of cardiovascular diseases, and in elderly patients it requires most careful use. The patient should be observed closely for hypoxia. Patients using a nasal catheter may breathe primarily by mouth and reduce oxygen intake. Although a face mask may remedy this problem, it does not guarantee sufficient oxygen inspiration. Older patients may not demonstrate cyanosis as the initial sign of hypoxia; instead, they may be restless, irritable, and dyspneic. These signs also can indicate high oxygen concentrations and consequent carbon dioxide narcosis, a particular risk to elderly patients receiving oxygen therapy. Blood gas levels will provide data to reveal these problems, and early correction is facilitated by keen nursing observation.

KEY CONCEPT
Instead of demonstrating cyanosis, older adults with hypoxia can become restless, irritable, and dyspneic.

Anorexia may accompany cardiovascular disease, and special nursing assistance may be necessary to help patients meet their nutritional needs. Several smaller meals throughout the entire day rather than a few large ones may compensate for poor appetite and reduce the work of the heart. Favorite foods, served attractively, can be effective. Patients should be encouraged to maintain a regular intake of glucose, the primary source of cardiac energy. Education may be necessary regarding low-sodium, low-cholesterol, and low-calorie diets. Therapeutic dietary modifications should attempt to incorporate ethnic food enjoyed by patients; patients may reject a prescribed special diet if they believe they must forfeit the foods that have been an important component of their lives for decades. It may be necessary to negotiate compromises; a realistic, although imperfect, diet with which patients are satisfied is more likely to be followed than an ideal one that patients cannot accept. The foods

included in the diets should be reviewed, and patients should be informed of the sodium, cholesterol, and caloric contents of these items. These foods can then be categorized as those that should be eaten "never," "occasionally or not more than once monthly," and "as desired." Patients should be taught to read labels of food, beverages, and drugs for sodium content; they must understand that carbonated drinks, certain analgesic preparations, commercial alkalizers, and homemade baking soda mixtures contain sodium.

KEY CONCEPT
To promote dietary compliance, foods should be categorized as those that should "never be eaten," "eaten occasionally," or "eaten as desired."

Straining from constipation, enemas, and removal of fecal impactions can cause vagal stimulation, a particularly dangerous situation for patients with cardiovascular disease. Measures to prevent constipation must be an integral part of the care plan for these patients; a stool softener may be prescribed. If bed rest is prescribed, range-of-motion exercises should be performed, because they will cause muscle contractions that compress peripheral veins and thereby facilitate the return of venous blood.

Patients who are weak or who fall asleep while sitting need to have their heads and necks supported to prevent hyperextension or hyperflexion of the neck. All elderly persons, not only those with cardiovascular disease, can suffer a reduction in cerebral blood flow from the compression of vessels during this hyperextension or hyperflexion. Those with CHF need good positioning and support. A semirecumbent position with pillows supporting the entire back maintains good body alignment, promotes comfort, and assists in reducing pulmonary congestion. Cardiac strain is reduced by supporting the arms with pillows or armrests. Footboards help prevent foot-drop contracture; patients should be instructed in how to use them for exercising.

If hepatic congestion develops, drugs may detoxify more slowly. Because the elderly may already have a slower rate of drug detoxification, nurses must be acutely aware of signs indicating adverse reactions to drugs. Digitalis toxicity particularly should be monitored and could present with a change in mental status, nausea, vomiting, arrhythmias, and a slow pulse. Because hypokalemia sensitizes the heart to the effects of digitalis, prevention through proper diet and the possible use of potassium supplements is advisable.

PROMOTING PERIPHERAL CIRCULATION

Nurses can play a significant role in preventing peripheral vascular problems. Health education for persons of all ages should reinforce the importance of exercise in promoting circulation; factors that can interfere with optimal circulation, such as crossing legs and wearing garters, should be reviewed. Weight control can be encouraged because obesity can interfere with venous return. Tobacco use should be discouraged because it may cause arterial spasms. Immobility and hypotension should be prevented to avoid thrombus formation. Exercises that may benefit patients with peripheral vascular disease are shown in Figure 24-4. Yoga and t'ai chi also can promote circulation. In addition, Buerger-Allen exercises (see Fig. 24-3) may be prescribed, and the patient and family members or caregivers will need to learn how they are done correctly and comfortably. Instruction in the correct use of support hose or special elastic stockings is important.

> **KEY CONCEPT**
> Circulation can be enhanced by exercise, support hose, and avoidance of obesity, immobility, hypotension, and obstructive clothing.

FOOT CARE

Persons with peripheral vascular disease must pay special attention to the care of their feet, which should be bathed and inspected daily. To avoid injury, patients should not walk in bare feet. Any foot lesion or discoloration should be brought promptly to the attention of the physician or nurse. These patients are at high risk of developing fungal infections from the moisture produced by normal foot perspiration; it is not unusual for the elderly to develop fungal infections under their nails, emphasizing the importance of regular, careful nail inspection. If untreated, a simple fungal infection can lead to gangrene and other serious complications. Placing cotton between the toes and removing shoes several times during the day will help keep the feet dry. Shoes should be large enough to avoid any pressure and safe enough to prevent any injuries to the feet; they should be aired after wearing.

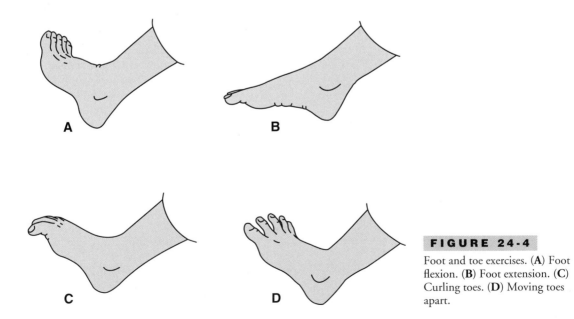

FIGURE 24-4

Foot and toe exercises. (**A**) Foot flexion. (**B**) Foot extension. (**C**) Curling toes. (**D**) Moving toes apart.

Laces should not be tied tightly because they can exert pressure on the feet. Colored socks may contain irritating dyes and would be best to avoid; socks should be changed regularly. Although the feet should be kept warm, the direct application of heat to the feet, as with heating pads, hot-water bottles, and soaks, can increase the metabolism and circulatory demand, thereby compounding the existing problem.

PROBLEMS ASSOCIATED WITH PERIPHERAL VASCULAR DISEASE

Ischemic foot lesions may be present in patients with peripheral vascular disease. If eschars are present, they should be loosened to allow drainage. Careful debridement is necessary to avoid bleeding and trauma; chemical debriding agents may be useful. Systemic antibiotic agents can be helpful in controlling cellulitis. Topical antibiotics usually are not used because epithelization must occur before bacterial flora can be destroyed. Analgesics may be administered to relieve associated pain. Good nutrition, particularly an adequate protein intake, and the maintenance of muscle strength and joint motion are essential. Various surgical procedures may be used in treating ischemic foot lesions, including bypass grafts, sympathectomies, and amputations.

Loss of a limb may represent a significant loss of independence to the elderly, regardless of the reality of the situation. With an altered body image, new roles may be assumed as other roles are forfeited. Patients and their families need opportunities to discuss their fears and concerns. Making them aware of the likelihood of a normal life and the availability of appliances that make ambulation, driving, and other activities possible may help reduce anxieties and promote a smoother adjustment to the amputation. The rehabilitation period can be long for the elderly and may necessitate frequent motivation and encouragement by nursing staff.

PROMOTING NORMALITY

An often unasked question of elderly patients relates to the impact of their cardiovascular condition on sexual activity. They may be reluctant to inquire because they fear being ridiculed or causing shock that "someone their age would still be interested in sex." They may resign themselves to forfeiting sexual activity under the misconception that they will further harm their hearts; research has demonstrated that pa-

tients often place unnecessary restrictions on sexual activities following heart attacks (Akdolun & Terakye, 2001). Nurses should encourage discussion of this subject and introduce the topic if patients seem unable to do so themselves. If there is fear of injuring the heart by resuming sexual activity, realistic explanations should be provided, including when sex can be resumed, how medications can affect sexual function, how to schedule medications for beneficial impact during sexual activity, and sexual positions that produce the least cardiac strain.

> **KEY CONCEPT**
> Nurses should offer patients realistic explanations about the relationship of cardiovascular conditions and sexual function.

Relaxation and rest are both important in the treatment of cardiovascular disease, and it is wise to remember that a patient who is at rest is not necessarily relaxed. The stresses from hospitalization, pain, ignorance, and fear regarding disability; alterations in lifestyle; and potential death can cause the patient to become anxious, confused, and irrational. Reassurance and support are needed, including full explanations of diagnostic tests, hospital or institutional routines, and other activities. Opportunities for patients and their families to discuss questions, concerns, and fears must be provided. Realistic explanations of any required restrictions and lifestyle changes should emphasize that patients need not become "cardiac cripples" just because they have a cardiac disease. Most patients can live a normal life and need to be reassured of this. (Refer to the resource list at the end of the chapter for names of organizations with resources to help patients live with cardiovascular disorders.)

Complementary Therapies

The benefits of digitalis (foxglove) in treating heart disease has stimulated interest in the use of other herbs for preventing and treating cardiovascular disorders. One such herb that shows promise is hawthorn berry, which has been found to dilate blood vessels to improve circulation to the heart, relieve spasms of the arterial wall, and produce a hypotensive effect (Mashour, Lin, & Frishman, 2000). Garlic, because it contains antioxidant sulfur compounds, has shown some value in dissolving clots (Fugh-Berman, 2000). Ginger has been shown to lower cholesterol. Patients are wise to discuss the use of medicinal herbs with their health care practitioners and to avoid exceeding recommended dosages.

Some of the nonconventional measures to facilitate deep relaxation and reduce stress can be effective in reversing heart disease. Meditation has been shown to increase blood flow and oxygen consumption (Canter, 2003). Biofeedback, guided imagery, t'ai chi, and yoga have been shown to lower blood pressure and heart rate (Astin et al., 2003). There is exploration into the use of acupuncture in conjunction with herbs to lower cholesterol levels, raise blood flow, and relieve angina (Bueno et al., 2001).

Some patients may find yoga beneficial to their circulation because the various asanas (postures) used in yoga increase circulation because of the effects on the endocrine glands and nerve plexuses. Acupressure massage techniques using rubbing, kneading, percussion, and vibration can improve circulation. The herb ginkgo biloba has shown promise as being effective in improving cerebral and peripheral circulation. The future may hold additional noninvasive measures to improve circulation.

Although the full benefits of complementary therapies are in the process of being discovered, these measures are less intrusive and less expensive than conventional treatments, and for the most part, carry minimal risk. Nurses should consider the use of these therapies to prevent heart disease and complement conventional treatments when pathology exists.

Critical Thinking Exercises

1. How does the lifestyle of the average American contribute to the risk of developing cardiovascular disease with age?
2. List the complications to the general health status of the older adult that can arise as a result of a cardiovascular disorder.
3. Outline general topical areas that you would teach to an older individual who is recovering from a myocardial infarction.
4. What measures could you advise young adults to incorporate into their health practices that would promote cardiovascular health in late life?

Web Connect

Explore the National Library of Medicine's *Clinician Guidelines for Cardiac Rehabilitation* at http://hstat.nlm.nih.gov/hq/Hquest/db/local.ahcpr.clin.crpc/screen/TocDisplay/s/44639/action/Toc.

● Resources

The following organizations provide educational materials on cardiovascular health and specific cardiovascular diseases:

American Heart Association
7320 Greenville Avenue
Dallas, TX 75231
(214) 750-5551, (800) 242-4596
www.amhrt.org

Mended Hearts (for patients with heart disease)
7272 Greenville Avenue
Dallas, TX 75231
(888) HEART99
www.mendedhearts.org

National Amputation Foundation
40 Church Street
Malvern, NY 11565
(516) 887-3600
www.nationalamputation.org

National Heart, Lung, and Blood Institute
Office of Information
Bethesda, MD 20205
www.nhlbi.nih.gov

● References

Akdolun, N., & Terakye, G. (2001). Sexual problems before and after myocardial infarction: patients' needs for information. *Rehabilitation Nursing, 26*(4), 152–158.

Astin, J. A., Shapiro, S. L., Eisenberg, D. M., & Forys, K. L. (2003). Mind-body medicine: State of the science, implications for practice. *Journal of the American Board Family Practice, 16*(2), 131–147.

Canter, P. H. (2003). The therapeutic effects of meditation. *British Medical Journal, 326*(7398), 1049–1050.

Frishman, W. H., Azer, V., & Sica, D. (2003). Drug treatment of orthostatic hypotension and vasovagal syncope. *Heart Disease, 5*(1), 49–64.

Fugh-Berman, A. (2000). Herbs and dietary supplements in the prevention and treatment of cardiovascular disease. *Preventive Cardiology, 3*(1), 24–32.

Koertge, J., Weidner, G., Elliott-Eller, M., Scherwitz, L., Merritt-Worden, T.A., et al. (2003). Improvement in medical risk factors and quality of life in women and men with coronary artery disease in the Multicenter Lifestyle Demonstration Project. *American Journal of Cardiology, 91*(11), 1316–1322.

Mashour, N. H., Lin, G. I., & Frishman, W. H. (2000). Herbal medicine for the treatment of cardiovascular disease. In P. B. Fontanarosa (Ed.), *Alternative medicine: An objective assessment* (p. 286). Chicago: American Medical Association.

Mukamal, K. J., Conigrave, K. M., Mittleman, M. A., Camargo, C. A., Stampfer, M. J., et al. (2003). Roles of drinking pattern and type of alcohol consumed in coronary heart disease in men. *New England Journal of Medicine, 348*(2), 109–111.

Ornish, D. (1996). *Dr. Dean Ornish's program for reversing heart disease.* New York: Ivy Books.

Ridker, P. M. (2003). Clinical application of C-reactive protein for cardiovascular disease detection and prevention. *Circulation, 107*(3), 363–369.

Yaes, R. J. (2003). Aspirin, clopidogrel, or both for secondary prevention of coronary disease. *New England Journal of Medicine, 348*(6), 560–563.

● Recommended Readings

Appel, L. J., Moore, T. J., Obarzanek, E., et al. (1997). A clinical trial of the effects of dietary patterns on blood pressure. *New England Journal of Medicine, 336*(16), 1117–1124.

Aronow, W. S. (2001). Therapy of older persons with congestive heart failure. *Annals of Long-Term Care, 9*(1), 23–29.

Bubien, R. S. (2000). A new beat on an old rhythm. *American Journal of Nursing. 100*(1), 42–51.

Bueno, E. A., Mamtani, R., & Frishman, W. H. (2001). Alternative approaches to the medical management of angina pectoris: Acupuncture, electrical nerve stimulation, and spinal cord stimulation. *Heart Disease, 3*(4), 236–241

Daviglus, M. L., Stamler, J., Orencia, A. J., et al. (1997). Fish consumption and the 30-year risk of fatal myocardial infarction. *New England Journal of Medicine, 336*(16), 1046–1053.

Furberg, C. D., & Psaty, B. M. (1995). Calcium antagonists: Antagonists or protagonists of mortality in elderly hypertensives? *Journal of the American Geriatric Society, 43*(8), 1309–1310.

Garcia-Palmieri, M. (2001). Cardiovascular disease prevention in the elderly. *Clinical Geriatrics, 9*(5), 69–77.

Gondek, M. C. (1999). Talking about sex: A post-MI script. *RN, 62*(7), 52–53.

Halm, M., & Penque, S. (1999). Heart disease in women. *American Journal of Nursing, 99*(4), 26–32.

Hazzard, W. R. (1999). *Principles of geriatric medicine* (4th ed.). New York: McGraw-Hill.

Horowitz, S. (1998). Cardiovascular health: Nondrug approaches. *Alternative and Complementary Therapies, 4*(6), 406–410.

Johns Hopkins Medical Institutions. (1999, September). Heart attack. *Health After 50,* p. 6.

Kaiser, F. E., & Morley, J. E. (1997). *Cardiovascular disease in older people.* New York: Springer.

Keaton, K. A., & Pierce, L. L. (2000). Cardiac therapy for men with coronary artery disease: The lived experience. *Journal of Holistic Nursing, 18*(1), 46–62.

Lai, S. C., & Cohen, M. N. (1999). Promoting lifestyle changes. *American Journal of Nursing, 99*(4), 63–64.

Lai, J. S., May, C., Wong, M. K., & Teng, S. H. (1995). Two-year trends in cardiorespiratory function among older t'ai chi chuan practitioners and sedentary subjects. *Journal of the American Geriatric Society, 43*(10), 1222–1227.

Lenhart, R. C. (1995). Pacemaker assessment and care plans in long-term care. *Geriatric Nursing, 16,* 276–280.

Lewandowski, D. M. (1999). Clinical snapshot: Myocarditis. *American Journal of Nursing, 99*(8), 44–45.

Luskin, F. M., Newell, M., Griffith, M., et al. (1998). A review of mind-body therapies in the treatment of cardiovascular disease: Implications for the elderly. *Alternative Therapies, 4*(3), 46–61.

Mann, S. J. (2000). The mind/body link in essential hypertension: Time for a new paradigm. *Alternative Therapies in Health and Medicine, 6*(2), 39–56.

Miller, C. (2002). Cardiovascular drugs: Reason for promise and vigilance. *Geriatric Nursing, 23*(1), 171–172.

Nunnelee, J. D., Kurgan, A., & Auer, A. I. (1995). Carotid endarterectomy in elderly vascular patients: Experience in a community hospital. *Geriatric Nursing, 16*(3), 121–123.

Pahor M., et al. Long-term survival and use of antihypertensive medications in older persons. *Journal of the American Geriatric Society, 43*(8), 1191–1197.

Park, K. C., Forman, D. E., & Wei, J. Y. (1995). Utility of beta-blockade treatment for older postinfarction patients. *Journal of the American Geriatric Society, 43*(7), 751–755.

Resnick, B. (1999). Atrial fibrillation in the older adult: Presentation and management issues. *Geriatric Nursing, 20*(4), 188–194.

Roberts, S. L., Johnson, L. H., & Keely, B. (1999). Fostering hope in the elderly: Congestive heart failure patient in critical care. *Geriatric Nursing, 20*(4), 195–199.

Robinson, A. W., & Sloan, H. L. (2000). Heart health and older women. *Journal of Gerontological Nursing, 26*(5), 38–45.

Rossi, M. S. (1995). Nursing grand rounds: The octogenarian cardiac surgical patient. *Journal of Cardiovascular Nursing, 9*(11), 75–95.

Satish, S., Freeman, D. H., Ray, L., & Goodwin, J. S. (2001). The relationship between blood pressure and mortality in the oldest old. *Journal of the American Geriatrics Society, 49*(4), 367–374.

Siomko, A. J. (2000). Demystifying cardiac markers. *American Journal of Nursing, 100*(1), 36–37.

Stanley, M. (1999). Congestive heart failure in the elderly. *Geriatric Nursing, 20*(4), 180–187.

U.S. Cardiac Rehabilitation Guideline Panel. (1995). *Cardiac rehabilitation.* Rockville, MD: U.S. Department of Health and Human Services.

Yen, P. K. (1998). Stopping heart disease with diet. *Geriatric Nursing, 19*(1), 50–51.

Yen, P. K. (1999). Diet lessons learned from aging hearts. *Geriatric Nursing, 20*(4), 223.

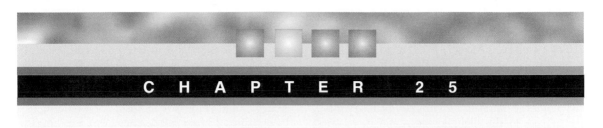

CHAPTER 25

Respiratory Conditions

■ *Learning Objectives*

After reading this chapter, you should be able to:

- list the impact of age-related changes on respiratory health
- describe measures to facilitate respiratory health in the elderly
- discuss the risks, symptoms, and care considerations associated with selected respiratory illnesses
- list interventions that can aid in preventing complications and promoting self-care in older persons with respiratory conditions

Effects of Aging on Respiratory Health

Respiratory health is vital to the elderly person's ability to maintain a physically, mentally, and socially active life. It can make the difference between a person maximizing opportunities to live life to the fullest and being too fatigued and uncomfortable to leave the confines of home. A lifetime of insults to the respiratory system from smoking, pollution, and infection takes its toll in old age, making respiratory disease a leading cause of disability and the fourth leading cause of death in persons over 70 years of age. However, positive health practices can benefit respiratory health at any age and minimize limitations imposed by problems.

The effects of aging create a situation in which respiratory problems can develop more easily and be more difficult to manage. Various connective tissues responsible for respiration and ventilation are weaker. The elastic recoil of the lungs during expiration is decreased because of less elastic collagen and elastin, and expiration requires the active use of accessory muscles. Alveoli are less elastic, develop fibrous tissue, and contain fewer functional capillaries. The loss of skeletal muscle strength in the thorax and diaphragm, combined with the loss of resilient force that holds the thorax in a slightly contracted position, contributes to the slight kyphosis and barrel chest seen in many older adults. The net effect of these changes is a reduction in vital capacity and an increase in residual volume—in other words, less air exchange and more air and secretions remaining in the lungs.

Further, age-related changes external to the respiratory system can affect respiratory health in significant ways. A reduction in body fluid and reduced fluid intake can cause drier mucous membranes, impeding the removal of mucus and leading to the development of mucous plugs and infection. Altered pain sensations can cause signals of respiratory problems to be unnoticed or mistaken for nonrespiratory disorders. Different norms for body temperature can cause fever to present at an atypically lower level, potentially being missed and allowing respiratory infections to progress. Loose, brittle teeth can dislodge or break, leading to lung abscesses, infections, and the aspiration of tooth fragments. Relaxed sphincters and slower gastric motility further contribute to the risk of aspiration. Impaired mobility, inactivity, and numerous medications associated with the highly prevalent diseases in the older population can decrease respiratory function, promote infection, interfere with early detection, and complicate treatment of respiratory problems. Astute assessment is essential to reducing the morbidity and mortality associated with these conditions (Display 25-1).

KEY CONCEPT

Pieces of brittle teeth can break off, be aspirated, and cause respiratory problems, reinforcing the importance of good oral health in late life.

Facilitating Respiratory Health

The high risk that every older person faces in developing respiratory disorders warrants the incorporation of preventive measures into all care plans. In addition to basic health practices, special attention to promoting respiratory activity is important. All older adults should be encouraged to do deep-breathing exercises several times daily. Keeping in mind that full expiration is more difficult than inspiration, these exercises should emphasize an inspiration ratio of 1:3. (See Chapter 15 for a full description of breathing exercises.) Even healthy, active people can benefit from including these exercises in their daily activities.

Smoking is the most important factor contributing to respiratory disease. Many elderly smokers started their habit at a time when the full effects of smoking were not realized and smoking was considered fashionable, sociable, and sophisticated. Although smokers may be aware of the health hazards associated with smoking, it is an extremely difficult habit to break. The effects on respiratory health initially may be so subtle and gradual that they are not realized. Unfortunately, by the time signs and symptoms become apparent, considerable damage to the respiratory system may have occurred. Smokers have twice the incidence of lung cancer, a higher incidence of all respiratory disease, more complications with respiratory problems, and commonly suffer from productive coughs, shortness of breath, and reduced breathing capacity. Although maximum benefit is obtained by not starting to smoke in the first place or quitting early in life, smoking cessation is beneficial at any age. Local chapters of the American Lung Association, health departments, clinics, and commercial agencies offer a wide range of smoking cessation approaches that may be useful.

Immobility is a major threat to pulmonary health, and the elderly frequently experience problems that decrease their mobility. Preventing fractures, pain, weakness, depression, and other problems that could decrease mobility is an essential goal. The elderly, family members, and caregivers all need to be educated about the multiple problems associated with immobility. It may be tempting for the older person to rest or for caring family to encourage that person to rest on days when arthritis or other discomforts are bothersome, unless it is understood that by doing so, more discomfort and disability can result. When immobility is unavoidable, hourly turning, coughing, and deep breathing will promote respiratory activity; blow bottles and similar equipment can also be beneficial. Persons who are chairbound may need the same attention to respiratory activity as the bedbound.

Assessment of Respiratory Conditions

General Observation

Much can be determined regarding the status of the respiratory system through careful observation of the following:

Color: coloring of the face, neck, limbs, and nail beds can be indicative of respiratory status. Ruddy, pink complexions often occur with chronic obstructive pulmonary disease (COPD) and are associated with hypoxia, which is caused by a high carbon dioxide level in the blood that inhibits involuntary neurotransmission from the pons to the diaphragm for inspiration. In the presence of chronic bronchitis, patients can have a blue or gray discoloration caused by the lack of oxygen binding to the hemoglobin.

Chest structure and posture: the anteroposterior chest diameter increases with age—significantly so in the presence of COPD. Abnormal spinal curvatures (eg, kyphosis, scoliosis, lordosis) should be noted.

Breathing pattern: the chest should be observed for symmetrical expansion during respirations, as well as the depth, rate, rhythm, and length of respirations. Decreased expansion of the chest can be caused by pain, fractured ribs, pulmonary emboli, pleural effusion, or pleurisy. The patient should be asked to change positions, walk, and cough to see if these activities result in any changes.

Interview

Some older persons can give unreliable accounts of their past respiratory symptoms or have grown so accustomed to living with their symptoms that they do not consider them unusual. Specific questions can assist in revealing disorders, such as the following:

"Do you ever have wheezing, chest pain, or a heavy feeling in your chest?"
"How often do you get colds? Do you get colds that keep returning? How do you treat them?"
"How far can you walk? How many steps can you climb before getting short of breath?"
"Do you have any breathing problems when the weather gets cold or hot?"
"How many pillows do you sleep on? Do breathing problems (eg, coughing, shortness of breath) ever awaken you from sleep?"
"How much do you cough during the day? During each hour? Can you control it?"
"Do you bring up sputum, phlegm, or mucus when you cough? How much? What color? Is it the consistency of water, egg white, or jelly?"
"How do you manage respiratory problems? How often do you use cough syrups, cold capsules, inhalers, vapors, rubs, or ointments?"
"Did you ever smoke? If so, for how long and when and why did you stop? How many cigarettes or cigars do you smoke daily? Do people you live with or spend a lot of time with smoke?"
"What kind of jobs have you had over your lifetime? Any in factories or chemical plants?"
"Do you live or have you lived near factories, fields, or high-traffic areas?"

More specific questions increase the likelihood of obtaining a full and accurate history of factors related to respiratory health. The dates of influenza and pneumonia vaccines should be ascertained and documented.

Physical Examination

The posterior chest is palpated to evaluate the depth of respirations, degree of chest movement, and presence of masses or pain. Normally there is bilateral movement during respirations and reduced expansion of the base of the lungs. Tactile fremitus is usually best felt in the upper lobes; increased fremitus in the lower lobes occurs with pneumonia and masses. COPD and pneumothorax can cause a lack of fremitus in the upper lobes.

Percussion of the lungs should produce a resonant sound. Auscultation of the lungs should reflect normal bronchial, vesicular, and bronchovesicular breath sounds; crackles, rhonchi, and wheezes are abnormal findings.

Assessment data should be reviewed for actual and potential nursing diagnoses that can be used in guiding the care plan.

> **KEY CONCEPT**
>
> The risk of insufficient respiratory activity in older adults who are bedbound is usually recognized and planned for; however, chairbound individuals may possess similar risks and require planned measures to promote adequate ventilation.

Older persons should be advised against treating respiratory problems themselves. Many over-the-counter cold and cough remedies can have serious effects in older adults and can interact with other medications being taken. These drugs also can mask symptoms of serious problems, thereby delaying diagnosis and treatment. The elderly should know that a cold lasting more than 1 week may not be a cold at all, but something more serious that requires medical attention.

All medications used by older persons should be reviewed for their impact on respiration. Decreased respirations or rapid, shallow breathing can be caused by many of the drugs commonly prescribed for this group; these drugs include analgesics, antidepressants, antihistamines, antiparkinson agents, synthetic antispasmodics, sedatives, and tranquilizers. As always, alternatives to drugs should be used whenever possible.

Environmental factors also influence respiratory health. Considerable attention has been paid to pollutants such as ozone, carbon monoxide, and nitrogen oxide that reduce the quality of the air we breathe outdoors. However, indoor air pollution can affect respiratory health as well. Synthetic or plastic building materials can emit gas; spores, animal dander, mites, pollen, plaster, bacteria, and viruses can be present in household dust; and cigarette smoke can add carbon monoxide and cadmium to indoor air. Conscious choices to minimize exposure to air pollution in the places where we reside, work, and play can help alleviate some of the stress to our respiratory systems. Furthermore, the quality of indoor air can be improved by:

- installing and maintaining air filters in heating and air conditioning systems
- vacuuming regularly (preferably using a central vacuum system or a water-trap vacuum that prevents dust from returning to the room)
- damp-dusting furnishings
- discouraging cigarette smoking

- opening windows to air out rooms
- maintaining green houseplants to help detoxify the air

> ✔ **Point to Ponder**
>
> *What sources of air pollution are you able to identify in your home and work environments? What can you do to correct these?*

Nurses should assist older adults in identifying and reducing sources of indoor pollutants. Housecleaning hints may be shared (eg, dusting with a damp cloth, airing out blankets, removing unnecessary stored paper and cloth objects); in some situations, helping older adults locate housecleaning services can prove beneficial to improving their respiratory health.

Finally, often overlooked in the prevention of respiratory problems is the significance of a healthy oral cavity. Infections of the oral cavity can lead to respiratory infections or can decrease appetite and facilitate a generally poor health status. As noted, teeth can break or dislodge, leading to lung abscesses, infections, and aspirated tooth fragments. Respiratory infections may decline when loose or diseased teeth are removed.

Selected Disorders

ASTHMA

Some older persons are affected with asthma throughout their lives; others develop it during old age. Its symptoms and management do not differ much from those of other age groups. Because of the added stress that asthma places on the heart, older asthmatics have a high risk of developing complications such as bronchiectasis and cardiac problems. The nurse should help detect causative factors (eg, emotions, mouth breathing, chronic respiratory infections) and educate the patient regarding early recognition of and prompt attention to an asthma attack when it does occur (Williams, Schmidt, Redd, & Storms, 2003).

Careful assessment of the aged asthmatic patient's use of aerosol nebulizers is advisable. Due to the difficulty some elders have in properly using inhalers, a spacer, or holding chamber, may be helpful to allow the inhalant medication to penetrate deep into the lungs. These systems consist of aerochambers that trap the medication or holding chambers that collapse and inflate during inhalation and expiration. Specific instructions are provided with each system. It is beneficial for the nurse to review the use of these devices as part of every assessment of patients who use them.

Cardiac arrhythmias leading to sudden death may be risked by the overuse of sympathomimetic bronchodilating nebulizers. Cromolyn sodium is one of the least toxic respiratory drugs that can be used, although several weeks of therapy may be necessary for benefits to be realized. Some of the new steroid inhalants are effective and carry a lower risk of systemic absorption and adverse reactions than older steroids.

CHRONIC BRONCHITIS

Many elderly persons demonstrate the persistent, productive cough; wheezing; recurrent respiratory infections; and shortness of breath caused by chronic bronchitis. These symptoms may develop gradually, sometimes taking years for the full impact of the disease to be realized, when, because of bronchospasm, the patient notices increased difficulty breathing in cold and damp weather. They experience more frequent respiratory infections and greater difficulty managing them. Episodes of hypoxia begin to occur because mucus obstructs the bronchial tree and causes carbon dioxide retention. As the disease progresses, emphysema may develop and death may occur from obstruction. The management of this problem, aimed at removing bronchial secretions and preventing obstruction of the airway, is similar for all age groups. Older patients may need special encouragement to maintain good fluid intake and expectorate secretions. The nurse can be most effective in preventing the development of chronic bronchitis by discouraging chronic respiratory irritation, such as from smoking, and by helping older adults prevent respiratory infections.

✔ **Point to Ponder**

Smoking-related respiratory diseases have an impact not only on the affected individual but also on society in terms of health care costs. What do you think about the costs to society that grow from an individual's personal decision to smoke? What incentives could be used by society to discourage this behavior?

EMPHYSEMA

Of increasing incidence in the older population is emphysema, a progressive chronic obstructive pulmonary disease (COPD). Factors causing this destructive disease include chronic bronchitis, chronic irritation from dusts or certain air pollutants, and morphologic changes in the lungs, which include distention of the alveolar sacs, rupture of the alveolar walls, and destruction of the alveolar capillary bed. Cigarette smoking also plays a major role in the development of emphysema. The symptoms are slow in onset and initially may resemble age-related changes in the respiratory system, causing many patients to experience delayed identification and treatment of this disease. Gradually, increased dyspnea is experienced, which is not relieved by sitting upright as it may have been in the past. A chronic cough develops. As more effort is required for breathing and hypoxia occurs, fatigue, anorexia, weight loss, and weakness are demonstrated. Recurrent respiratory infections, malnutrition, congestive heart failure, and cardiac arrhythmias are among the more life-threatening complications the elderly can experience from emphysema.

Treatment usually includes postural drainage, bronchodilators, the avoidance of stressful situations, and breathing exercises, which are an important part of patient education. Cigarette smoking definitely should be stopped. The older patient may have insufficient energy to consume sufficient food and fluid; nurses need to assess for this and arrange for dietary interventions that can facilitate intake (eg, frequent small feedings and high-protein supplements). If oxygen is used, it must be done with extreme caution and close supervision. It must be remembered that for these patients, a low oxygen level rather than a high carbon dioxide level stimulates respiration. The older patient with emphysema is a high-risk candidate for the development of carbon dioxide narcosis. Respiratory infections should be prevented, and any that do occur, regardless of how minor they may seem, should be promptly reported to the physician. Sedatives, hypnotics, and narcotics may be contraindicated because the patient will be more sensitive to these drugs. It may be useful to consult with patients' physicians regarding the possibility of lung volume reduction surgery (a procedure in which the most severely diseased portions of the lung are removed to allow remaining tissues and respiratory muscles to work better). Patients with emphysema need a great deal of education and support to be able to manage this disease. It is difficult for the patient to adjust to the presence of a serious chronic disease requiring special care or even a lifestyle change. The patient must learn to pace activities, avoid extremely cold weather, administer medications correctly, and recognize symptoms of infection. Display 25-2 outlines a sample care plan for the patient with emphysema.

LUNG CANCER

It is uncertain whether the increased incidence of lung cancer in the aged population is due to more cases of lung cancer actually occurring or improved diagnostic tools and greater availability of medical care. Lung cancer occurs more frequently in men, although the rate among women is rising. The mortality rate from lung cancer is higher among whites. Cigarette smokers have twice the incidence as nonsmokers. A high incidence occurs among individuals who are chronically exposed to agents such as asbestos, coal gas, radioactive dusts, and chromates. This emphasizes the significance of obtaining thorough information regarding a patient's occupational history as part of the nursing assessment. Although conclusive evidence is unavailable, some association has been reported between the presence of lung scars, such as those resulting from tuberculosis and pneumonitis, and lung cancer.

> **KEY CONCEPT**
> Chronic exposure to cigarette smoke, asbestos, coal gas, radioactive dusts, and chromates can contribute to the development of lung cancer.

The individual may have lung cancer long before any symptoms develop. Thus, people at high risk should be screened regularly and periodic roentgenograms should be obtained to detect this disease in an early stage. Dyspnea, coughing, chest pain, fatigue, anorexia, wheezing, and recurrent upper respiratory infections are part of the symptomatology seen as the disease progresses. Diagnosis is confirmed through chest roentgenogram, sputum cytology, bronchoscopy, and biopsy. Treatment may consist of surgery, chemotherapy, or radiotherapy, requiring the same type of nursing care as that for patients of any age with this diagnosis.

LUNG ABSCESS

A lung abscess may result from pneumonia, tuberculosis, a malignancy, or trauma to the lung. Aspiration of foreign material can also cause a lung abscess; this may be a particular risk to aged persons who have decreased pharyngeal reflexes. Symptoms, which resemble those of many other respiratory problems, include anorexia, weight loss, fatigue, temperature elevation, and a chronic cough. Sputum production may occur, but this is not always demonstrated in older persons. Diagnosis and management are the same as that for other age groups. Modifications for postural drainage, an important component of the treatment, are discussed later in this chapter. Because protein can be lost through the sputum, a high-protein, high-calorie diet should be encouraged to maintain and improve the nutritional status of the older patient. (Refer to Chapter 23 for a discussion of influenza, pneumonia, and tuberculosis.)

Nursing Considerations

PREVENTING COMPLICATIONS

Once respiratory diseases have developed, close monitoring of the patient's status is required to minimize disability and prevent mortality. Close nursing observation can prevent and detect respiratory complications and should include checking the following:

- respiratory rate and volume
- pulse (eg, a sudden increase can indicate hypoxia)
- blood pressure (eg, elevations can occur with chronic hypoxia)
- temperature (eg, not only to detect infection but also to prevent stress on the cardiovascular and respiratory systems as they attempt to meet the body's increased oxygen demands imposed by an elevated temperature)
- neck veins (eg, for distention)
- patency of airway
- coughing (eg, frequency, depth, productivity)
- quality of secretions
- mental status

Inappropriate oxygen administration can have serious consequences for older persons, necessitating that nurses strictly adhere to proper procedures when it is

D I S P L A Y 2 5 · 2

Sample Care Plan for the Patient With Emphysema

Nursing Diagnoses

> *Impaired gas exchange related to chronic tissue hypoxia*
>
> *Risk for infection related to pooling of secretions in lungs*

Goals

The patient
> maintains a patent airway
> expectorates secretions from lungs
> is free from respiratory infections

Actions

- Determine impact of respiratory symptoms on activities of daily living (ADL), identify actual or potential deficits in engaging in ADL, and provide assistance to compensate for deficits or interventions to increase self-care ability
- Schedule rest periods between activities.
- Teach breathing exercises to increase inspiratory to expiratory ratio using the following guidelines:
  - slowly inhale to the count of 5
  - lean forward (30–40°) and slowly exhale to the count of 10; use pursed-lip breathing for expiration
  - repeat several times, breathing slowly and rhythmically
- Teach abdominal breathing to assist with expiration using the following guidelines:

In a lying position

- Place a book or small pillow on the abdomen
- Push out the abdomen during inspiration; observe the book or pillow rise
- Exhale slowly through pursed lips while pulling in the abdomen

In a sitting position

- Hold a book or small pillow against the abdomen
- Push out the abdomen against the book or pillow during inspiration
- Lean forward, exhale slowly through pursed lips and

pull in the abdomen, pressing the book or pillow against the abdomen
- Instruct patient to cough and breath deeply at least once every 8 hours. Coughing can be stimulated by deep expiration and could be planned following breathing exercises.
- Perform postural drainage exercises as ordered; allow rest periods between position changes and be careful to avoid forceful pounding as elderly with brittle bones could experience a fracture.
- If antibiotics are prescribed, ensure that they are administered on time to maintain a constant blood level.
- Control contact with persons who have signs of respiratory infection.
- Note signs of respiratory infection and promptly report to the physician.
- Maintain a stable room temperature of 75°F.
- If oxygen is prescribed, administer with caution and close observation to prevent carbon dioxide narcosis (see Figure 25-1).
- Ensure that influenza and pneumococcal vaccines have been administered, unless contraindicated.

Desired Outcomes

The patient
> maintains a patent airway
> expectorates secretions
> is free from respiratory infection

Nursing Diagnosis

Activity intolerance related to chronic hypoxia

Goal

> The patient performs ADLs without becoming fatigued or experiencing respiratory symptoms

Actions

- Identify factors that contribute to activity intolerance (eg, interruptions to sleep due to coughing, lack of knowledge of ways to schedule activities to preserve energy) and control or improve as possible.

(Continued)

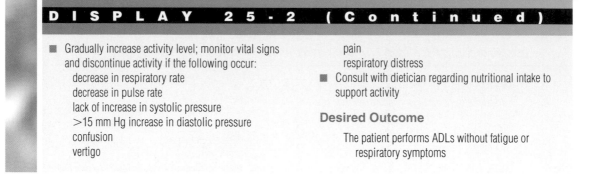

DISPLAY 25-2 (Continued)

■ Gradually increase activity level; monitor vital signs and discontinue activity if the following occur:
  decrease in respiratory rate
  decrease in pulse rate
  lack of increase in systolic pressure
  >15 mm Hg increase in diastolic pressure
  confusion
  vertigo
  pain
  respiratory distress

■ Consult with dietician regarding nutritional intake to support activity

Desired Outcome

The patient performs ADLs without fatigue or respiratory symptoms

---

used (Fig. 25-1). The gauge should be checked frequently to ensure that it is set at the prescribed level; the oxygen flow should be checked for any interruption or blockage from an empty tank, kinked tubing, or other problem. Nurses should evaluate and recommend the method of administration that will be most effective for the individual patient. Older patients who breathe by mouth or have poor control in keeping their lips sealed most of the time may not receive the full benefit of a nasal cannula. An emaciated person whose facial structure does not allow for a tight seal of a face mask may lose a significant portion of oxygen through leakage. A patient who is insecure and anxious inside an oxygen tent may spend oxygen for emotional stress and not gain full therapeutic benefit. The patient's nasal passages should be regularly cleaned to maintain patency. Indications of insufficient oxygenation must be closely monitored; some older persons will not become cyanotic when hypoxic, so other signs must be evaluated. With increasing numbers of patients being discharged from hospitals on oxygen for home use and with the realization that many elderly people lack capabilities, knowledge, and caregiver support, realistic appraisals of the patient's ability to use home oxygen safely are crucial. Information must be reinforced and supervision through home health agencies or other community resources used until the patient or caregiver is comfortable and competent with this treatment. The home environment must be evaluated for safety. Consideration must be given to the impact of oxygen on the patient and family's total lifestyle; whether home oxygen results in the family having a new lease on life or becoming prisoners in their home can be

influenced by the assistance and support they are given.

Postural drainage often is prescribed for removing bronchial secretions in certain respiratory conditions. The basic steps for this procedure are the same as those for other adults, with some slight modifications. If aerosol medications are prescribed, they should be administered before the postural drainage procedure. The position for postural drainage depends on the individual patient and on the portion of the lung involved. The older patient needs to change positions slowly and be allowed a few minutes to rest between position changes to adjust to the new position. The usual last position for postural drainage—lying face down across the bed with the head at floor level—may be stressful for the older person and have adverse effects. The nurse can consult with the physician regarding the advisability of this position and possible alterations to meet the needs of the individual patient. Cupping and vibration facilitate drainage of secretions; it must be emphasized that old tissues and bones are more fragile and may be injured more easily. The procedure should be discontinued immediately if dyspnea, palpitation, chest pain, diaphoresis, apprehension, or any other sign of distress occurs. Thorough oral hygiene and a period of rest should follow postural drainage. Documentation of the tolerance of the procedure and the amount and characteristic of the mucus drained is essential.

Coughing to remove secretions is important in the management of respiratory problems; however, nonproductive coughing may be a useless expenditure of energy and stressful to the older patient. Various measures can be used to promote productive cough-

pectorants also may be prescribed to loosen secretions and make coughing more productive. A basic, although extremely significant, measure to reinforce is good fluid intake. Patients should be advised to use paper tissues, not cloth handkerchiefs, for sputum expectoration. Frequent handwashing and oral hygiene are essential and have many physical and psychological benefits.

> **KEY CONCEPT**
> Nonproductive coughing can be a useless expenditure of energy and stressful to an older adult.

COMPLEMENTARY THERAPIES

Some herbs are believed to affect respiratory health. Mullein, marshmallow, and slippery elm have mucus-secreting effects and can soothe irritated respiratory linings. Lobelia, coltsfoot, and sanguinaria have been used as expectorants. Aromatherapy using eucalyptus, pine, lavender, and lemon may prove useful. Prior to introducing any herbal remedy, research for possible interactions with medications the patient is using and discuss with the physician.

Hot, spicy foods (eg, garlic, onion, chili peppers) are recommended to open air passages, whereas mucus-forming foods, such as dairy products and processed foods, are ill advised. Vitamins A, C, E, and B_6, zinc; and proteolytic enzymes are suggested as dietary supplements.

Acupuncture, under a trained therapist, is used for the management of asthma, emphysema, and hay fever. Acupressure is being used with some benefit by persons with asthma, bronchitis, and emphysema. Yoga can promote deep breathing and good oxygenation of tissues. Rolfing (a technique using pressure applied with the fingers, knuckles, and elbows to release fascial adhesions and realign the body into balance) and massage can free the rib cage and improve breathing. Growing numbers of Americans are using complementary therapies for the prevention and management of respiratory conditions. Although the efficacy of these methods may not be fully established, nurses should keep an open mind; if the therapy does no harm and is believed by the individual to be of benefit, positive outcomes could be achieved by combining complementary with traditional treatments.

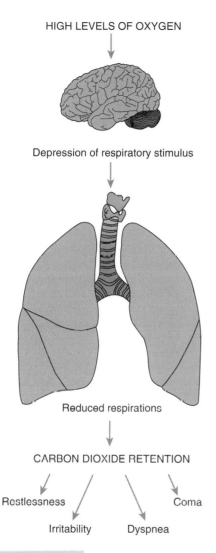

HIGH LEVELS OF OXYGEN → Depression of respiratory stimulus → Reduced respirations → CARBON DIOXIDE RETENTION → Restlessness, Irritability, Dyspnea, Coma

FIGURE 25-1

Oxygen must be administered to older people carefully. Chronic high levels of oxygen can depress the respiratory stimulus in the brain, thereby reducing respiration and promoting carbon dioxide retention.

ing. Hard candy and other sweets increase secretions, thereby helping to make the cough productive. The breathing exercises discussed earlier can also be beneficial. A variety of humidifiers can be obtained without prescription for home use; the patient needs to be taught the correct, safe use of such an apparatus. Ex-

PROMOTING SELF-CARE

Bronchodilators may be prescribed in pocket nebulizer form for the treatment of bronchial asthma and other conditions causing bronchospasm, such as chronic bronchitis or emphysema. Effective use of these devices depends on the ability of the individual to manipulate the apparatus and coordinate the spray with inhalation—areas that can be problematic for older persons with slower responses, poorer coordination, arthritic joints, or general weakness. Before an inhaler is prescribed, the ability of the patient to use it correctly must be assessed. If the patient is able to manage the skills required for use, instructions and precautions should be reviewed in depth. The patient and caregivers must understand the serious cardiac effects of excessive use. Normally, one or two inhalations are sufficient to relieve symptoms for 4 hours. To ensure that the inhaler does not become empty unexpectedly and leave the person without medication when needed, the fullness of the inhaler should be evaluated periodically by placing it in a bowl of water. When full, the inhaler will sink; when empty, it will float—varying levels in between indicate partial levels of fullness.

> **KEY CONCEPT**
> The effective use of inhalers requires the ability of the user to manipulate the apparatus and coordinate the spray with inhalation—tasks that can be difficult for some older persons.

Not long ago, patients on ventilator support were found in intensive care units of acute hospitals. Today, growing numbers of ventilator-dependent persons are being managed at home or in long-term care facilities. Each ventilator has unique features, and nurses should seek the guidance of a respiratory care specialist to ensure a thorough understanding and correct use of the equipment. Whether in their own homes or in an institutional setting, these patients need strong multidisciplinary support to assist with the complex web of physical, emotional, and social care needs they may present. Nurses can play a significant role in providing a realistic assessment of the abilities of patients and family caregivers to manage ventilator-related care. It makes little sense to use a ventilator to save a patient's life and then threaten that life by sending the person home with a family who cannot meet care needs. Special attention also must be paid to the quality of life of the ventilator-dependent patient; counseling, sensory stimulation, expressive therapies, and other resources should be used.

Polyvalent influenza vaccines and pneumococcal vaccines can benefit most elderly persons and are particularly advisable for those with respiratory disease. Patients should be encouraged to discuss these vaccines with their physicians, and when patients are unable to take this initiative, nurses should plan to do so.

Respiratory problems are frightening and produce anxiety. Patients with these conditions require psychological support and reassurance, especially during periods of dyspnea. Patients need a complete understanding of their disease and its management to help reduce their anxiety. Repeated encouragement may be required to assist the patient in meeting the demands of a chronic disease. Some patients may find it necessary to spend most of their time indoors to avoid the extremes of hot and cold weather; some may have to learn to transport oxygen with them as they travel outside their homes; some may need to move to a different climate for relief. These changes in lifestyle may have a significant impact on their total lives. As with any persons having chronic diseases, patients with respiratory problems can benefit from being assisted to live the fullest life possible with their conditions, rather than become prisoners to them.

Critical Thinking Exercises

1. What self-imposed and environmentally imposed risks to younger adults can contribute to the development of respiratory conditions in later life?
2. In what ways can age-related changes affect the development, recognition, and management of respiratory conditions?
3. What key points would you include in an educational program for the promotion of respiratory health in senior citizens?
4. Describe the precautions that must be taken when oxygen is administered to older adults.

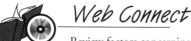

Web Connect

Review factors concerning air pollution and respiratory health at www.cdc.gov/nceh/airpollution.

● Resources

American Lung Association
1740 Broadway
New York, NY 10019
(212) 315-8700
www.lungusa.org

Asthma and Allergy Foundation of America
19 West 44th Street
New York, NY 10036
(212) 921-9100
www.aafa.org

National Heart, Lung, and Blood Institute Information Center
P.O. Box 30105
Bethesda, MD 20824
(301) 592-8573
www.nhlbi.nih.gov

Office on Smoking and Health
Centers for Disease Control and Prevention
4770 Buford Highway NE
Atlanta, GA 30341
(800) 232-1311
www.cdc.gov/tobacco

● Reference

Williams, S. G., Schmidt, D. K., Redd, S. C., & Storms, W., and the National Asthma Education and Prevention Program. (2003). Key clinical activities for quality asthma care. Recommendations of the National Asthma Education and Prevention Program. *MMWR Recommendations Report, March 28*(52)(RR-6), 1–8.

● Recommended Readings

Barnes, P. J. (2001). Modern management of COPD in the elderly. *Annals of Long-Term Care, 9*(5), 51–56.

Janowiak, J. J., & Hawthorne, D. C. (1999). A comprehensive approach to controlling allergies and asthma. *Alternative and Complementary Therapies, 5*(5), 251–253.

McBride, S., Graydon, J., Sidani, S., & Hall, L. (1999). The therapeutic use of music for dyspnea and anxiety in patients with COPD who live at home. *Journal of Holistic Nursing, 17*(5), 229–250.

Monahan, K. (1999). A joint effort to affect lives: The COPD wellness program. *Geriatric Nursing, 20*(4), 200–208.

Rosenberg, H., & Resnick, B. (2003). Exercise intervention in patients with chronic obstructive pulmonary disease. *Geriatric Nursing, 24*(2), 90–98.

Wynd, C. A. (1997). Smoking cessation. In B. M. Dossey (Ed.), *Core Curriculum for Holistic Nursing* (pp. 220–225). Gaithersburg, MD: Aspen.

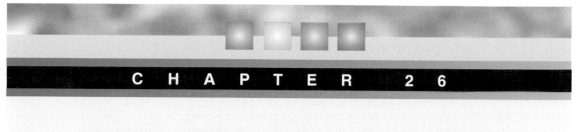

Gastrointestinal Conditions

■ Learning Objectives

After reading this chapter, you should be
able to:

• describe the scope of gastrointestinal
problems in the older population

• discuss measures to promote
gastrointestinal health

• list symptoms and management of
selected gastrointestinal disorders

Scope and Impact of Gastrointestinal Problems in Late Life

Significantly fewer older people die from gastrointestinal problems than from diseases of other major body systems; however, these problems often are the source of many complaints and discomforts in this age group. Indigestion, belching, diarrhea, constipation, nausea, vomiting, anorexia, weight gain or loss, and flatulence are among the bothersome problems that increasingly occur, even in the absence of organic cause. Gallbladder disease and various cancers of the gastrointestinal tract increase in incidence in later life. In addition, poor nutrition, medications, emotions, inactivity, and a variety of other factors influence the status of gastrointestinal health.

Usually, older adults are aware of their gastrointestinal discomforts and use various measures to manage symptoms of these problems. In some situations, misinformation can interfere with good gastrointestinal health (eg, assuming that tooth loss is normal or believing a daily laxative is essential); in other circumstances, self-treatment can delay the diagnosis of pathologies (eg, using antacids to mask symptoms of stomach cancer). Astute assessment can reveal problems that patients may have omitted sharing with their physicians and can identify practices that interfere with good health. Assessment considerations and potential nursing diagnoses for gastrointestinal problems are described in Display 26-1 and Nursing Diagnosis Table 26-1, respectively.

Facilitating Gastrointestinal Health

A variety of gastrointestinal problems can be avoided by good health practices. Good dental hygiene and regular visits to the dentist can prevent disorders that can threaten nutritional intake, general health, comfort, and self-image. The proper quantity and quality of foods can enhance general health and minimize the risk of indigestion and constipation. (Refer to Chapter 16 for more specific information on ways to promote nutritional health.) Knowledge of the relationship of medications to gastrointestinal health is also important.

Selected Disorders

ANOREXIA

Anorexia can be related to a variety of conditions, including medication side effects, inactivity, physical illness, or age-related changes, such as decreased taste and smell sensations, reduced production of the hormone leptin, and gastric changes that cause satiation with smaller volumes of food intake. In the elderly particularly, losses and challenges (eg, death of loved ones, financial worries, and living with effects of chronic conditions) could cause anxiety and depression that could affect appetite. The initial step in managing this problem is to identify its cause. Depending on the cause, treatment could consist of a high-calorie diet, referral to social programs, tube feeding, hyperalimentation, psychiatric therapy, or medications. Some stimulation to the appetite can be achieved through the use of certain herbs, such as ginger root, ginseng, gotu kola, and peppermint. Intake, output, and weight should be monitored; weight loss greater than 5% within a 1-month period and 10%

within a 6-month period are considered significant and require evaluation.

DRY MOUTH (XEROSTOMIA)

Saliva serves several important functions, such as lubricating soft tissues, assisting in remineralizing teeth, promoting taste sensations, and helping to control bacteria and fungus in the oral cavity. Reduced saliva, therefore, can have significant consequences.

Dry mouth can be caused by a variety of factors in addition to age-related slight declines in saliva secretion. Many of the medications used by the elderly (eg, diuretics, antihypertensives, anti-inflammatories, and antidepressants) can affect salivation. Sjögren's syndrome, a disease of the immune system, can reduce salivary gland function and cause severe dryness of the mucous membrane. Mouth breathing and altered cognition contribute to this problem, also.

Persons with dry mouth benefit from frequent oral hygiene, not only because of the comfort obtained, but also to reduce the higher risk of dental disease related to dry mouth. Saliva substitutes (eg, Salivart Synthetic Saliva) are available as gels and rinses; however, sipping water to relieve dryness and stimulating saliva production with hard sugarless candy and gum are effective for many individuals.

DENTAL PROBLEMS

Dental care is important throughout an individual's life. Dental examination can be instrumental in the early detection and prevention of many problems that affect other body systems. Poor teeth can restrict food intake, which can cause constipation and malnourishment; they also detract from appearance, which can affect socialization, and this can result in a poor appetite, which also can lead to malnourishment. Periodontal disease can predispose the aged to systemic infection. Although dental care is important in preventing these problems, financial limitations prevent many older persons from seeking dental attention. Some have the misconception that dentures eliminate the need for regular visits to the dentist; others, like many younger persons, fear the dentist. The nurse should encourage regular dental examination and promote dental care, explaining that serious diseases can be detected by the dentist and helping patients

D I S P L A Y   2 6 - 1

Assessment of Gastrointestinal Conditions

General Observations

General appearance: Pallor can be associated with blood loss from gastrointestinal bleeding. Weakness and fatigue can be due to malnutrition, fluid and electrolyte imbalances, or bleeding. Obesity or unusual thinness should be noted.

Odors. Unusual breath odors can be associated with disorders. Halitosis can indicate poor oral hygiene practices, disease of the oral cavity or esophagus, lung abscess or infection, liver disease, or uremia.

Skin. Dry, poorly turgored skin can indicate dehydration; scaling, itching, discolored skin, or skin eruptions can result from a variety of nutritional deficiencies.

Interview

Carefully structured questions can reveal hidden problems, particularly in older adults who accept some gastrointestinal symptoms as normal or who have lived with these symptoms for so long that they no longer consider them abnormalities. Questions should review topics such as the following:

Status of teeth or dentures. "When was your last dental exam? How do you care for your teeth or dentures? When did you get your dentures; how do they fit? Do you have any pain, bleeding, or other symptoms?"

Taste, appetite. "Does food taste differently to you than it did in the past? What do you do to make food taste better? How is your appetite; how does it compare to earlier years?"

Symptoms. "Do you ever have a sore mouth, difficulty swallowing, choking, a sense that something has 'gone down the wrong hole,' nausea, vomiting, bleeding from your mouth, blood in your vomitus or stool, pain or burning in your stomach or intestines, diarrhea, constipation, gas, bleeding from your rectum?" Specific questions should be asked to explore each positive response.

Weight. "Have you noticed any recent changes in your weight? Have you been trying to gain or lose weight?"

Digestion. "How often do you have indigestion? What seems to cause it and how is it managed? Is there a sense of fullness or discomfort in the chest after meals? Does regurgitation or belching ever occur?"

Elimination. "How often do you have a bowel movement? Do you have to take special measures to move your bowels? If so, what are they? Do you strain to have a bowel movement? Is there ever blood in your stools or on the toilet tissue? What are the color and consistency of your bowel movements?"

Diet. "Describe what and when you eat in a typical day. Do foods have a different taste to you? Can you shop for and cook meals on your own? Has your eating pattern changed?"

Further questions may be necessary in response to certain problems that emerge through the interview.

Physical Examination

Inspection, auscultation, percussion, and palpation aid in validating problems identified through the interview and in detecting undisclosed disorders. A systematic examination of the gastrointestinal system would review the following:

Lips. Note symmetry, color, moisture, and general condition. Because capillaries are abundant in the lips, a bluish discoloration could reflect poor oxygenation. Cracks and fissures can be associated with riboflavin deficiencies; jagged teeth or poorly fitting dentures also can be responsible for cuts and cracks on the lips.

(Continued)

Oral cavity. With a tongue depressor and flashlight, inspect the mouth. The mucous membrane should be moist and pink. Black persons may have a pigmented mucosa. Excessive dryness of the mucosa or tongue can indicate dehydration. Note lesions or areas of irritation, which could be caused by teeth, dentures, or pathologic conditions. White beads in the oral cavity can be a sign of moniliasis infections and should be cultured. Bleeding, swollen gums are most commonly associated with periodontal disease. Swollen gums also can result from phenytoin therapy or leukemia. Lead poisoning causes a bluish black line along the edge of the gums, but only if teeth are present. Older persons can develop lead poisoning due to occupational exposure or contact within their home environment.

Tongue. Examine the top and bottom surface of the tongue. A coating on the tongue can be associated with poor hygiene or dehydration. A smooth, red tongue occurs with iron, vitamin B12, or niacin deficiencies.

Thick, white patches can indicate leukoplakia, which could be precancerous. Attention should be given to lesions on the tongue that have been present for several weeks because they can be cancerous; they more frequently occur on the bottom surface than on the top of the tongue. Varicosities on the undersurface of the tongue are not unusual findings.

Pharynx. During normal swallowing, the vagus nerve causes the soft palate to rise and block the nasopharynx so that aspiration is prevented. To test this function, press a tongue depressor on the middle of the tongue, but not so far back that gagging results, and ask the patient to say "ah." The soft palate should rise when "ah" is said. If soreness, redness, or white patches are present in the throat, a culture is warranted.

Abdomen. Have the patient lie supine on a firm surface and inspect the abdomen. Have the patient void first. Ask about any scars that are present; the patient may have forgotten to mention an appendectomy that occurred 50 years ago. Striae, or stretch marks, are pink or blue if newly developed and silvery white if old; they can result from obesity, ascites, pregnancy, or tumors. Rashes, indentations and other findings should be noted. Both sides of the abdomen should be symmetrical with no bulging areas. A symmetrical distention most commonly is due to obesity, although it also can be associated with ascites or tumors. Central, lower-abdominal (ie, below the umbilicus) distention occurs with bladder distention or tumors of the uterus or ovaries. Central, upper abdominal distention may result from gastric dilation or pancreatic tumors. The abdomen should rise and fall in conjunction with respirations. Peristaltic activity may be observed; sometimes, gently flicking a finger on the abdomen will stimulate peristalsis. With the diaphragm of the stethoscope, bowel sounds can be heard about once every 5 to 15 seconds; they usually are irregular. If no bowel sounds are heard, try stimulating them by flicking a finger on the abdomen. No sounds for at least 5 minutes can indicate the absence of bowel sounds, and medical evaluation would be warranted. Loud, gurgling sounds indicate increased peristaltic activity. Palpation of the abdomen should normally reveal no masses.

Rectum. A rectal examination can be performed with the patient in a standing position, bent over the examination table, or in a left lateral position with the right hip and knee flexed. Inspect the perianal area first. Flaccid skin sacs around the anus are hemorrhoids. Fissures, tumors, inflammation, and poor hygienic practices may be noted. Ask the patient to bear down, which could make additional hemorrhoids or rectal prolapse visible. Ask the patient to bear down again and inset a lubricated gloved finger into the anal canal. Assure the patient that it is normal to feel as if a bowel movement is imminent. The sphincter should tighten around the finger. Masses or other abnormalities along the rectal wall should be noted. A hard mass that prevents full palpation of the rectum may be a fecal impaction. Impactions may or may not be movable. If it is a fecal impaction, fecal material will be found on the glove or a discharge will occur when the examining finger is withdrawn.

Stool. A stool specimen should be obtained; fecal material withdrawn during the rectal examination can give clues to problems. Black, tarry stools can be associated with the ingestion of iron preparations or iron-rich foods or can indicate upper gastrointestinal bleeding; bright-red blood accompanies bleeding from the lower bowel or hemorrhoids; pale, fatty stool can occur with absorption problems; gray or tan stool is caused by obstructive jaundice; and mucus in the stool may result from inflammation.

ND *Nursing Diagnosis*

TABLE 26-1 ● *Nursing Diagnoses Related to Gastrointestinal Problems*

Causes or Contributing Factors	Nursing Diagnosis
Anemia, constipation, obesity, vitamin and mineral deficiencies, dehydration	Activity Intolerance
Anorexia, obesity, hemorrhoids, lack of roughage in diet, dehydration, habitual laxative use	Constipation
Medications, peptic ulcer, gastritis, ulcerative colitis, diverticulitis, diabetes, fecal impaction, tube feedings, stress	Diarrhea
Indigestion, constipation, hemorrhoids, flatus	Acute Pain
Uncontrolled diabetes, infection, peritonitis, diarrhea, vomiting, blood loss, insufficient fluid intake, high-solute tube feedings	Deficient Fluid Volume
Diabetes, malnutrition, hemorrhoids	Risk for Infection
Intestinal obstruction, anorexia, nausea, vomiting, poor dental status, altered taste sensations, constipation	Imbalanced Nutrition: Less Than Body Requirements
Altered taste sensations, ethnic preferences, inactivity, lack of motivation to eat well	Imbalanced Nutrition: More Than Body Requirements
Diabetes, cancer, gingivitis, periodontal disease, jagged teeth, poorly fitting dentures, dehydration, malnutrition, dry mouth	Impaired Oral Mucous Membrane

find free or inexpensive dental clinics. Understanding how modern dental techniques minimize pain can alleviate fears. Although older persons may not have had the benefit of fluoridated water or fluoride treatments when younger, topical fluoride treatments are as beneficial to the teeth of the aged as they are to younger teeth. Patients should be instructed to inform their dentists about health problems and medications they take to help them determine how procedures need to be modified, what healing rate to expect, and which medications cannot be administered.

Dental problems can be caused by altered taste sensation, a poor diet, or a low-budget carbohydrate diet with excessive intake of sweets, which can cause tooth decay. Deficiencies of the vitamin B complex and calcium, hormonal imbalances, hyperparathyroidism, diabetes, osteomalacia, Cushing disease, and syphilis can be underlying causes of dental problems, and certain drugs, such as phenytoin, which can cause gingivitis or antihistamines, and antipsychotics, which cause severe dry mouth, can play a part. The aging process itself takes its toll on teeth. Surfaces are commonly worn down from many years of use, varying degrees of root absorption occur, and loss of tooth enamel increase the risk of irritation to deeper dental tissue. Although be-

nign neoplastic lesions develop more frequently than malignant ones, cancer of the oral cavity, especially in men, increases in incidence with age, as does moniliasis, which is often associated with more serious problems, such as diabetes or leukemia. It should not be assumed that all white lesions found in the mouth are moniliasis; biopsy is important to make sure they are not cancerous. Periodontal disease, which damages the soft tissue surrounding teeth and supporting bones, has a high incidence among the elderly. Dental caries occur less frequently in older people, but they remain a problem.

KEY CONCEPT
With age, the teeth experience a wearing down of the surfaces, decrease in the size and volume of pulp, increased brittleness, varying degrees of root absorption, and a loss of enamel.

Good oral hygiene is especially important to the aged, who already may be having problems with anorexia or food distaste. Teeth, gums, and tongue should be brushed regularly using a soft toothbrush, which also can be used in gentle gum massage for people with dentures. Daily flossing of natural teeth should be performed, and brushing is superior to using swabs, even for the teeth of unconscious patients. Because the buccal mucosa is thinner and less vascular with age, trauma to the oral cavity should be avoided. The nurse should notify the dentist and physician of an atonic or atrophic tongue, lesions, mucosa discoloration, loose teeth, soreness, bleeding, or any other problem identified during inspection and care of the oral cavity.

DYSPHAGIA

The incidence of swallowing difficulties increases with age. As swallowing depends on complex mechanisms involving several cranial nerves and the muscles of the mouth, face, pharynx, and esophagus, anything that impacts those structures can cause dysphagia. Gastroesophageal reflux disease (GERD) is a common cause, as are stroke and structural disorders. Dysphagia can be oropharyngeal, characterized by difficulty transferring food from the mouth into the pharynx and esophagus, or esophageal, involving transfer of food down the esophagus.

A careful assessment and observation assists in diagnosing the cause of the problem. Patients with dysphagia should be asked:

* when the problem began
* what other symptoms accompany the dysphagia (chest pain, nausea, or coughing)
* what types of foods are most problematic (eg, solids or liquids)
* if the problem is intermittent or present with every meal

An observation of food intake can offer insights into the nature of the problem. Referral to a speech-language pathologist is essential to developing an effective plan of care.

Prevention of aspiration and promotion of adequate nutritional status are major goals in the care of patients with dysphagia. Follow the recommendations of the speech-language therapist closely. Patients with dysphagia should eat in an upright position, ingesting small bites in an unhurried manner. Offer verbal cues as needed. An easily-accessible suction machine is beneficial in the event of choking. Food intake and weight are important to monitor.

HIATAL HERNIA

The incidence of hiatal hernia increases with age, affecting about half of the people over age 50, and is of greater incidence in older women. There is some thought that the low-fiber diets of Americans contributes to the high prevalence of this condition. The two types of hiatal hernia are sliding (axial) and rolling (paraesophageal). The sliding type is the most common and occurs when a part of the stomach and the junction of the stomach and esophagus slide through the diaphragm. Most patients with GERD have this type of hiatal hernia. In the rolling or paraesophageal type, the fundus and greater curvatures of the stomach roll up through the diaphragm. Heartburn, dysphagia, belching, vomiting, and regurgitation are common symptoms associated with hiatal hernia. These symptoms are especially problematic when the patient is recumbent. Pain, sometimes mistaken for a heart attack, and bleeding may also occur. Diagnosis is confirmed by a barium swallow and esophagoscopy. A majority of patients are managed medically. If the patient is obese, weight reduction can minimize the problem. A bland diet may be recommended, as may the use of milk and antacids for symptomatic relief. Several small meals each day rather than three large ones help improve hiatal hernias and may be advantageous to the aged in coping with other age-related gastrointestinal problems. Eating before bedtime should be discouraged. Some patients may find it helpful to sleep in a partly recumbent position. H2 blockers, such as ranitidine, cimetidine, or nizatidine, and proton-pump inhibitors like lansoprazole and omeprazole, often are prescribed. Display 26-2 offers a sample care plan for the patient with hiatal hernia.

> **KEY CONCEPT**
> Several small meals throughout the day, rather than three large ones, not only assist in the management of hiatal hernia but also can benefit the gastrointestinal health of all elders.

Most persons affected by cancer of the esophagus are elderly. This disease commonly strikes between the ages of 50 and 70 years and is of higher incidence in men, black people, and alcoholic persons. Poor

DISPLAY 26-2

Sample Care Plan for the Patient With Hiatal Hernia

Nursing Diagnosis

Pain

Goal

The patient is free from discomfort related to hiatal hernia.

Actions

- Assist patient in identifying situations that cause discomfort (eg, bending, bedtime snacking); advise patient to avoid them.
- Teach and support low-calorie diet if obesity is a problem.
- Advise patient to eat 5 to 6 small-portioned meals during the day rather than 3 large meals; in a hospital or institutional setting, consult with dietician to arrange this meal plan.
- Instruct patient to eat meals slowly and to sit upright while eating and for at least 1 hour thereafter.
- Discourage consumption of spicy foods, caffeinated beverages, carbonated beverages, and alcohol.
- Advise patient to stop smoking if patient has this habit; refer to smoking cessation program as needed.
- Advise patient against consuming food for at least 2 hours prior to bed time or nap.
- Instruct patient to avoid heavy lifting, bending, wearing girdles or tight pants, and coughing or sneezing strenuously.
- Prevent constipation to avoid straining during bowel movements.
- Elevate upper portion of bed by placing blocks under the head of the bed (this is preferable to raising upper portion of mattress due to risk of shearing force).

- Administer antacids as prescribed.

Desired Outcome

The patient
  is free from pain and pressure
  maintains weight within the desired range
  consumes the prescribed diet

Nursing Diagnosis

Imbalanced nutrition

Goals

The patient
  consumes the prescribed diet
  is free from abdominal discomfort

Actions

- Consult with nutritionist and physician to develop diet plan appropriate for the patient.
- Instruct patient to eat 5 or 6 small-portioned meals rather than 3 large ones.
- Identify foods that increase symptoms and instruct patient to omit these from diet; offer foods of equal nutritive value to replace food eliminated from diet if necessary.
- Record and monitor weight and dietary intake.

Desired Outcomes

The patient
  maintains weight within desired range
  ingests the prescribed diet in 5 to 6 small meals daily

oral hygiene and chronic irritation from tobacco, alcohol, and other agents contribute to the development of this problem. Barrett's esophagus, a condition in which the normal lining of the esophagus is replaced by a type of lining usually found in the intestines (intestinal metaplasia) is associated with an increased risk of developing cancer (Peters, 2003); the risk of developing adenocarcinoma is 30 to 125 times higher in people who have Barrett's esophagus than in people who do not (National Institute of Diabetes and Digestive and Kidney Disease, 2002). Dysphagia, weight loss, excessive salivation, thirst, hiccups, anemia, and chronic bleeding are symptoms of the disease. Barium swallow, esophagoscopy, and biopsy are performed as diagnostic measures. Treatment usually consists of surgical resection and a poor prognosis is common among aged patients. Benign tumors of the esophagus are rare in the elderly.

PEPTIC ULCER

Although peptic ulcers occur most frequently at younger ages, the incidence of this problem is on the rise for older persons. In addition to stress, diet, and genetic predisposition as causes, particular factors are believed to account for the increased incidence of ulcers in the aged, including longevity, more precise diagnostic evaluation, and the fact that ulcers can be a complication of chronic obstructive pulmonary disease, which is increasingly prevalent. Drugs commonly prescribed for the elderly that can increase gastric secretions and reduce the resistance of the mucosa include aspirin, reserpine, tolbutamide, phenylbutazone, colchicine, and adrenal corticosteroids.

Peptic ulcers tend to present with more acute symptoms in the elderly, such as pain, bleeding, obstruction, and perforation. Diagnostic and therapeutic measures resemble those used for younger adults. The nurse should be alert to complications associated with peptic ulcer, which may be especially threatening to the geriatric patient, such as constipation or diarrhea caused by antacid therapy and pyloric obstruction resulting in dehydration, peritonitis, hemorrhage, and shock.

> ✔ **Point to Ponder**
>
> *In what ways do diet, activity, emotions, and other factors affect your appetite, diet, digestion, and bowel elimination? Do you notice any patterns that you could correct, and, if so, how?*

CANCER OF THE STOMACH

The incidence of gastric cancer increases with age, occurring most frequently in people between 50 and 70 years of age. It is more prevalent among men, black people, and poor socioeconomic groups. Adenocarcinomas account for most gastric malignancies. Anorexia, epigastric pain, weight loss, and anemia are symptoms of gastric cancer; these symptoms may be insidious and easily mistaken for indigestion problems. Bleeding and enlargement of the liver may occur. Symptoms related to pelvic metastasis may also develop. Diagnosis is confirmed by barium swallow and gastroscopy with biopsy. Surgical treatment consisting of a partial or total gastrectomy is preferred. Unfortunately, older people with gastric cancer have a poor prognosis.

> 🔑 **KEY CONCEPT**
> Symptoms of gastric cancer can be insidious and easily mistaken for indigestion.

DIVERTICULAR DISEASE

Multiple pouches of intestinal mucosa in the weakened muscular wall of the large bowel, known as diverticulosis, are common among the elderly. Chronic constipation, obesity, hiatal hernia, and atrophy of the intestinal wall muscles with aging contribute to this problem. The low-fiber, low-residue diets that are common in Western societies are a major reason for diverticulosis being common in this country but rare in many Third World countries. Most cases involve the sigmoid colon; many cases are asymptomatic. If symptoms are present, they can include slight bleeding, as well as a change in bowel habits (constipation, diarrhea, or both) and tenderness on palpation of the left lower quadrant. Usually a barium enema identifies the problem. Surgery is not performed unless severe bleeding develops. Medical management is most common and includes an increase in dietary fiber intake, weight reduction, and avoidance of constipation.

Bowel contents can accumulate in the diverticula and decompose, causing inflammation and infection; this is known as diverticulitis. Although fewer than half the patients with diverticulosis develop diverticulitis, most patients who do are elderly. Older men tend to experience this problem more than any other group.

Overeating, straining during a bowel movement, alcohol, and irritating foods may contribute to diverticulitis in the patient with diverticulosis. Abrupt onset of pain in the left lower quadrant, similar to that of appendicitis but over the sigmoid area, is a symptom of this problem. Nausea, vomiting, constipation, diarrhea, low-grade fever, and blood or mucus in the stool may also occur. These attacks can be severely acute or slowly progressing; although the acute attacks can cause peritonitis, the slower forms can also be serious because of the possibility of lower bowel obstruction resulting from scarring and abscess formation. In addition to the mentioned complications, fistulas to the bladder, vagina, colon, and intestines can develop. During the acute phase, efforts are focused on reducing infection, providing nutrition, relieving discomfort, and promoting rest. Usually nothing is ingested by mouth, and intravenous therapy is used. When the acute episode subsides, the patient is taught to consume a low-residue diet. Surgery, performed if medical management is unsuccessful or if serious complications occur, may consist of a resection or temporary colostomy. Continued follow-up should be encouraged.

CANCER OF THE COLON

Cancer at any site along the large intestine is common in the elderly and affects both sexes equally. The sigmoid colon and rectum tend to be frequent sites for carcinoma; in fact, colorectal cancer is the second most common malignancy in the United States. Although the pattern of symptoms frequently varies for each person, some common symptoms include:

- bloody stools
- change in bowel function
- anorexia
- nausea
- epigastric pain
- jaundice

Some older patients ignore bowel symptoms, believing them to be from constipation, poor diet, or hemorrhoids. The patient's description of bowel problems is less reliable than a digital rectal examination, which detects half of all carcinomas of the large bowel and rectum. Fecal occult blood testing is effective for early detection of colonic tumors. The standard diagnostic tests, including barium enema and sigmoidoscopy with biopsy, are used to confirm the diagnosis. Surgical resection with anastomosis or the

formation of a colostomy is usually performed. Medical-surgical nursing textbooks can provide information on this surgery, and nurses should consult them for specific guidance on caring for patients with this condition.

> **KEY CONCEPT**
> An annual stool occult blood test and digital rectal examination are recommended because they can detect many cancers of the large bowel and rectum. In addition, a flexible sigmoidoscopy every 5 years or a colonoscopy every 10 years is advised as an important test to detect colon cancer.

It is important to realize that a colostomy can present many problems for the aged. In addition to having to adjust to many bodily changes with age, a colostomy presents a major adjustment and a threat to a good self-concept. Older adults may feel that a colostomy further separates them from society's view of normal. Socialization may be impaired by the patient's concern over the reactions of others or by fear of embarrassing episodes. Reduced energy reserves, arthritic fingers, slower movement, and poorer eyesight are among the problems that may hamper the ability to care for a colostomy, thus causing dependency on others to assist with this procedure. This need for assistance may be perceived as a significant loss of independence for elders. Tactful, skilled nursing intervention can promote psychological as well as physical adjustment to a colostomy. Continued follow-up is beneficial to assess the patient's changing ability to engage in this self-care activity, identify problems, and provide ongoing support and reassurance.

ACUTE APPENDICITIS

Although acute appendicitis does not occur frequently in older persons, it is important to note that it may present with altered signs and symptoms if it does occur. The severe pain that occurs in younger persons may be absent in elders, whose pain may be minimal and referred. Fever may be minimal, and leukocytosis may be absent. These differences often cause a delayed diagnosis. Prompt surgery will improve the patient's prognosis. Unfortunately, delayed or missed diagnosis and the inability to improve the general status of the patient before this emergency surgery can lead to greater complications and mortality in older persons with appendicitis.

CHRONIC CONSTIPATION

It is not uncommon for elders to be bothered by and concerned about constipation, and many factors can contribute to this problem, including:

- an inactive lifestyle
- low fiber and fluid intake
- depression
- laxative abuse
- certain medications, such as opiates, sedatives, and aluminum hydroxide gels
- dulled sensations that cause the signal for bowel elimination to be missed
- failure to allow sufficient time for complete emptying of the bowel (there may not be full emptying of the bowel during one movement in elders, and it is not unusual for a second bowel movement to be required half an hour after the initial defecation)

A diet high in fiber and fluid and regular activity can promote bowel elimination, and particular foods that patients find effective (eg, prunes or chocolate pudding) can be incorporated into the regular diet. A mixture of raisins, prunes, dates, and currants can be a nourishing, tasty snack that promotes bowel elimination. (For individuals with chewing impairments, this can be blended with yogurt or applesauce.) Providing a regular time for bowel elimination is often helpful; mornings tend to be the best time for the elderly to empty their bowels. Sometimes rocking the trunk from side to side and back and forth while sitting on the toilet will stimulate a bowel movement. Only after these measures have failed should medications be considered.

> **KEY CONCEPT**
>
> Measures to promote bowel elimination include scheduling a regular time for it, incorporating high-fiber foods into the diet, and rocking the trunk from side to side and back and forth while sitting on the toilet.

Older persons may need education concerning bowel elimination. The safe use of laxatives should be emphasized to prevent laxative abuse. The patient should be aware that diarrhea resulting from laxative abuse may cause dehydration, a serious threat to life. Dandelion root, cascara sagrada, senna, and rhubarb are herbs that stimulate bowel movement and can be taken to prevent constipation.

Older adults in a hospital or nursing home may benefit from an elimination chart that reflects the time, amount, and characteristics of bowel movements. This chart can help the nurse prevent constipation and impaction by providing easily accessible data regarding bowel elimination. Even older persons in the community can benefit from the use of an elimination record that they can maintain themselves.

Chronic constipation that does not improve with the usual measures may require medical evaluation, including anal, rectal, and sigmoid examinations, to determine the presence of any underlying cause.

INTESTINAL OBSTRUCTION

Partial or complete impairment of flow of intestinal contents in the large intestines most often occurs due to cancer of the colon; adhesions and hernias are the primary cause of obstructions in the small intestine. Other causes of blockage include diverticulitis, ulcerative colitis, hypokalemia, vascular problems, and paralytic ileus, a mechanical obstruction that can occur following surgery due to nerves being affected by the extended lack of peristaltic activity.

Symptoms vary depending on the site and cause of the obstruction:

- Small bowel obstruction causes upper and midabdominal pain in rhythmic recurring waves related to the small intestine's attempt to push the contents through the obstruction. Vomiting occurs and may bring some relief.
- Obstructions occurring past the ileum cause abdominal distension so severe that the raised diaphragm can inhibit respirations. Vomiting is more severe than with small bowel blockages and initially is composed of semidigested food and later, contains bile and is more watery.
- Obstruction of the colon causes lower abdominal pain, altered bowel habits, distension, and a sensation of the need to defecate. Vomiting usually does

not occur until late, when the distension reaches the small intestine.

Symptoms must be thoroughly reviewed. Bowel sounds should be noted; bowel obstruction can cause high-pitched peristaltic rushes to be heard on auscultation.

Timely intervention is essential to prevent bowel strangulation and serious complications. X-rays and blood evaluation typically are done to determine the cause and extent of the problem. Intestinal intubation is the major treatment and often helps to decompress the bowel and allow the obstruction to be broken. If medical management is unsuccessful or if the cause is due to vascular or mechanical obstructions, surgery is required. In addition to supporting the medical or surgical treatment plan, nurses need to promote the patient's comfort and ensure that fluid and electrolyte balance is restored and maintained.

FECAL IMPACTION

Constipation frequently leads to fecal impaction in older adults. An absence or insufficient amount of stool should create suspicion of an impaction. What may appear to be diarrhea can be a result of the oozing of liquid feces around the impaction. While taking a rectal temperature, the nurse may detect resistance to the thermometer and find feces on the thermometer when it is withdrawn. A movable mass may be palpated by digital examination. The best approach to fecal impactions is to prevent them from developing; the preventive measures discussed with constipation should be exercised. Once the impaction has developed, it must be softened, broken, and removed.

Because policies may vary, nurses should review the permissive procedures of their employing agency to ensure that removal of a fecal impaction is an acceptable nursing action. An enema, usually oil retention, may be prescribed to assist in the softening and elimination process. Manual breaking and removal of feces with a lubricated gloved finger will promote removal of the impaction. Sometimes, injecting 50 mL hydrogen peroxide through a rectal tube will cause breakage of the impaction as the hydrogen peroxide foams. Care should be taken not to traumatize or overexert the patient during these procedures.

FECAL INCONTINENCE

Involuntary defecation, fecal incontinence, is most often associated with fecal impaction in older adults who are institutionalized or physically or cognitively impaired. For this reason, the initial step is to assess for the presence of an impaction. If an impaction is not present, other causes must be assessed; possible causes of fecal incontinence include decreased contractile strength, impaired automaticity of the puborectal and external anal sphincter (secondary to age-related muscle weakness or injury to the pudendal nerve), and reduced reservoir capacity (secondary to surgical resection or the presence of a tumor). Proctosigmoidoscopy, proctography, and anorectal manometry are among the diagnostic tests used to evaluate this disorder. The cause of the incontinence dictates the treatment approach, which could include bowel retraining (Display 26-3), drugs, surgery, or biofeedback.

CANCER OF THE PANCREAS

Pancreatic cancer is difficult to detect until it has reached an advanced stage. Anorexia, weakness, weight loss, and wasting are generalized symptoms easily attributed to other causes. Dyspepsia, belching, nausea, vomiting, diarrhea, constipation, and obstructive jaundice may occur as well. Fever may or may not be present. Epigastric pain radiating to the back may be experienced. This pain is relieved when the patient leans forward and is worsened when a recumbent position is assumed. Surgery is performed to treat this problem. Unfortunately, the disease is generally so advanced by the time diagnosis is made that the prognosis is usually poor.

BILIARY TRACT DISEASE

The incidence of gallstones increases with age and affects women more frequently than men. Pain is the primary symptom associated with this problem. Treatment measures include nonsurgical therapies, such as rotary lithotrite treatment and extracorporeal shock wave lithotripsy, and the standard surgical procedures. Obstruction, inflammation, and infection are potential outcomes of gallstones and should be monitored.

Cancer of the gallbladder primarily affects older persons, especially women. Fortunately, this disease does not occur frequently. Pain in the right upper quadrant,

D I S P L A Y   2 6 · 3

Bowel Retraining for the Patient With Incontinence

Overview

Bowel incontinence refers to the inability to voluntarily control the passage of stool. It can result from decreased anal muscle tone, disturbances in the neural innervation of the rectum, loss of cortical control, rectal prolapse, diarrhea, constipation with overflow related to impaction, or altered cognition.

Goal

To control bowel elimination

Actions

Record and evaluate patient's bowel elimination pattern.
Establish consistent time to toilet based on pattern.
Position patient in best physiologic position for bowel movement: sitting with normal posture.
Have patient lean forward or prop feet on stool to increase intra-abdominal pressure.
Instruct patient to bear down and attempt to defecate.
Record results; ensure patient does not develop fecal impaction.
If necessary, stimulate anorectal reflex with glycerin suppository 30 to 45 minutes before scheduled bowel movement.
Supplement toilet activities with exercise and good fluid (minimally 1500 mL/d) and fiber intake unless contraindicated.

anorexia, nausea, vomiting, weight loss, jaundice, weakness, and constipation are the usual symptoms. Although surgery may be performed, the prognosis for the patient with cancer of the gallbladder is poor.

Gastrointestinal symptoms, although common, can indicate serious medical problems and need to be taken seriously. The diagnosis of these problems can be difficult because of atypical symptomatology and easy confusion with disorders of other systems. Therefore, the nurse should add as much information as possible to the patient's history to increase the likelihood of prompt, appropriate treatment.

Critical Thinking Exercises

1. Discuss the potential impact of anorexia on physical, mental, and social health.
2. Describe the changes in dental care that have occurred since today's elderly were children and the way in which this will affect dental health of future generations of elders.
3. What preventive measures could be recommended to older adults to promote bowel elimination?
4. Mr. Clark is a 75-year-old participant in an adult day-care program. In interviewing him, you learn that he had a cerebrovascular accident 2 years ago that left him with some right-sided weakness. His medical record indicates that he also has a history of hiatal hernia, depression, hypertension, and osteoarthritis. He is taking antihypertensive, antidepressant, and nonsteroid anti-inflammatory drugs.

   What threats to gastrointestinal health exist for Mr. Clark? How would you determine whether indications of those threats existed and what measures could be taken to reduce those threats?

Web Connect

Explore the Colorectal Cancer Network website at www.colorectal-cancer.net to learn about resources for patients, treatment options, and news pertaining to colorectal cancer.

● **Resources**

National Foundation for Ileitis and Colitis
295 Madison Avenue
New York, NY 10017
(212) 685-3440

National Oral Health Information Clearinghouse
1 NOHIC Way
Bethesda, MD 20892
(301) 402-7364
www.nohic.nidcr.nih.gov

United Ostomy Association
2001 West Beverly Boulevard
Los Angeles, CA 90057
(213) 413-5510
www.uoa.org

● **References**

National Institute of Diabetes and Digestive and Kidney Disease. (2002). *Barrett's esophagus.* Bethesda, MD: National Digestive Diseases Information Center. NIH Publication No. 02-4546.
Peters, J. H. (2003). Barrett's esophagus: Now what? *Annals of Surgery, 237*(3), 299–300.

● **Recommended Readings**

Arnaudm, M. J., & Vellas, B. J. (1998). *Hydration and aging.* New York: Springer.
Bartlett, S. (1998). *Geriatric nutrition handbook.* New York: Chapman and Hall.
Benton, J. M., O'Hara, P. A., Chen, H., Harper, D. W., & Johnson, S. F. (1997). Changing bowel hygiene practice successfully: A program to reduce laxative use in a chronic care hospital. *Geriatric Nursing, 18,* 12–17.
Chernoff, R. (2003). *Geriatric nutrition. The health professionals handbook* (2nd ed.). New York: Jones and Bartlett.
Coleman, P. (2002). Improving oral health care for the frail elderly: A review of widespread problems and best practices. *Geriatric Nursing, 23*(1), 189–197.
Cooper, J., & Wade, W. E. (1998). *Gastrointestinal drug therapy in the elderly.* New York: Pharmaceutical Products Press.
Dunmore, F. (2002). Care models for the older adult with gastroesophageal reflux disease. *Geriatric Nursing, 23*(2), 212–216.
Gaspar, P. M. (1999). Water intake of nursing home residents. *Journal of Gerontological Nursing, 25*(4), 23–29.
Hurwitz, A., Brady, D. A., Schaal, S. E., Samloff, I. M., Dedon, J., & Ruhl, C. E. (1997). Gastric acidity in older adults. *Journal of the American Medical Association, 278*(8), 659–662.
Kasahara, M., Faacks, N., & Shelton, D. (1995). Occasional fecal incontinence among community-dwelling older adults. *Journal of the American Geriatrics Society, 43*(7), 834.
Kayser-Jones, J., & Pengilly, K. (1999). Dysphagia among nursing home residents. *Geriatric Nursing, 20*(2), 7–8.
Liebmann, L. J. (1998). Patterns of nursing home referrals to consultant dieticians. *Geriatric Nursing, 19*(5), 284–286.
Meletis, C. D. (1998). Gastrointestinal integrity and good health: Key nutrients for maintaining the balance of life. *Alternative and Complementary Therapies, 4*(6), 411–413.
Miceli, B. V. (1999). Nursing unit meal management maintenance program: Continuation of safe swallowing and feeding beyond skilled therapeutic intervention. *Journal of Gerontological Nursing, 25*(8), 22–36.
Ratnaike, R., & Hatherly, S. (2002). Dysphagia in older persons, Part I: Oropharyngeal dysphagia. *Clinical Geriatrics, 10*(3), 19–31.
Shanley, C., & O'Loughlin, G. (2000). Dysphagia among nursing home residents: An assessment and management protocol. *Journal of Gerontological Nursing, 28*(8), 35–48.
Sheehy, C., & Hall, G. R. (1998). Rethinking the obvious: A model for preventing constipation. *Journal of Gerontological Nursing, 24*(3), 38–44.
Syngal, S., Schrag, D., Falchuk, M., Tung, N., Farraye, F. A., et al. (2003). Colorectal cancer test use among persons aged ≥50 years. *Journal of the American Medical Association, 289,* 2492–2493.
Thjodleifsson, B., & Jonsson, P. V. (2001). Management of gastroesophageal reflux disease in the elderly patient. *Clinical Geriatrics, 9*(6), 50–57.
Walsh, J. M. E., & Terdiman, J. P. (2003). Colorectal cancer screening: Scientific Review. *Journal of the American Medical Association, 289*(10), 1288–1296.

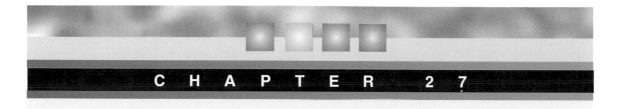

Musculoskeletal Conditions

■ Learning Objectives

After reading this chapter, you should be able to:

- list measures that promote good musculoskeletal function

- describe factors contributing to, symptoms of, and related nursing care for fractures, osteoarthritis, rheumatoid arthritis, osteoporosis, and gout

- discuss pain management measures

- identify risks associated with musculoskeletal problems

- describe measures to facilitate independence in persons with musculoskeletal problems

*I*t is the rare older individual who does not experience some degree of discomfort, disability, or deformity from musculoskeletal disorders. In fact, musculoskeletal diseases are the leading cause of functional impairment in older adults. Stiff and aching joints, muscle cramps, reduced range of motion, and greater ease of fracturing bones are challenges that must be confronted in the elderly. Because activity and mobility are vital to the total health of elders, musculoskeletal problems that limit functional capacity can have devastating effects. The assessment for musculoskeletal problems should consider not only the presence of these conditions but also the effect they have on the older adult's function (Display 27-1). Prevention of these problems and aggressive intervention to minimize their impact if they are present should be integral parts of gerontological nursing care.

Facilitating Musculoskeletal Function

A good diet is important in preventing and managing musculoskeletal problems. A well-balanced diet rich in proteins and minerals will help maintain the structure of the bones and muscles. A minimum of 1500 mg calcium should be included in the diet daily for elderly men and women who are not taking estrogen (1000 mg if taking estrogen). Table 27-2 details good sources of calcium. If dietary intake of calcium does not meet the daily requirement, supplements should be taken to supplement for the deficient amount (ie, if a person who is supposed to consume 1500 mg daily only derives an average of 1000 mg from his or her diet, a 500-mg supplement should be taken).

In addition to the quality of the diet, attention also must be paid to its quantity. Obesity places strain on the joints, which aggravates conditions such as arthritis. Weight reduction frequently will ease musculoskeletal discomforts and reduce limitations and should be promoted as a sound health practice for persons of all ages.

Activity promotes optimum musculoskeletal function and reduces the many complications associated with immobility. Fear of reinjuring a healing bone or causing pain could cause an unnecessary limitation of activities. Realistic explanations describing the healing process or the benefit of exercise to aching joints are most important (Fig. 27-1). Patients and their families can benefit from an understanding of the hazards arising from immobility; sympathetic family members who believe they are helping their elderly relatives by allowing them to be inactive may be more willing to encourage activity if they are aware of the harm that immobility can cause. Continued support, encouragement, and positive reinforcement by nurses can help patients considerably.

> 🔑 **KEY CONCEPT**
> Some older adults may limit activities for fear of reinjuring a healing bone or causing pain.

Selected Disorders

FRACTURES

Trauma, cancer metastasis to the bone, osteoporosis, and other skeletal diseases contribute to fractures in older persons. The neck of the femur is a common site for fractures in elders, especially in older women, and most of these fractures result from falls. Colles' fracture (break at the distal radius) is one of the most frequent upper extremity fractures that occurs when attempting to stop a fall with an outstretched hand. Elders also are at risk for compression fractures of the vertebrae, resulting from falls or lifting heavy objects. Not only do the more brittle bones of older persons fracture more easily, but also their rate of healing is slower than in younger persons, potentially predisposing older adults to the many complications associated with immobility.

Knowing that the risk of fracture and its multiple complications is high among the elderly, the gerontological nurse must aim toward prevention, drawing on the effectiveness of basic common sense measures. Because their coordination and equilibrium are poorer, older people should be advised to avoid risky activities (eg, climbing on ladders or chairs to reach high places). To prevent dizziness and falls resulting from postural hypotension, older individuals should rise from a kneeling or sitting position slowly. Safe, properly fitting shoes with a low, broad heel can prevent stumbling and loss of balance, and hand rails for climbing stairs or rising from the bath tub provide support and balance. Placing both feet near the edge of a curb or bus before stepping up or down is safer than a poorly balanced stretch of the legs (Fig. 27-2). Older persons should be reminded to be careful where they are walking to avoid tripping in holes and

DISPLAY 27-1

Assessment of Musculoskeletal Problems

General Observation

Assessment of the musculoskeletal system can begin even before the formal examination by noting the patient's actions, such as transfer activities, ambulation, and use of hands.

Observations that should be noted include the following:

- abnormal gait (Table 27-1)
- abnormality of structure
- dysfunction of a limb
- favoring of one side
- tremor
- paralysis
- weakness
- atrophy of a limb
- redness, swelling of a joint
- use of cane, walker, wheelchair

Interview

Although it may seem tedious, it is best to go from head to toe and question the patient about limited function or discomfort in specific parts of the body. Examples of questions could include the following:

"Does your jaw ever get stiff or hurt when you chew?"

"Do you get a stiff neck?"

"Does your shoulder ever tighten?"

"Do your hips hurt after you have walked for a while?"

"Are your joints stiff in the morning?"

"Do you have muscle cramps?"

"How far are you able to walk?"

"Are you able to take care of your home, get in and out of a bathtub, and climb stairs?"

Specific inquiry should be made into how the patient manages musculoskeletal pain, particularly in reference to the use of analgesics, heat, and topical preparations.

Physical Examination

The active and passive range of motion of all joints should be examined. Note the degree of movement with and without assistance. Specific areas to review include the following:

Shoulder. The patient should be able to lift both arms straight above the head. With arms straight at the sides, the patient should be able to lift them laterally above the head (ie, 180°) with hands supine and 110° with hands prone. The patient should be able to extend the arms 30° behind the body from the sides.

Neck. The patient should be able to turn the head laterally and to flex and extend the head approximately 30° in all directions.

Elbow. The patient should be able to open the arms fully and flex the joint enough to allow the hand to touch the shoulder.

Wrist. The patient should be able to bend the wrist 80° in the palmar direction and 70° in the dorsal direction. With a hand-waving motion, the patient should be able to bend the wrist laterally 108 toward the radial or thumb side and 60° in the direction of the ulnar side. The patient should be able to move the hand to 90° in the prone and supine positions.

Finger. The patient should be able to bend the distal joint of the finger approximately 45° and the proximal joint 90°. Hyperextension of 30° should be possible.

Hip. While lying down, the patient should be able to abduct and adduct the leg 45°. With the patient lying on his back, the leg should be able to be lifted 90° with the knee straight and 125° with the knee bent.

Knee. While lying on the stomach, the patient should be able to flex the knee approximately 100°.

Ankle. The patient should be able to point the toes 10° toward the head and 408 toward the foot of the bed or examining table. There should be a 35° inversion and a 25° eversion.

(Continued)

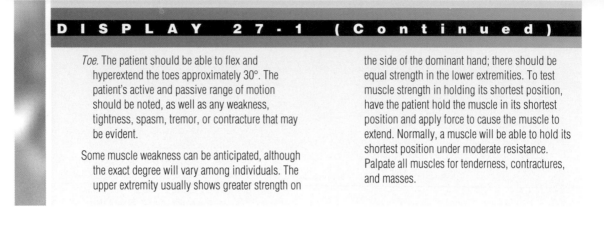

D I S P L A Y   2 7 - 1   (C o n t i n u e d)

Toe. The patient should be able to flex and hyperextend the toes approximately 30°. The patient's active and passive range of motion should be noted, as well as any weakness, tightness, spasm, tremor, or contracture that may be evident.

Some muscle weakness can be anticipated, although the exact degree will vary among individuals. The upper extremity usually shows greater strength on the side of the dominant hand; there should be equal strength in the lower extremities. To test muscle strength in holding its shortest position, have the patient hold the muscle in its shortest position and apply force to cause the muscle to extend. Normally, a muscle will be able to hold its shortest position under moderate resistance. Palpate all muscles for tenderness, contractures, and masses.

on damaged sidewalks or slipping on pieces of ice. Older eyes are more sensitive to glare, so sunglasses may be helpful for improving vision outdoors. A nightlight is extremely valuable in preventing falls during night visits to the bathroom. Loose rugs and clutter on floors and stairs should be removed. Because even the healthiest older person can experience some confusion when waking during the night, bed rails can be used to prevent falls from bed and attempts at sleepwalking, whether at home or away. Putting the bed against a wall with a straight chair at the other side is an effective substitute.

TABLE 27-1 ● *Gait Disturbances*

Gait Pattern	Associated Disorder
Ataxic Unsteady, uncoordinated, feet raised high while stepping and then dropped flat on floor	Cerebellum disease Intoxication
Foot slapping Wide based, feet raised high while stepping and then slapped down against floor, no staggering or weaving	Lower motor neuron disease Paralysis of pretibial and peroneal muscles
Hemiplegic Unilateral foot drop and foot dragging, leg circumducted, arm flexed and held close to side	Unilateral upper motor neuron disease
Parkinsonian Trunk leans forward, slight flexion of hip and knees, no arm swing while stepping, short and shuffling steps, starts slowly and then increases in speed	Parkinsonism
Scissors Slow, short steps; legs cross while stepping	Spastic paraplegia Dementia Cerebral palsy
Spastic Uncoordinated, jerking gait; legs stiff; toes drag	Spastic paraplegia Spinal cord tumor Multiple sclerosis

TABLE 27-2 ● *Good Sources of Calcium*

Source	Portion	Calcium (mg)
Plain low-fat yogurt	1 cup	250–400
Sardines	½ cup	375
Fruit juice, calcium fortified	1 glass	300
Skim milk	1 cup	302
Buttermilk	1 cup	300
Instant, enriched cooked farina	1 cup	200
Swiss cheese	1 ounce	272
Ice cream	1 cup	175
Low-fat (2%) cottage cheese	1 cup	155
Cooked turnip greens	½ cup	150
Tofu	½ cup	150
Broccoli	1 cup	136

The high prevalence and ease of fractures in elders warrant that this injury be suspected whenever older adults fall or otherwise subject their bones to trauma. Symptoms include pain, change in the shape or length of a limb, abnormal or restricted motion of a limb, edema, spasm of surrounding tissue, discoloration of tissue, and bone protruding through the tissue. The absence of these symptoms does not negate the possibility of a fracture. Overt signs and symptoms can be absent; in addition, the position of the fracture can prevent it from being apparent on the initial roentgenogram. As the patient is transported for evaluation, immobility of the injured site and control of bleeding are essential.

> 🔑 **KEY CONCEPT**
> The absence of typical signs of fracture does not guarantee that a bone is not broken; therefore, close nursing observation is essential whenever a bone has been subjected to trauma.

Fractures heal more slowly in older adults, and the risk of complications is greater. Pneumonia, thrombus formation, pressure ulcers, renal calculi, fecal impaction, and contractures are among the complications that special nursing attention can help prevent. Activity within the limits determined by the physician should be promoted, including deep-breathing and coughing exercises, isometric and range-of-motion exercises, and frequent turning and position changes. Fluids should be encouraged, and the characteristics of urine output noted. Good nutrition will

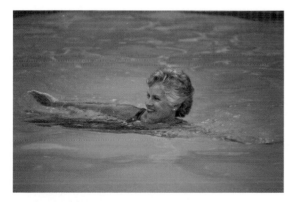

FIGURE 27-1

Exercise is essential to the musculoskeletal health of aging persons.

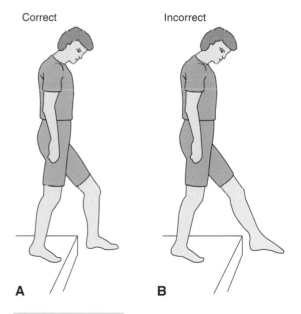

FIGURE 27-2

(**A**) The correct method for stepping to or from a curb is to place both feet near the edge of the curb before stepping up or down. (**B**) The incorrect method is to stretch the legs apart before stepping.

facilitate healing, increase resistance to infection, and decrease the likelihood of other complications. Joint exercise and proper positioning can prevent contractures. Correct body alignment can be maintained with the use of foot boards, trochanter rolls, and sandbags. Keeping the skin dry and clean, preventing pressure, stimulating circulation through massage, and frequently turning the patient may reduce the risk of decubiti. Sheepskin, water beds, and alternating-pressure mattresses are beneficial, but they are not substitutes for good skin care and frequent position changes.

The patient should be mobilized as early as possible. Because the patient may fear using the fractured limb and avoid doing so, explanations and reassurance are required to help the individual understand that the healed limb is safe to use. Progress in small steps may be easier for the patient to tolerate physically and psychologically; the first attempt at ambulation may be to stand at the bedside, the next to walk to a nearby chair, and the next to walk to the bathroom. Initially, it may be helpful for two people to assist the patient with ambulation, especially because weakness and dizziness are common. The principles of nursing management for specific types of fractures are available in medical-surgical nursing textbooks, and the nurse is advised to explore that literature for more detailed information.

OSTEOARTHRITIS

Osteoarthritis is the deterioration and abrasion of joint cartilage, with the formation of new bone at the joint surfaces. This problem is increasingly seen with advanced age and affects women more than men; it is the leading cause of physical disability in elders. Unlike rheumatoid arthritis, osteoarthritis does not cause inflammation, deformity, and crippling—a fact that is reassuring to the affected individual who fears the severe disability often seen in persons with rheumatoid arthritis. For many years, it was believed that the wear and tear of the joints as an individual ages were responsible for the development of osteoarthritis; however, greater insights into the pathophysiology of the condition have afforded a new understanding of this condition. Disequilibrium between destructive (matrix metalloprotease enzymes) and synthetic (tissue inhibitors of matrix metalloprotease) elements lead to a lack of homeostasis necessary to maintain cartilage, causing the joint changes. Excessive use of the joint,

trauma, obesity, low vitamin D and C levels, and genetic factors may also predispose an individual to this problem. Patients with acromegaly have a high incidence of osteoarthritis. Usually, osteoarthritis affects several joints rather than a single one. Weight-bearing joints are most affected, the common sites being the knees, hips, vertebrae, and fingers.

> **KEY CONCEPT**
> Osteoarthritis is the leading cause of physical disability in older people.

Systemic symptoms do not accompany osteoarthritis. Crepitation on joint motion may be noted, and the distal joints may develop bony nodules (ie, Heberden nodes). The patient may notice that the joints are more uncomfortable during damp weather and periods of extended use. Although isometrics and mild exercises are beneficial, excessive exercise will cause more pain and degeneration.

Analgesics may be prescribed to control pain. Acetaminophen is the first drug of choice because of its safety over nonsteroidal antiinflammatory drugs. Because individual response to analgesics varies, nurses should assess the effectiveness of various analgesics for the patient. Rest, heat or ice, ultrasound, and gentle massage will help relieve joint aches. Acupuncture has been shown to bring about short-term relief. Splints, braces, and canes provide support and rest to the joints. The importance of maintaining proper body alignment and using good body mechanics should be emphasized when educating the patient. Cold water fish and other foods high in the essential fatty acids have anti-inflammatory effects and should be abundant in the diet. Vitamins A, B, B_6, C, and E and zinc, selenium, niacinamide, calcium, and magnesium are among the nutritional supplements that could prove useful in controlling symptoms. The over-the-counter supplements glucosamine and chondroitin have proved helpful for some people. Weight reduction may improve the obese patient's status and should be encouraged. It is beneficial if a homemaker service or other household assistance relieves the patient of strenuous activities that cause the joints to bear weight. Occupational and physical therapists can be consulted for assistive devices to promote independence in self-care activities. Display 27-2 presents a sample care plan for the patient with osteoarthritis.

D I S P L A Y 2 7 - 2

Sample Care Plan for the Patient With Osteoarthritis

Nursing Diagnosis

Chronic pain related to joint inflammation, stiffness, and fluid accumulation

Goals

The patient

expresses relief or control of pain
is unrestricted by pain to engage in activities of daily living
is free from adverse effects of analgesics

Actions

- Ask patient to self-evaluate pain on a scale of 0 to 10 (0 = no pain, 10 5 most severe); monitor daily.
- Review with patient factors that precipitate, worsen, or relieve pain, incorporate this information into care to prevent and control pain.
- Apply heat as ordered to relieve discomfort and promote mobility. Encourage patient to use socks, blankets, and adequate clothing to keep muscles and joints warm.
- Administer analgesics as ordered or instruct patient in proper self-administration. Monitor effectiveness, tolerance, side effects.
- Assist patient in maintaining good body alignment and posture.
- Assess impact of pain on ability to fulfill activities of daily living (ADL). Consult with physical and occupational therapists regarding exercises and assistive devices that can promote independence.
- Instruct patient in ways to minimize stress to joints and muscles.
- Instruct patient in use of guided imagery, biofeedback, and relaxation techniques; offer massages and other forms of therapeutic touch.

Desired Outcomes

The patient

expresses relief or improved control of pain

participates in ADL to the maximum degree possible
achieves maximum benefit and no adverse effects from analgesics

Nursing Diagnosis

Impaired physical mobility related to pain and limited joint movement

Goals

The patient

maintains or achieves functional positions of joints
maintains or achieves optimal joint mobility
is free from flexion contractures

Actions

- Assess range of joint motion on admission or at first visit and regularly thereafter; note for each joint: swelling, warmth, tenderness, and structural or functional abnormalities.
- Instruct or assist patient in maintaining proper body alignment, good posture, correct use of joints.
- Advise patient to avoid stressing joints (eg, heavy lifting, running, hammering).
- Schedule analgesic administration and other pain relief measures before activities.
- During exacerbation of pain, provide adequate rest for joints and assist patient in positioning joints in functional alignment.
- Consult with rehabilitation specialists regarding appropriate exercise to improve muscle strength, tone, and mobility, and possible use of assistive devices and mobility aids (eg, canes, walkers, customized eating utensils, dressing aids).
- Encourage or assist patient to perform range-of-motion exercises at least twice daily.
- Provide warm-up of muscles and joints prior to activities and exercises and a cool-down period afterwards.

(Continued)

D I S P L A Y   2 7 - 2   (C o n t i n u e d)

Desired Outcomes

The patient

maintains joints in functional positions
moves joints to maximum capacity is free from joint
deformity and injury
and other complications of immobility

Nursing Diagnosis

*Potential self-care deficit related to pain or joint
immobility*

Goals

The patient

is able to eat, bathe, dress, transfer, ambulate, and
toilet independently
Uses assistive aids properly and effectively

Actions

■ Assess the patient's ability to eat, bathe, dress, transfer,
ambulate, and toilet independently. Identify deficits in
independently meeting ADL and plan measures to
compensate for deficits; identify risks and potential
deficits and plan measures to prevent loss of
independent function.

■ Allow patient maximum independence and
participation in care activities.

■ Educate patient as to proper management of condition
and measures that can reduce risk of losing
independence (eg, exercise to maintain mobility, use of
assistive devices).

■ Encourage patient to express feelings about actual or
potential dependency; provide realistic explanations
and emotional support.

Desired Outcomes

The patient

performs ADL and self-care activities with maximum
independence

uses assistive aids properly and effectively
is free from declines in independence

Nursing Diagnoses

*Body image disturbance related to joint abnormality,
immobility, altered self-care ability*
*Self-esteem disturbance related to changes in body
appearance and function*

Goals

The patient

expresses acceptance of and realities associated with
chronic condition
expresses feelings regarding body changes
develops effective mechanisms to cope with body
changes
identifies constructive ways to function with body
changes
is free from complications associated with body
image and self-esteem disturbances

Actions

■ Assess impact of altered function and appearance on
patient.

■ Encourage patient to express concerns, fears, and
feelings.

■ Help patient identify effective coping measures (eg,
effective measures used to cope with problems in the
past, counseling, development of new interests).

■ Help patient identify and focus on capabilities rather
than limitations.

Desired Outcomes

The patient

verbalizes acceptance of realistic body changes
uses effective coping mechanisms
identifies and engages in meaningful activities
is free from depression, withdrawal, and other
complications associated with body image and
self-esteem disturbances

RHEUMATOID ARTHRITIS

Rheumatoid arthritis affects many persons, particularly those 20 to 40 years old; it is a major cause of arthritic disability in later life as a result. Fortunately, the incidence decreases after 65 years of age; most older patients with this disease developed it earlier in life. Specifically, the deformities and disability associated with this disease primarily begin during early adulthood and peak during middle age; in old age, greater systemic involvement occurs. This disease occurs more frequently in women and in persons with a family history of the problem.

In rheumatoid arthritis, the synovium becomes hypertrophied and edematous with projections of synovial tissue protruding into the joint cavity. The affected joints are extremely painful, stiff, swollen, red, and warm to the touch. Joint pain is present during rest and activity. Subcutaneous nodules over bony prominences and bursae may be present, as may deforming flexion contractures. Systemic symptoms include fatigue, malaise, weakness, weight loss, wasting, fever, and anemia.

Encouraging patients to rest and providing support to the affected limbs are helpful measures. Limb support should be such that decubiti and contractures are prevented. Splints are commonly made for the patient in an effort to prevent deformities. Range-of-motion exercises are vital to maintain musculoskeletal function; the nurse may have to assist the patient with active exercises. Physical and occupational therapists can provide assistive devices to promote independence in self-care activities, and heat, gentle massage, and analgesics can help control pain. Patients with rheumatoid arthritis may be prescribed antiinflammatory agents (particularly prostaglandins), corticosteroids, antimalarial agents, gold salts, and immunosuppressive drugs. The nurse should be familiar with the many toxic effects of these drugs and detect them early if they occur.

Some patients with rheumatic heart disease are sensitive to the "nightshade" foods: potatoes, peppers, eggplant, tomatoes, and other solanines; eliminating these from the diet could prove beneficial. Herbs that could improve symptoms include turmeric, ginger, skullcap, and ginseng.

Patients with rheumatoid arthritis and their families need considerable education to be able to manage this condition. Patient education should include a knowledge of the disease, treatments, administration of medications, identification of side effects, exercise regimens, use of assistive devices, methods to avoid and reduce pain, and an understanding of the need for continued medical supervision. Accepting this chronic disease is not an easy task for either the patient or the family. Finally, the patient may be a prime target for salespeople offering a quick cure or relief for arthritis and should be advised to consult a nurse or physician before investing many dollars on useless fads. **(Visit the Connection website to learn how guided imagery can be used for pain management.)**

OSTEOPOROSIS

Osteoporosis is the most prevalent metabolic disease of the bone; it primarily affects adults in middle to later life, with some groups being at higher risk than others (Display 27-3). Demineralization of the bone occurs, evidenced by a decrease in the mass and density of the skeleton. Any health problem associated with inadequate calcium intake, excessive calcium loss, or poor calcium absorption can cause osteoporosis. Many of the following potential causes are problems commonly found among older persons.

> *Inactivity or immobility.* A lack of muscle pull on the bone can lead to a loss of minerals, especially calcium and phosphorus. This particularly may be a problem for limbs in a cast.
>
> *Diseases.* Cushing syndrome, an excessive production of glucocorticosteroids by the adrenal gland, is believed to inhibit the formation of bone matrix. The increased metabolic activity of hyperthyroidism causes more rapid bone turnover and the faster rate of bone resorption to bone formation causes osteoporosis. Excessive diverticulitis can interfere with the absorption of sufficient amounts of calcium. Although the direct relationship is uncertain at this time, diabetes mellitus can contribute to the development of osteoporosis. The percentage of cases of osteoporosis that result secondary to other diseases is relatively small.
>
> *Reduction in anabolic sex hormones.* Decreased production or loss of estrogens and androgens may be responsible for insufficient bone calcium; therefore, postmenopausal women are at high risk of developing this problem.

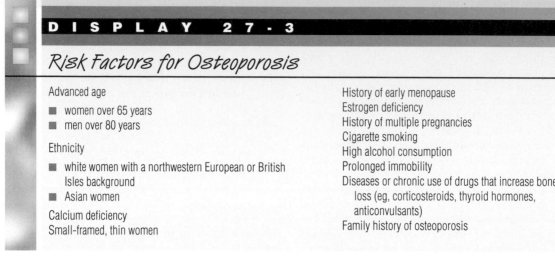

DISPLAY 27·3

Risk Factors for Osteoporosis

Advanced age
- women over 65 years
- men over 80 years

Ethnicity
- white women with a northwestern European or British Isles background
- Asian women

Calcium deficiency
Small-framed, thin women

History of early menopause
Estrogen deficiency
History of multiple pregnancies
Cigarette smoking
High alcohol consumption
Prolonged immobility
Diseases or chronic use of drugs that increase bone loss (eg, corticosteroids, thyroid hormones, anticonvulsants)
Family history of osteoporosis

Diet. An insufficient amount of calcium, vitamin D, vitamin C, protein, and other nutrients in the diet can cause osteoporosis. Excessive consumption of caffeine or alcohol decreases the body's absorption and retention of calcium.

Drugs. Heparin, furosemide, thyroid supplements, corticosteroids, tetracycline, and magnesium- and aluminum-based antacids can lead to osteoporosis.

✔ **Point to Ponder**
To what risk factors for osteoporosis are you subject, and what can you do to reduce them?

Osteoporosis may cause kyphosis and a reduction in height. Spinal pain can be experienced, especially in the lumbar region. The bones may tend to fracture more easily. Usually patients are asymptomatic, however, and unaware of the problem until it is detected by radiography. Bone mass can be assessed through several different types of noninvasive techniques, including single-photon absorptiometry (SPA), dual-photon absorptiometry (DPA), quantitative computed tomography (CT), and dual-energy x-ray absorptiometry (DEXA), which is the most widely used and recommended method (Placide & Martens, 2003).

Treatment depends on the underlying cause of the disease and may include calcium supplements, vitamin D supplements, progesterone, estrogen, anabolic agents, fluoride, or phosphate. A relatively recent drug that has been shown beneficial in producing modest increases in bone mass is a synthetic form of calcitonin, a hormone produced in the thyroid that is a powerful inhibitor of osteoclastic activity (the cells that continuously reabsorb bone). Biophosphonates are another beneficial new category of drugs that are primarily antiresorptive (ie, they prevent or significantly slow the normal osteoclastic activity responsible for the resorption of bone). A diet rich in protein and calcium is encouraged. Braces may be used to provide support and reduce spasms. A bed board is also beneficial and should be recommended. The patient must be advised to avoid heavy lifting, jumping, and other activities that could result in a fracture. Persons providing care for these patients must remember to be gentle when moving, exercising, or lifting them because fractures can occur easily. Compression fractures of the vertebrae are a potential complication of osteoporosis. Range-of-motion exercises and ambulation are important to maintain function and prevent greater damage.

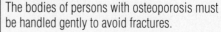

KEY CONCEPT
The bodies of persons with osteoporosis must be handled gently to avoid fractures.

GOUT

Gout is a metabolic disorder in which excess uric acid accumulates in the blood. As a result, uric acid crystals are deposited in and around the joints, causing severe pain and tenderness of the joint and warmth, redness, and swelling of the surrounding tissue. Attacks can last from weeks to months, with long remissions between attacks possible.

Treatment aims to reduce sodium urate through a low-purine diet (eg, avoidance of bacon, turkey, veal, liver, kidney, brain, anchovies, sardines, herring, smelt, mackerel, salmon, and legumes) and the administration of drugs. Alcohol should also be avoided because it increases uric acid production and reduces uric acid excretion. Colchicine or phenylbutazone can be used to manage acute attacks; long-term management could include colchicine, allopurinol, probenecid, or indomethacin. Gout attacks can be precipitated by the administration of thiazide diuretics, which raise the uric acid level of the blood. Vitamin E, folic acid, and eicosapentaenoic acid (EPA) can be useful dietary supplements. Herbs such as yucca and devil's claw reduce symptoms in some persons.

PODIATRIC CONDITIONS

By age 65, nearly 90% of all people have some type of foot problem that causes some degree of discomfort or dysfunction. Not surprisingly then, the foot problems of old age have commanded a specialty of their own:

podogeriatrics. Lifelong foot problems, changes in gait, diseases that affect the feet (eg, gout, diabetes, and peripheral vascular disease), and age-related loss of fat padding of the foot contribute to foot conditions. Because of the impact of these problems on mobility and independence, podiatric conditions need to be effectively identified and treated. Some of the common conditions include (Fig. 27-3) the following.

Calluses. Calluses are caused by friction and irritation on the feet that create layers of thickened skin. The dryness of the skin and poor fitting shoes contribute to callus formation. They usually appear on the heels and soles and, although not painful, can be unsightly. Furthermore, there is the risk that people will attempt to shave or cut off calluses from their feet and risk injuring their skin. Massaging the feet with lotions and oils can aid in preventing calluses.

Corns. Corns are cone-shaped layers of thick, dry skin that form over a bony prominence. Pressure on the area causes discomfort as the tip of the cone presses into the tissue. Additional pressure increases the size of the corn and, consequently, the pain. U-shaped corn pads and loosely wrapping the toe in lamb's wool are superior to oval or round corn pads, which can restrict circulation. As with calluses, patients should be advised not to attempt to remove corns on their own.

Bunions (Hallux valgas). A bunion or bursa is a bony prominence over the first metatarsal head.

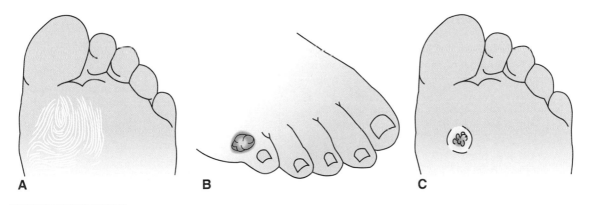

FIGURE 27-3

Foot disorders. (**A**) Callus. (**B**) Corn. (**C**) Plantar wart.

There is a medial deviation of the first metatarsal with abduction of the great toe in relation to that metatarsal. Bunions occur more often in women—not surprising when women's shoe styles that commonly have tight toe fit and the tight hosiery that pull toes together are considered. Some bunions are hereditary in nature. The increased width of the foot caused by the bunion can cause difficulty in finding properly fitting shoes. Shoe repair shops can stretch shoes to accommodate bunions; custom-made shoes are beneficial, also. Surgery may be indicated for some cases.

Hammer toe (Digiti Flexus). A hyperextension at the metatarsophalangeal joint with flexion and often corn formation at the proximal interphalangeal joint. The toe begins to resemble the shape of the hammers inside a piano, thus its name. Although the joint itself is not painful, pressure to the area results in discomfort. Orthotics can provide symptomatic relief, but surgery is necessary for correction.

Plantar fascitis. A common cause of heel pain, often mistaken for a spur, is plantar fascitis. The plantar fascia is a thick ligamentous band in the bottom of the foot that runs from the ball of the foot to the heel, where it is attached. Poor alignment of the foot that causes pronation or supination of the foot during walk, results in stretching and stress of the plantar fascia. Plantar fascitis is an inflammation of this band at its heel attachment. Pain is the primary symptom and occurs in the center or the inner side of the heel. Pain is worse after a period of rest; most people experience the most pain in the morning. After walking, the pain may subside but tends to increase as pressure is put on the heel from walking or standing. Pain can radiate to the ankle or arch of the foot if nerves become irritated secondary to the swollen plantar fascia. Symptomatic treatment can include stretching exercises of the foot (pulling up on the ball of the foot), applying ice to the heel for 30-minute periods, and wearing cushions in the heel and shoes with heels elevated about 2 inches. The most effective means of relieving pain and preventing inflammation is to have the foot realigned through the use of custom-made orthotics. Patients need to be advised that it may take several months before improvement is noted after treatment is initiated.

Infections. Housing of the foot in shoes, particular ones made from synthetic materials, creates a warm, moist environment that facilitates fungus and bacterial growth. *Onychomycosis* is a fungal infection of the nail or nail bed in which the toenail appears enlarged, thick, brittle, and flaky. As the fungus forms under the nail and displaces it up, the sides of the nail are pushed into the skin and cause pain. Antifungal preparations assist in eliminating the infection, although they are stubborn to treat. *Tinea pedis,* better known as athlete's foot, is a fungal infection of the foot that can cause burning and itching; the skin surface will peel, crack, and be red, often with vesicle eruptions. The breaks in the skin surface provide easy entry for bacteria.

Ingrown nails (Onychocryptosis). Ingrown nails can occur due to tight fitting shoes or cutting the nail excessively short. As the nail grows its edge cuts into the tissue, leading to inflammation. Soaks and topical antibiotics may be prescribed; usually, a podiatrist can correct this problem by removing the ingrown portion and cleaning the area.

The elderly's own shaving, cutting, and chemical treatment of podiatric conditions can result in serious complications; therefore, patients should be referred to podiatrists for treatment of foot conditions. Nurses should teach older adults about proper foot care (eg, keeping feet clean and dry, wearing safe and proper-fitting shoes, exercising feet, and cutting nails straight across and even with the top of the toe) and the importance of seeking professional podiatric care for problems. Nurses can offer foot massages because they can aid in stimulating circulation, reducing edema, and promoting comfort. (Be aware that foot massages may be contraindicated in patients with peripheral vascular disease or lesions, so consult with the physician first.)

Nursing Considerations

MANAGING PAIN

Pain often accompanies musculoskeletal problems. Degenerative changes in the tendons and arthritis often are responsible for painful shoulders, elbows, hands, hips, knees, and spines. Cramps, especially during the night, commonly are experienced in calves, feet, hands, hips, and thighs. Joint strain and damp weather more frequently cause musculoskeletal pain in the elderly than in the young.

Pain relief is essential in promoting optimal physical, mental, and social function. Unrelieved pain can interfere with older persons' abilities to engage in self-care, manage their households, and maintain social contact. To enrich the quality of life, every effort should be made to minimize or eliminate pain. Often, heat will relieve muscle spasms, and a warm bath at bedtime accompanied by blankets and clothing to keep the extremities warm can reduce spasms and cramps throughout the night and promote uninterrupted sleep. Because older adults are at high risk for burns, care must be taken to avoid injury if heat applications or soaks are used. Passive stretching of the extremity can be helpful in controlling muscle cramps. Excessive exercise and musculoskeletal stress should be avoided, as well as situations known to cause pain, such as heavy lifting or damp weather. Back rubs using slow, long, rhythmic strokes can promote relaxation and comfort. Pain in the weight-bearing joints can be alleviated by resting those joints, supporting painful joints during transfers, and using a walker or cane (Fig. 27-4). Correct positioning, whereby all body parts are in proper alignment, can help prevent and manage pain. Accidental bumping against the patient's bed or chair and rough handling of the patient during care activities must be prevented. Nurses may also need to emphasize to other caregivers the need for extra gentleness in turning and lifting older patients.

> **KEY CONCEPT**
> Unrelieved pain can significantly affect an older person's independence and quality of life.

Diversional activities are useful in preventing the patient's preoccupation with pain. Acupuncture, acupressure, and chiropractic therapy are among the alternative therapies that may help some patients control pain. The goal is to aid the patient in achieving the maximum level of activity with the least degree of pain (Nursing Diagnosis Table 27-1).

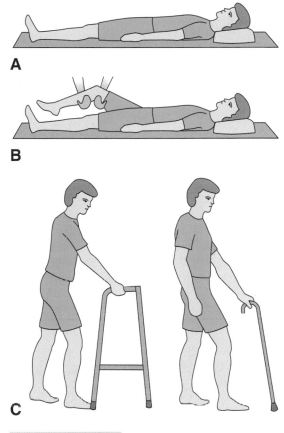

FIGURE 27-4

Methods for reducing musculoskeletal pain. (**A**) Good body alignment. (**B**) Support of parts of the limb adjacent to the painful joint when moving or lifting. (**C**) Use of a walker or cane.

> **KEY CONCEPT**
> Alternative therapies, such as acupuncture, acupressure, guided imagery, massage, therapeutic touch, and chiropathy, can prove helpful in controlling pain.

PREVENTING INJURY

Safety considerations are essential for all elderly persons because of their high incidence of accidents and musculoskeletal injuries and the prolonged

ND Nursing Diagnosis

TABLE 27-1 ● Nursing Diagnoses Related to Musculoskeletal Problems

Causes or Contributing Factors	Nursing Diagnosis
Muscle fatigue, pain, deformity	Activity Intolerance
Pain, fear of injury	Anxiety
Inactivity or immobility from pain or disability	Constipation
Fracture, contracture, spasms, arthritis	Pain (Acute, Chronic)
Change or loss of function or appearance	Fear
Arthritis, contracture, pain, impaired range of motion	Impaired Home Maintenance
Unsteady gait, pain, improper use of heat	Risk for Injury
Spasms, atrophy, pain, deformity	Impaired Physical Mobility
Impaired self-care capacity	Powerlessness
Immobility, pain, deformity	Self-Care Deficit
Change in body structure or function, pain, immobility, increased dependency	Disturbed Body Image
Pain, fatigue, positioning difficulties, altered body image	Sexual Dysfunction
Pain, spasms, cramps	Disturbed Sleep Pattern
Change in body structure or function, altered self-concept, pain	Impaired Social Interaction
Immobility, pain, disfigurement	Social Isolation

time required for healing. Prevention includes paying attention to the area where one is walking; climbing stairs and curbs slowly; using both feet for support as much as possible; using railings and canes for added balance; wearing properly fitting, safe shoes for good support; and avoiding long trousers, nightgowns, or robes. The importance of the safe use of heat has already been mentioned; it is useful for patients to learn how to measure water temperature and use hot-water bottles and heating pads safely. Patients with peripheral vascular disease must be warned that the local application of heat can cause circulatory demands that their body will be unable to meet; they should be informed that other means of pain relief may be more beneficial to them. Warm baths can reduce muscle spasm and provide pain relief, but they also can cause hypotensive episodes leading to dizziness, fainting, and serious injury.

Carelessly turning patients so that legs hit the bed rail, dropping them into a chair during a transfer, restraining them in an unaligned position, roughly handling a limb, or attempting to use force to straighten a contracture can lead to muscle strain and fractures. Gentle handling will prevent unnecessary musculoskeletal discomfort and injury.

PROMOTING INDEPENDENCE

Any loss of independence associated with the limitations imposed by musculoskeletal problems has a serious impact on physical, emotional, and social well-being. Therefore, nurses must explore all avenues to help patients minimize limitations and strengthen capacities, thereby promoting the highest possible level of independence. Canes, walkers, and other assistive devices can often provide significant aid in compensating for handicaps and should be used when feasible (Figs. 27-5, 27-6, and 27-7). Physical and occupational therapists can be valuable resources in determining appropriate assistive devices for use with specific deficits.

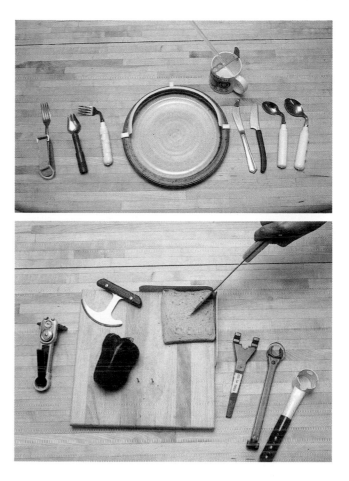

FIGURE 27-5

Self-care devices can help the client achieve the maximum independence possible. (*Top*) Assistive feeding devices help the client to grasp and get food on the utensils. (*Bottom*) Assistive food preparation devices aid in opening containers and cutting and preparing food. (Craven, R.F. & Hirnle, C.J. [2003]. *Fundamentals of nursing: Human health and function* [4th ed., p. 737]. Philadelphia: Lippincott Williams & Wilkins.)

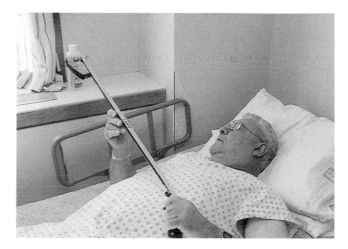

FIGURE 27-6

A reacher is a handy device for the client with mobility restrictions. (Craven, R.F. & Hirnle, C.J. [2003]. *Fundamentals of nursing: Human health and function* [4th ed., p. 803]. Philadelphia: Lippincott Williams & Wilkins.)

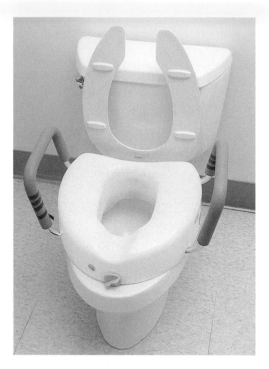

FIGURE 27-7

A raised toilet seat allows a client with mobility problems to safely use the toilet at home. (Craven, R.F. & Hirnle, C.J. [2003]. *Fundamentals of nursing: Human health and function* [4th ed., p. 738]. Philadelphia: Lippincott Williams & Wilkins.)

Critical Thinking Exercises

1. What are some factors that cause people to reduce their physical activity with age?
2. What major points should be included in a program to educate senior citizens on measures to reduce their risk of fractures?
3. Describe the impact of arthritis on psychosocial well-being.
4. Discuss nonpharmacologic measures to control musculoskeletal pain.
5. What situations could an older adult encounter during an acute hospitalization that could increase the risk for sustaining a fracture?
6. What resources are available in your community to assist patients in the management of their musculoskeletal problems?

Web Connect

Search for "aquatics for arthritis" in your state to learn of local programs that can benefit individuals with arthritis.

● Resources

Arthritis Foundation
1314 Spring Street NW
Atlanta, GA 30309
(800) 283-7800
www.arthritis.org

**National Arthritis and Musculoskeletal and Skin
 Diseases Information Clearinghouse**
NAMSIC AMS Circle
National Institutes of Health
Bethesda, MD 20892
(301) 495-4484
www.nih.gov/niams/

National Osteoporosis Foundation
1150 17th Street NW
Suite 500
Washington, DC 20036
(800) 624-2663
www.nof.org

Rheumatoid Disease Foundation
5106 Old Harding Road
Franklin, TN 37064
www.mall-net.com/arth/

● Reference

Placide, J., & Martens, M. G. (2003). Comparing screening methods for osteoporosis. *Current Women's' Health Report, 3*(3), 207–210.

● Recommended Readings

Birdwood, G. F. B. (1996). *Understanding osteoporosis and its treatment: A guide for physicians and their patients.* Pearl River, NY: Parthenon Publishing Group.

Bourgon, R. (1998). The nutritional approach to treating rheumatoid arthritis. *Alternative and Complementary Therapies, 4*(3), 187–194.

Capezuti, E., Strumpf, N. E., Evans, L. K., Grisso, J. A., & Maislin, G. (1998). The relationship between physical restraint removal and falls and injuries among nursing home residents. *Journal of Gerontology: Medical Sciences, 53A*, M47–M52.

Chang, R. W. (Ed.). (1996). *Rehabilitation of persons with rheumatoid arthritis.* Gaithersburg, MD: Aspen.

Davis, G. C., & White, T. L. (2000). Planning an osteoporosis education program for older adults in a residential setting. *Journal of Gerontological Nursing, 26*(1), 16–23.

Dharmarajan, T. S., Ahmed, S., & Russell, R. O. (2001). Recurrent falls from severe hypocalcemia resulting in nursing home placement: A preventable geriatric problem. *Annals of Long-Term Care, 9*(7), 65–68.

Dowd, R., & Cavalieri, R. J. (1999). Help your patient live with osteoporosis. *American Journal of Nursing, 99*(4), 55–62.

Feldt, K. S., & Finch, M. (2002). Older patients with hip fractures: Treatment of pain following hospitalization. *Journal of Gerontological Nursing, 28*(8), 27–35.

Field-Munves, E. (2001). Evidence-based decisions for the treatment of osteoporosis. *Annals of Long-Term Care, 9*(3), 70–79.

Gaines, J. M., Talbot, L. A., & Metter, E. J. (2002). The relationship of arthritis self-efficacy to functional performance in older men and women with osteoarthritis of the knee. *Geriatric Nursing, 23*(1), 167–170.

Galsworthy, T. D., & Wilson, P. L. (1996). Osteoporosis: It steals more than bone. *American Journal of Nursing, 96*(6), 26–34.

Gates, R., & Whipple, B. (2003). Outwitting osteoporosis: The smart woman's guide to bone health. New York: Beyond Words Publication.

Holt, S. (1998). Bone and joint health: Dietary supplements. *Alternative and Complementary Therapies, 4*(3), 195–204.

Horan, M. A., & Little, R. A. (1998). *Injury in the aging.* New York: Cambridge University Press.

Kaufman, D. L. (1997). *Injuries and illness in the elderly.* St. Louis: Mosby.

Kessenich, C. R. (2000). Update on osteoporosis in elderly men. *Geriatric Nursing, 21*(5), 242–244.

Loeb, J. L. (1999). Pain management in long-term care. *American Journal of Nursing, 99*(2), 48–53.

Luskin, F. M., Newell, K. A., Griffith, M., Holmes, M., Telles, S., et al. (2000). A review of mind/body therapies in the treatment of musculoskeletal disorders with implications for the elderly. *Alternative Therapies in Health and Medicine, 6*(2), 46–56.

Maki, B. E. (1997). Gait changes in older adults: Predictors of falls or indicators of fears? *Journal of the American Geriatrics Society, 45*, 313–320.

Marcus, R. (1996). *Osteoporosis.* San Diego, CA: Academic Press.

McCarry, K. A., & Cyr, M. G. (2001). Prevention of bone loss and fractures in postmenopausal osteoporosis. *Clinical Geriatrics, 9*(13), 47–56.

Meyer, G., Warnke, A., Bender, R., et al. (2003). Effect on hip fractures of increased use of hip protectors in nursing homes. *British Medical Journal, 326*(1), 76–80.

Norton, R., Campbell, A. J., Lee-Joe, T., Robinson, E., &

Butler, M. (1997). Circumstances of falls resulting in hip fractures among older people. *Journal of the American Geriatrics Society, 45,* 1108–1112.

Ramsburg, K. L. (2000). Rheumatoid arthritis. *American Journal of Nursing, 100*(11), 40–43.

Rothfeld, G. S., & LeVert, S. (1996). *Natural medicine for back pain.* Emmaus, PA: Rodale Press.

Sears, J. R., & Ganger, P. M. (2000). Antibiotics to treat RA. *RN, 63*(1), 41–42.

Thomas, E., Richardson, J. C., Irvine, A., Hassel, A. B., & Hay, E. M. (2003). Osteoporosis: What are the implications of DEXA scanning 'high risk' women in primary care? *Family Practice, 20*(3), 289–293.

Tideiksaar, R. (1996). *Falling in old age* (2nd ed.). New York: Springer.

Trivedi, D. P., Doll, R., & Khaw, K. T. (2003). Effect of four monthly oral Vitamin D3 (Cholecalciferol) supplementation on fractures and mortality in men and women living in the community. *British Medical Journal, 2003*(2), 469–474.

Tsai, P., & Tak, S. (2003). Disease-specific pain measures for osteoarthritis of the knee or hip. *Geriatric Nursing, 24*(2), 106–109.

Young, D. M., Mentes, J. C., & Titler, M. G. (1999). Acute pain management protocol. *Journal of Gerontological Nursing, 25*(6), 10–21.

Genitourinary Conditions

■ Learning Objectives

After reading this chapter, you should be able to:

- list measures that promote genitourinary health

- outline factors to consider in assessing genitourinary health

- describe the incidence, symptoms, and management of selected genitourinary disorders

- outline a care plan for the patient who is incontinent

- discuss measures to promote a positive self-concept in the patient with a genitourinary disorder

*G*enitourinary problems, although bothersome, frequent, and potentially life-threatening, are disorders not easily discussed by older adults. Some feel embarrassment or believe it is inappropriate to talk about these problems; others fear societal reactions to an older person's concern about sexual function; still others may associate genitourinary problems with sexual "wrongdoing" and feel guilty over the development of these disorders; and some individuals accept symptoms of genitourinary disorders as a normal part of aging. These factors, along with reluctance to obtain gynecologic and urologic examinations, often delay early detection and treatment. Untreated, these problems can jeopardize total body health and profoundly affect psychosocial well-being. Nurses are in ideal positions to develop close relationships with geriatric patients, which can help them to more comfortably discuss problems of the urinary tract and reproductive system. By demonstrating sensitivity, acceptance, and understanding of patients' problems, nurses can facilitate prompt, appropriate intervention.

A complete history and examination are essential to pinpoint specific areas that require further investigation; however, obtaining data about genitourinary function and problems can be difficult. Because older persons may feel embarrassment, distaste, or guilt about discussing these problems, a comfortable tone should be set and sensitivity displayed during the assessment to facilitate good data collection. Some of the areas to include in assessing the genitourinary system are described in Display 28-1; Nursing Diagnosis Table 28-1 outlines some of the nursing diagnoses that could be identified.

✔ Point to Ponder

How comfortable are you hearing someone old enough to be your parent or grandparent discuss sexual problems? What contributed to your attitudes about this?

Facilitating Genitourinary Health

Basic health practices, which are easily incorporated into the daily schedule, can prevent a variety of urinary tract problems. For instance, a good fluid intake can reduce the amount of bacteria in the bladder. An acidic urine, beneficial in preventing infection, can be enhanced by the intake of vitamin C and foods such as cranberries, prunes, plums, eggs, cheese, fish, and grains. Activity can eliminate urinary stasis, and frequent toileting can prevent urinary retention (Fig. 28-1). Catheterization significantly increases the risk of infection and should be avoided.

Another way to facilitate genitourinary health is to stress the value of regular examinations of the repro-

ductive system. An annual gynecologic examination, including a Pap smear, is essential for the older woman; she should also be knowledgeable about self-examination of the breasts. The American Cancer Society and the American Urological Association recommend annual prostate-specific antigen (PSA) testing for older men. Although useful in discovering some cancers in earlier stages, PSA tests can produce false positive and false negative results (Sriprasad et al., 2001). Men with prostatic hypertrophy should be examined at least every 6 months to ensure that a malignancy has not developed. Finally, the nurse should ensure that older men know how to perform testicular self-examination. Chapter 13 discusses nursing considerations in fostering sexual function in older adults.

🔑 KEY CONCEPT

It is important to ensure that older women know how to perform breast self-examination and that older men know how to perform testicular self-examination.

Selected Disorders

PROBLEMS OF THE URINARY TRACT

Urinary Incontinence

A common and bothersome disorder of elders that requires skillful nursing attention is the involuntary loss of urine, or urinary incontinence. Studies have shown that urinary incontinence is present in 30% of the community-based elderly, 50% of the institutionalized aged, and 30% of hospitalized older adults; this problem is twice as prevalent in women as compared to men (Durrant and Snape, 2003; Landi, Cesari, Russo, Onder, Lattanzio, & Bernabei, 2003). The following are various types of incontinence.

Stress: caused by weak supporting pelvic muscles. When pressure is placed on the pelvic floor (eg, from laughing, sneezing, or coughing), urine is involuntarily lost.

Urgency: caused by urinary tract infection (UTI), enlargement of the prostate, diverticulitis, or pelvic or bladder tumors. Irritation or spasms of the bladder wall cause a sudden elimination of urine.

Assessment of the Genitourinary System

Interview

The interview should include a review of function, signs, and symptoms. Questions should be asked pertaining to the following:

Frequency of voiding. "How often do you need to urinate during the day and during the night? Has there been any recent change in that pattern?"

Continence. "Do you ever lose control of your urine? Do you experience a steady stream of urine dribbling at all times or at certain times? Is urine released when you cough or sneeze? How soon do you need to toilet after getting the urge to void before you lose control?"

Retention. "Do you ever feel that you have not fully emptied your bladder after you have voided? Do you have a sense of fullness in your bladder after voiding?"

Pain. "Does it burn when you void? Do you experience pain in your lower abdomen or anywhere else? Is there any tenderness, discomfort, itching, or pain anywhere along your genital area?"

Discharge. "Do you ever have secretions, blood, or other discharge from your genitals?"

Urine. "Have you ever seen crystals or particles in your urine? Is your urine ever pink, bloody, or discolored? Is it as clear as tap water or as dark as rusty water? Does your urine ever have a strong odor? If so, what is that odor like?"

Sexual dysfunction. "Can you obtain an erection and hold it through intercourse? What are your ejaculations like? Is your vagina sensitive or overly dry during intercourse? Do you feel extra pressure or that your partner's penis is hitting a blockage during intercourse? Can you have satisfying orgasms? Has there been any change in your sexual pattern?"

Urine Sample

A urinalysis can provide basic information about this system. The specific gravity should range from 1.005 to 1.025, and the pH from 4.6 to 8. Although alkaline urine is most often associated with infections, it can be present if the specimen has been sitting for a few hours. Normally the urine should be free of glucose and protein, but renal changes in the older adult cause proteinuria and glycosuria to be less reliable findings. It is beneficial to note characteristics of the urine sample such as the following:

Color. Examination of the urine's color can yield insight into the presence of health problems. Dark colors can indicate increased urine concentration. Red or rust color usually is associated with the presence of blood. Yellow-brown or green-brown color can be caused by an obstructed bile duct or jaundice. Orange urine results from the presence of bile or the ingestion of phenazopyridine. Very dark brown urine is associated with hematuria or carcinoma.

Odor. A faint aromatic odor of the urine is normal. Strong odor, which can indicate concentrated urine associated with dehydration, should be noted. Ammonia-like odor can accompany infections.

Physical Examination

Inspect, percuss, and palpate the abdomen for bladder fullness, pain, or abnormalities. Test women for stress incontinence by doing the following:

Have the patient drink at least one full glass of fluid and wait until she senses fullness of the bladder.

Instruct the patient to stand. If this is not possible, have her sit as upright as possible.

Ask the patient to hold a 4 × 4 gauze at her perineum.

Instruct the patient to cough vigorously.

The test is negative if no leakage or leakage of only a few drops occurs. If residual urine is a problem, a postvoid residual may be ordered in which the patient is catheterized within 15 minutes of voiding to determine the volume of urine remaining in the bladder.

(Continued)

D I S P L A Y   2 8 - 1   (C o n t i n u e d)

If incontinence is present, the patient should be referred for a comprehensive evaluation; it can prove useful to maintain a record or have the patient maintain a diary of each occurrence of incontinence and factors associated with these incidents.

The genitalia should be inspected for lesions, sores, breaks, or masses. Note bleeding, discharges, odors, and other abnormalities. If the patient has not had a gynecologic examination or mammogram within the past year, she should be referred accordingly. Likewise, the male patient should receive a prostate-specific antigen (PSA) test and prostate examination if one has not been done within the past year.

The breasts should be palpated for masses. The procedure for self-examination of the breasts should be reviewed and instruction provided if the patient is unskilled in this technique.

Overflow: associated with bladder neck obstructions and medications (eg, adrenergics, anticholinergics, and calcium channel blockers). Bladder muscles fail to contract or periurethral muscles do not relax, leading to an excessive accumulation of urine in the bladder.

Neurogenic (reflex): arising from cerebral cortex lesions, multiple sclerosis, and other disturbances along the neural pathway. There is an inability to sense the urge to void or control urine flow.

Functional: caused by dementia, disabilities that prevent independent toileting, sedation, inaccessible bathroom, medications that impair cognition, or any other factor interfering with the ability to reach a bathroom.

Mixed incontinence: incontinence can be due to a combination of these factors.

Nurses should not assume that individuals with incontinence, even long-term incontinence, have necessarily had this problem identified and evalu-

Nursing Diagnosis

ND TABLE 28-1 ● *Nursing Diagnoses Associated With Genitourinary Problems*

Causes or Contributing Factors	Nursing Diagnosis
Sexual dysfunction, pain, embarrassment over symptoms or treatments	Anxiety
Infection, cancer, retention	Pain
Concentrated urine, immobility, more alkaline urine, more alkaline and fragile vaginal canal, prostatic hypertrophy, catheterization	Risk for Infection
Falls on urine puddles, fragile vaginal tissue	Risk for Injury
Immobility, dementia, weakness	Toileting Self-Care Deficit
Incontinence, sexual dysfunction	Body Image Disturbance
Infection, pain, altered structures, embarrassment	Sexual Dysfunction
Incontinence, vaginitis	Impaired Skin Integrity
Nocturia, retention, dysuria	Sleep Pattern Disturbance
Embarrassment over symptoms, odor, frequency, discomfort	Impaired Social Interaction
Infection, retention, calculi, prostatic enlargement, vaginitis, strictures, incontinence	Impaired Urinary Elimination

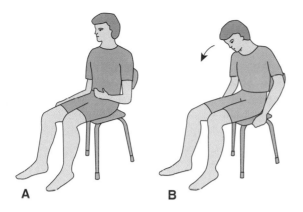

A   **B**

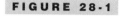

FIGURE 28-1

Measures to facilitate voiding. (**A**) Massaging bladder area. (**B**) Rocking back and forth.

ated. Embarrassment in discussing this disorder or the belief that incontinence is a normal outcome of aging can lead to unreported incontinence. This reinforces the importance of questioning about incontinence during every routine assessment. In addition to referring the patient for a comprehensive medical evaluation, nurses can help identify the cause and determine appropriate treatment measures through the process of nursing assessment. Display 28-2 lists some of the factors to consider in assessing the incontinent individual. The initial goal for incontinent individuals is to have the cause of the incontinence identified; thereafter, treatment goals are developed based on the underlying cause. Kegel exercises, biofeedback, and medications (eg, estrogen or anticholinergics) may be useful for the improvement of stress incontinence; in some circumstances, surgery may be warranted. Urgency incontinence can be aided by adherence to a toileting schedule, Kegel exercises, biofeedback, and medications (eg, anticholinergics or adrenergic antagonists). Overflow incontinence may benefit from adherence to a toileting schedule, the use of the Crede method, intermittent catheterization, and medications (eg, parasympathomimetics). Interventions to assist with functional incontinence could range from improvement of mobility to provision of a bedside commode. Display 28-3 presents a sample care plan for the incontinent patient.

> **KEY CONCEPT**
> Nurses cannot assume that persons with long-standing incontinence have received a comprehensive evaluation of this problem.

Inconsistency on the part of the nursing staff will be destructive to the progress of patients and denigrating to their efforts to regain bladder control. Conversely, positive reinforcement and encouragement are most beneficial to the patient during this difficult program. Indwelling catheters should be used only in special circumstances and certainly never for the convenience of staff. Half of patients will develop bacteriuria within the first 24 hours of being catheterized; 35% to 40% of all nosocomial infections are catheter-associated UTIs (Foxman, 2003). In addition, the risk of developing urinary calculi is high when indwelling catheters are present. (Urinary tract infections are discussed in Chap. 23.)

Bladder Cancer

The incidence of bladder cancer increases with age, and older men have twice the rate of older women. Chronic irritation of the bladder, exposure to dyes, and cigarette smoking, avoidable factors, are among the risk factors associated with bladder tumors. Some of the symptoms resemble those of a bladder infection, such as frequency, urgency, and dysuria. A painless hematuria is the primary sign and characterizes cancer of the bladder. Standard diagnostic measures for this disease are used with the aged patient, including cystoscopic examination. Treatment can include surgery or radiation, depending on the extent and location of the lesion. The nurse should use the nursing measures described in medical-surgical nursing literature. Observation for signs indicating metastasis, such as pelvic or back pain, is part of the nursing care for patients with bladder cancer.

Renal Calculi

Renal calculi occur most frequently in middle-aged adults. In older adults, the formation of stones can be

DISPLAY 28-2

Factors to Review When Assessing the Patient Who is Incontinent

Medical History

Note diagnoses that could contribute to incontinence, such as delirium, dementia, cerebrovascular accident, diabetes mellitus, congestive heart failure, urinary tract infection.

Medications

Review all prescription and nonprescription drugs used for those that can affect continence, such as diuretics, antianxiety agents, antipsychotics, antidepressants, sedatives, narcotics, antiparkinsonism agents, antispasmodics, antihistamines, calcium channel blockers, and a-blockers and a-stimulants.

Functional Status

Assess activities of daily living (ADL) and impaired ADL capacities; ask about recent changes in function; determine degree of dependency on others for mobility, transfers, toileting.

Cognition

Test cognitive function; review symptoms such as depression, hallucinations; ask about recent changes in mood or intellectual function.

Neuromuscular Function in Lower Extremity

Test patient's ability to keep leg lifted against your efforts to gently push it down; touch various areas along both legs with pin point and smooth side of safety pin to determine patient's ability to detect and differentiate sensations.

Urinary Control and Retention

Test for stress incontinence in women; determine postvoid residual.

Bladder Fullness and Pain

Inspect, percuss, and palpate the bladder for distention, discomfort, and abnormalities.

Elimination Pattern

Record bladder and bowel elimination patterns and associated factors for several days; inquire about changes to elimination pattern; note frequency, pattern, amount, and relationship to other factors.

Fecal Impaction

Palpate the rectum for the presence of fecal impaction (unless contraindicated).

Symptoms

Ask about urgency, burning, vaginal itching, pain, pressure in bladder area, fever.

Diet

Assess intake of potential bladder irritants: caffeine, alcohol, citrus fruits/juices, tomatoes, spicy foods, artificial sweeteners

Reactions to Incontinence

Explore how incontinence has affected activities, lifestyle, self-concept; determine patient's appraisal of problem.

caused by immobilization, infection, changes in the pH or concentration of urine, chronic diarrhea, dehydration, excessive elimination of uric acid, and hypercalcemia. Pain, hematuria, and symptoms of urinary tract infection are associated with this prob-lem, and gastrointestinal upset may also occur. Standard diagnostic and treatment measures are used for the aged, and the nurse can assist by preventing urinary stasis, providing ample fluids, and facilitating prompt treatment of urinary tract infections.

DISPLAY 28-3

Sample Care Plan for the Patient With Incontinence

Nursing Diagnosis

Impaired urinary elimination

Goals

The patient
    achieves partial or complete restoration of bladder
        control
    effectively contains expelled urine

Actions

- Ensure that a comprehensive evaluation has been conducted to identify cause of incontinence and potential for regained bladder control.
- Identify individual voiding pattern: frequency, sensation of signal to void, time between signal being received and inability to hold urine, amount voided, and symptoms.
- If potential for bladder control exists, initiate bladder retraining program.
- Monitor intake and output; estimate urine lost on clothing and linens (1 inch diameter is approximately equal to 10 mL of urine).
- Ensure that bathroom is easily accessible; provide bedside commode or bedpan if needed.
- Offer at least 1500 mL liquids daily unless contraindicated.
- Encourage patient to lean forward while sitting on commode and to press on lower abdomen (Crede method) to promote optimal bladder emptying.
- Teach patient methods to stimulate voiding reflex: pouring warm water over perineum, stroking abdomen and inner thigh, drinking water while sitting on commode.
- Instruct female patient in Kegel exercises. Provide urinary sheaths, condom catheters, adult briefs, sanitary pads, or incontinence pants to contain urine.
- Avoid indwelling catheter use.
- When incontinent episodes occur, discuss cause with patient in a matter-of-fact manner.

- Modify environment to accommodate incontinence (eg, protect mattress and furniture, provide good ventilation, use room deodorizer, keep bathroom well-lighted).

Desired Outcomes

The patient

    has cause of incontinence identified
    achieves partial or complete urinary continence
    engages in usual patterns of activities and social
        interactions without restrictions related to
        incontinence

Nursing Diagnosis

*Risk for impaired skin integrity related to
incontinence*

Goals

The patient

    maintains skin integrity
    is dry and odor free

Actions

- Check patient for wetness every 2 hours; change clothing and linen as necessary.
- Thoroughly cleanse and dry patient's skin after incontinent episodes.
- Assess skin status daily.

Desired Outcomes

The patient

    is free from skin redness, irritation, and breaks in
        integrity
    is free from urine odor

Nursing Diagnosis

Risk for injury related to incontinence

(Continued)

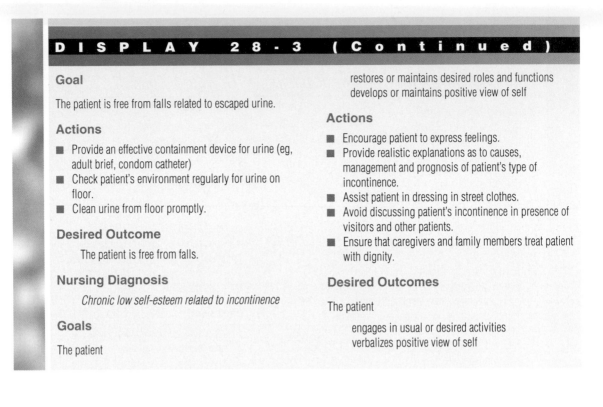

D I S P L A Y   2 8 - 3   (C o n t i n u e d)

Goal

The patient is free from falls related to escaped urine.

Actions

- Provide an effective containment device for urine (eg, adult brief, condom catheter)
- Check patient's environment regularly for urine on floor.
- Clean urine from floor promptly.

Desired Outcome

The patient is free from falls.

Nursing Diagnosis

Chronic low self-esteem related to incontinence

Goals

The patient

restores or maintains desired roles and functions
develops or maintains positive view of self

Actions

- Encourage patient to express feelings.
- Provide realistic explanations as to causes, management and prognosis of patient's type of incontinence.
- Assist patient in dressing in street clothes.
- Avoid discussing patient's incontinence in presence of visitors and other patients.
- Ensure that caregivers and family members treat patient with dignity.

Desired Outcomes

The patient

engages in usual or desired activities
verbalizes positive view of self

Glomerulonephritis

Most frequently, chronic glomerulonephritis already exists in older persons who develop an acute condition. The symptoms of this disease may be so subtle and nonspecific that they are initially unnoticed. Clinical manifestations include fever, fatigue, nausea, vomiting, anorexia, abdominal pain, anemia, edema, arthralgias, elevated blood pressure, and an increased sedimentation rate. Oliguria may occur, as can moderate proteinuria and hematuria. Headache, convulsions, paralysis, aphasia, coma, and an altered mental status may be consequences of cerebral edema associated with this disease. Diagnostic and treatment measures do not differ significantly from those used for the young. Antibiotics, a restricted sodium and protein diet, and close attention to fluid intake and output are basic parts of the treatment plan. If the elder is receiving digitalis, diuretics, or antihypertensive drugs, close observation for cumulative toxic effects resulting from compromised kidney function must be maintained. The patient should be evaluated periodically after the acute illness is resolved for exacerbations of chronic glomerulonephritis and signs of renal failure.

PROBLEMS OF THE FEMALE REPRODUCTIVE SYSTEM

Infections and Tumors of the Vulva

The vulva loses hair and subcutaneous fat with age. Accompanying these changes is a flattening and folding of the labia. General atrophy occurs as well. These changes cause the vulva to be more fragile and more easily susceptible to irritation and infection. Senile vulvitis is the term used to describe vulvar infection associated with hypertrophy or atrophy. Vulvar problems in the aged may reflect serious disease processes such as diabetes, hepatitis, leukemia, and pernicious anemia.

> **KEY CONCEPT**
> Age-related changes cause the vulva to be more fragile and more easily susceptible to irritation and infection.

Incontinence and poor hygienic practices can also be underlying causes of vulvitis. Pruritus is the primary symptom associated with vulvitis. Patients who are confused and noncommunicative may display restlessness, and the nurse may discover that they are suffering from irritation and thickening of the vulvar tissue as a result of scratching. Initially, treatment aims to find and manage any underlying cause. Good nutritional status helps improve the condition, as does special attention to cleanliness. Sitz baths and local applications of saline compresses or steroid creams may be included in the treatment plan. Special attention is required to keep the incontinent patient clean and dry as much as possible.

Although pruritus is commonly associated with vulvitis, it may be a symptom of a vulvar tumor. Pain and irritation also may be associated with this problem. Any mass or lesion in this area should receive prompt attention and be biopsied. The clitoris is commonly the site of a vulvar malignancy. Cancer of the vulva, the fourth most common gynecologic malignancy in later life, may be manifested by large, painful, and foul-smelling fungating or ulcerating tumors. The adjacent tissues may also be affected. A radical vulvectomy is usually the treatment of choice and tends to be well tolerated by the older woman. Less commonly used is radiation therapy, which is not tolerated as well as surgery. Counseling regarding self-care practices, body image, and sexual activity should be provided. Early treatment, before metastasis to inguinal lymph nodes, improves prognosis.

Atrophic Vaginitis

The postmenopausal woman experiences a variety of changes that affect the vaginal canal, including reduction in collagen and adipose tissue, shortening and narrowing of the vaginal canal, decreased elasticity, less vaginal lubrication, and a more alkaline vaginal pH as a result of lower estrogen levels. The vagina is more fragile and easily irritated as a result of these changes, which heightens the risk for vaginitis. Itching, foul-smelling discharge, and postcoital bleeding are symptoms associated with vaginal infection. Treatment could include topical estrogen creams and estrogen replacement therapy. Nurses should advise the older woman to avoid douches and the use of perfumed soaps and sprays to the genitalia, wear cotton underwear, keep the genital area clean and dry, and to use lubricants (eg, K-Y jelly, vitamin E oil, and aloe vera gel) when engaging in intercourse. (Chapter 23 offers an additional discussion of vaginitis.)

Cancer of the Vagina

Cancer of the vagina is rare in older women; it results more frequently from metastasis than from the vaginal area as a primary site. All vaginal ulcers and masses detected in aged women should be viewed with suspicion of malignancy and be biopsied. Because chronic irritation can predispose women to vaginal cancer, those who have chronic vaginitis or who wear a pessary should obtain frequent Pap smears. Treatment is similar to that used for younger women and may consist of irradiation, topical chemotherapeutic agents, or surgery, depending on the extent of the carcinoma.

Problems of the Cervix

With age, the cervix becomes smaller, and this is accompanied by an atrophy of the endocervical epithelium. Occasionally the endocervical glands can seal over, causing the formation of nabothian cysts. As secretions associated with these cysts accumulate, fever and a palpable tender mass may be evident. It is important, therefore, for the older woman to receive regular gynecologic examinations in which the patency of the cervix is checked.

Cancer of the Cervix

The incidence of cervical cancer peaks in the fifth and sixth decades of life and thereafter declines. Although most endocervical polyps are benign in older women, they should be viewed with suspicion until biopsy confirms such a diagnosis. Vaginal bleeding and leukorrhea are signs of cervical cancer in aged women. Pain does not usually occur. As the disease progresses, the patient can develop urinary retention or incontinence, fecal incontinence, and uremia. Treatment of cervical cancer can include radium or surgery. The National Cancer Institute (2003) states that women 65 to 70 years of age who have had at least three normal Pap tests and no abnormal Pap tests in the last 10 years may decide, upon consultation with their healthcare provider, to stop cervical cancer screening.

Problems of the Uterus

The uterus decreases in size with age, becoming so small in some older women that it cannot be palpated on examination. The endometrium continues to respond to hormonal stimulation.

Cancer of the Endometrium

Cancer of the endometrium is not uncommon in the older woman and is of higher incidence in obese, diabetic, and hypertensive women. Any postmenopausal bleeding should give rise immediately to suspicion of this disease. Dilation and curettage usually are done to confirm the diagnosis because not all cases can be detected by Pap smears alone. Treatment consists of surgery, irradiation, or a combination of both. Early treatment can prevent metastasis to the vagina and cervix. Endometrial polyps can also cause bleeding and should receive serious attention because they could be indicative of early cancer.

Problems of the Fallopian Tubes and Ovaries

Although masses are occasionally detected in the fallopian tubes, they rarely present any significant problem to the older woman. The primary changes the fallopian tubes undergo with age are shortening, straightening, and atrophy. The ovaries also atrophy with age, becoming smaller and thicker. They may not be palpable during the gynecologic examination because of their decreased size. Ovarian cancer is responsible for only 5% of malignant disease in older women, although it is the leading cause of death from gynecologic malignancies. Early symptoms are nonspecific and can be confused with gastrointestinal discomfort. As it progresses, the clinical manifestations of this disease include bleeding, ascites, and the presence of multiple masses. Treatment may consist of surgery or irradiation. Benign ovarian tumors commonly occur in older women, and surgery is usually required to differentiate them from malignant ones.

> **KEY CONCEPT**
> Although ovarian cancer is less common than endometrial or cervical cancer, it is more deadly when it does occur.

Perineal Herniation

As a result of the stretching and tearing of muscles during childbirth and of the muscle weakness associated with advanced age, perineal herniation is a common problem among older women. Cystocele, rectocele, and prolapse of the uterus are the types most likely to occur. Associated with this problem are lower back pain, pelvic heaviness, and a pulling sensation. Urinary and fecal incontinence, retention, and constipation may also occur. Sometimes the woman is able to feel pressure or palpate a mass in her vagina. These herniations can make intercourse difficult and uncomfortable. Although rectoceles do not tend to worsen with age, the opposite is true for cystoceles, which will cause increased problems with time. Surgical repair is the treatment of choice and can be successful in relieving these problems.

Dyspareunia

Dyspareunia is a common problem among older women but is not necessarily a normal consequence of aging. Nulliparous women experience this problem more frequently than women who have had children. Because vulvitis, vaginitis, and other gynecologic problems can contribute to dyspareunia, a thorough gynecologic examination is important, and any lesions or infections should be corrected to alleviate the problem. All efforts should be made to help the older woman achieve a satisfactory sexual life. (Chapter 13 presents a more detailed discussion of sexual problems.)

> **KEY CONCEPT**
> Dyspareunia is a common, although not necessarily normal, finding in older women.

Problems of the Breast

The breasts atrophy with age, sagging more and hanging at a lower level. Some retraction of the nipples may occur as a result of shrinkage and fibrotic changes. Firm linear strands may develop on the breasts from fibrosis and calcification of the terminal ducts.

Cancer of the Breast

Decreased fat tissue and atrophy in older women's breasts can cause tumors, possibly present for many years, to become more evident. Because breast cancer is a leading cause of cancer deaths in aged as well as younger women, regular breast examinations should be encouraged. Unfortunately, although the incidence of breast cancer increases with age, the older the woman is the less likely she is to perform self-examination of breasts or receive a yearly mammogram or breast examination by a health care professional. Diagnostic and treatment measures for women with breast cancer are the same at any age.

KEY CONCEPT

Although the incidence of breast cancer rises with age, older women are the least likely group to receive mammograms and breast examinations by a professional or to perform self-examinations of breasts.

PROBLEMS OF THE MALE REPRODUCTIVE SYSTEM

Benign Prostatic Hyperplasia

A majority of older men have some degree of benign prostatic hyperplasia, which causes approximately 1 in 4 of them to have dysuria. Symptoms of this problem progress slowly but continuously; they begin with hesitancy, decreased force of urinary stream, frequency, and nocturia as a result of obstruction of the vesical neck and compression of the urethra that causes a compensatory hypertrophy of the detrusor muscle and subsequent outlet obstruction. Dribbling, poor control, overflow incontinence, and bleeding may occur. As the hyperplasia progresses the bladder wall loses its elasticity and becomes thinner, leading to urinary retention and an increased risk of urinary infection. Unfortunately, some men are reluctant or embarrassed to seek prompt medical attention and may develop kidney damage by the time symptoms are severe enough to motivate them to be evaluated. Treatment can include prostatic massage, the use of urinary antiseptics and, if possible, the avoidance of diuretics, anticholinergics, and antiarrhythmic agents. The herb saw palmetto can help some men reduce the size of the prostate, improving urinary flow and decreasing nocturia. The most common prostatectomy approach used for older men with prostatism is transurethral surgery. The patient should be reassured

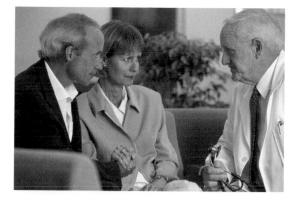

FIGURE 28-2

Men benefit from realistic explanations of the effects of treatments on sexual function.

that this surgery will not guarantee impotence. On the other hand, realistic explanations are needed so the patient understands that this surgery will not cause a sudden rejuvenation of sexual performance (Fig. 28-2) (Display 28-4). (Prostatitis is discussed in Chapter 23.)

Cancer of the Prostate

Prostatic cancer increases in incidence with age. In fact, more than half of men over 70 years of age have histologic evidence of prostate cancer, although less than 3% will die from the disease (National Cancer Institute SEER, 2003). Often, this disease can be asymptomatic; however, a majority of prostatic cancers can be detected by digital rectal examination, which emphasizes the importance of regular physical examinations. Benign hypertrophy should be followed closely because it is thought to be associated with prostatic cancer, the symptoms of which can be similar. Symptoms such as back pain, anemia, weakness, and weight loss can develop as a result of metastasis. If metastasis has not occurred, treatment may consist of irradiation or a radical prostatectomy; the latter procedure will result in impotency. Estrogens may be used to prevent tumor dissemination. Palliative treatment, used if the cancer has metastasized, includes irradiation, transurethral surgery, orchiectomy, and estrogens. General principles associated with these therapeutic measures are applicable to the

D I S P L A Y   2 8 - 4

The Patient Recovering From Prostate Surgery

Mr. K is a 73-year-old man who is a patient on a surgical unit. He works as a part-time salesman in a family business and has recently married a 50-year-old woman with whom he enjoys a good relationship. His health was good until several months ago when he developed nocturia, urinary hesitancy, and dribbling after urination. Physical examination revealed moderate benign prostatic hypertrophy for which a transurethral resection prostatectomy was performed. Mr. K is recovering well from the surgery and will have his urinary catheter removed in preparation for his discharge.

Mr. K informs you that his physician has instructed him to "take it easy for a couple of weeks, drink a lot of fluids, schedule a follow-up appointment, and call if there are any problems." Although he did not address these issues with his physician, Mr. K is concerned that he doesn't know what type of problems to look for or if it is all right for him to return to work. As he continues to talk, he express concern about his wife's reactions to his "inability to have sex now that he has had prostate surgery." Based on this brief contact, the nurse could anticipate some care planning needs:

Nursing Diagnosis

Risk for injury and infection related to surgery

Goals

The patient

is free from injury
is free from infection

Action

- Advise patient to avoid strenuous activities for 3 to 4 weeks.
- Advise patient to prevent constipation. Recommend dietary adjustments as needed; advise patient to consult with physician regarding use of stool softener if bowel movements are strained or irregular.
- Teach patient to avoid Valsalva maneuver.
- Encourage high fluid intake unless contraindicated.

- Teach patient to observe for and promptly report signs of complications, including bright red blood in urine, elevated temperature, severe pain, weakness.

Desired Outcomes

The patient

is free from injury
is free from infection

Nursing Diagnoses

Sexual dysfunction related to surgery
Deficient knowledge related to effect of surgery on sexual function

Goals

The patient

expresses realistic understanding of effect of surgery on sexual function
resumes satisfying sexual relationship

Action

- Consult with physician regarding sexual restrictions; discuss with patient. (Typically, sexual intercourse is avoided for about 1 month postoperatively, after which time patient can usually return to previous sexual function. It is not unusual for complete return of sexual function to take as long as 1 year.)
- Assess patient's understanding of impact of surgery on sexual function; clarify misinformation as needed.
- Listen to patient's concerns and provide support.
- Discuss anticipated return of sexual function with patient's wife, if acceptable to patient.
- Prepare patient for possibility of retrograde ejaculation (dry climax), which will make urine appear milky.
- Discuss with couple the potential for anxiety and other psychological factors related to illness and surgery to interfere with sexual function.
- Encourage couple to share other forms of intimacy until intercourse can be resumed.

(Continued)

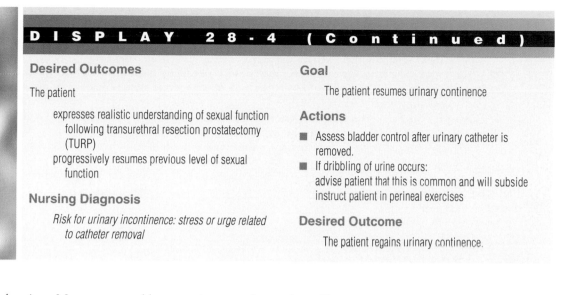

DISPLAY 28-4 (Continued)

Desired Outcomes

The patient

expresses realistic understanding of sexual function following transurethral resection prostatectomy (TURP)
progressively resumes previous level of sexual function

Nursing Diagnosis

Risk for urinary incontinence: stress or urge related to catheter removal

Goal

The patient resumes urinary continence

Actions

■ Assess bladder control after urinary catheter is removed.
■ If dribbling of urine occurs:
advise patient that this is common and will subside
instruct patient in perineal exercises

Desired Outcome

The patient regains urinary continence.

---

aged patient. Many men are able to continue sexual performance after orchiectomy and during estrogen therapy; the physician should be consulted for specific advice concerning the expected outcomes for individual patients.

Tumors of the Penis, Testes, and Scrotum

Cancer of the penis is rare and appears as a painless lesion or wartlike growth on the prepuce or glans. The resemblance of this growth to a chancre can cause a misdiagnosis or a reluctance on the part of the patient to seek treatment. A biopsy should be done of any penile lesion. Treatment may consist of irradiation and local excision for small lesions and partial or total penile amputation for extensive lesions.

Testicular tumors are uncommon in the aged but are usually malignant when they do occur; testicular enlargement and pain and enlargement of the breasts are suspicious symptoms. Chemotherapy, irradiation, and orchiectomy are among the treatment measures. As part of the assessment, nurses should ascertain the patient's knowledge of testicular self-examination and provide education on this procedure if necessary; the American Cancer Society can provide educational materials that could be used for this instruction.

Scrotal masses, usually benign, can be caused by conditions such as hydrocele, spermatocele, varico-

cele, and hernia. Symptoms and treatment depend on the underlying cause and are the same as for younger men. As with any genitourinary problem, counseling regarding self-care practices, body image, and sexual activity is important.

Additional Nursing Considerations

PROMOTING A POSITIVE SELF-CONCEPT

Nurses need sensitivity in dealing with patients' genitourinary problems. In addition to being areas that are considered taboo for discussion for some persons, these disorders may raise fears and anxieties that tales of becoming incontinent and sexless in old age perhaps are valid. Realistic explanations and a committed effort to correcting these disorders are vital. All levels of staff need to be reminded of the importance of discretion and dignity in managing these problems. Staff members should not check to see if a patient's pants are wet in front of others, allow someone to sit on a bedside commode in a hallway, bring in a group of students without the patient's permission to show them his orchitis, or scold the patient for having an accident in bed. Every effort should be made to minimize embarrassment and promote a positive self-concept.

Critical Thinking Exercises

1. What are the factors that would be reviewed in assessing urinary incontinence and what barriers could arise in reviewing them and obtaining accurate answers from older adults?
2. What can be done to reduce each of the major causes of urinary incontinence in the elderly?
3. Describe the factors that can affect sexual function in old age and actions that can be taken to promote healthy sexual activity.
4. Discuss reasons for older adults not performing breast and testicular self-examinations and measures nurses could take to promote older adults performing these examinations.
5. What actions could be taken to promote a positive self-concept of an individual with urinary incontinence?
6. Identify resources in your community to assist patients with incontinence or cancer of the reproductive system.

Web Connect

Review a comprehensive consumer fact sheet on *Incontinence in Women prepared by the National Kidney and Urologic Disease Information Clearinghouse at http://www.niddk.nih.gov/health/urolog/pubs/uiwomen/ uiwomen.htm.*

● Resources

American Foundation for Urologic Disease
1128 North Charles Street
Baltimore, MD 21201
(800) 242-2383
www.afud.org

National Association for Continence
P.O. Box 8310
Spartanburg, SC 29305
(800) 252-3337
www.nafc.org

National Kidney Foundation
30 East 33rd Street
New York, NY 10016
(800) 622-9010
www.kidney.org

National Kidney and Urologic Disease Information Clearinghouse
Box NKUDIC
Bethesda, MD 20892
(310) 468-6345
www.niddk.nih.gov/health/urolog/urolog.htm

Procter and Gamble (incontinence care products)
Procter and Gamble Plaza

Cincinnati, OH 45202
(800) 428-8363
www.pg.com

Simon Foundation for Continence
P.O. Box 835
Wilmette, IL 60091
(800) 23-SIMON
www.simonfoundation.org

Women's Suffrage for Prostate Cancer Awareness and Support
2139 Courtside Circle
Carson City, NV 89703
(888) 776-2262
info@pcawomen.org

● References

Durrant, J., & Snape, J. (2003). Urinary incontinence in nursing homes for older people. *Age and Ageing, 32*(1), 12–18.

Foxman, B. (2003). Epidemiology of urinary tract infections: incidence, morbidity, and economic costs. *Disease a Month, 49*(2), 53–70.

Landi, F., Cesari, M., Russo, A., Onder, G., Lattanzio, F., & Bernabei, R. (2003). Potentially reversible risk factors and urinary incontinence in frail older people living in community. *Age and Ageing, 32*(2), 194–199.

National Cancer Institute. (2003). Task force announces new cancer screening guidelines. *Cancer.gov News Center,* Posted January 22, 2003. Retrieved April 2, 2004, from www.cancer.gov/newscenter/pressreleases/cervicalscreen.

National Cancer Institute, SEER (Surveillance Epidemiology and End Results) (2003). *Prevalence: Prostate cancer.* Retrieved May 30, 2003, from http://seer.cancer.gov/faststats/html/pre_prost.html.

Sriprasad, S., Dew, T. K., Muir, G. H., Thompson, P. M., Mulvin, D., et al. (2001). Validity of PSA, free/total PSA ratio and complexed/total PSA ratio measurements in men with acute urinary retention. *Prostate Cancer and Prostatic Disease, 4*(3), 167–172.

● Recommended Readings

American Journal of Nursing. (2003). The state of the science on urinary incontinence. A summary of the July 2002 symposium. *American Journal of Nursing, 103*(3), 45–49.

Bassett, S., & Smyer, T. (2003). Health screening practices in rural long-term care facilities. *Journal of Gerontological Nursing, 29*(4), 42–49.

Baum, N., & Lipp, A. (2001). PSA for the primary care physician. *Clinical Geriatrics, 9*(8), 32–38.

Beduschi, R., Beduschi, M. C., & Osterling, J. E. (1998). Benign prostatic hyperplasia: Use of drug therapy in primary care. *Geriatrics, 53*(3), 24–40.

Ben-Tovim, D. I., Dougherty, M. L., Stapleton, A. M., & Pinnock, C. B. (2002). Coping with prostate cancer: a quantitative analysis using a new instrument, the centre for clinical excellence in urological research coping with cancer instrument. *Urology, 59*(3), 383–388.

Bradway, C., Hernly, S., & the NICHE Faculty. (1998). Urinary incontinence in older adults admitted to acute care. *Geriatric Nursing, 19,* 98–101.

Brandeis, G. H., Baumann, M. M., Hossain, M., Morris, J. N., & Resnick, N. M. (1997). The prevalence of potentially remediable urinary incontinence in frail older people: A study using the minimum data set. *Journal of the American Geriatrics Society, 45,* 179–184.

Bruner, D. W., Pickett, M., Joseph, A., & Burggraf, V. (2000). Prostate cancer elder alert: Epidemiology, screening, and early detection. *Journal of Gerontological Nursing, 26*(1), 6–15.

Burgio, K. L., Goode, P. S., Locher, J. L., et al. (2002). Behavioral training with and without biofeedback in the treatment of urge incontinence in older women: A randomized controlled trial. *Journal of the American Medical Association, 288,* 2293–2299.

Carbone, D. J., & Seftel, A. D. (2002). Erectile dysfunction: Diagnosis and treatment in older men. *Geriatrics, 57*(9), 18–24.

Chasens, E. R., & Umlauf, M. G. (2003). Nocturia: A problem that disrupts sleep and predicts obstructive sleep apnea. *Geriatric Nursing, 24*(2), 76–81.

Cooper, J. (1997). *Urinary incontinence in the elderly: Pharmacotherapy treatment.* New York: Pharmaceutical Products Press.

Dowling-Castronovo, A. (2001). Urinary incontinence assessment. *Journal of Gerontological Nursing, 27*(5), 6–7.

Evans, F. (1999). Indwelling catheter care: Dispelling the misconceptions. *Geriatric Nursing, 20*(2), 8.

Faubert, P. F., & Porush, J. G. (1998). *Renal disease in the elderly* (2nd ed.). New York: Marcel Dekker.

Frenchman, I. B. (2001). Cost of urinary incontinence in two skilled nursing facilities: A prospective study. *Clinical Geriatrics, 9*(1), 49–52.

Gray, M. (2000). Urinary retention management in the acute care setting. Part 1. *American Journal of Nursing, 100*(7), 40–48.

Gray, M. (2000). Urinary retention management in the acute care setting. Part 2. *American Journal of Nursing, 100*(8), 36–44.

Gray, M. (2003). The importance of screening, assessing, and managing urinary incontinence in primary care. *Journal of the American Academy of Nursing Practice, 15*(3), 102–107.

Holt, S. (1999). Natural approaches to promote sexual function: Part 2: Stimulants and dietary supplements. *Alternative and Complementary Therapies, 5*(5), 279–285.

Kantor, D. E., & Houlden, A. (1999). Breast cancer in older women: Treatment, psychosocial effects, interventions, and outcomes. *Journal of Gerontological Nursing, 25*(7), 19–25.

Klingman, L. (1999). Assessing the male genitalia. *American Journal of Nursing, 99*(7), 47–51.

Luft, J., & Vriheas-Nichols, A. A. (1998). Identifying the risk factors for developing incontinence: Can we modify individual risk? *Geriatric Nursing, 19,* 66–70.

Mackenzie, D. L. (1999). When *E. coli* turns deadly. *RN, 62*(7), 28–32.

Maloney, C. (2002). Estrogen and recurrent UTI in postmenopausal women. *American Journal of Nursing, 102*(8), 44–54.

Mather, K. F., & Bakas, T. (2002). Nursing assistants' perception of their ability to provide continence care. *Geriatric Nursing, 23*(1), 76–81.

Mount Sinai School of Medicine. (1999). Postmenopausal? See your gynecologist anyway! *Focus on Healthy Aging, 2*(11), 1, 6.

Mueller, C., & Cain, H. (2002). Comprehensive management of urinary incontinence through quality improvement efforts. *Geriatric Nursing, 23*(1), 82–87.

Pickett, M., Bruner, D. W., Joseph, A., & Burggraf, V. (2000). Prostate cancer elder alert: Living with treatment choices and outcomes. *Journal of Gerontological Nursing, 26*(2), 22–34.

Smith, D. B. (1998). A continence care approach for long-term care facilities. *Geriatric Nursing, 19,* 81–86.

Taft, C. (1999). A team approach to managing urinary incontinence, *Geriatric Nursing, 20*(2), 94–97.

Urinary Incontinence Guideline Panel. (1996). *Managing acute and chronic urinary incontinence: Clinical practice guideline update.* (AHCPR Pub. No. 96–0686). Rockville, MD: Agency for Health Care Policy and Research, Public Health Service, U.S. Department of Health and Human Services.

Vanderford, V. (1999). Older women and mammography: Factors influencing their attitudes. *Geriatric Nursing, 20*(5), 255–259.

Walsh, P. C., & Worthington, J. F. (1997). *The prostate: A guide for men and the women who love them.* Baltimore, MD: Johns Hopkins University Press.

Weber, B. A., Roberts, B. L., & McDougall, G. J. (2000). Exploring the efficacy of support groups for men with prostate cancer. *Geriatric Nursing, 21*(5), 250–253.

Zaccagnini, M. (1999). Clinical snapshot: Prostate cancer. *American Journal of Nursing, 99*(4), 34–35.

CHAPTER 29

Neurologic Conditions

Chapter Outline

Facilitating neurologic health
Controlling risk factors
Recognizing symptoms early
Selected disorders
Parkinson's disease
Transient ischemic attacks
Cerebrovascular accidents
Nursing interventions related to
neurologic problems
Promoting independence
Preventing injury

Learning Objectives

After reading this chapter, you should be able to:

- list risk factors for neurologic problems
- identify signs and symptoms of neurologic disorders
- describe the symptoms, unique features, and related nursing care for Parkinson's disease, transient ischemic attacks, and cerebrovascular accidents
- discuss actions that promote independence in persons with neurologic problems
- describe measures to reduce the risk of injury

The nervous system has a profound influence on our interaction with the world. A healthy system enables us to sense the pleasures around us, protect ourselves from harm, solve problems, derive intellectual stimulation, and communicate our needs, thoughts, and desires. Every aspect of our basic activities of daily living depends on a good neurologic status. Dysfunction of this system has a ripple effect on other systems and can profoundly affect health, safety, normalcy, and general well-being. Astute nursing assessment (Display 29-1) can help reveal problems that warrant intervention and identify nursing diagnoses (Nursing Diagnosis Table 29-1).

Facilitating Neurologic Health

Many neurologic disorders occur for reasons beyond our control, but some can be prevented or minimized. For instance, cigarette smoking, obesity, ineffective stress management, elevated cholesterol, and hypertension are significant risk factors for neurovascular disease. The risk of injury to the head and spinal column is increased with unsafe actions, such as failure to use seatbelts, incompetent driving skills, alcohol and drug abuse, and falls. Infections of the ear or sinus and sexually transmitted diseases can lead to neurologic dysfunction. Most of these factors are within an individual's control. Nurses should educate

D I S P L A Y   2 9 - 1

Assessment of Neurologic Function

General Observations

Keen observation while interviewing the patient can aid in detecting a variety of neurologic problems. On initial inspection of the patient, asymmetry, deformity, weakness, paralysis, and other abnormalities can be seen. If such problems are noted, inquire into their origin, length of time present, and resulting limitations or problems. Explore the presence of symptoms of neurologic disorders, such as pain, tingling sensations, numbness, blackouts, headaches, twitching, seizures, dizziness, distortions of reality, weakness, and changes in mental status.

Speech

During something as basic as simple introductions, speech disorders can become evident. If speech problems exist, it is important to differentiate problems with articulation (ie, dysarthria) and problems with the use of symbols (ie, dysphagia). With dysarthria, the symbols, in this case, words, are used correctly, but speech may be slurred or distorted as a result of poor motor control. Subtle dysarthrias can be disclosed by asking the patient to pronounce the following syllables:

- me, me, me (to test the lips)
- la, la, la (to test the tongue)
- ga, ga, ga (to test the pharynx).

Dysphasias can be receptive, expressive, or a combination of both. To test for a receptive aphasia, ask the patient to follow a command (eg, pick up the pencil); the patient's inability to understand what these symbols mean will prevent the command from being followed. The patient with expressive aphasia will be able to understand commands but will not be able to put symbols together into an intelligent speech form. Point to several objects and ask the patient to name them; mild dysphasias (ie, paraphasia) may be noted if the patient substitutes a close, although inaccurate, word for the right one, such as calling a shoe a boot or a watch a clock. The ability to understand and express oneself through the written word is important to evaluate also. Ask the patient to write a short sentence that you dictate and to read a sentence from a newspaper. Ensure that the patient has the educational and visual abilities to fulfill these demands.

Physical Examination

One component of the physical assessment of the nervous system involves the test of sensations. To help document areas where problems are identified, a figure drawing may prove useful. Ask the patient to close his or her eyes and to describe the sensations felt. Touch various parts of the body (eg, forehead, cheeks, arms, hands, legs, feet) lightly with your finger or a cotton wisp and note if the patient is able to feel the sensations. Compare analogous areas on both sides of the body and distal and proximal areas on the same extremity. If these primary sensations are intact, test the patient's ability to identify two simultaneous stimuli (eg, touch the right cheek and the left forearm). To test cortical sensation (ie, sterognosis), have the patient, again with closed eyes, identify various objects placed in each hand (eg, key, marble, coin). The inability to sense these objects is known as astereognosis.

Several simple measures are used for coordination and cerebellar testing. Hold up your finger and ask the patient to touch it and then touch his nose; have the patient continue this action as you move your fingers to different areas. Do this point-to-point testing with both the patient's arms, and note uneven, jerking movements and the inability to touch your finger or his nose. To test coordination in the lower extremity, have the patient lie down and run the heel of one foot against the shin of the other leg. The ability to make rapid alternating movements can be tested by having the patient rapidly tap his index finger on the thigh or a table surface. Tandem walking, in which the patient walks heal to toe as though walking a tightrope. also tests coordination; patients with arthritic deformities may not be able to perform this test. Have weak or poorly coordinated patients hold your hand during the tandem walking test.

(Continued)

Nurses can perform some tests of reflexes. To test the corneal reflex, gently touch the cornea with a wisp of clean cotton. Tissue and gauze are too rough and can cause corneal abrasions. Normally, the eye should blink. The Babinski reflex (ie, plantar response) is tested by stroking the sole of the patient's foot. Normally the toes should flex; an abnormal response is extension and fanning of the toes.

Each of the cranial nerves can be tested to identify further problems. Lumbar puncture, cerebral angiography, pneumoencephalography, and computed tomography scans are among other screening devices used to evaluate neurologic problems. A review of mental status is included in the assessment of the nervous system. (For information on mental status examination, refer to Chap. 34.)

persons of all ages in preventive measures that promote neurologic health in late life.

KEY CONCEPT
Some neurologic problems can be prevented by maintaining weight within a normal range, avoiding cigarette smoking, effectively managing stress, driving safely, and controlling infections.

The close relationship and regular contact nursing staff have with patients puts them in an ideal position to detect new or subtle symptoms of neurologic diseases that otherwise may be missed (Display 29-2). Recognizing symptoms and taking prompt action to ensure that patients are evaluated in a timely manner can help prevent irreversible or serious dysfunction.

Point to Ponder
Review your health status and lifestyle for risk factors for neurologic disorders. If risks are present, how can you reduce them?

Selected Disorders

PARKINSON'S DISEASE

Parkinson's disease affects the ability of the central nervous system (CNS) to control body movements. It is more common in men and occurs most frequently after the fifth decade of life. The incidence rises with age but peaks at age 75 years. Although its exact cause is unknown, this disease is thought to be associated with a history of metallic poisoning, encephalitis, and cerebrovascular disease, especially arteriosclerosis. A finding in people with Parkinson's disease compared with individuals who have other causes of tremors is the presence of the Lewy body, an intracellular inclusion body, in the brain. The death of substantia nigra cells within the basal ganglia leads to a significant reduction in dopamine, which is responsible for the symptoms.

A faint tremor in the hands or feet that progresses over a long time may be the first clue of Parkinson's disease (Fig. 29-1). The tremor is reduced when the patient attempts a purposeful movement. Muscle rigidity and weakness develop, evidenced by drooling, difficulty in swallowing, slow speech, and a monotone voice. The face of the patient assumes a mask-like appearance, and the skin is moist. Bradykinesia (slow movement) and poor balance occur. Appetite frequently increases, and emotional instability may be demonstrated. A characteristic sign is a shuffling gait while leaning forward at the trunk. The rate of movement increases as the patient walks, and the patient may not be able to voluntarily stop walking. As the disease progresses, the patient may become entirely unable to ambulate. Secondary symptoms include depression, sleep disturbances, dementia, forced eyelid closure, drooling, dysphagia, constipation, shortness of breath, urinary hesitancy, urgency, and reduced interest in sex.

A variety of measures are used to control the tremors and maintain the highest possible level of independence. Anticholinergics may be prescribed to decrease the patient's symptoms. Nurses need to be aware that anticholinergics can exacerbate glaucoma,

ND *Nursing Diagnosis*

TABLE 29-1 ● *Nursing Diagnoses Related to Neurologic Problems*

Causes or Contributing Factors	Nursing Diagnosis
Impaired sensory or motor function, fatigue, pain, depression, need for equipment or aids that use energy	Activity Intolerance
Altered self-concept, inability to communicate, dependency	Anxiety
Inability to sense signal, lack of motor control, immobility	Constipation
Poor positioning, pressure on brain, neuritis	Pain
Dysphasia, dysarthria, altered mental status	Impaired Verbal Communication
Altered body structure or function, dependency	Ineffective Coping
Barriers from disabilities	Deficient Diversional Activity
Demands, dependency, and role changes due to patient's illness	Interrupted Family Processes
Altered body structure and function, dependency	Fear
Loss of function, lifestyle change	Anticipatory Grieving
Dependency, disability, altered self-concept	Ineffective Health Maintenance
Disability, dependency, pain, impaired mental status	Impaired Home Maintenance
Immobility, lack of sensation	Risk for Infection
Impaired sensory function, fatigue, altered mental status, improper use of aids, altered mobility or coordination	Risk for Injury
Paralysis, weakness, vertigo, poor coordination	Impaired Physical Mobility
Swallowing disorder, inability to feed self or express desires, depression, altered taste, anorexia	Imbalanced Nutrition: Less Than Body Requirements
Inability to provide adequate oral hygiene	Impaired Oral Mucous Membrane
Dependency, disability, impaired communication, role change	Powerlessness
Weakness, paralysis, poor coordination, visual disorders	Self-Care Deficit
Altered body structure or function, dependency, role change	Chronic Low Self-Esteem
Decreased or lost sensory function, cerebral vascular accident, sensory deprivation	Disturbed Sensory Perception
Impaired nerve supply, disability, altered self-image, depression	Ineffective Sexual Patterns
Altered ability to feel pressure or pain, immobility	Impaired Skin Integrity
Altered body structure or function, dysphasia, dysarthria, visual or hearing deficits, depression, altered self-concept	Impaired Social Interaction
Inability to communicate, disability, impaired mobility	Social Isolation
Cerebrovascular accident, depression, anxiety, fear, altered cerebral function	Disturbed Thought Processes
Lack of sensory awareness to void or ability to control bladder emptying, inability to communicate needs or toilet self	Impaired Urinary Elimination

warranting close monitoring of the condition when it is present. Also, anticholinergics can cause temporary anuria. Close monitoring during drug therapy is important. While they are taking levodopa, patients should avoid foods that are high in vitamin B_6, such as avocados, lentils, and lima beans, because they will counteract the drug; dietary restrictions are not necessary if the patient is taking Sinemet. The herb passion flower is believed to reduce passive tremors when used alone or in combination with levodopa (Libster, 2002). New technology to control symptoms, such as pulse generators that send electrical impulses that

DISPLAY 29-2

Subtle Indications of Neurologic Problems

- New headaches that occur in early morning or interrupt sleep
- Change in vision (eg, sudden decreased acuity, double vision, blindness in portion of visual field)
- Sudden deafness, ringing in ears
- Mood, personality changes
- Altered cognition or level of consciousness
- Clumsiness, unsteady gait
- Numbness, tingling of extremity
- Unusual sensation or pain over nerve

block tremor-causing brain signals, drug infusion systems, and gene therapy, may be able to benefit some people who have Parkinson's disease (Aebischer & Pralog, 2003); the neurologist should be consulted regarding the potential usefulness to the patient.

Joint mobility is maintained and improved by active and passive range-of-motion exercises; warm baths and massage may facilitate these exercises and relieve muscle spasms caused by rigidity. Contractures are a particular risk of elders with Parkinson's disease. Physical and occupational therapists should be actively involved in the exercise program to help the patient find devices that increase self-care ability. Surgical intervention is rare for aged patients because they do not tend to respond well.

Tension and frustration will aggravate the patient's symptoms; therefore, it is important for the nurse to offer psychological support and minimize emotional upsets. Teaching helps patients and their families gain realistic insight into the disease. The nurse should emphasize that the disease progresses slowly and that therapy can minimize disability. Although intellectual functioning is not impaired by this disease, the speech problems and helpless appearance of patients may cause others to underestimate their mental ability; this can be extremely frustrating and degrading to the patient, who may react by becoming depressed or irritable. Continuing support by the nurse can help the family maximize the patient's mental capacity and understand personality changes that may occur. Communication and mental stimulation should be encouraged on a level that the patient always enjoyed. As the disease progresses, the patient requires increased assistance. Skillful nursing assessment is essential to ensure that the demands for assistance are met while the maximum level of patient independence is preserved.

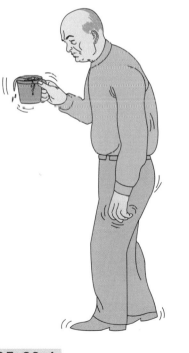

FIGURE 29-1

Tremors and shuffling gait characteristic of Parkinson's disease.

TRANSIENT ISCHEMIC ATTACKS

Transient ischemic attacks (TIAs), or temporary episodes of CNS dysfunction, can be caused by any situation that reduces cerebral circulation. Hyperextension and flexion of the head, such as when an individual falls asleep in a chair, can impair cerebral blood flow. Reduced blood pressure resulting from anemia and certain drugs (eg, diuretics and antihypertensives) and cigarette smoking, due to its vasoconstrictive effect, will also decrease cerebral circulation, as will sudden standing from a prone position. Hemiparesis, hemianesthesia, aphasia, unilateral loss of vision, diplopia, vertigo, nausea, vomiting, and dysphagia are among the manifestations of a TIA, depending on the location of the ischemic area. These signs can last from minutes to hours, and complete recovery is usual within a day. Treatment may consist of correction of the underlying cause, anticoagulant therapy, or vascular reconstruction. A significant concern regarding TIAs is that they increase the patient's risk of sustaining a cerebrovascular accident (CVA).

KEY CONCEPT

Good alignment and support of the head and neck can prevent hyperextension and flexion of the head that can lead to impaired cerebral blood flow.

CEREBROVASCULAR ACCIDENTS

Older persons with hypertension, severe arteriosclerosis, diabetes, gout, anemia, hypothyroidism, silent myocardial infarction, TIAs, and dehydration and those who smoke are among the high-risk candidates for a CVA, the third leading cause of death in this age group. Although a ruptured cerebral blood vessel could be responsible for this problem, most CVAs in elders are caused by partial or complete cerebral thrombosis. Light-headedness, dizziness, headache, drop attack (feeling of being strongly and suddenly pulled to the ground), and memory and behavioral changes are some of the warning signs of a CVA. A drop attack is a fall caused by a complete muscular flaccidity in the legs but with no alteration in consciousness. Patients describing or demonstrating these symptoms should be referred for prompt medical evaluation. Because nurses are in a key position to first learn of these signs, they can be instrumental in helping the patient avoid disability or death from a stroke. CVAs can occur without warning, however, and show highly variable signs and symptoms, depending on the

area of the brain affected. Major signs tend to include hemiplegia, aphasia, and hemianopsia.

Although older adults have a higher mortality rate from CVAs than the young, those who do survive have a good chance of recovery. Good nursing care can improve the patient's chance of survival and minimize the limitations that impair a full recovery. In the acute phase, nursing efforts have the following aims:

- Maintain a patent airway.
- Provide adequate nutrition and hydration.
- Monitor neurologic and vital signs.
- Prevent complications associated with immobility.

In addition, unconscious patients need good skin care and frequent turning because they are more susceptible to pressure ulcer formation. If an indwelling catheter is not being used, it is important for the nurse to examine the patient for indications of an overdistended bladder and promptly remedy the situation if it occurs. The eyes of the unconscious patient may remain open for a long time, risking drying, irritation, and ulceration of the cornea. Corneal damage can be prevented by eye irrigations with a sterile saline solution followed by the use of sterile mineral oil eye drops. Eye pads may be used to help keep the eyelids closed; these are changed daily and frequently checked to make sure the lids are actually closed. Regular mouth care and range-of-motion exercises are also standard measures.

☑ **Point to Ponder**

How would your life and the lives of your family members be affected if you suffered a stroke?

When consciousness is regained and the patient's condition stabilizes, more active efforts can focus on rehabilitation. It may be extremely difficult for patients to understand and participate in their rehabilitation because of speech, behavior, and memory problems. Although these problems vary depending on the side of the brain affected, some general observations can be noted. Attention span is reduced and long, complicated directions may be confusing. Memory for old events may be intact, whereas recent events or explanations are forgotten, a characteristic demonstrated by many aged persons without a history of CVA. Patients may have difficulty transferring information from one situation to another. For example, they may be able to remember the steps in lifting from the bed to the wheelchair but be unable to apply the same principles in moving from the wheelchair to an armchair. Confusion, restlessness, and irritability may arise from sensory deprivation. Emotional lability may also be a problem. To minimize the limitations imposed by these problems, the nurse may find the following actions helpful:

- Talk to the patient during routine activities.
- Briefly explain the basics of what has occurred, the procedures being performed, and the activities to expect.
- Speak distinctly but do not shout.
- Devise an easy means of communication, such as a picture chart to which one can point.
- minimize environmental confusion, noise, traffic, and clutter.
- Aim for consistency of those providing care and of care activities.
- Use objects familiar to patients (eg, their own clothing, clock, etc.).
- Keep a calendar or sign in the room showing the day and date.
- Supply sensory stimulation through conversation, radio, television, wall decorations, and objects for patients to handle.
- Provide frequent positive feedback; even a minor task may be a major achievement for the patient.
- Expect and accept errors and failures.

The reader is advised to consult general medical-surgical textbooks for more detailed guidance in the care of patients who have suffered a stroke. Local chapters of the American Heart Association also provide much useful material for the nurse, the patient, and the family on the topic of stroke.

Nurses should promote activities that reduce patients' risk of stroke. Managing hypertension is important in decreasing fatal and nonfatal strokes in the elderly. Likewise, smoking cessation is helpful. Elderly persons who stop smoking could improve cerebral perfusion levels, which is an important measure in preventing strokes.

> **KEY CONCEPT**
> Managing hypertension is important in reducing the risk of stroke in the elderly.

Display 29-3 provides a sample care plan for the patient who has experienced a stroke.

Nursing Interventions Related to Neurologic Problems

PROMOTING INDEPENDENCE

Older patients with neurologic problems face limitations imposed both by the disease and those resulting from the aging process. Skillful and creative nursing assistance can help patients achieve maximum levels of independence. Some self-help devices—rails in the hallways, grab bars in bathrooms, and numerous other household modifications—can extend the time that patients can live independently in the community. Periodic home visits by a nurse, regular contact with a family member or friend, and a daily call from a local telephone reassurance program can help the patient feel confident and protected, which promotes independence. Although these patients may perform tasks awkwardly and slowly, family members need to understand that allowing independent function is physically and psychologically more beneficial than doing tasks for them. Continuing patience, reassurance, and encouragement are essential to maximize patients' capacities for independence.

Personality changes often accompany neurologic problems. Patients may become depressed as they realize their limitations or become frustrated by their need to be dependent on others. Their reactions may be displaced and evidenced by irritability toward others, often their loved ones or immediate caregivers. Family members and caregivers may need help in understanding the reasons for this behavior and in learning effective ways of dealing with it. Getting offended or angry at such patients may only serve to anger or frustrate them further. Understanding, patience, and tolerance are needed.

>
> **KEY CONCEPT**
> Caregivers should be prepared for the personality changes experienced by many individuals who have neurologic disorders.

Sample Care Plan for the Patient Convalescing From a Cerebrovascular Accident

Nursing Diagnoses

Self-care deficits related to sensory or motor impairment, visual deficits, fatigue, aphasia

Activity intolerance related to depression, poor motivation, prolonged immobility, fatigue

Goal

The patient progressively increases independence in activities of daily living (ADL)

Actions

- Assess patient's independence-dependence in each of the ADL.
- Assess cognition and emotional status; repeat monthly or whenever there is a change in physical or mental status.
- Consult with physical therapist (PT) and develop plans for exercises, transfer techniques, and mobility aids.
- Consult with occupational therapist (OT) and develop plans for measures to improve independence in ADL and adaptive or assistive equipment.
- Ensure that patient properly uses mobility aids and adaptive or assistive equipment.
- Encourage patient to use existing capabilities and recognize efforts to be independent.
- Offer assistance with ADL as needed; ensure that caregivers provide adequate time for tasks to be performed by patient when possible.
- Monitor nutritional status, intake, and output.
- Review patient's progress regularly with multidisciplinary team, patient, and family.

Desired Outcomes

The patient

performs ADL with increasing levels of independence
engages in self-care activities without fatigue,
   shortness of breath, or
significant change in vital signs
is free from self-care deficits

Nursing Diagnosis

Impaired physical mobility related to altered sensory and motor function

Goals

The patient

is free from complications related to immobility
progressively increases independent mobility

Actions

- Determine active and passive range of motion of every joint; reassess at least monthly.
- Guide patient through range-of-motion exercises at least three times each day; provide assistance as needed.
- Use isometric, resistance, muscle-setting exercises if possible.
- Ensure that patient is properly positioned and maintained in proper alignment.
- Establish the amount of time patient can remain in one position before showing indications of pressure. To do this, check the patient's skin after he or she has been in the same position for half an hour; if no redness is noted, increase amount of time patient remains in position by half hour increments up to 2 hours. A repositioning schedule is developed based on the amount of time the patient has been assessed to be able to remain in a position without redness of tissues.
- Instruct patient to cough and deep breathe at least every 2 hours.
- Encourage adequate fluid intake and a high-fiber intake, unless contraindicated.
- Use massage, lotion, or protective padding as needed to protect skin integrity.
- Assist patient with proper use of mobility aids.
- Consult with PT regarding ways to increase mobility.
- Monitor progress and give feedback to patient.

(Continued)

D I S P L A Y   2 9 - 3   (C o n t i n u e d)

Desired Outcomes

The patient

> progressively increases independence
> is free from complications secondary to immobility
> uses mobility aids consistently and safely

Nursing Diagnoses

> *Ineffective role performance related to loss of body function, physical changes, role changes*
> *Interrupted family process related to changes in function, dependency on family for caregiving, ineffective coping*

Goals

The patient

> expresses acceptance of altered lifestyle and functions
> develops or maintains satisfying interactions with family

Actions

■ Interview patient and family to identify patient's previous interests, roles, and functions; assess patient's ability or readiness to resume activities.

■ Identify and implement measures to enable patient to engage in previous interests, roles, and functions with modifications.

■ Acknowledge patient's frustrations with altered capabilities; encourage expression of feelings.

■ Encourage patient to participate in family and social functions in community; assist patient and family in identifying measures and aids to facilitate activities.

■ Monitor patient's mood; intervene if problems are noted.

■ Confer with family regarding their feelings and needs; plan accordingly.

Desired Outcomes

The patient

> engages in satisfying activities with family and friends
> verbalizes positive attitude toward necessary lifestyle changes
> participates in activities and fulfills roles to maximum degree possible

PREVENTING INJURY

Protecting patients with a neurologic disorder from hazards is particularly important. Uncoordinated movements, weakness, and dizziness are among the problems that cause these patients to be at high risk for accidents. Whether in an institutional setting or the patient's own home, the environment should be scrutinized for potential sources of mishaps, such as loose carpeting, poorly lit stairwells, clutter, ill-functioning appliances, and the lack of fire warning systems, fire escapes, tub rails, nonslip tub surfaces, and other safeguards. Safety considerations also include the prevention of contractures, pressure ulcers, and other risks to health and well-being. It is an injustice to the patient to allow preventable complications to hamper progress and compound disability.

Critical Thinking Exercises

1. Outline the content of a health education program to instruct older adults on practices that could reduce their risks of neurologic problems.
2. Mr. J, aged 68, experienced a stroke 1 week ago that left him with right-sided weakness, aphasia, and incontinence. His wife is eager to have him discharged from the hospital and care for him at home. You have heard her state to Mr. J that he "needn't worry about a thing because she'll do everything that needs to be done and all he has to do is stay in bed and take it easy." Based on the information provided, what problems face Mr. and Mrs. J? Develop a care plan to address their needs.
3. What factors will worsen the symptoms of the patient with Parkinson's disease? What suggestions could you give caregivers to promote maximum function of this patient?
4. What resources exist in your community to assist patients with Parkinson's disease, stroke, or other neurologic disorders?

Web Connect

Keep abreast of the latest neuroscience news at the website for the National Institute of Neurological Disorders and Stroke at www.ninds.nih.gov/index.htm.

●Resources

American Heart Association Stroke Connection
7320 Greenville Avenue
Dallas, TX 75231
(800) 553-6321
www.strokeassociation.org

American Parkinson's Disease Association
1250 Hylan Boulevard
Suite 4B
Staten Island, NY 10305
(800) 223-2732
www.apdaparkinson.org

Epilepsy Foundation of America
4351 Garden City Drive
Landover, MD 20785
(301) 459-3700
www.efa.org

National Institute of Neurological Disorders and Stroke
9000 Rockville Pike
Building 31, Room BA16
Bethesda, MD 20892
(800) 352-9424
www.ninds.nih.gov

National Multiple Sclerosis Society
733 Third Avenue
New York, NY 10017
(800) 344-4861
www.nmss.org

National Parkinson Foundation
1501 Northwest 9th Avenue
Miami, FL 33136
(800) 327-4545
www.parkinson.org

National Stroke Association
8480 East Orchard Road
Suite 1000
Englewood, CO 80111
(800) STROKES
www.stroke.org

Paralyzed Veterans of America
801 18th Street
Washington, DC 20006
(800) 424-8200
www.pva.org

Parkinson's Disease Foundation
710 West 168th Street
New York, NY 10032
(800) 457-6676
www.parkinsons-foundation.org

United Parkinson Foundation
833 West Washington Boulevard
Chicago, IL 60607
(312) 733-1893
www.aoa.dhhs.gov/aoa/dir/221.html

● References

Aebischer, P., & Pralog, W. (2003). Gene therapy approaches for Parkinson's disease. *Journal of Neurochemistry, 85*(6 Suppl 2), 8.

Libster, M. (2002). *Delmar's integrative herb guide for nurses* (p. 590). Albany, NY: Delmar.

Stodghill, R. (1997, March 24). A jolt of relief from Parkinson's disease. *Business Week,* p. 34.

● Recommended Readings

Birkett, P. D. (1996). *The psychiatry of stroke.* Washington, DC: American Psychiatric Press.

Boysen, G. (2001). Prevention of recurrent stroke in the elderly. *Annals of Long-Term Care, 9*(9), 21–26.

Bruno, A. (Ed.). (1996). *Stroke in the elderly.* New York: Springer.

Easton, K. L. (1999). The poststroke journey: From agonizing to owning. *Geriatric Nursing, 20*(2), 72–75.

Goldsmith, C. (1999). Clinical snapshot: Parkinson's disease. *American Journal of Nursing, 99*(2), 46–47.

Hilton, E. L. (2002). The meaning of stroke in elderly women: A phenomenological investigation. *Journal of Gerontological Nursing, 28*(7), 19–26.

Kalra, L. (2001). Approaches to organization of stroke care: A review. *Clinical Geriatrics, 9*(13), 33–42.

Kayser-Jones, J., & Pengilly, K. (1999). Dysphagia among nursing home residents. *Geriatric Nursing, 20*(2), 75–79.

Miller, J. L. (2002). Parkinson's disease primer. *Geriatric Nursing, 23*(1), 69–73.

Miller, R. M., & Woo, D. (1999). Stroke: Current concepts of care. *Geriatric Nursing, 20*(2), 68–72.

O'Hanlon-Nichols, T. (1999). Neurological assessment. *American Journal of Nursing, 99*(6), 44–55.

Shastry, B. S. (2002). Therapeutic options for Parkinson's disease. *Drugs Today, 38*(6), 445–451.

Tinter, R., & Jankovic, J. (2001). Assessment and treatment of Parkinson's disease in the elderly. *Clinical Geriatrics, 9*(1), 62–74.

Wang, E., & Snyder, D. S. (1998). *Handbook of the aging brain.* San Diego, CA: Academic Press.

Williams, M. E. (1995). *The American Geriatrics Society's complete guide to aging and health* (pp. 159–186). New York: Harmony Books.

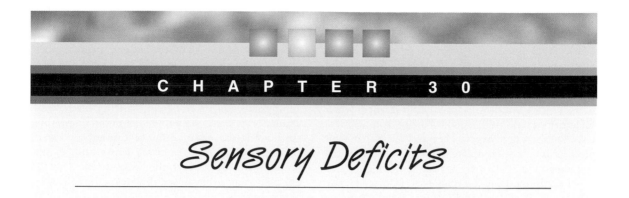

CHAPTER 30

Sensory Deficits

■ *Learning Objectives*

After reading this chapter, you should be able to:

- describe the importance of good sensory function and the impact of sensory deficits
- list measures to promote healthy sensory function
- identify signs of and nursing interventions for cataracts, glaucoma, macular degeneration, detached retina, corneal ulcers, and hearing impairment

Importance of Good Sensory Function

Good sensory function is an extremely valuable asset that often is taken for granted. For instance, people are better able to protect themselves from harm when they can see, hear, smell, touch, and express danger. The reduced ability to protect oneself from hazards because of sensory deficits can result in serious falls from unseen obstacles, missed alarms and warnings, ingestion of hazardous substances from not recognizing their taste, an inability to detect the odor of smoke or gas, and burns and skin breakdown because of decreased cutaneous sensation of excessive temperature and pressure.

Intact senses also facilitate accurate perception of the environment. The environment is perceived with distortion when sensory function is impaired (eg, people might suspect they are being talked about if they are unable to hear the conversation of those around them). Impaired sensory function affects everyday experiences. For example, reading the newspaper and recognizing a familiar face on the street can be hampered by poor eyesight. Food tastes bland without properly functioning taste buds. Freshly cut flowers lose their fragrances when olfactory functioning is poor. Finally, communication, the sharing of experiences, and the exchange of feelings are more complete when all the senses can participate.

Alterations during the aging process, excessive use and abuse of certain medications, and the disease processes that affect all age groups contribute to the sensory problems of elders. Sensory deficits compound the other problems that threaten the health and well-being of older persons—their increased vulnerability to accidents, their social isolation and declining physical function, and many other limitations regarding self-care activities. Because it is the rare older individual who does not suffer from some sensory deficit, it behooves the nurse working with the aged to be skilled in assessing sensory function (Display 30-1), ensure that sensory problems are properly evaluated, and implement associated assistive techniques. Nursing Diagnosis Table 30-1 lists some of the nursing diagnoses associated with sensory deficits.

✔ **Point to Ponder**

How would being blind or deaf affect your daily life? What reactions do you think you would experience?

Facilitating Optimal Sensory Function

VISION

Despite age-related changes, the majority of older persons have sufficient visual capacity to meet normal self-care demands with the assistance of corrective lenses. Serious visual problems can develop, however, and should be recognized early to prevent significant visual damage. Routine eye examinations by an ophthalmologist are important in detecting and treating eye problems early in elders. Frequently, people postpone eye examinations because their present corrective lenses are still functional, the need is not apparent, or they have limited finances. The gerontological nurse can be instrumental in ensuring appropriate visual care by emphasizing that eye examinations are necessary to detect problems, despite apparent need. It is important to inform people that, although an optician prepares lenses and an optometrist fits the lenses to the visual deficit, only the ophthalmologist diagnoses and treats the full range of eye diseases.

In addition to annual eye examinations, prompt evaluation is required for any symptom that could indicate a visual problem, including burning or pain in the eye, blurred or double vision, redness of the conjunctiva, spots, headaches, and any other change in vision. The diet should be reviewed to ensure an adequate intake of nutrients that promote good vision (Display 30-2). A variety of disorders can threaten the elder's vision. For instance, arteriosclerosis and diabetes can cause damage to the retina, and nutritional deficiencies and hypertension can result in visual impairment. The reader can refer to the sections of this book that describe these diseases to understand the pathophysiology involved.

HEARING

Gerontological nurses have a responsibility to help aging persons protect and preserve their hearing as well. Some hearing deficits in old age can be avoided by good care of the ears throughout life. Such care should include:

- prompt and complete treatment of ear infections
- prevention of trauma to the ear (eg, from a severe blow or a foreign object in the ear)
- removal of cerumen or particles by irrigating the external auditory canal rather than by using cotton-tipped applicators, hairpins, and similar devices (avoid using a forceful stream of solution during this procedure because it can cause perforation of the eardrum)
- protection from exposure to loud noises, such as those associated with factory and construction work, vehicles, loud music, and explosions (earplugs or other sound-reducing devices should be used when exposure is unavoidable)
- regular audiometric examinations

Assessment of Sensory Function

General Observations

During interactions with the patient, signs of hearing deficits can be noted such as missed communication, requests to have words repeated, reliance on lip reading, and cocking of the head to one side in an effort to hear better. Eye problems can be identified by noticing if the patient uses eyeglasses, demonstrates difficulty seeing (eg, bumping into objects, unable to see small print), or possesses eye abnormalities such as drooping eyelids, discolored sclera, excess tearing, discharge, and unusual movements of the eyes. Foul odors (eg, associated with incontinence or vaginitis) that do not seem to bother the patient could reflect diminished olfactory function; cigarette burns on finger or unrecognized pressure ulcers may indicate that the patient has reduced ability to sense pressure and pain.

Interview

The patient should be asked about the date and type of the last ophthalmic and audiometric examinations (eg., Where was the examination done? Was an ophthalmologist or optometrist seen? Did the eye examination include tonometry? Was a full audiometric evaluation or basic hearing screening done?). If eyeglasses or hearing aids are used, questions should be asked about where, when, and how these appliances were obtained (eg, reading glasses purchased from the local pharmacy versus prescription glasses; hearing aid obtained via television advertisement). Questions can be asked to disclose the presence of sensory problems, such as the following:

"Has there been any change in your vision? Please describe."

"Are your glasses as useful to you as they were when you first obtained them?"

"Do you experience pain, burning, or itching in the eyes?"

"Do you ever see spots floating across your eyes? How often does this happen and how large and numerous are the spots?"

"Do you ever see flashes of light or halos?"

"Are your eyes ever unusually dry or watery?"

"Do you have difficulty with vision at night, in dimly lit areas, or in bright areas?"

"Does anyone in your family have glaucoma or other eye problems?"

"Have you noticed any change in your ability to hear? Please describe."

"Are certain sounds more difficult for you to hear than others?"

"Do you ever experience pain, itching, ringing, or a sense of fullness in your ears?"

"Do your ears accumulate a lot of wax? How do you manage this?"

"Is there ever drainage from your ears?"

"Is your sense of smell as keen as it was in earlier years? Describe any differences."

"Do you have any problems or have you noticed changes in your ability to feel pain, pressure, or different temperatures?"

Physical Examination

Inspect the eyes for unusual structure, drooping eyelids, discoloration, and abnormal movement. Loss of elasticity around the eyes, indicated by bags, is a common finding. Black-skinned persons may normally have a slight yellow discoloration of the sclera. Palpation of the eyeballs with the eyelids closed can reveal hard-feeling eyes with extremely elevated intraocular pressure and spongy-feeling eyes with fluid volume deficits. Lesions on the lids should be noted.

A gross evaluation of visual acuity can be done by having the patient read a Snellen chart or various-sized lettering on a newspaper. If the patient is unable to see letters on the chart or newspaper, an estimation of the extent of the visual limitation can be obtained by determining if the patient is able to see fingers held up before him or can merely make out figures.

(Continued)

DISPLAY 30-1 (Continued)

If the patient has restrictions in seeing all portions of the visual field, the exact nature of this problem should be reviewed. A blind spot in the visual field (ie, scotoma) can occur with macular degeneration, a narrowing of the peripheral field may be associated with glaucoma, and blindness in the same half of both eyes (ie, homonymous hemianopia) can be present in persons who have experienced a cerebrovascular accident.

Extraocular movements are tested by having the patient follow the nurse's finger as it is moved to various points, horizontally and vertically. Irregular, jerking movements can result from disturbances in cranial nerves III, IV, or VI.

Inspection of the ears usually shows cerumen accumulation, increased hair growth, and atrophy of the tympanic membrane, which causes it to appear white or gray. Cerumen impactions should be noted and removed. A small, crusted, ulcerated lesion on the pinna can be a sign of basal or squamous cell carcinoma.

A gross evaluation of hearing can be made by determining the patient's ability to hear a watch ticking. Both ears should be checked. In addition to presbycusis and conductive hearing losses, ear or upper respiratory infections, ototoxic drugs, and diabetes can be responsible for diminishing hearing.

Nursing Diagnosis

ND **TABLE 30-1** ● *Nursing Diagnoses Associated with Sensory Deficits*

Causes or Contributing Factors	Nursing Diagnosis
Sensory deprivation or overload, impaired communication	Activity Intolerance
Impaired communication, altered self-concept, reduced ability to protect self	Anxiety
Acute glaucoma, corneal ulcer, detached retina	Acute Pain
Hearing deficit	Impaired Verbal Communication
Impaired vision or hearing	Diversional Activity Deficit
Visual deficits, inability to protect self	Impaired Home Maintenance
Reduced tactile sensations	Risk for Infection
Inability to see, hear, smell, or feel hazards	Risk for Injury
Inability to protect self, care for self, communicate	Powerlessness
Visual disorders	Self-Care Deficit
Dependency, impaired interactions, altered self-concept	Disturbed Body Image
Impairment of any of the sensory organs	Sensory-Perceptual Alterations
Reduced tactile sensations	Impaired Skin Integrity
Misperception of environment	Disturbed Sleep Pattern
Visual or hearing deficits	Impaired Social Interaction
Visual or hearing deficits, frustration of patient or others in attempting to communicate	Social Isolation
Misperceptions or sensory deprivation due to altered sensory function	Disturbed Thought Processes

D I S P L A Y   3 0 - 2

Nutrients Beneficial to Vision

Nutrient	Benefit to Vision
Zinc	Promotes normal visual capacity and adaptation to dark; supplementation can reduce visual loss in macular degeneration; deficiency can facilitate cataract development
Selenium	May aid in preventing cataracts; supplementation with vitamin E can reduce visual loss in macular degeneration
Vitamin C	Promotes normal vision; supplementation may improve vision in persons with cataracts
Vitamin A	Maintains healthy rods and cones in retina
Vitamin E	May aid in preventing cataracts; supplementation in large doses can prevent macular degeneration
Riboflavin	Aids in preventing cataracts
Ginkgo biloba	May prevent degenerative changes in eye
Flavonoid	Improves night vision and adaptation to dark; promotes visual acuity; improves capillary integrity to reduce hemorrhage risk in diabetic retinopathy

Visual Deficits and Related Nursing Interventions

CATARACTS

A *cataract* is a clouding of the lens or its capsule that causes the lens to lose its transparency. Cataracts are common in older people because everyone develops some degree of lens opacity as they age. Exposure to ultraviolet B increases the risk of developing cataracts, emphasizing the importance of wearing proper sunglasses to protect the eyes. Most elders do have some degree of lens opacity with or without the presence of other eye disorders.

KEY CONCEPT
Everyone develops some degree of lens opacity with age, although it is more severe in persons who have high exposure to sunlight.

No discomfort or pain is associated with cataracts. At first, visual acuity is not affected, but as opacification continues, vision is distorted, night vision is decreased, and objects appear blurred. People may have trouble seeing street signs while driving and feel that there is a film over the eye. Eventually, lens opacity and vision loss are complete. Glare from sunlight and bright lights is extremely bothersome to the affected person; this is due to the cloudy lens causing light to scatter more than it would in a clear lens. Nuclear sclerosis develops, causing the lens of the eye to become yellow or yellow-brown; eventually the color of the pupil changes from black to a cloudy white. Some individuals may report an improvement in the ability to see small print and objects ("second sight"), which is due to changes in the lens that increase nearsightedness.

Surgery to remove the lens is the only cure for a cataract. Cataracts affect people differently; therefore, the need for surgery needs to be assessed based on an individual's unique situation. Patients with a single cataract may not necessarily undergo surgery if vision in the other eye is good, and these individuals should concentrate on strengthening their existing visual capacity, reducing their limitations, and using the safety measures applicable to any visually impaired person (Fig. 30-1). Sunglasses, sheer curtains over windows, furniture placed away from bright light, and several soft lights instead of a single bright

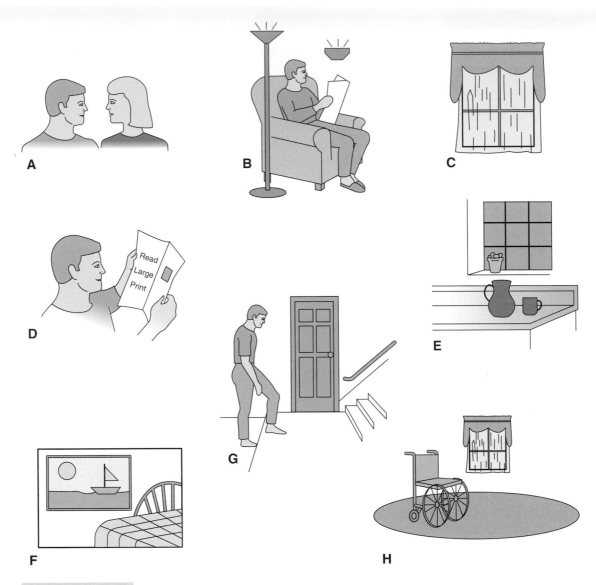

FIGURE 30-1

Compensating for visual deficits in the aged. (**A**) Face the person when speaking. (**B**) Use several soft indirect lights instead of a single glaring one. (**C**) Avoid glare from windows by using sheer curtains or stained windows. (**D**) Use large-print reading material. (**E**) Have frequently used items within the visual field. (**F**) Avoid the use of low-tone colors and attempt to use bright ones. (**G**) Use contrasting colors on doorways and stairs and for changes in levels. (**H**) Identify personal belongings and differentiate the room and wheelchair with a unique design rather than by letters or numbers.

light source minimize annoyance from glare. It is beneficial to place items within the visual field of the unaffected eye, a consideration when preparing a food tray and arranging furniture and frequently used objects. Regular evaluations of the patient by an ophthalmologist are essential to detect changes or a new problem in the unaffected eye.

Cataract Surgery

For most patients, surgery improves vision. Cataract surgery is an outpatient procedure and elders withstand it well. Gerontological nurses are in a position to reassure older patients and their families that age is no deterrent to cataract surgery. Patients typically can resume nonstrenuous activities within a day. The simple surgical procedure and several weeks of rehabilitation can result in years of improved vision and, consequently, a life of higher quality. Two types of surgical procedures are used for removing the lens. Intracapsular extraction is the surgical procedure of choice for the aged patient with cataracts and consists of removing the lens and the capsule. Extracapsular extraction is a simple surgical procedure in which the lens is removed and the posterior capsule is left in place. A common problem with this type of surgery is that a secondary membrane may form, requiring an additional procedure for discission of the membrane.

The most common method of replacing the surgically removed lens is the insertion of an intraocular lens at the time of cataract surgery. For older patients, this method has been more successful than adjusting to a contact lens or special cataract glasses. The intraocular lens tends to distort vision less than cataract glasses do and does not require the care of a contact lens. Some patients do develop complications with a lens implant, such as eye infection, loss of vitreous humor, and slipping of the implant.

GLAUCOMA

Glaucoma is a degenerative eye disease in which the optic nerve is damaged from an above-normal intraocular pressure (IOP). It ranks after cataracts as a major eye problem in the aged and is the major cause of blindness in this population, accounting for 10% of all blindness in the United States. Glaucoma tends to occur in people over age 40 and increases in prevalence with age. Black individuals tend to develop glaucoma at earlier ages than whites, and women have a higher incidence than men. Although the exact cause is unknown, glaucoma can be associated with increased size of the lens, iritis, allergy, endocrine imbalance, emotional instability, and a family history of this disorder. Drugs with anticholinergic properties can exacerbate glaucoma due to their effects of dilating the pupil. An increase in IOP occurs rapidly in acute glaucoma and gradually in chronic glaucoma.

Acute Glaucoma

With acute, or closed-angle, glaucoma, the patient experiences severe eye pain, headache, nausea, and vomiting. In addition to the rapid increased tension within the eyeball, edema of the ciliary body and dilation of the pupil occur. Vision becomes blurred, and blindness will result if this problem is not corrected within a day. Diagnosis is confirmed by placing a tonometer on the anesthetized cornea to measure IOP (Fig. 30-2). The normal pressure is within 20 mm Hg. A reading between 20 to 25 mm Hg is considered potential glaucoma. Another diagnostic test (ie, gonioscopy) uses a contact lens and a binocular microscope to allow direct examination of the anterior chamber and differentiate closed-angle from open-angle glaucoma. In the past, if IOP did not decline within 24 hours, surgical intervention would be necessary. However, medications are now effective in treating the acute attack (eg, carbonic anhydrase inhibitors, which reduce the formation of aqueous solution; mannitol, urea, or glycerin, which reduce fluid because of their ability to increase osmotic tension in the circulating blood). An iridectomy may be performed after the acute attack to prevent future episodes of acute glaucoma.

Chronic Glaucoma

Chronic, or open-angle, glaucoma is more common than acute glaucoma. It often occurs so gradually that affected individuals are unaware that they have a visual problem. Peripheral vision becomes slowly but increasingly impaired so that people may not realize for a long time why they bump or knock over items at their side. They may need to change eyeglasses frequently. As the impairment progresses, central vision is affected. People may complain of a tired feeling in their eyes, headaches, misty vision, or seeing halos

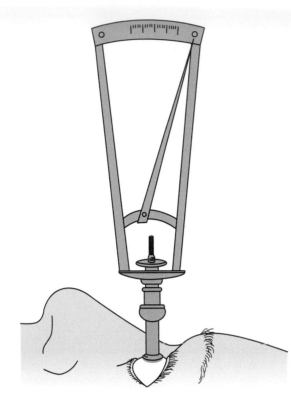

FIGURE 30-2

Measuring intraocular pressure by use of a tonometer.

around lights—symptoms that tend to be more pronounced in the morning. The cornea may have a cloudy appearance, and the iris may be fixed and dilated. Although this condition usually involves one eye, both eyes can become affected if treatment is not sought. The same procedures as mentioned with acute glaucoma are used to diagnose this problem. Treatment, aimed toward reducing the IOP, may consist of a combination of a miotic and a carbonic anhydrous inhibitor or of surgery to establish a channel to filter the aqueous fluid (eg, iridectomy, iridencleisis, cyclodialysis, corneoscleral trephining).

> **KEY CONCEPT**
> Open-angle glaucoma, the most common form, can be asymptomatic until an advanced stage; therefore, glaucoma screening is important.

Care and Prevention of Complications

Vision lost due to glaucoma cannot be restored. However, additional damage can be prevented by avoiding any situation or activity that increases IOP. Physical straining and emotional stress should be prevented. Miotics may be instilled into the eye; acetazolamide may be used. Because many individuals have difficulty getting all of the eye drops into the eye, an administration technique called tear duct occlusion (Display 30-3) is recommended. This technique can increase the amount of medication the eye absorbs by 50% (Johns Hopkins Medical Institutions, 2000). Mydriatics, stimulants, and agents that elevate the blood pressure must not be administered. It may benefit patients to carry a card or wear a bracelet indicating their problem to prevent administration of these medications in situations in which they may be unconscious or otherwise unable to communicate. Abuse and overuse of the eyes must also be prevented. Periodic evaluation by an ophthalmologist is an essential part of the continued care of the patient with glaucoma. Display 30-4 presents a sample care plan for the patient with open-angle glaucoma.

Patient compliance with treatment for glaucoma can be challenging. The silent nature of this condition, difficulties with instilling eyedrops, and the cost of medications contribute to a lack of adherence to the plan of care. Nurses need to teach patients about the disease and its care and counsel them about the importance of compliance. The care plan for these patients needs to include ongoing reinforcement of self-care measures for disease management.

MACULAR DEGENERATION

Macular degeneration involves damage or breakdown of the macula, which results in a loss of central vision. The most common form is involutional macular degeneration, which is associated with the aging process, although macular degeneration can also result from injury, infection, or exudative macular degeneration. Routine ophthalmic examinations can identify macular degeneration, again emphasizing the importance of annual eye examinations.

> **KEY CONCEPT**
> A loss of central vision accompanies macular degeneration.

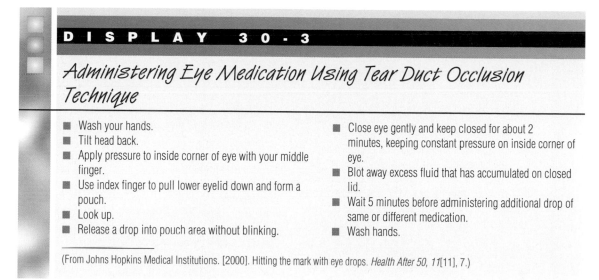

DISPLAY 30-3

Administering Eye Medication Using Tear Duct Occlusion Technique

- Wash your hands.
- Tilt head back.
- Apply pressure to inside corner of eye with your middle finger.
- Use index finger to pull lower eyelid down and form a pouch.
- Look up.
- Release a drop into pouch area without blinking.

- Close eye gently and keep closed for about 2 minutes, keeping constant pressure on inside corner of eye.
- Blot away excess fluid that has accumulated on closed lid.
- Wait 5 minutes before administering additional drop of same or different medication.
- Wash hands.

(From Johns Hopkins Medical Institutions. [2000]. Hitting the mark with eye drops. *Health After 50, 11*[11], 7.)

Laser therapy has been used for the treatment of some forms of macular degeneration, but the involutional type does not respond well to this procedure. Magnifying glasses, high-intensity reading lamps, and other aids can prove helpful to patients with this condition.

DETACHED RETINA

Older persons may experience detachment of the retina, a forward displacement of the retina from its normal position against the choroid. The symptoms, which can be gradual or sudden, include the perception of spots moving across the eye, blurred vision, flashes of light, and the feeling that a coating is developing over the eye. Blank areas of vision progress to complete loss of vision. The severity of the symptoms depends on the degree of retinal detachment. Prompt treatment is required to prevent continued damage and eventual blindness. There does not tend to be pain. Initial measures most likely to be prescribed, bed rest and the use of bilateral eye patches, can be frightening to the older patient, who may react with confusion and unusual behavior. The patient should be made to feel as secure as possible; frequent checks and communication, easy access to a call light or other means of assistance, and full, honest explanations will help provide a sense of well-being. After

time has been allowed for the maximum amount of "reattachment" of the retina to occur, surgery may be planned. Several surgical techniques are used in the treatment of detached retinas. Electrodiathermy and cryosurgery cause the retina to adhere to its original attachment; scleral buckling and photocoagulation decrease the size of the vitreous space. Eye patches remain on the patient for several days after surgery. Specific routines vary according to the type of surgery performed. The patient needs frequent verbal stimuli to minimize anxiety and enhance psychological comfort. Physical and emotional stress must be avoided. Approximately 2 weeks after surgery, the success of the operation can be evaluated. A minority of patients must undergo a second procedure. It is important for the patient to understand that periodic examination is important, especially because some patients later suffer a detached retina in the other eye.

CORNEAL ULCER

Inflammation of the cornea, accompanied by a loss of substance, causes the development of a corneal ulcer. Febrile states, irritation, dietary deficiencies, lowered resistance, and cerebrovascular accident tend to predispose the individual to this problem. Corneal ulcers, which are extremely difficult to treat in older persons, may scar or perforate, leading to destruction

D I S P L A Y   3 0 · 4

The Patient With Open-Angle Glaucoma

Mr. Clark is a 76-year-old black man who has been diagnosed with open-angle glaucoma during his opthalmologic examination today. He was discovered to have a significant reduction in peripheral vision bilaterally. On questioning Mr. Clark, the nurse learns that although he denies noticing any change in vision, he did describe that his eyes occasionally felt tired and "aching," and that he did see halos around light; he did admit to having "a lot of headaches."

The medical record indicates that Mr. Clark has a history of hypertension and arthritis that significantly limits the mobility of his fingers. His hypertension is controlled without the use of any medication; he uses ibuprofen for his arthritic pain. In reviewing his medication schedule the nurse discovers that Mr. Clark uses an albuteral inhaler for bronchial asthma; he states that he "forgot to tell the eye doctor about this." He contributes that he "gets colds often," which he cures himself "with over-the-counter cold remedies." Also, he claims to have problems with bowel elimination, passing stool every 3 to 4 days with considerable straining and effort.

Mr. Clark lives alone in a basement apartment. He has no family in the state, but enjoys a close relationship with a young couple who live in the same building. Mr. Clark is concerned that he will go blind and will be unable to care for himself.

The ophthalmologist has ordered pilocarpine hydrochloride eye drops and a return visit for 3 months from today.

In reviewing Mr. Clark's history the nurse develops the following care plan:

Nursing Diagnosis

Deficient knowledge related to management of disease

Goals

The patient

learns facts about glaucoma and related care
administers eye drops correctly

Actions

■ Assess patient's knowledge about disease in relation to:
what it is
care required
symptoms to note and report
precautions
■ Clarify misunderstandings and provide instruction as necessary.
■ Ensure that the patient understands importance of regular administration of eye drops.
■ Evaluate patient's ability to manipulate dropper and instill drops (particularly in light of arthritic hands). Instruct as necessary. If patient is unable to independently use dropper and instill drops, determine ability of neighbor to assist and provide instruction to neighbor.
■ Instruct patient to discuss asthma condition with physician as pilocarpine hydrochloride should be used with caution in persons with asthma. Reinforce importance of patient sharing complete medical history with every health care provider with whom he has contact. (Follow up to ensure that the patient remembers to discuss this condition with physician and reinforce any advice given.)
■ Prepare patient for side effects from pilocarpine hydrochloride, such as blurring of vision for 1 to 2 hours after administration; review related safety considerations.
■ Teach patient to avoid situations that can increase intraocular pressure, such as aggressive coughing, sneezing, and straining during defecation.
■ Advise patient to avoid self-medication for treatment of colds because cold remedies can contain mydriatic agents that can increase intraocular pressure.
■ Discuss chronic nature of glaucoma and need for lifetime administration of medications and attention to precautions and recognition of symptoms that should be reported. Reinforce that although lost vision cannot be restored, additional loss usually can be avoided with control of the disease.

(Continued)

DISPLAY 30-4 (Continued)

Desired Outcomes

The patient

accurately describes nature of disease, symptoms, precautions, and related care

demonstrates ability to instill eye drops or has reliable arrangement for caregiver to administer them

Nursing Diagnosis

Risk for injury related to impaired vision and risks associated with glaucoma

Goals

The patient

is free from injury related to impaired vision

uses preventive measures to avoid complications associated with glaucoma

Actions

- Explain impact of reduced peripheral vision and related safety precautions, such as placing frequently used objects in visual field, keeping clutter off floor, turning head to fully see objects to the side, avoiding driving.
- Instruct patient to avoid situations that could damage vision by increasing intraocular pressure, such as aggressive coughing, sneezing, straining to have a bowel movement, strenuous exercise, emotional stress.
- Encourage patient to keep bathroom and hallways well lit because vision may be impaired at night or in dimly lit areas as a result of pilocarpine hydrochloride use.
- Advise patient to avoid activities for several hours following administration of eye drops to accommodate blurred vision that could occur during this time.
- Assist patient in obtaining medical identification bracelet to assure others are informed of his condition in the event he is unable to communicate.

Desired Outcomes

The patient

is free from injury related to glaucoma

is free from complications related to glaucoma

Nursing Diagnosis

Anxiety and fear related to loss of vision

Goals

The patient

lives a satisfying lifestyle with effective management of disease

is free from anxiety and fear

Actions

- Encourage patient to express feelings regarding loss of vision and impact on function. Listen and offer support.
- Clarify misconceptions; offer realistic explanations.
- Determine activities that are important to patient and those that are at risk of being threatened by condition. Develop strategies to preserve and promote these activities.
- Assist patient in locating resources that can promote function, independence, and enjoyment. Contact local offices of agencies for the visually impaired for assistance.

Desired Outcomes

The patient

expresses satisfaction with lifestyle

functions in apartment independently or with partial assistance

is free from anxiety and fear

Nursing Diagnosis

Constipation

Goal

The patient

eliminates feces without straining at least every 2 to 3 days

Actions

- Assess bowel elimination pattern; if no problem exists, reinforce current practices; if constipation is a problem, initiate measures to promote regular bowel elimination, such as increasing fiber in diet, establishing regular time for bowel elimination, using stool softener.

Desired Outcome

The patient

has a bowel movement without straining at least once every 2 to 3 days

of the cornea and blindness. The affected eye may appear bloodshot and show increased lacrimation. Pain and photophobia are also present. Nurses should advise patients to seek prompt assistance for any irritation, suspected infection, or other difficulty with the cornea as soon as it is identified. Early care is often effective in preventing the development of a corneal ulcer and preserving visual capacity. Cycloplegics, sedatives, antibiotics, and heat may be prescribed to treat a corneal ulcer. Sunglasses will ease the discomfort associated with photophobia. It is important that the underlying cause be treated—an infection, abrasion, or presence of a foreign body. Corneal transplants are occasionally done for more advanced corneal ulcers.

Hearing Deficits and Related Nursing Interventions

CAUSES OF HEARING DEFICITS

A significant number of older people, including a majority of those residing in nursing homes, have some degree of hearing loss, resulting from a variety of factors other than aging. Exposure to noise from jets, traffic, heavy machinery, and guns cause cell injury and loss. The higher incidence of hearing loss in men may be associated with their more frequent employment in occupations that subject them to loud noises (eg, truck driving, construction work, and heavy factory work). Recurrent otitis media and trauma can damage hearing. Certain drugs may be ototoxic, including aspirin, bumetanide, ethacrynic acid, furosemide, indomethacin, erythromycin, streptomycin, neomycin, karomycin, and Rauwolfia derivatives; the delayed excretion of these drugs in many older persons may promote this effect. Diabetes, tumors of the nasopharynx, hypothyroidism, syphilis, other disease processes, and psychogenic factors can also contribute to hearing impairment.

Particular problems affect the ears of the older person (Fig. 30-3). Vascular problems, viral infections, and presbycusis are often causes of inner ear damage. In otosclerosis, an osseous growth causes fixation of the foot plate of the stapes in the oval window of the cochlea. This may be a middle ear problem; it is more common among women and can progress to complete deafness. Infections of the middle ear are less common in older individuals; they usually accompany more serious disorders, such as tumors and diabetes. The external ear can be affected by dermatoses, furunculosis, cerumen impaction, cysts, and neoplasms. **(Visit the Connection website to learn how to correct cerumen impaction.)**

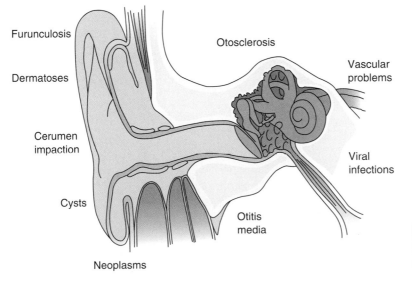

FIGURE 30-3

Problems affecting the ears of older adults.

PATIENT CARE

The first action in caring for someone with a hearing deficit should be to encourage audiometric examination. Hearing impairment should not be assumed to be a normal consequence of aging and ignored. It would be most sad and negligent if the cause of the hearing problem were easily correctable (eg, removal of cerumen or a cyst) but allowed to limit the life of the affected individual. Advise elders against purchasing a hearing aid without a complete audiometric evaluation. Many older persons invest money for a hearing aid from their limited budget to discover that their particular hearing deficit cannot be improved by this means.

> **KEY CONCEPT**
> Patients should be advised to avoid purchasing a hearing aid without a complete audiometric examination.

Sometimes the underlying cause of the hearing problem can be corrected. Frequently, however, elders must learn to live with varying degrees of hearing deficits. Helping older adults live with such deficits is a challenge in gerontological care. It is not unusual for individuals with a hearing impairment to demonstrate emotional reactions to their hearing deficits. Unable to hear conversation, patients may become suspicious of those around them and accuse people of talking about them. Anger, impatience, and frustration can result from repeatedly unsuccessful attempts to understand conversation. Patients may feel confused or react inappropriately on receiving distorted verbal communications. Being limited in the ability to hear danger and protect themselves, may make them feel insecure. Being self-conscious of their limitation, may make them avoid social contact to escape embarrassment and frustration. Social isolation can be a serious threat, because people sometimes avoid an older person with a hearing deficit because of the difficulty in communication. Even telephone contact may be threatened. Approximately 10% of elders have difficulty hearing telephone conversations. Physical, emotional, and social health can be seriously affected by this deficit.

A neighbor should be alerted to the individual's hearing problem so that he or she can be protected in an emergency. In an institutional setting, such patients should be located near the nurse's station. People with hearing loss should be advised to request explanations and instructions in writing so that they receive the full content.

Those working with elders can minimize the limitations caused by hearing deficits. When talking with individuals with high-frequency hearing loss, the speaker should talk slowly, distinctly, and in a low-frequency voice. Raising the voice or shouting will only raise the sounds to a higher frequency and compound the deficit. Methods for promoting more accurate and complete communication include talking into the less impaired ear, facing the individual when talking, using visual speech (eg, sign language, gestures, and facial expressions), allowing the person to lip read, using a stethoscope to amplify sounds (speaking into the diaphragm while the earpieces are in the patient's ears), and using flash cards, work lists, and similar aids and devices.

HEARING AIDS

The otologist can determine whether a hearing aid would be valuable for the given individual and recommend the particular aid best suited to the patient's needs. The nurse is in a key position to educate the older individual on the importance of consulting an otologist before purchasing a hearing aid (Fig. 30-4). Patients must understand that, even with a hearing aid, their problems will not be solved. Although hearing will improve, it will not return to normal. Speech may sound distorted through the aid because when speech is amplified, so are all environmental noises, which can be most uncomfortable and disturbing to the individual. Sounds may be particularly annoying in areas where reverberation can easily occur (eg, a church or large hall). Some persons never make the adjustment to a hearing aid and choose not to wear the appliance rather than to tolerate these disturbances and distortions. **(Visit the Connection website to learn about living with a hearing aid.)**

Local chapters of hearing and speech associations and organizations serving the deaf can provide assistance and educational materials to those affected by and interested in hearing problems.

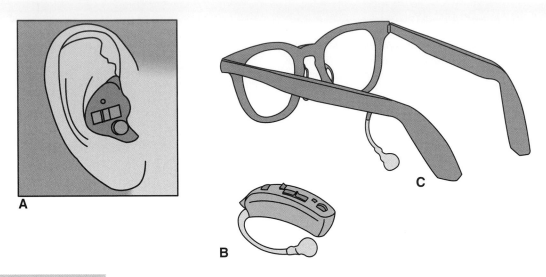

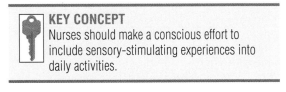

FIGURE 30-4

Types of hearing aids. (**A**) In-the-ear model. (**B**) Behind-the-ear model. (**C**) Eyeglass model.

Other Sensory Deficits and Related Nursing Interventions

Sight and hearing are not the only senses affected by the aging process; other sensations are also reduced with age. The number of functioning taste buds may be significantly decreased, especially those responsible for sweet and salty flavors. Pain and pressure are not sensed as easily in late life. Age-related effects on tactile sensation may also be noted by the difficulty some older persons have in discriminating between temperatures. Some loss of olfactory function may be noted as well.

To compensate for the multiple sensory deficits older persons may experience, special attention must be paid to stimulation of all the senses during routine daily activities. The diet can be planned to include a variety of flavors and colors. Perfumes, fresh flowers, and scented candles, safely used, can provide interesting fragrances. In an institutional setting, having a pot brewing fresh coffee in the patients' area can provide a pleasant and familiar aroma during the early morning hours; likewise, a tabletop oven can allow for cookie baking and other cooking activities in the patients' area, providing a variety of stimuli. Different textures can be used in upholstery and clothing

fabrics. Clocks that chime, music boxes, and wind chimes can vary environmental sounds. The design of facilities for the elderly should take into consideration the use of different shapes and colors. Intellectual stimulation, through conversation, music, and books, for instance, is also vital.

> **KEY CONCEPT**
> Nurses should make a conscious effort to include sensory-stimulating experiences into daily activities.

Touch is not only a means of sensory stimulation but also an expression of warmth and caring. Too frequently, the nurse may touch the patient only during specified procedures. It is easy for patients to begin to feel that others perceive them only in terms of tasks rather than as total human beings. How often are patients referred to as "a complete bath," "a dressing change," or "a feed?" How often are these labels nonverbally communicated when the nurse's only encounters with the patient are for the sake of these activities? Holding a hand, rubbing a cheek, and patting a shoulder, basic as they may seem, can convey a message to patients that they are still valued as unique human beings. Acceptance of the patient's efforts to touch is also important. The universal language of touch can often communicate a friendship, warmth, and caring that overcomes the most severe sensory deficit.

> **KEY CONCEPT**
> Patients need to be touched at times other than when treatments are administered.

Critical Thinking Exercises

1. What can be done to prevent vision and hearing losses with aging?
2. Why are older adults unaware of the signs of glaucoma?
3. Outline a teaching plan for a patient with newly diagnosed glaucoma.
4. Outline modifications to the average home that could benefit a person with impaired vision.
5. List assistive devices to promote the independent function of persons with impaired vision or hearing.
6. Locate resources in your community to assist persons with visual and hearing impairments.

Web Connect

Locate state agencies specializing in visual impairment, sources of financial assistance for eye care, and other resources for people with visual impairment at the website of the American Macular Degeneration Foundation at www.macular.org/.

● Resources

Alexander Graham Bell Association for the Deaf
3417 Volta Place, NW
Washington, DC 20007
(202) 337-5220
www.agbell.org

American Council of the Blind
1211 Connecticut Avenue, NW
Suite 506
Washington, DC 20036
(202) 833-1251
www.acb.org

American Humane Association Hearing Dog Program
63 Inverness Drive East
Englewood, CO 80110
(866) 242-1877
www.americanhumane.org

American Speech-Language-Hearing Association
10801 Rockville Pike
Rockville, MD 20852

(800) 498-2071
www.asha.org

Blinded Veterans Association
1735 DeSales Street, NW
Washington, DC 20036
(202) 347-4010
www.bva.org

Guide Dogs for the Blind
P.O. Box 1200
San Rafael, CA 94902
(415) 479-4000
www.guidedogs.com

Guiding Eyes for the Blind
250 East Hartsdale Avenue
Hartsdale, NY 10530
(914) 723-2223
www.guiding-eyes.org

Independent Living Aids
200 Robbins Lane
Jericho NY 11753
(800) 537-2118
www.indepenedentliving.com

Leader Dogs for the Blind
1039 South Rochester Road
Rochester, MN 48063
(313) 651-9011
www.leaderdog.org

Lighthouse National Center for Vision and Aging
111 East 59th Street
New York, NY 10022
(212) 821-9200
www.lighthouse.org

National Association for the Deaf
814 Thayer Avenue
Silver Spring, MD 20910
(301) 587-1788
www.nad.org

National Association for the Visually Handicapped
305 East 24th Street
New York, NY 10010
(212) 899-3141
www.navh.org

National Braille Association
3 Townline Circle
Rochester, NY 14623
(716) 427-8260
http://members.aol.com/nbaoffice

National Association of the Deaf Law Center
814 Thayer Avenue
Silver Spring, MD 20910
(301) 587-7730
www.healthfinder.gov/orgs/HR1053.htm

National Federation of the Blind
National Center for the Blind
1800 Johnson Street
Baltimore, MD 21230
(410) 659-9314
www.nfb.org/

National Information Center on Deafness
Gallaudet College
T-6, 800 Florida Avenue, NE
Washington, DC 20002
(202) 651-5109
www.gallaudet.edu

National Library Service for the Blind and Physically Handicapped
Library of Congress
1291 Taylor Street, NW
Washington, DC 20542
(202) 287-5100
www.lcweb.loc.gov/nls

Recorded Periodicals
919 Walnut Street
Philadelphia, PA 19107
(215) 627-0600
www.libertynet.org/asbinfo/mags.html

Recordings for the Blind and Dyslexic
20 Roszel Road
Princeton, NJ 08540
(866) RFBD-585
www.rfbd.org

Self-Help for Hard of Hearing People
7910 Woodmont Avenue
Suite 1200
Bethesda, MD 20814
(301) 657-2248
www.shhh.org

● Reference

Johns Hopkins Medical Institutions. (2000). Hitting the mark with eye drops. *Health After 50, 11*(11), 7.

● Recommended Readings

Demers, K. (2001). Hearing screening. *Journal of Gerontological Nursing, 27*(11), 8–9.

Dowling, J. S., & Bright, M. A. (1999). A collaborative research project on therapeutic touch. *Journal of Holistic Nursing, 17*(3), 296–307.

Gerdner, L. A. (1999). Individualized music intervention protocol. *Journal of Gerontological Nursing, 25*(10), 10–15.

Houde, S. C., & Huff, M. A. (2003). Age-related vision loss in older adults: A challenge for gerontological nurses. *Journal of Gerontological Nursing, 29*(4), 25–33.

Hutchinson, C. P. (1999). Healing touch: An energetic approach. *American Journal of Nursing, 99*(4), 43–54.

Jupiter, T., & Spivey, V. (1997). Perception of hearing loss and hearing handicap on hearing aid use by nursing home residents. *Geriatric Nursing, 18*(5), 201–208.

Kerr, M. (2003). Silent strokes spur cognitive decline, dementia. *Caring for the Ages, 4*(5), 56

Kerr, M. (2003). Stroke deaths to double in next 30 years. *Caring for the Ages, 4*(5), 56.

Kessler, S. (2000). A kiss. *RN, 63*(2), 43–45.

Kohl, M. (1998). Prevention: The best treatment for macular degeneration. *Alternative and Complementary Therapies, 4*(6), 414–416.

Kupfer, C. (1995). Ophthalmologic disorders. In W. B. Abrams & R. Berkow (Eds.), *The Merck manual of geriatrics* (2nd ed., p. 1055). Rahway, NJ: Merck Sharp & Dohme Research Laboratories.

Mahoney, D. F. (1996). Cerumen impaction and hearing impairment among nursing home residents: Nursing implications. In V. Burggraf & R. Barry (Eds.), *Gerontological nursing: Current practice and research* (pp. 159–168). Thorofare, NJ: Slack.

Melore, G. G. (Ed.). (1997). *Treating vision problems in the older adult.* St. Louis: Mosby.

O'Brien, B. (1997). Experiences with aromatherapy in the elderly. *Journal of Alternative and Complementary Medicine, 3*(3), 211.

Orr, A. L. (1998). *Issues in aging and vision: A curriculum for university programs and inservice training.* New York: AFB Press.

Pinkerton, J. (1996). *The sound of healing.* New York: Alliance Books.

Scheiman, M. (Ed.). (1997). *Understanding and managing vision deficits: A guide for occupational therapists.* Thorofare, NJ: Slack.

Stone, C. M. (1999). Preventing cerumen impaction in nursing facility residents. *Journal of Gerontological Nursing, 25*(5), 43–45.

Tesch-Romer, C. (1997). Psychological effects of hearing aid use in older adults. *Journal of Gerontology: Psychological Sciences, 52B*(3), 127–138.

Dermatologic Conditions

■ Learning Objectives

After reading this chapter, you should be able to:

- list practices that promote good skin health
- describe signs of and nursing care for pruritus, keratosis, seborrheic keratosis, malignant melanoma, stasis dermatitis, and pressure ulcer
- discuss measures that help patients with skin problems feel normal
- identify alternative therapies that promote good skin health

Perhaps the most obvious effects of growing old are the changes involving the integumentary system. Lines and wrinkles, thicker nails, and graying hair are constant reminders of the aging process. Past health practices largely influence the status of the integument in old age; its status in old age, in turn, influences older persons' general health. In other words, problems involving other body systems can result from an unhealthy integumentary system.

The direct contact between nursing staff and patients allows nursing staff to detect skin problems that may not be apparent to other health care professionals. It is important for nurses to regularly assess patients' skin status (Display 31-1) and identify nursing diagnoses (Nursing Diagnosis Table 31-1) and problems in need of referral for medical attention. Because serious complications, such as new pressure ulcers, can result from undetected skin problems, astute attention to skin status is crucial.

Facilitating Good Skin Status

Some general measures can help to prevent and manage dermatologic problems in older persons. It is important to avoid drying agents, rough clothing, highly starched linens, and other items irritating to the skin. Good skin nutrition and hydration can be promoted by activity, bath oils, lotions, and mas-

D I S P L A Y   3 1 - 1

Assessment of Skin Status

General Observations

One of the positive features of assessing the integumentary system is that its status is evident to the naked eye. A quick observation can assist in evaluating skin color, moisture, and cleanliness; the presence of lesions; hair condition and grooming; and the condition of the nails. Signs such as pallor or flushing can provide clues to health problems.

Interview

The patient should be asked about itching, burning sensations on the skin surface, hair loss, increased fragility of nails, and other symptoms associated with integumentary system problems. This opportunity also can be used to review bathing and shampooing practices.

Physical Examination

The entire skin surface should be examined from head to toe, including behind the ears, within skin folds, under the breasts, and between the toes. Bathing and massages are good opportunities to inspect the skin. Lesions should be described as specifically as possible in regard to their color (eg, purple, black, hypopigmented), configuration (eg, linear, separate, confluent, annular), size (eg, measurement of depth and diameter), drainage, and type. Terms used to describe types of lesions include the following:

Macule: a small nonpalpable spot or discoloration
Papule: a discoloration < 1/2 cm in diameter with palpable elevation
Plaque: a group of papules
Nodule: a lesion 1/2 to 1 cm in diameter with palpable elevation; the skin may or may not be discolored
Tumor: a lesion > 1 cm with palpable elevation; the skin may or may not be discolored
Wheal: a red or white palpable elevation that may occur in variable sizes
Vesicle: a lesion < 1/2 cm in diameter that contains fluid and has a palpable elevation
Bulla: a lesion > 1/2 cm in diameter that contains fluid and has a palpable elevation
Pustule: a lesion containing purulent fluid; of variable size and palpable elevation
Fissure: a groove in the skin
Ulcer: an open depression in the skin that may occur in variable sizes.

Many persons of African, Asian, or Native American backgrounds have mongolian spots. These are irregular, dark areas (resembling bruises) that may be found on the buttocks, lower back, and to a lesser extent on the arms, abdomen, and thighs.
Skin turgor can be tested by gently pinching various areas of the skin. Skin turgor tends to be poor in most older adults; however, the areas over the sternum and forehead do experience less of an age-related reduction in turgor and are good areas for turgor assessment.
Pressure tolerance can be assessed by inspecting a pressure point after the patient has been in the same position for half an hour; if redness is present, the patient must be on a turning schedule of every half an hour. If redness is not present, allow the patient to remain in the same position for 1 hour and inspect; if redness is not apparent increase increments by half an hour up to 2 hours.
By using the back of the hands and touching various areas, the nurse can obtain a gross assessment of skin temperature. Coldness or temperature inequalities between the extremities should be noted.

ND Nursing Diagnoses

TABLE 31-1 ● *Nursing Diagnoses Related to Dermatologic Problems*

Causes or Contributing Factors	Nursing Diagnosis
Altered body appearance	Anxiety
Pruritus, infection, ulcer	Pain
Ulcer, fragile skin	Risk for Infection
More fragile skin	Risk for Injury
Age-related changes to skin, hair, and nails; pain	Disturbed Body Image
Altered self-concept due to age-related changes, more fragile vaginal epithelium	Sexual Dysfunction
Fragile skin, immobility	Impaired Skin Integrity
Altered self-concept due to age-related changes to integument	Impaired Social Interaction
Pressure sites, ulcers	Ineffective Tissue Perfusion

sages. Although skin cleanliness is important, excessive bathing may be hazardous to the skin; daily partial sponge baths and complete baths every third or fourth day are sufficient for the average older person. Early attention to and treatment of pruritus and skin lesions are advisable for preventing irritation, infection, and other problems.

Exposure to ultraviolet rays damages the skin, causing a condition known as *solar elastosis,* or *photoaging.* Loss of elasticity and wrinkling of the skin are characteristic of this sun-induced premature aging of the skin. Fair-skinned individuals who easily burn when in the sun are at particularly high risk of this condition. Sun-screening lotions are beneficial in protecting the skin; the sun protection factor (SPF) required will depend on the ease at which the skin burns and could range from a SPF of 15 or more in highly sensitive persons to a SPF of 4–6 in people who seldom burn and tan dark brown easily. Patients need to be reminded that skin damage can occur on overcast days because ultraviolet rays can penetrate clouds.

All persons should be encouraged to look their best and make the most of their appearance. However, efforts to avoid the normal outcomes of the aging process can be fruitless and frustrating. Money that could be applied to more basic needs is sometimes invested in attempts to defy reality. The nurse should emphasize to persons young and old that no cream, lotion, or miracle drug will remove wrinkles and lines or return youthful skin. While clarifying misconceptions regarding rejuvenating products, the nurse can encourage the use of cosmetics to protect the skin and maintain an attractive appearance; many benefits may be derived from this practice. Because increasing numbers of aging individuals are seeking cosmetic surgery, gerontological nurses will find it beneficial to be informed of the various types of surgical interventions and help patients locate competent cosmetic surgeons. Patients need to be aware that not all surgeons are skilled in cosmetic surgery, and some unfortunate complications have resulted from unskilled physicians performing cosmetic surgery or injecting patients with collagen or silicone. Nurses should explore patients' reasons for seeking cosmetic surgery to ensure that it is a rational decision rather than a symptom of an underlying problem, such as depression or a neurotic disorder; counseling and therapy may be a more pressing need than surgical intervention in some circumstances. Perhaps as society achieves a greater acceptance and understanding of the aging process, the masking of the effects of aging with cosmetics and surgery will be replaced by an appreciation of the natural beauty of age.

✓ **Point to Ponder**

How much of your self-concept is based on your physical appearance? How do you anticipate reacting to the physical manifestations of aging?

Selected Conditions

PRURITUS

The most common dermatologic problem among elders is pruritus. Although atrophic changes alone may be responsible for this problem, pruritus can be precipitated by any circumstance that dries the person's skin, such as excessive bathing and dry heat. Diabetes, arteriosclerosis, hyperthyroidism, uremia, liver disease, cancer, pernicious anemia, and certain psychiatric problems can also contribute to pruritus. If not corrected, the itching may cause traumatizing scratching, leading to breakage and infection of the skin. Prompt recognition of this problem and implementation of corrective measures are, therefore, essential. If possible, the underlying cause should be corrected. Careful assessment is required to assure conditions such as scabies are not present that would demand special precautions. Bath oils, moisturizing lotions, and massage are beneficial in treating and preventing pruritus. Vitamin supplements and a high-quality, vitamin-rich diet may be recommended. The topical application of zinc oxide has been effective in controlling itching in some individuals. Antihistamines and topical steroids may also be prescribed for relief.

> **KEY CONCEPT**
> Excessive bathing and dry heat dry the skin and can promote pruritus.

KERATOSIS

Keratoses, also referred to as actinic or solar keratoses, are small, light-colored lesions, usually gray or brown, on exposed areas of the skin. Keratin may be accumulated in these lesions, causing the formation of a cutaneous horn with a slightly reddened and swollen base. Freezing agents and acids can be used to destroy the keratotic lesions, but electrodesiccation or surgical excision ensures a more thorough removal. Close nursing observation for changes in keratotic lesions is vital because they are precancerous.

SEBORRHEIC KERATOSIS

It is not uncommon for older persons to have several dark, wartlike projections on various parts of their bodies. These lesions, called *seborrheic keratoses,* may be as small as a pinhead or as large as a quarter. They tend to increase in size and number with age. In the sebaceous areas of the trunk, face, and neck and in persons with oily skin, these lesions appear dark and oily; in less sebaceous areas, they are dry in appearance and of a light color. Normally, seborrheic keratoses will not have swelling or redness around their base. Sometimes abrasive activity with a gauze pad containing oil will remove small seborrheic keratoses. Larger, raised lesions can be removed by freezing agents or by a curettage and cauterization procedure. Although these lesions are benign, medical evaluation is important to differentiate them from precancerous lesions. In addition, the cosmetic benefit of removal should not be overlooked for the older patient.

> **KEY CONCEPT**
> The dark, wartlike projections known as seborrheic keratoses can be as small as a pinhead or as large as a quarter.

MALIGNANT MELANOMA

Although responsible for a small percentage of total deaths from cancer, malignant melanoma is significant because it is a highly metastatic and fatal skin cancer. The incidence of melanomas has been rising in the United States, probably due to sun exposure. Fair-skinned individuals are at higher risk for melanomas than the general population, and the incidence increases with age.

Melanomas can be classified as follows.

Lentigo maligna melanoma. This black, brown, white, or red pigmented flat lesion occurs predominately on sun-exposed areas of the body. With time it enlarges and becomes progressively irregularly pigmented. The mean age at diagnosis is 67.

Superficial spreading melanoma. Most melanomas are of this type. The lesion appears as variable-pigmented plaque with an irregular border. It can occur on any area of the body. Its incidence peaks in middle age and continues to be high through the eighth decade.

Nodular melanoma. This melanoma can be found on any body surface and presents as a darkly pigmented papule that increases in size over time.

Suspicious lesions should be evaluated and biopsied. Usually, melanomas are excised with removal of some of the surrounding tissue and subcutaneous fat. Some physicians recommend removal of all palpably enlarged lymph nodes. The prognosis depends on the depth of the melanoma rather than the type.

Patients should be taught to inspect themselves for melanomas, identify moles that demonstrate changes in pigmentation or size, and seek evaluation of suspicious lesions. Early detection improves the prognosis.

VASCULAR LESIONS

Age-related changes can weaken the walls of the veins and reduce the veins' ability to respond to increased venous pressure. This problem is compounded by obesity and hereditary factors. Weakened vessel walls cause varicose veins. The poor venous return and congestion that results lead to edema of the lower extremities, which leads to poor tissue nutrition. As the poorly nourished legs accumulate debris, inadequately carried away with the venous return, the legs gain a pigmented, cracked, and exudative appearance. Subsequent scratching, irritation, or other trauma (which can result from tight elastic-band stockings) that occurs with stasis dermatitis can then easily result in the formation of leg ulcers. These ulcers, known as stasis ulcers, often appear on the medial aspect of the tibia above the malleolus and prior to actual skin breakdown, present as a dark discoloration of the skin.

Stasis ulcers need special attention to facilitate healing. Infection must be controlled and necrotic tissue removed before healing will occur. Good nutrition is an important component of the therapy, and a diet high in vitamins and protein is recommended. Once healing has occurred, concern should be given to avoiding situations that promote stasis dermatitis. The patient may need instruction regarding a diet for weight reduction or the planning of high-quality meals. Venous return can be enhanced by elevating the legs several times a day and by preventing interferences to circulation, such as standing for long periods, sitting with legs crossed, and wearing garters.

Elastic support stockings may be prescribed and, although effective, can be a challenge for some older adults to apply. The ability of patients to properly put on these stockings needs to be assessed and instruction provided as needed. Some patients may require ligation and stripping of the veins to prevent further episodes of stasis dermatitis.

PRESSURE ULCER

Tissue anoxia and ischemia resulting from pressure can cause the necrosis, sloughing, and ulceration of tissue. This is commonly known as a pressure ulcer, or decubitus ulcer. Any part of the body can develop a pressure ulcer, but the most common sites are the sacrum, greater trochanter, and ischial tuberosities (Fig. 31-1). Older adults are at high risk for pressure ulcers because they:

- have skin that is fragile and damages easily
- often are in a poor nutritional state
- have reduced sensation of pressure and pain
- are more frequently affected by immobile and edematous conditions, which contribute to skin breakdown

In addition to developing more easily in older persons, pressure ulcers require a longer period to heal than in younger people. Therefore, the most important nursing measure is to prevent their formation; to do this, it is essential to avoid unrelieved pressure. Encouraging activity or turning the patient who cannot move independently is necessary. The patient's individual pressure tolerance (see Display 31-1) determines the frequency of turning; a turning schedule of every 2 hours may not be sufficient for every patient, and pressure ulcers can develop under that turning schedule. Shearing forces that cause two layers of tissue to move across each other should be prevented by not elevating the head of the bed more than 30°, not allowing patients to slide in bed, and lifting instead of pulling patients when moving them. Pillows, flotation pads, alternating-pressure mattresses, and water beds can be used to disperse pressure from bony prominences. It must be emphasized that these devices do not eliminate the need for frequent position changes. When they are sitting in a chair, patients should be urged to move and should be assisted with shifting their weight at certain intervals. Lamb's wool and heel protectors are useful in preventing irri-

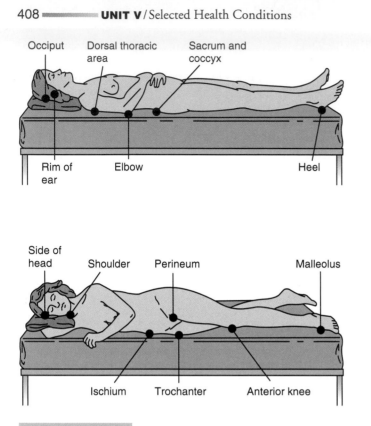

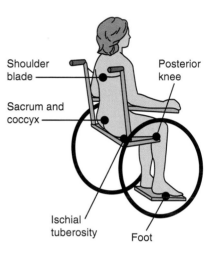

FIGURE 31-1

Common locations for pressure sores when supine and sitting.

tation to bony prominences. Sheets should be kept wrinkle free, and the bed should be checked frequently for foreign objects, such as syringes and utensils, which the patient may be lying on unknowingly.

A high-protein, vitamin-rich diet to maintain and improve tissue health is also essential to avoid formation of pressure ulcers. Good skin care is another essential ingredient in prevention. Skin should be kept clean and dry, and blotting the patient dry will avoid irritation from rubbing the skin with a towel. Bath oils and lotions, used prophylactically, will help keep the skin soft and intact. Massage of bony prominences and range-of-motion exercises promote circulation and help keep the tissues well nourished. The person who is incontinent should be thoroughly cleansed with soap and water and dried after each episode to avoid skin breakdown from irritating excreta.

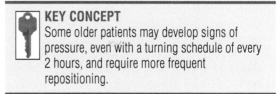

KEY CONCEPT
Some older patients may develop signs of pressure, even with a turning schedule of every 2 hours, and require more frequent repositioning.

Once evidence of an ulcer is noted, aggressive intervention is necessary to avoid the multiple risks associated with this impairment of skin integrity. It is useful to determine the state of the pressure ulcer because various treatments are effective for different stages. The various stages of pressure ulcers may be recognized by the following signs and relieved by the following measures.

Hyperemia. Redness of the skin appears quickly and can disappear quickly if pressure is removed.

There is no break in the skin and the underlying tissues remain soft. Relieving the pressure by the use of a square of adhesive foam is useful; it is advisable to protect the skin with a product such as DuoDerm (Squibb) or Tegasorb (3M) before applying the adhesive.

Ischemia. Redness of the skin develops from up to 6 hours of unrelieved pressure and is often accompanied by edema and induration. It can take several days for this area to return to its normal color, during which the epidermis may blister. Skin should be protected with Vigilon, which contains water and is soothing to the area. If the skin surface is broken, it should be cleansed daily with normal saline or the product suggested by your agency.

Necrosis. Unremitting pressure extending over 6 hours can cause ulceration with a necrotic base. This type of sore requires a transparent dressing that protects from bacteria but is permeable to oxygen and water vapor. Thorough irrigation is essential during dressing changes. Sometimes topical antibiotics are used. It may take weeks to months for full healing to occur.

Ulceration. If pressure is not relieved, necrosis will extend through the fascia and potentially to the bone. Eschar, a thick, coagulated crust, is frequently present, and bone destruction and infection may occur. Unless eschar is removed, the underlying tissue will continue to break down, so debridement is essential.

A recommended system for describing the stages of ulcers, and one that is used in the Minimum Data Set tool for assessing nursing home residents, is described in Display 31-2.

Because the risk of pressure ulcer formation is high among older patients, it is wise for gerontological nurses to assess patients' risk for pressure ulcers upon admission or first contact. Several tools that have been used for several decades can assist in objective assessment of pressure ulcer risk, such as the Braden scale (Bergstrom, Allman & Carlson, 1994) and the Norton scale (Norton, McLaren, & Exton-Smith 1962). The Pressure Sore Status Tool (PSST) (Bates-Jensen, 1996) is an instrument that offers a means for assessing and monitoring existing pressure ulcers using 13 indexes (eg, size, exudate, necrotic tissue, edema, and granulation). Depending on the patient population served and types of clinical setting, agencies and facilities may find that they need to develop their own tools to assess risk and monitor pressure ulcers.

Nursing Considerations

PROMOTING NORMALCY

Psychological support can be especially important to the patient with a dermatologic problem. Unlike res-

---

D I S P L A Y   3 1 - 2

Stages of Pressure Ulcers

- **Stage 1**—a persistent area of skin redness (without a break in the skin) that does not disappear when pressure is relieved
- **Stage 2**—a partial thickness loss of skin layers involving the epidermis that presents clinically as an abrasion, blister, or shallow crater
- **Stage 3**—a full thickness of skin is lost extending through the epidermis and exposing the subcutaneous tissues; presents as a deep crater with or without undermining adjacent tissue
- **Stage 4**—a full thickness of skin and subcutaneous tissue is lost, exposing muscle, bone, or both; presents as a deep crater that may include necrotic tissue, exudate, sinus tract formation, and infection

piratory, cardiac, and other disorders, dermatologic problems are often visibly unpleasant to the patient and others. Visitors and staff may unnecessarily avoid touching and being with the patient in reaction to his or her skin problems. The nurse can reassure visitors regarding the safety of contact with the patient and provide instruction for any special precautions that must be followed. The most important fact to emphasize is that the patient is still normal, with normal needs and feelings, and will appreciate normal interactions and contact.

USING ALTERNATIVE THERAPIES

For centuries, various herbs have been used to treat skin problems. Today the use continues, as evidenced by creams, lotions, and shampoos containing aloe, chamomile, and other plant products. Aloe vera has emollient properties when used externally, and many people find it useful for treating minor cuts and burns. The external application of chamomile extract is used for skin inflammation. Witch hazel has long been used for its astringent effects and is applied externally for the treatment of bruises and swelling.

Essential oils are also increasingly used for the prevention and treatment of skin problems, including thyme oil as an antiseptic, thyme-linalol and rosewood oil for topical acne, rosemary oil for cell regeneration, and the oils of basil, cinnamon, garlic, lavender, lemon, sage, savory, and thyme for bites or stings. Topical application of peppermint oil can have an anti-inflammatory effect and speed the healing of wounds and mild burns.

Some homeopathic and naturopathic remedies are being used to treat skin eruptions, as is acupuncture. Biofeedback, guided imagery, and relaxation exercises can help control the symptoms of some dermatologic disorders.

There is belief that nutritional supplements can also be beneficial for skin disorders; those most commonly recommended are zinc, magnesium, essential fatty acids, and vitamins A, B complex, B_6, and E. Patients should be urged to discuss the use of alternative therapies with their physician.

Critical Thinking Exercises

1. Discuss the psychosocial implications of pressure ulcers and malignant melanoma.
2. Describe the method for determining an individualized turning schedule.
3. What are the benefits and risks associated with cosmetic surgery?
4. Develop a protocol for the prevention of pressure ulcers.

Web Connect

Review pamphlets about various facial plastic surgery procedures by visiting the website of the American Academy of Facial and Reconstructive Plastic Surgery at www.aafprs.org/patient/procedures/proctypes.html.

● Resources

American Cancer Society
1599 Clifton Road NE
Atlanta, GA 30329
(800) 227-2345
www.cancer.org

National Arthritis and Musculoskeletal and Skin Diseases Information Clearinghouse
NAMSIC AMS Circle
National Institutes of Health
Bethesda, MD 20892
(301) 495-4484
www.nih.gov/niams

● References

Bates-Jensen, B. M. (1996). *Why and how to assess pressure ulcers.* Presented at the Ninth Annual Symposium on Advanced Wound Care, Atlanta, April 20, 1996.

Bergstrom, M., Allman, R. M., & Carlson, E. D. (1994). *Treatment of Pressure Ulcers.* Clinical Practice Guideline No. 15, AHCPR Pub No 95-0652. Rockville, MD: U.S. Department of Health and Human Services, Public Health Service, Agency for Health Care Policy and Research.

Norton, D., McLaren, R., & Exton-Smith, A. N. (1962) *An investigation of geriatric nursing problems in the hospital.* London: National Corporation for the Care of Old People.

● Recommended Readings

Ayello, E. A., & Braden, B. (2001). Why is pressure ulcer risk assessment so important? *Nursing 2001, 31*(11), 75–79.

Ayello, E. A. (1999). Predicting pressure ulcer sore risk (try this). *Journal of Gerontological Nursing, 25*(10), 7–9.

Bryant, R. A. (Ed.) (2000). *Acute and chronic wounds: Nursing management* (2d ed.). St. Louis: Mosby.

Consortium for Spinal Cord Medicine. (2000). *Pressure ulcer prevention and treatment following spinal cord injury: A clinical practice guideline for health care professionals.* Guideline available at *www.pvs.org.* Washington, D.C.: Paralyzed Veterans of America.

Dunn, L. B., Damesyn, M., Moore, A. A., Reuben, D. B., & Greendale, G. A. (1997). Does estrogen prevent skin aging? *Archives of Dermatology, 133,* 339–342.

Hardy, M. A. (1996). What can you do about your patient's dry skin? *Journal of Gerontological Nursing, 22*(5), 10–18.

Hess, C. T. (2000). *Nurse's clinical guide to wound care* (3rd ed.). Springhouse, PA: Springhouse.

Johns Hopkins Medical Institutions. (2000). Diabetes complications: More than skin deep. *Health After 50, 11*(11), 6.

Krasner, D. L., Rodeheaver, G. T., & Sibbald, R. G. (Eds.). (2001). *Chronic wound care: A clinical source book for healthcare professionals* (3rd ed.). Wayne, PA: HMP Communications.

Maklebust, J., & Sieggreen, M. (2001). *Pressure ulcers: Guidelines for prevention and nursing management* (3rd ed.). Springhouse, PA: Springhouse.

Morison, M. J. (Ed). (2001). *The Prevention and treatment of pressure ulcers.* St. Louis: Mosby, 2001.

Norman, R. A. (2001). Causes and management of xerosis and pruritus in the elderly. *Annals of Long-Term Care, 9*(12), 35–40.

Rosenberg, C. J. (2002). New checklist for pressure ulcer prevention. *Journal of Gerontological Nursing, 28*(8), 7–12.

Sprigle, S., Linden, M., McKenna, D., Davis, K., & Riordan, B. (2001). Clinical skin temperature measurement to predict incipient pressure ulcers. *Advances in Skin and Wound Care, 14*(3), 133–137.

Sussman, C., & Bates-Jensen, B. M. (2001). *Wound care: A collaborative practice manual for physical therapists and nurses* (2nd ed.). Gaithersburg, MD: Aspen Publishers.

Thompson, J. (2000). A practical guide to wound care. *RN, 63*(1), 48–49.

Vap, P. W., & Dunaye, T. (2000). Pressure ulcer risk assessment in long-term care nursing. *Journal of Gerontological Nursing, 26*(6), 37–45.

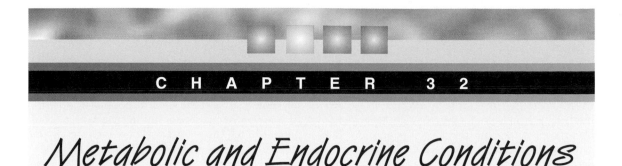

Metabolic and Endocrine Conditions

■ Learning Objectives

After reading this chapter, you should be able to:

* describe unique manifestations of diabetes in the elderly
* outline a teaching plan for the older person with diabetes
* list symptoms of hypothyroidism and hyperthyroidism
* describe lifestyle changes helpful in reducing elevated cholesterol levels

*T*he endocrine system enables the body to grow and develop, reproduce, metabolize energy, maintain homeostasis, and respond to stress and injury. This complex system consists of glands that synthesize and secrete hormones—substances that are transported from glands through the blood to targeted tissues where they exert specific effects either directly or indirectly by interacting with specific cell receptors. There are two major classes of hormones: steroids and thyronines, which are lipid soluble, and polypeptides and catecholamines, which are water soluble.

With aging, the endocrine system experiences changes that can be diverse and interrelated in that some changes are compensatory responses for others. Knowledge of these changes and their effects is beneficial in interpreting symptoms and advising elders regarding practices to promote optimal health.

Diabetes

A blend of various knowledge and skills is required when caring for older adults who have diabetes. Diabetes, the seventh leading cause of death among older adults, has a particularly high prevalence among black people and people 65 to 74 years of age. Consequently, nurses must be adequately informed of how the detection and management of diabetes in elders differs from that in other age groups.

GLUCOSE INTOLERANCE

Glucose intolerance is a common occurrence among older adults; several explanations are offered for this.

Research has shown that a physiologic deterioration of glucose tolerance occurs with increasing age. Also, diagnostic techniques have been improved, enabling more persons with the condition to be detected. Finally, some believe that the high prevalence of glucose intolerance is a result of an increase in the incidence of diabetes throughout the general population. Regardless of the reason, it is agreed that different standards must be applied in evaluating glucose tolerance in the elderly.

> **KEY CONCEPT**
> The high prevalence of hyperglycemia in the elderly population is believed to be related to physiologic deterioration of glucose tolerance with age, improved diagnostic tests, and a general increase in the prevalence of diabetes in the population as a whole.

DIAGNOSIS

Early diagnosis of diabetes in older persons often is difficult. The classic symptoms of diabetes may be absent, leaving nonspecific symptoms as the only clues. Some indications of diabetes in elders include orthostatic hypotension, periodontal disease, stroke, gastric hypotony, impotence, neuropathy, confusion, glaucoma, Dupuytren contracture, and infection. Laboratory tests, as well as symptoms, may be misleading. Because the renal threshold for glucose increases with age, older individuals can be hyperglycemic without evidence of glycosuria, thus limiting the validity of urine testing for glucose.

Among all the diagnostic measures, the glucose tolerance test is the most effective. To avoid a false-positive diagnosis, more than one test should be performed. The American Diabetes Association recommends that a minimum of 150 g carbohydrate be ingested daily for several days before the test; older, malnourished individuals may be prescribed 300 g. Recent periods of inactivity, stressful illness, and inadequate dietary intake should be communicated to the physician because these situations can contribute to glucose intolerance. In such circumstances, more accurate results can be obtained if the test is postponed for a month after the episode. Nicotinic acid, ethacrynic acid, estrogen, furosemide, and diuretics can decrease glucose tolerance and should not be administered before testing. Monoamine oxidase in-

hibitors, propranolol, and high dosages of salicylates may lower blood sugar levels and also interfere with testing.

Usual nursing measures are applied during glucose tolerance testing of the aged. If unusual symptoms, such as confusion, develop during the test, it is important to tell the physician. Those interpreting the glucose tolerance test may find it beneficial to use age-related gradients. Typically, for each decade after age 55 years, 10 mg/dL is added to the standard values at the first, second, and third hours. Thus, a glucose level that would be significantly elevated for a 35-year-old person may be within normal limits for an 85-year-old individual.

> **KEY CONCEPT**
> A glucose level that would be abnormal for a young adult could fall within the normal range for an older individual.

The diagnosis of diabetes usually is established if one of three criteria exists:

1. Random plasma glucose concentrations are greater than or equal to 200 mg/dL.
2. Fasting blood glucose concentrations are greater than or equal to 136 mg/dL on two occasions.
3. Plasma glucose concentrations after oral glucose intake are greater than or equal to 200 mg/dL.

PATIENT EDUCATION

Once the diagnosis has been confirmed, the nurse should establish a teaching plan (Fig. 32-1 and Display 32-1). Diabetes is known as a serious and chronic problem to most lay individuals, and its diagnosis can be frightening. Fear and anxiety can interfere with the learning process for older people with newly diagnosed diabetes, who may have witnessed the crippling or fatal effects of diabetes in others and anticipate such occurrences in themselves. Having lived through a period in which diabetes was not successfully managed and was often severely disabling or fatal, the older individual may not be aware of the advances in diabetic management.

Elderly people may be depressed or angry that this disease threatens to decrease further the quality of the remainder of their lives; they may question the value of exchanging an unrestricted lifestyle for a potentially

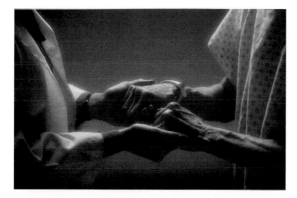

FIGURE 32-1

The teaching–learning process is highly individualized.

longer but restricted one. Concerns may arise about how a special diet and medications will be afforded on an already limited budget. Social isolation may develop from fear of becoming ill in public or facing restrictions that make them different from their peers. They may question their ability to manage their diabetes independently and worry that institutionalization will be necessary. Such concerns must be recognized and dealt with by the nurse to reduce the risk of other limitations and promote the individual's self-care capacities (Nursing Diagnosis Table 32-1). Reassurance, support, and information can reduce barriers to learning about and managing diabetes. The steps described in Display 32-2, helpful in any patient education situation, offer guidance in teaching the older diabetic patient.

DISPLAY 32-1

Content for Diabetic Patient Education

General Overview

Definition and description of diabetes mellitus
Basic anatomy and physiology
Basic metabolism of nutrients
Impact of advanced age on glucose metabolism, presentation of symptoms, complications

Nutrition

Food groups, food exchange system
Dietary requirements
Consistent pattern of food intake
Menu plans
Understanding food labels
Flexibility of diet

Activity and Exercise

Coordination and goal setting with healthcare provider
Planning exercise in relation to glucose levels
Precautions
Monitoring glucose, vital signs
Recognizing complications
Importance of good fluid intake

Medications

Actions
Dosage

Proper administration
Precautions
Adverse effects
Interactions

Monitoring

Purpose, goals
Types
Procedure

Recognizing Hypoglycemia and Hyperglycemia

Description and definition of hypoglycemia and hyperglycemia
Prevention

Recognition of Symptoms

Actions to take for each
Signs that warrant contacting healthcare provider

Prevention of Complications

Foot care
Eye examinations
Adjustments for diabetes care during illnesses
Recognition of complications (eg, infections, neuropathies)

Nursing Diagnosis

ND **TABLE 32-1** ● *Nursing Diagnoses Related to Diabetes Mellitus*

Causes or Contributing Factors	Nursing Diagnosis
Fear of disease's impact	Anxiety
High risk for loss of body part or function	Fear
Hyperglycemia	Risk for Infection
Decreased sensations, confusion, or dizziness from hypoglycemia	Risk for Injury
Diagnostic tests, care demands, denial	Deficient Knowledge
Lack of knowledge, self-care limitation	Noncompliance
Insufficient calories to meet energy, insulin demands	Imbalanced Nutrition: Less Than Body Requirements
Caloric intake in excess of energy, insulin coverage	Imbalanced Nutrition: More Than Body Requirements
Inability to meet therapeutic demands, feeling that disease is controlling life	Powerlessness
Peripheral neuropathies, retinopathy	Disturbed Sensory Perception
Peripheral neuropathy, vaginitis	Sexual Dysfunction
Susceptibility to fungal infections, pruritus from hyperglycemia	Impaired Skin Integrity
Urinary frequency	Disturbed Sleep Pattern
Altered neurovascular function secondary to neuropathies	Ineffective Tissue Perfusion

MANAGEMENT OF THE ILLNESS

One factor that must be considered in the management of the older person with diabetes is the patient's ability to handle a syringe and vial of insulin. Several repeat demonstrations of this skill should be performed during the hospitalization, especially on days when arthritis discomfort is present.

 KEY CONCEPT
Several repeat demonstrations of the older person's ability to self-inject insulin are advisable to evaluate competence in self-administration.

More specifically, because most elderly persons have some degree of visual impairment, their ability to read the calibrations on an insulin syringe must be evaluated. The yellowing of the lens with age tends to filter out low-tone colors such as blues and greens; because these colors are frequently used to identify various levels of glycosuria in urine testing kits, it is important to assess the older individual's ability to discriminate between these shades. Older people may

also be limited in their ability to purchase and prepare adequate meals because of financial, energy, or social limitations. This can interfere with management of the illness. Meals on Wheels, food stamps, the assistance of a neighbor, and other appropriate resources should be used to assist the individual.

Altered tubule reabsorption of glucose may lead to inaccurate results from urine testing. The older individual can be hyperglycemic without being glycosuric. On the other hand, higher blood glucose levels are common in elders, and minimal or mild glycosuria usually is not treated with insulin. Although nurses are not responsible for prescribing insulin coverage, they need to be aware that the insulin requirements of older patients are individualized. Responses to various insulin levels should be carefully observed and communicated to the physician.

Many diabetic patients must perform blood glucose level testing using a finger-prick method. Patients must be instructed in this technique and demonstrate competence in its performance. The finger-prick technique will most likely be replaced in the near future by an infrared device that determines the blood glucose level by measuring how light is absorbed by the body. The patient sticks a finger into a small meter that

DISPLAY 3 2 - 2

General Guidelines for Patient Education

Assess Readiness to Learn

Discomfort, anxiety, and depression may block learning and the retention of knowledge. Relieving these symptoms, and allowing time for patients to develop to the point where they desire and can cope with information, may be necessary.

Assess Learning Capacities and Limitations

This includes consideration of educational level, language problems, literacy, present knowledge, willingness to learn, cultural background, previous experience with the illness, memory, vision, hearing, speech, and mental status.

Outline Content of Presentation

Your outline should not only be specific and clear but should also consider learning priorities. Nurses sometimes feel obligated to teach every detail about an illness, condensing a multitude of new facts and procedures into a short time frame. Most people need time to receive, absorb, sort, and translate new information into behavioral changes; the elderly are no different. Altered cerebral function or slower responses may further interfere with learning in the aged. Patients and their families should have a role in setting teaching priorities; the most vital information should be given first, followed by other relevant material. Visiting nurses and other resources should be used after hospital discharge to continue the teaching plan if the proposed outline is not completed during the hospitalization.

Alter the Teaching Plan in View of Capacities and Limitations

The nurse may feel that an explanation of the physiologic effects of diabetes is significant for new diabetics. However, the older person who tends to be confused or has a poor memory may not have long-range benefit from this type of information.

It may be better to use that time to reinforce diet information or to make sure the most significant information required for self-care is retained.

Prepare the Patient for the Teaching-Learning Session

Patients should understand that education is an integral part of care. Whenever possible, a specific time should be arranged in advance to avoid conflict with other activities and to allow the family to be present if desired.

Provide Environment Conducive to Learning

An area that is quiet, clean, relaxing, and free from odors and interference will help to create a good atmosphere for learning. Distraction should be minimal, especially in view of the aged's reduced capacity to manage multiple stimuli.

Use the Most Effective Individualized Educational Material

The nurse must recognize the limitations of standard teaching aids and the importance of individualized methods. An aid that was successful for one person may not be effective for another. The variety of sophisticated audiovisual aids that are commercially prepared and available in many agencies as resources for nurses are impressive, but they may not necessarily be effective for the given patient. The quality of an audio cassette may be excellent, but it is of little benefit to the older person with a hearing problem. A slide presentation, even slowly paced, may present facts more rapidly than can be absorbed by an older person with delayed response time. The print on a commercial pamphlet may appear minute to older eyes. The language used in many commercial materials may not be one to which the person is accustomed. Original handmade aids suited for the individual's unique needs may have a value equal to or greater than commercially prepared ones. Selectivity in methodology is essential.

(Continued)

DISPLAY 32-2 (Continued)

Use Several Approaches to the Same Body of Knowledge

The greater the number of different exposures to new material, the higher the probability that the material will be learned. Combine verbal explanation with charts, diagrams, pamphlets, demonstrations, discussions with other patients, and audiovisual resources.

Leave Material With the Patient for Later Review

Often, it is helpful to summarize the teaching session in writing, using language familiar to the patient. This provides concrete material that the patient can review independently later and share with the family.

Reinforce Key Points

Reinforcement should be regular and consistent, with all staff members supporting the teaching plan. For example, if the objective of the nurse caring for the patient has been to increase competency in self-injection of insulin, then the person substituting on the nurse's day off should comply with the established objectives rather than administering the insulin for the individual. Informal reinforcement of information during other daily activities should also be planned.

Obtain Feedback

Evaluate whether the patient and family have received and understood accurately the information communicated. This can be done by observing return demonstrations, asking questions, and listening to discussions among patients.

Reevaluate Periodically

To ascertain retention and effectiveness of the teaching sessions, informally reevaluate at a later time. Remember that retention of information may be especially difficult for the older individual.

Document

Describe specifically what was taught, when, who was involved, what methodology was used, the patient's reaction and understanding, and future plans for remaining learning needs. This assists the staff caring for patients during their hospitalization and serves as a guide for those providing continued care after discharge.

---

shines an infrared light through the skin. The infrared method should make glucose testing more convenient and pain free for diabetic persons.

Regular exercise is important for older diabetic patients and provides multiple health benefits. Physical activity can improve the patient's response to insulin during the period in which the exercise regimen is done, if the exercise is sufficient to lower the resting heart rate. In the diabetic individual, however, a vigorous exercise program or changes in an exercise program must be reviewed with the physician to prevent adverse consequences. For example, moderate-to-vigorous exercise increases the absorption of insulin and heightens the use of glucose by the exercising muscles, potentially leading to hypoglycemia.

Attempts should be made to maintain a consistent daily food intake because an insulin dosage is prescribed to cover a specific amount of food. This may be problematic if the elderly person has a minimal food intake during the week when alone but an increased intake when visiting with family on weekends or if the patient skimps on meals when financial resources are low. Psychosocial factors can influence consistent food intake as much as physical factors. The nurse and physician must carefully assess, plan, and manage insulin needs in view of the individual's unique problems and lifestyle. Special attention must also be paid to elders in a hospital or nursing home setting to ensure that food intake is regular and adequate.

> **KEY CONCEPT**
> Psychosocial factors can alter food intake from day to day and affect insulin requirements.

A diet high in complex carbohydrates and fibers controls the release of glucose into the bloodstream and can reduce insulin requirements. Nutritional supplements can reduce the risk of complications; such supplements include vitamin B$_6$, folic acid, riboflavin (B$_2$), magnesium, zinc, and chromium. Herbs with hypoglycemic properties include bilberry, fenugreek, garlic, ginseng, and mulberry leaves.

Some individuals require only oral hypoglycemic agents to control their diabetes. Those on insulin therapy who have lost weight or have not been ketoacidotic may have their insulin substituted by oral hypoglycemic agents. Still others will need periodic changes in their insulin dosages to meet changing demands. These factors, combined with other management difficulties in the older diabetic person, necessitate frequent reevaluation of the patient's status. The continuation of health supervision is an essential part of diabetic management.

> ✔ **Point to Ponder**
>
> *Consider your schedule of eating, exercise, sleep, and rest. How consistent a pattern do you have from day to day, and what adjustments would you need to make if you had to live with a condition such as diabetes?*

COMPLICATIONS

Older people are subject to a long list of complications from diabetes and have a greater risk of developing these complications than younger adults. Hypoglycemia seems to be a greater threat to older patients than ketoacidosis, and this is especially problematic because of the possible presentation of a different set of symptoms. Classic symptoms such as tachycardia, restlessness, perspiration, and anxiety may be totally absent in the older individual with hypoglycemia. Instead, any of the following may be the first indication of the problem: behavior disorders, convulsions, somnolence, confusion, disorientation, poor sleep patterns, nocturnal headache, slurred speech, and unconsciousness. Uncorrected hypoglycemia can cause tachycardia, arrhythmias, myocardial infarctions, cerebrovascular accident, and death.

> 🔑 **KEY CONCEPT**
> Rather than the classic symptoms of hypoglycemia that one would anticipate in younger adults, older individuals instead may experience confusion, abnormal behavior, altered sleep patterns, nocturnal headache, and slurred speech.

Peripheral vascular disease is a common complication in the older individual who has diabetes and is influenced by the poorer circulation and atherosclerosis often associated with increased age. Symptoms may range from numbness and weak pulses to infection and gangrene. The nurse should identify and promptly communicate to the physician symptoms of peripheral vascular disease. Educating the patient in proper foot care and in the early detection of foot problems can help reduce the risk of this problem; referral to a podiatrist also can prove beneficial. (Foot problems of the person with diabetes are discussed in Chap. 32.) (**Visit the Connection website to learn about an inexpensive tool that can be used to identify reduced sensitivity of the foot.**)

Another significant vascular problem of older patients with diabetes is retinopathy with consequent blindness. Individuals who are hypertensive or who have had diabetes for a long time have a greater risk of developing this complication. Hemorrhage, pigment disturbances, edema, and visual disorders are manifested with this problem.

Drug interactions can be a major source of complications for older diabetic patients. Many elders with diabetes use other drugs that have the potential to interact with their antidiabetic therapy. Nurses should review all medications the patient is taking to identify those drugs that may interact with antidiabetic medications. Consideration also must be given to asking about the use of herbal remedies that could affect blood glucose levels.

A variety of additional complications can affect older individuals who are living with diabetes. Cognitive impairment can be a complication. Older persons may develop neuropathies, demonstrated through tingling sensations progressing to stinging or stabbing pain; carpal tunnel syndrome; paresthesias; nocturnal diarrhea; tachycardia; and postural hypotension. They have twice the mortality rate from coronary artery disease and cerebral arteriosclerosis and a higher incidence of urinary tract infections. They also have a higher risk of problems developing in virtually every body system. Early detection of complications is essential and can be facilitated by nursing intervention and patient education. Competent management of the older patient with diabetes is a vital activity that requires considerable skill and poses a great challenge and responsibility to the practice of nursing. The recognition of differences in symptomatology, diagnosis, management, and complications is crucial. Display 32-3 lists some potential care plan goals. Resources of benefit to patients with diabetes are listed at the end of this chapter.

Hypothyroidism

Thyroxine (T_4) and triiodothyronine (T_3) are essential hormones produced by the thyroid gland. Aging affects the thyroid gland in several ways, including moderate atrophy, fibrosis, increasing colloid nodules, and some lymphocytic infiltration. Although production of T_4 declines with age, this is believed to be a compensatory process related to decreased tissue use of the hormone; serum levels of thyroid hormones do not significantly change.

A subnormal concentration of thyroid hormone in the tissues is known as *hypothyroidism*. This condition rises in prevalence with age and is more common in women than men. Hypothyroidism can take the form of *primary*, which results from a disease process that destroys the thyroid gland, or *secondary*, which is caused by insufficient pituitary secretion of thyroid-stimulating hormone (TSH). Primary hypothyroidism is characterized by low free T_4 or free T_4 index with an elevated TSH level; secondary hypothyroidism displays low free T_4 or free T_4 index and low TSH. A subclinical hypothyroidism can exist in which the person is asymptomatic but has an elevated TSH level and normal T_4. If symptoms are present but TSH, T_3, and T_4 levels are normal, it could be beneficial for the patient to have the thyrotropin-releasing hormone (TRH) level checked because this is more sensitive than the other thyroid levels and could help reveal subnormal thyroid function.

SYMPTOMS

Symptoms can be easily missed or attributed to other conditions and include:

- fatigue, weakness, and lethargy
- depression and disinterest in activities
- anorexia
- weight gain
- impaired hearing
- periorbital or peripheral edema
- constipation
- cold intolerance

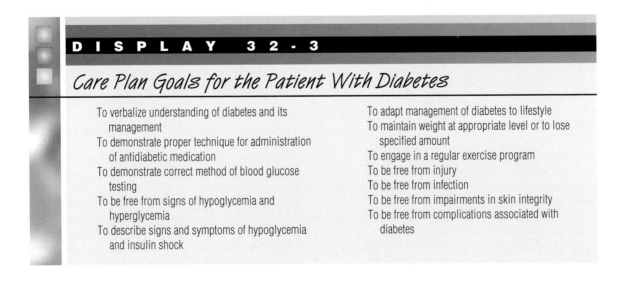

D I S P L A Y   3 2 - 3

Care Plan Goals for the Patient With Diabetes

To verbalize understanding of diabetes and its management

To demonstrate proper technique for administration of antidiabetic medication

To demonstrate correct method of blood glucose testing

To be free from signs of hypoglycemia and hyperglycemia

To describe signs and symptoms of hypoglycemia and insulin shock

To adapt management of diabetes to lifestyle

To maintain weight at appropriate level or to lose specified amount

To engage in a regular exercise program

To be free from injury

To be free from infection

To be free from impairments in skin integrity

To be free from complications associated with diabetes

- myalgia, paresthesia, and ataxia
- dry skin and coarse hair

TREATMENT

Treatment includes replacement of thyroid hormone using a synthetic T_4 (eg, Synthroid, thyroxine). Initially, a low dose is recommended to avoid exacerbation of asymptomatic coronary artery disease that could occur from rapid replacement. Desiccated thyroid preparations are avoided. Regular monitoring will provide feedback for the need for dosage adjustments.

KEY CONCEPT
Initially, thyroid replacement is prescribed at a low dose and gradually increased under close supervision to prevent cardiac complications.

Nursing measures should support the treatment plan and assist patients with the management of symptoms (eg, prevention of constipation and provision of extra clothing to compensate for cold intolerance). It is important that patients understand that thyroid replacement will most likely be a lifelong requirement.

Hyperthyroidism

At the other extreme from hypothyroidism is a condition known as *hyperthyroidism*. In this disorder, the thyroid gland secretes excess amounts of thyroid hormones. Hyperthyroidism is less prevalent than hypothyroidism in older adults; it affects women more than men.

Diagnostic testing can be challenging because blood tests do not always reflect hyperthyroidism. This is particularly true in malnourished elders, whose T_3 levels will be reduced due to their nutritional status; thus, the excess secretion will cause the T_3 to fall within a normal range. Diagnosis relies on evaluation of T_4 and free T_4, TSH, and increased uptake of radionuclide thyroid scans.

SYMPTOMS

Classic symptoms of hyperthyroidism include diaphoresis, tachycardia, palpitations, hypertension, tremor, diarrhea, stare, lid lag, insomnia, nervousness, confusion, heat intolerance, increased hunger, proximal muscle weakness, and hyperreflexia. However, like hypothyroidism, hyperthyroidism can present with atypical symptoms in older adults. For example, increased perspiration may not occur, and for the person with a history of chronic constipation, diarrhea may be displayed by now having regular bowel movements.

TREATMENT

Treatment of hyperthyroidism depends on the cause. In *Graves' disease,* an autoimmune disorder that leads to the production of an antibody to the TSH receptor that stimulates thyroid growth and overproduction of thyroid hormone, or when there is a *single autonomous nodule,* treatment typically includes antithyroid medications or radioactive iodine. If *toxic multinodular goiter* is the underlying cause, surgery may be preferred due to the delayed and incomplete response to medications. Hypothyroidism can develop as a complication in persons who have had surgery or radioactive iodine therapy.

Patients with a history of thyroid disease need special monitoring when experiencing an acute illness, surgery, or trauma because this can precipitate extreme thyrotoxicosis (thyroid storm). Hospitalization may be required to return their thyroid level to a normal range.

Hyperlipidemia

The risk of coronary artery disease associated with elevated total cholesterol increases with age, primarily because of increases in low-density lipoprotein (LDL). In addition to age, older persons may have conditions that can cause lipoprotein disorders, such as uncontrolled diabetes, hypothyroidism, uremia, and nephrotic syndrome, or be using corticosteroids, thiazide diuretics, and other drugs that increase the risk.

DIAGNOSIS

In evaluating the patient, a full lipid profile rather than just a plasma total cholesterol level should be obtained. Because cholesterol values can change from day to day, no single laboratory value should be used to classify a patient. Triglyceride levels are sensitive to food; therefore, a definitive screening test requires that the patient fast for 12 hours prior to testing. A high-density lipoprotein (HDL) level greater than 60 mg/dL is desirable; triglycerides greater than 200 mg/dL are borderline and greater than 240 mg/dL are high. An LDL less than 100 mg/dL is recommended for people with coronary heart disease or diabetes; a level less than 130 mg/dL is advised for persons without coronary heart disease or diabetes who have two or more coronary risk factors and less; LDL less than 160 mg/dL is desirable for persons without coronary heart disease or diabetes who have one or no risk factors.

If secondary causes of lipoprotein disorders (eg, diet high in saturated fat or cholesterol, excessive alcohol intake, exogenous estrogen supplementation, poorly controlled diabetes, uremia, use of β-blockers or corticosteroids) can be ruled out, a primary or familial lipoprotein disorder may be present. The most common familial lipoproteinemias are transmitted as autosomal dominant traits, so children of elders affected by this condition should be screened and counseled regarding lifestyle practices that can prevent hypercholesterolemia.

TREATMENT

Dietary changes and exercise are the initial approaches to treating this condition. The American Heart Association's (AHA) step 1 diet is recommended for initial treatment. If the patient is following a diet similar to the step 1 diet already, a step 2 diet will be prescribed. The gerontological nurse should refer patients to a nutritionist for guidance on these diets. As mentioned in Chapter 32, the Dean Ornish diet is more restrictive than the AHA diet and has been shown to improve LDL levels. Some general dietary guidelines are shown in Display 32-4. Other lifestyle practices that can assist include reducing weight and limiting alcohol intake. A variety of medications can be used if diet and lifestyle modifications alone do not bring about results. These can include bile acid sequestrants (cholestyramine, colestipol), nicotinic acid (niacin [Nicolar]), 3-hydroxy-3-methylglutaryl-coenzyme A (HMG CoA) reductase inhibitors (pravastatin, fluvastatin, simvastatin), fibric acid derivatives (gemfibrozil, clofibrate), and omega-3 fatty acids (fish oils).

> **KEY CONCEPT**
> Dietary and lifestyle changes required to reduce cholesterol levels can be difficult to make.

Some alternative and complementary therapies have also proven beneficial in reducing cholesterol levels, such as water-soluble fiber (oats, guar gum, pectin, mixed fibers) garlic supplements, green tea, and antioxidant vitamins A, C, and E and β-carotene.

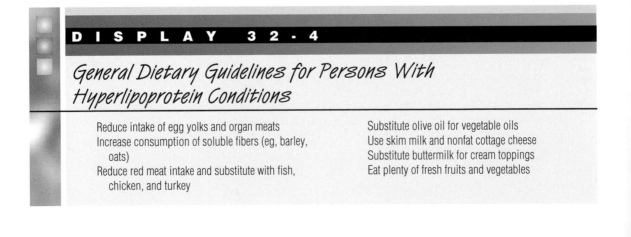

DISPLAY 32-4

General Dietary Guidelines for Persons With Hyperlipoprotein Conditions

Reduce intake of egg yolks and organ meats
Increase consumption of soluble fibers (eg, barley, oats)
Reduce red meat intake and substitute with fish, chicken, and turkey

Substitute olive oil for vegetable oils
Use skim milk and nonfat cottage cheese
Substitute buttermilk for cream toppings
Eat plenty of fresh fruits and vegetables

Critical Thinking Exercises

1. Discuss reasons for different norms to be used to interpret the outcomes of glucose tolerance tests in the elderly.
2. Describe the challenges to physical and psychosocial well-being faced by the older diabetic patient.
3. In what ways do age-related changes affect the presentation of symptoms and risks associated with diabetes and thyroid disease?
4. Outline a teaching plan for the person with hyperlipidemia that includes natural and alternative/complementary therapies.

Web Connect

Review the American Heart Association's recommendations for cholesterol screening at www.americanheart.org/presenter.jhtml?identifier=4504.

●Resources

American Diabetes Association
1701 North Beauregard Street
Alexandria, VA 22311
(800) 342-2383
www.diabetes.org

American Heart Association
7272 Greenville Avenue
Dallas, TX 75231
(800) 242-8721
www.americanheart.org

National Diabetes Information Clearinghouse
1 Information Way
Bethesda, MD 20892
(301) 654-3327
www.niddk.nih.gov/health/diabetes/ndic.html

●Recommended Readings

American Diabetes Association. (2002). *American Diabetes Association complete guide to diabetes: Ultimate home reference from the diabetes experts.* New York: McGraw Hill.

Brownstein, D. (2002). *Overcoming thyroid disorders.* New York: Medical Alternatives Press.

Cameron, B. L. (2002). Making diabetes management routine. *American Journal of Nursing, 102*(2), 26–33.

Cuchel, M., & Rader, D. J. (2003). The value of raising HDL cholesterol in the elderly. *University of Pennsylvania Institute on Aging,* Winter 2003, pp. 8–10.

Duvoisen, R. (2003) *Diabetes sourcebook: Basic consumer health information about type 1 diabetes, type 2 diabetes, gestational diabetes, and related disorders* (3rd ed.). Detroit: Omnigraphics.

Fleming, D. R. (1999). Challenging traditional insulin injection practices. *American Journal of Nursing, 99*(2), 72–74.

Helfand, M., & Redfern, C. C. (1998). Screening for thyroid disease: An update. *Annals of Internal Medicine, 129,* 144–158.

Johns Hopkins Medical Institutions. (2000). Diabetes complications: More than skin deep. *Health After 50, 11*(11), 6.

Kennedy, J. W., & Caro, J. F. (1996). The ABCs of managing hyperthyroidism in the older patient. *Geriatrics, 51*(5), 22–24, 27, 31–32.

LaRosa, J. C. (1996). Dyslipidemia and coronary artery disease in the elderly. *Clinics in Geriatric Medicine, 12*(1), 33–40.

Lindeman, R. D., Yau, C. L., Baumgartner, R. N., Morley, J. E., & Garry, P. J. (2003). Longitudinal study of fasting serum glucose concentrations in healthy elderly: The New Mexico aging process study. *Journal of Nutrition, Health, and Aging, 7*(3), 172–177.

Mealey, B. L., & Rethman, M. P. (2003). Periodontal disease and diabetes mellitus. Bidirectional relationship. *Dentistry Today, 22*(4), 107–113.

Mount Sinai School of Medicine. (2000). Exercise lowers diabetes risk. *Focus on Health Aging, 3*(2), 2.

Rahman, K. (2001). Historical perspective on garlic and cardiovascular disease. *Journal of Nutrition, 131*(3s), 977S–979S.

Shoback, D., & Jaffe, M. (1996). Thyroid disease and disorders of calcium and phosphorus balance. In E. T. Lonergan (Ed.), *Geriatrics* (pp. 166–182). Stamford, CT: Appleton & Lange.

Sinha, B., & Nattrass, M. (2001). Efficacy of new drug therapies for diabetes in the elderly. *Annals of Long-Term Care, 9*(6), 23–29.

Tkacs, N. C. (2002). Hypoglycemia unawareness. *American Journal of Nursing, 102*(2), 34–40.

Yen, P. (2002). Treating diabetes with diet. *Geriatric Nursing, 23*(5), 175–176.

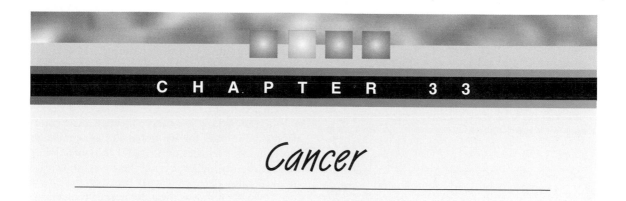

CHAPTER 33

Cancer

■ *Chapter Outline*

■ *Learning Objectives*

After reading this chapter, you should be
able to:

- discuss the prevalence and risks of
  cancer in the elderly

- describe reasons for cancer being
  more complex in the elderly

- list factors that increase the risk of
  cancer

- outline measures that can reduce the
  risk of cancer

- describe risks of older adults receiving
  conventional cancer treatment

- discuss reasons for patients' choice to
  use complementary and alternative
  medicine (CAM)

- list issues to be evaluated in the selection of CAM
- discuss nursing considerations in caring for older patients with cancer

Caring for elders with cancer is a nearly inescapable aspect of gerontological nursing. Cancer is a disease of older people, being the second leading cause of death in persons age 65 years and older (National Center for Health Statistics, 2001). Most new cases are diagnosed in older adults, and the probability of developing this disease dramatically increases with advancing age. The National Cancer Institute acknowledges that age is the single most important risk factor for cancer. Cancer rates increase from childhood on, with the most dramatic increases being in late life (Table 33-1). The rates peak at age 80–84 for males and at age 85 and above for females, the rates for white and black females do not increase as rapidly as those for their male counterparts. The rates for white females are similar to those for black females until age 70 and older, when they are slightly higher. Even if there was no increase in cancer rates, the prevalence of cancer in the elderly will rise in the future as the older population continues to grow.

> **KEY CONCEPT**
> More than half of persons diagnosed with cancer are over age 65.

TABLE 33-1 ● *Percentage* of Population Diagnosed With Cancer in the Previous 10 Years*

Men						Women					
Age	All ages	50–59	60–69	70–79	80+	Age	All ages	50–59	60–69	70–79	80+
Site/Rate/Ethnicity											
All sites	2	2	7	14	14	*All sites*	1.9	4	6	7	7
Whites	2	2.5	7.5	14	14	Whites	2	4	6	8	7.5
Blacks	2.5	2.9	9	15	13.5	Blacks	1.5	3	4	6	6
Hispanic	1.5	1	5	9	8.5	Hispanic	1	2	4	4.5	4
Asian/Pacific Islander	1.5	1	4	9	11	Asian/Pacific Islander	1	3	4	5	5
Colon and rectum	.3	.3	.8	1.5	1.9	*Colon and rectum*	.2	.2	.6	1	1.6
Whites	.3	.3	.8	1.5	1.9	Whites	.2	.2	.6	1	1.6
Blacks	.3	.4	.9	1.3	1.6	Blacks	.2	.3	.7	1.1	1.4
Hispanic	.2	.2	.6	1	1	Hispanic	.1	.2	.4	.6	.8
Asian/Pacific Islander	.3	.3	.8	1.5	2	Asian/Pacific Islander	.2	.2	.5	.9	1.3
Lung and bronchus	.1	.1	.4	.7	.4	*Lung and bronchus*	.08	.1	.3	.4	.3
Whites	.1	.1	.4	.6	.4	Whites	.08	.1	.3	.5	.3
Blacks	.1	.2	.6	.7	.4	Blacks	.08	.1	.3	.4	.2
Hispanic	.05	.06	.2	.3	.2	Hispanic	.03	.04	.1	.2	.1
Asian/Pacific Islander	.1	.1	.3	.7	.4	Asian/Pacific Islander	.04	.06	.2	.2	.2
Prostate	1	.8	4	8	8	*Breast*	.8	2.5	2.5	3	3
Whites	1	.7	4	8	8	Whites	.09	3	3	3	3
Blacks	2	1	6	11	10	Blacks	.7	2	2	2	2
Hispanic	.7	.4	2.4	6	5	Hispanic	.5	1.5	1.5	2	1
Asian/Pacific Islander	.6	.2	1.5	5	6	Asian/Pacific Islander	.6	2	2	2	2

*Rounded to nearest whole number.
Source: U.S. Bureau of the Census. (1999). Estimated percent population diagnosed with cancer in the previous 10 years by age at prevalence, site, and race/ethnicity. Table 29, Washington, D.C.: Bureau of the Census.

Cancer in any age group presents many clinical challenges; however, in older adults, the complexities grow. Despite having the highest rate of most cancers, the elderly have the lowest rate of receiving early detection tests, thus their disease may be in an advanced stage when diagnosed (Walker & Covinsky, 2001). In addition, it is the rare older adult who doesn't have another health condition (eg, heart disease, diabetes mellitus, arthritis, or chronic obstructive pulmonary disease [COPD]) present when diagnosed with cancer. The presence of multiple health conditions elevates the risk of complications, disability, and death for older patients diagnosed with cancer. Further, concern regarding how the older patient's already compromised organs will tolerate chemotherapy and other cancer therapies could impact treatment decisions. Survival rates for older adults are lower than in younger persons for most types of cancer, even if they are diagnosed at the same stage.

Gerontological nurses have a significant role to play in the prevention, diagnosis, and treatment of cancer. By encouraging healthy lifestyle habits in persons of all ages, the risk factors for developing cancer can be reduced. Educating patients about cancer screening and facilitating their efforts to obtain tests can enable cancers to be detected in early stages, thereby increasing survival rates. Creative, holistic, and skillful nursing interventions that offer support—physical, emotional, and spiritual—to individuals diagnosed with cancer and their significant others promote the best possible quality of life in the presence of the disease.

Aging and Cancer

As mentioned, cancer primarily is a disease of old age, but why is that so? There are two major theories that attempt to explain the increased incidence of cancer with age. The first has to do with biological changes that impair the ability to resist diseases. This is supported by decreases in the mitochondrial activity of the cell that reduces its ability to resist cancer. Changes in the immune system (reduced T-cell activity, interleukin-2 levels, and mitogen responsiveness) impair the body's ability to recognize cancerous cells and destroy them.

Prolonged exposure to carcinogens over the years is another explanation for the rising incidence of cancer with age. This is demonstrated by the growth of melanomas on the skin of persons who have had chronic exposure to damaging ultraviolet rays and the development of lung cancer in industrial workers who regularly breathed toxic substances. Although the extent of responsibility that either age-related changes or exposure has in the development of cancer cannot be clearly stated at this time, it is evident that aging adults face an increased risk of developing cancer; therefore, the reduction of risk factors is beneficial.

> **KEY CONCEPT**
> The increased incidence of cancer with age could result from age-related changes that reduce the ability to resist the disease or prolonged exposure to carcinogens.

Cancer Risk Factors

HEREDITY

Inherited alterations in the genes called BRCA1 and BRCA2 (short for *breast cancer 1* and *breast cancer 2*) are involved in many cases of hereditary breast and ovarian cancer. The risk that BRCA1 or BRCA2 is associated with these cancers is highest in women with a family history of multiple cases of breast cancer; with at least one family member having two primary cancers at different sites, or who are of Eastern European (Ashkenazi) Jewish background. (Breast Cancer Linkage Consortium, 1999; Brekelmans et al., 2001).

> **KEY CONCEPT**
> As many as 10% of women carry the gene for the hereditary form of breast cancer.

DIET

There is a link between a high-fat diet and certain cancers, such as cancer of the breast, colon, uterus, and prostate. Obesity increases the rates of cancer of the prostate, pancreas, uterus, colon, and ovary and to breast cancer in older women. Conversely, a diet rich in fiber and antioxidants can offer protection against some types of cancer.

Research has shown that cooking certain meats at high temperatures creates chemicals that are not present in uncooked meats, and a few of these chemicals may increase cancer risk. In addition, researchers have discovered that people who ate diets high in animal fat had higher rates of stomach cancer than those who ate low animal fat diets (Palli et al., 2000). Additional studies have shown that an increased risk of developing colorectal, pancreatic, and breast cancer is associated with high intakes of well-done, fried, or barbecued meats. Microwaving meats at least 2 minutes before cooking can reduce the risk (Thomas, 2003).

> **KEY CONCEPT**
> Eating foods as close to their natural form as possible is a good health habit and could have benefits in reducing the risk of cancer.

Many people fear that food additives, which now number in the thousands, are causing a variety of conditions, ranging from attention deficit disorder to cancer. However, there is no clear evidence that food additives are risk factors for cancer. The government claims that the careful laboratory screening of these substances before they are introduced to the market assures safety. (Information about food additives is available from the U.S. Food and Drug Administration's Center for Food Safety and Applied Nutrition, Direct Additives Branch, 200 C Street SW, Washington, DC 20204; 202-205-4314).

NITRATES

The contamination of drinking water from nitrate, a chemical used in fertilizers, has been associated with an increased risk of non-Hodgkin's lymphoma (Ward et al., 2000). The risk is directly correlated to the level of nitrates consumed and is particularly high in rural areas. Interestingly, vegetables high in nitrate content, such as spinach, beets, and lettuce, did not carry the same risk.

Although the correlation between higher rates of brain cancer and the use of aspartame gave rise to suspicion that artificial sweeteners are a risk factor in the development of cancer, the link between artificial sweeteners and cancer has not been proven (Butchko et al., 2002).

Coffee was believed to contribute to cancer, but the National Cancer Institute has not proved any link. Solvents (eg, ethylene chloride [dichloromethane], ethyl acetate, and trichloroethylene) once used in the process of decaffeinating coffee were suspected as having a role in cancer development; however, coffee makers now use alternative solvents that are considered without risk.

FLUORIDATED WATER

Considerable debate has gone on regarding the role of fluoridated water in the development of cancer. However, numerous studies have not shown that fluoride increases the risk of cancer, and the National Cancer Institute (2003) supports this position.

TOBACCO

Cigarette smoking is the most significant cause of lung cancer and the leading cause of lung cancer death in both men and women. Smoking is also responsible for one third of all cancer deaths and for most cancers of the larynx, oral cavity, and esophagus. It is highly associated with the development of, and deaths from, bladder, kidney, pancreatic, and cervical cancers (American Health Foundation, 2003).

> **KEY CONCEPT**
> Environmental exposure to secondhand smoke increases the risk of lung cancer to nonsmokers.

ALCOHOL

Heavy alcohol consumption increases the risk of cancer of the mouth, throat, esophagus, larynx, and liver. It is wise to limit alcoholic beverages to no more than two drinks per day.

RADIATION

Periodically, through the media or questions from consumers, nurses may hear concern that the radiation emitted from handheld cellular phones can increase the risk of cancer. Although no studies to date have shown a definite relationship, the long-term health effects of cellular phone use is yet to be known

(Inskip et al., 2001; Trichopoulos & Adami, 2001; Warren, Prevatt, Daly, & Antonelli, 2003).

Before the 1950s, x-rays were used to treat acne, ringworm of the scalp, and enlarged thymus, tonsils, and adenoids. This exposure to radiation increased the risk for thyroid cancer. It is important to ask about these treatments in the health assessment of older adults so that special attention can be given to examination of their thyroid gland.

ULTRAVIOLET RADIATION

Repeated exposure to ultraviolet rays from the sun, sunlamps, and tanning beds can increase the risk of skin cancer, particularly in persons with fair skin. Blocking the sun's rays with hats and long-sleeved clothing and using sunscreens rated between 15 and 30 sun protection factor (SPF) are useful protective measures.

KEY CONCEPT
It is important to advise younger people that the tanning they subject their skin to today could cost them in an increased risk of cancer as they grow older.

OCCUPATIONAL EXPOSURE TO CARCINOGENS

Exposure to asbestos, nickel, cadmium, uranium, radon, vinyl chloride, benzene, and other substances can increase the risk of cancer. This reinforces the importance of obtaining a full occupational history during the assessment to identify potential health risks.

RADON

Radon is an invisible, odorless, and tasteless gas that seeps up through the ground and diffuses into the air. It can enter homes through cracks in the foundation. Outdoors, radon gas exists at harmless levels, but in areas without adequate ventilation, radon can accumulate to levels that substantially increase the risk of lung cancer (Duckworth, Frank-Stromborg, Oleckno, Duffy, & Burns, 2002). This happens because when radon decays, it emits tiny radioactive particles that damage the lungs when inhaled. Inexpensive

testing kits are available to determine the radon level in a home. If high radon levels are detected, special measures can be taken to reduce them. (More information can be obtained through state and local government agencies and from the National Safety Council's radon hotline at 1-800-SOS-RADON (1-800-767-7236).

SPECIAL RISKS FOR WOMEN

A variety of factors have been associated with increased breast and ovarian cancer risk (Martin & Weber, 2000). Because most of these cancers occur in women over age 50 years (except those cancers related to an altered BRCA1 or BRCA2 gene in women who often develop breast or ovarian cancer before age 50), increased age is a factor (Turchetti, Cortesi, Federico, Romagnoli, & Silingardi, 2002). Women who had their first menstrual period before the age of 12 or experienced menopause after age 55 have a slightly increased risk of breast cancer, as do women who had their first child after age 30. Women who have a first-degree relative (mother, sister, or daughter) or other close relative with breast and/or ovarian cancer may be at increased risk for developing these cancers. Women whose mothers took diethylstilbestrol (DES) during pregnancy have an increased risk of vaginal cancer (Li et al., 2003). In addition, women with relatives who have had colon cancer are at increased risk of developing ovarian cancer. Excess estrogen is suspected to contribute to breast cancer because of its natural role in stimulating breast cell growth. Long-term hormonal replacement therapy may increase a woman's risk of breast and ovarian cancer, although research is inconclusive at this time. Exercise could decrease the risk of breast cancer.

Point to Ponder
What are your risks for developing cancer?
What can you do to reduce them?

OTHER CONTRIBUTING FACTORS

A variety of additional factors have been speculated to have a role in cancer. For instance, some people think that because stress and other "toxic" emotions can depress immune function, they also can contribute to cancer. Evidence currently does not conclusively support this relationship. Some people have theorized that dental conditions could influence the development of breast cancer because they block the flow of energy through the acupuncture meridian on which the breast lies. The theories continue to grow. Gerontological nurses need discretion to sort through these theories and while promoting positive health habits, not alarm patients with unsupported claims.

Prevention

A review of the risk factors for cancer offer insights into some of the preventive measures that could prove useful in avoiding this disease. Display 33-1 offers some useful preventive measures that can be incorporated into health education and counseling.

> **KEY CONCEPT**
> Many cancers can be prevented by healthy lifestyle practices that minimize risks.

Screening

Early detection can improve prognosis of cancer and should be encouraged for persons of all ages. Medicare does provide reimbursement for screening tests for breast, cervical, colorectal, and prostate cancers. Some of the recommended tests are outlined in Display 33-2.

> **Point to Ponder**
> *What would be your primary concerns if you faced treatment for cancer?*

Treatment

CONVENTIONAL

The plan of treatment depends on the specific cancer; however, most conventional forms of treatment include surgery, radiation, chemotherapy, and biologic therapy. Although the same basic care measures will apply to older patients undergoing these treatments as to adults of any age, there are some unique risks. Persons over age 70 have a higher risk of mortality and complications from all surgeries, and this risk is heightened with emergency or unplanned surgeries, as can occur with an unexpected detection of a mass. Advanced age can affect the pharmacokinetics and pharmacodynamics of cytotoxic drugs and increase the risk of complications (eg, cardiotoxicity, neurotoxicity, and myelodepression). Doses need to be adjusted carefully to account for altered glomerular filtration rates and other differences. Fortunately, there is no significant difference between the elderly and adults of other ages in the ability to tolerate radiation therapy.

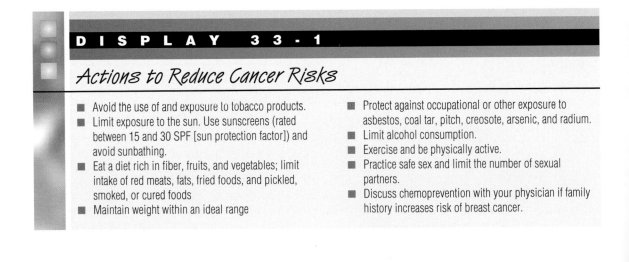

DISPLAY 33-1

Actions to Reduce Cancer Risks

- Avoid the use of and exposure to tobacco products.
- Limit exposure to the sun. Use sunscreens (rated between 15 and 30 SPF [sun protection factor]) and avoid sunbathing.
- Eat a diet rich in fiber, fruits, and vegetables; limit intake of red meats, fats, fried foods, and pickled, smoked, or cured foods
- Maintain weight within an ideal range

- Protect against occupational or other exposure to asbestos, coal tar, pitch, creosote, arsenic, and radium.
- Limit alcohol consumption.
- Exercise and be physically active.
- Practice safe sex and limit the number of sexual partners.
- Discuss chemoprevention with your physician if family history increases risk of breast cancer.

DISPLAY 33-2

Recommended Cancer Screening for Older Adults

- Annual check-up that examines oral cavity, thyroid, breasts, ovaries, testicles, and skin
- Annual mammogram
- Annual fecal occult blood test
- Flexible sigmoidoscopy every 5 years
- Double contrast barium enema every 5 years
- Colonoscopy every 10 years
- Pap test: every 2–3 years if there have been three consecutive normal tests; the American Cancer Society suggests that women 70 years of age or older who

have had three consecutive normal Pap tests and no abnormal Pap tests in the last 10 years may choose to discontinue cervical screening
- Annual endometrial biopsy for women at high risk for hereditary nonpolyposis colon cancer
- Annual prostate-specific antigen (PSA) and digital rectal examination beginning at age 50 (African-American men or those who have a first-degree relative diagnosed with prostate cancer at an early age should begin annual testing at age 45)

Based on recommendations of the American Cancer Society.

> **Point to Ponder**
>
> *Why would you seek complementary and alternative therapies if you or a loved one were diagnosed with cancer?*

COMPLEMENTARY AND ALTERNATIVE MEDICINE

Complementary and alternative therapies (CAM; see Display 33-3) are used by nearly half of all Americans and by more than 80% of people with cancer (Richardson, Sanders, Palmer, Greisinger, & Singletary, 2000). These therapies include special diets, psychotherapy, spiritual practices, vitamin supplements, and herbal remedies.

CAM therapies often are attractive to patients with cancer because of the healing philosophies and approaches used. CAM practitioners tend to have a holistic orientation. They are concerned with treating the disease but also likely to be equally, if not more, concerned with caring for the whole person. CAM practitioners offer:

- *Relationship-centered care:* They invest the time in learning about the unique characteristics of patients and enter a unique journey with each patient.

- *Support:* Learning to live with cancer is challenging and demanding. Even if the malignant cells are eliminated, emotional and spiritual pain may be present. CAM practitioners provide unconditional acceptance and understanding of patients "where they are"
- *Healing partnerships:* CAM practitioners honor patients' rights to control their care and their lives, seeing their role as empowering, facilitating, and supporting patients in the healing process.
- *Comfort:* Many CAM therapies are high touch and relieve stress and discomfort. Psychological comfort is provided as practitioners take the time to listen, to reassure, and to be emotionally available.
- *Hope:* Particularly when conventional medicine has exhausted its treatments, CAM practitioners provide options that can offer hope and encouragement through knowing that *something* is being attempted. Patients can heal—that is, feel a sense of wholeness and live the best possible quality of life—despite having an incurable disease.

Although CAM can contribute to a patient's care, it is unwise for patients to use these therapies without carefully weighing risks and benefits. The labels *natural* or *holistic* do not assure safety or that the therapy is the best option for the patient for his or her given circumstances. Display 33-4 offers some questions that nurses can use in assisting patients in evaluating

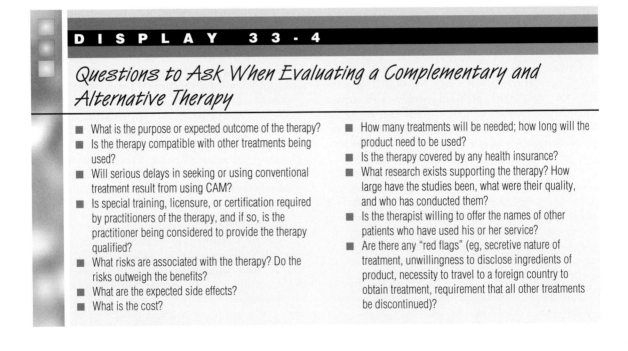

DISPLAY 33-3

Categories of Complementary and Alternative Therapies

The National Center for Complementary and Alternative Medicine (NCCAM) classifies CAM therapies into five groups or domains:

- alternative medical systems (eg, homeopathic medicine and traditional Chinese medicine)
- mind-body interventions (eg, visualizations and relaxation)
- manipulative and body-based methods (eg, chiropractic and massage)
- biologically based therapies (eg, vitamins and herbal products)
- energy therapies (eg, qi gong and therapeutic touch)

CAM. Nurses can provide a useful service to patients in helping them to research claims made by promoters of therapies and products to treat cancer. The National Cancer Institute and National Center for Complementary and Alternative Medicine (see Resource listings) can offer assistance in evaluating CAM claims.

Knowledge about CAM is rapidly growing, and today's hypotheses could be proved or disproved tomorrow. Nurses are challenged to stay current of this expanding field so that they can integrate CAM into their practice safely and effectively.

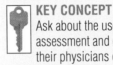 **KEY CONCEPT**
Ask about the use of CAM during every assessment and encourage patients to inform their physicians of all therapies and products being used.

DISPLAY 33-4

Questions to Ask When Evaluating a Complementary and Alternative Therapy

- What is the purpose or expected outcome of the therapy?
- Is the therapy compatible with other treatments being used?
- Will serious delays in seeking or using conventional treatment result from using CAM?
- Is special training, licensure, or certification required by practitioners of the therapy, and if so, is the practitioner being considered to provide the therapy qualified?
- What risks are associated with the therapy? Do the risks outweigh the benefits?
- What are the expected side effects?
- What is the cost?

- How many treatments will be needed; how long will the product need to be used?
- Is the therapy covered by any health insurance?
- What research exists supporting the therapy? How large have the studies been, what were their quality, and who has conducted them?
- Is the therapist willing to offer the names of other patients who have used his or her service?
- Are there any "red flags" (eg, secretive nature of treatment, unwillingness to disclose ingredients of product, necessity to travel to a foreign country to obtain treatment, requirement that all other treatments be discontinued)?

Other chapters of this book can be consulted for information about other cancers, eg, cancer of the colon (Chap. 26), breast (Chap. 28), prostate (Chap. 28), lung (Chap. 25), stomach (Chap. 26), testes (Chap. 28), and pancreas (Chap. 26).

Nursing Considerations

Gerontological nurses have a commitment to promoting healthy aging. One means of demonstrating this is to increase awareness of measures that can prevent cancer (Display 33-1). Opportunities for educating individuals can range from teaching formal group classes to discussing options for change when risk factors are identified during individual assessments. This education need not be limited to elders. Cancer prevention to younger people can promote a healthier senior population in the future.

Assure that patients understand the warning signs of cancer. The American Cancer Society's (2002) use of the word CAUTION, in which each letter represents the first letter of a warning sign, provides a useful way to remember them:

- **C**hange in bowel or bladder habits
- **A** sore that does not heal
- **U**nusual bleeding or drainage
- **T**hickening or lump in the breast or elsewhere
- **I**ndigestion or swallowing difficulty
- **O**bvious change in a wart or mole
- **N**agging persistent cough or hoarseness

In addition, assess patients' knowledge of self-examination for cancer (eg, breast examination, testicular examination, skin inspection); provide instruction as needed. For patients who are unable to perform self-examinations, develop a plan for caregivers to perform these examinations for these patients on a regular schedule. Inquire about dates of last cancer screening tests and refer for testing as needed.

When the diagnosis of cancer is made, help patients to obtain the best possible care. Some oncology centers may specialize in a particular cancer and be able to offer more options to patients than other facilities. Also, as appropriate, assist patients in contacting the National Cancer Institute to learn about clinical trials that may be beneficial.

The diagnosis of cancer can be considerably overwhelming and stressful to many patients. Older adults may recall the grim experiences of people with cancer they have known throughout their lives—people who were diagnosed years ago when treatment options were considerably more limited than today—and fear that their outlook will be similar. They may fear that they will experience pain, deformity, and lost independence. The cost of treatment could present significant burdens to patients and their families. Plans and pursuits may have to be forfeited as treatment of the disease takes center stage. Patients will need strong support during this time. Consult with the physician to learn about the patient's diagnosis, treatment plan, and prognosis. Assess the patient's understanding; clarify misconceptions and offer explanations where needed. Provide ample opportunity for the patient to express feelings.

Remember that the diagnosis of cancer touches lives beyond the patient's. Family and significant others may share the patient's concerns and have additional ones of their own. For example, a wife may worry that the cost of her husband's treatment or his death will place her in a financially vulnerable position. Or a daughter may grieve that her parent may not survive to see her marry. They, too, need support. (Local chapters of the American Cancer Society can provide information on support groups for people with cancer and their loved ones.)

Patients may experience a variety of reactions as they cope with their disease, including depression, grief, guilt, anger, bargaining, and acceptance. Similar to the grief experienced with the dying process, they may float in and out of various stages at different times. Sensitivity to the patient's emotional and spiritual status during each encounter is essential. Remember that family members may experience these same fluctuations in emotions

Older adults receiving radiation and chemotherapy require the same basic care and face the same general risks as adults of any age who undergo these treatments; oncology nursing literature should be consulted for guidance. The challenges with older adults may be increased because of common age-related factors that contribute to increased risks for malnutrition, dehydration, constipation, immobility, impaired skin integrity, and infection. Close monitoring and taking actions to prevent complications (eg, reporting changes in vital signs or increased fatigue) are essential.

A significant fear associated with cancer is pain. Patients need to be assured that pain can be managed.

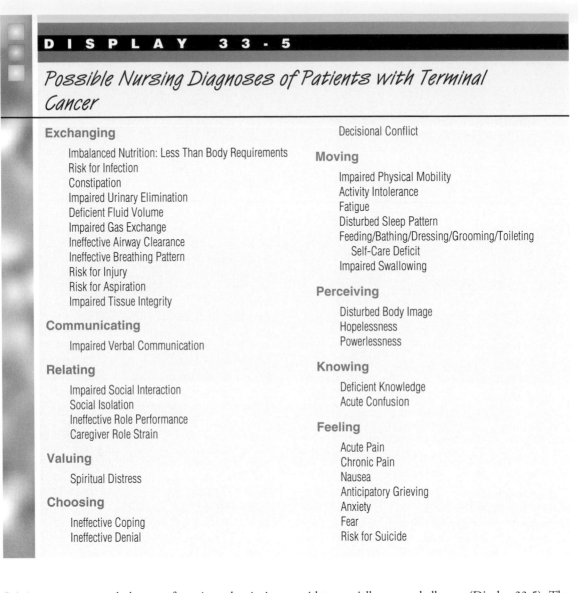

DISPLAY 33-5

Possible Nursing Diagnoses of Patients with Terminal Cancer

Exchanging

  Imbalanced Nutrition: Less Than Body Requirements
  Risk for Infection
  Constipation
  Impaired Urinary Elimination
  Deficient Fluid Volume
  Impaired Gas Exchange
  Ineffective Airway Clearance
  Ineffective Breathing Pattern
  Risk for Injury
  Risk for Aspiration
  Impaired Tissue Integrity

Communicating

  Impaired Verbal Communication

Relating

  Impaired Social Interaction
  Social Isolation
  Ineffective Role Performance
  Caregiver Role Strain

Valuing

  Spiritual Distress

Choosing

  Ineffective Coping
  Ineffective Denial

  Decisional Conflict

Moving

  Impaired Physical Mobility
  Activity Intolerance
  Fatigue
  Disturbed Sleep Pattern
  Feeding/Bathing/Dressing/Grooming/Toileting
    Self-Care Deficit
  Impaired Swallowing

Perceiving

  Disturbed Body Image
  Hopelessness
  Powerlessness

Knowing

  Deficient Knowledge
  Acute Confusion

Feeling

  Acute Pain
  Chronic Pain
  Nausea
  Anticipatory Grieving
  Anxiety
  Fear
  Risk for Suicide

It is important to regularly assess for pain and assist in developing a plan to prevent and manage pain. (See Chap. 17 for a fuller discussion of comfort measures.)

Physical, emotional, and spiritual support are required by patients with terminal cancer as they cope with potentially many challenges (Display 33-5). The needs of these patients and their families can change and demand regular reassessment and adjustment to the plan of care. Chapter 41 offers guidelines for end-of-life care that are applicable to patients with terminal cancer.

Critical Thinking Exercises

1. Develop an outline of the content for a health education program for a senior citizen group on "Cancer Prevention, Risks, and Diagnosis."
2. Describe current lifestyle factors that may affect the risk of cancer in future generations of elders.
3. Develop a plan of care for an older adult diagnosed with lung cancer that integrates conventional and CAM therapies.
4. What actions could nurses take in their communities to reduce cancer risks?

Web Connect

Learn about cancer research priorities and clinical trials and obtain general information about cancer at the National Cancer Institute's website, www.cancer.gov/.

● Resources

Sources of National Cancer Institute Information

Cancer Information Service
Toll-free: 1-800-4-CANCER (1-800-422-6237)
TTY (for deaf and hard of hearing callers): 1-800-332-8615

NCI Online
Use http://cancer.gov to reach NCI's website.

The National Center for Complementary and Alternative Medicine Clearinghouse
This organization offers fact sheets and other publications, and responds to inquiries from the public

NCCAM Clearinghouse
P.O. Box 7923
Gaithersburg, MD 20898-7923
Telephone: 1-888-644-6226 (toll free)
Fax: 1-866-464-3616
Website: http://nccam.nih.gov

● References

American Cancer Society. (2002). *Cancer Facts and Figures 2002*. Atlanta, GA: American Cancer Society.

American Health Foundation. (2003). Cancer etiology and prevention. Retrieved May 29, 2003, from http://www.ahf.org/research/research03.html.

The Breast Cancer Linkage Consortium. (1999)Cancer risks in BRCA2 mutation carriers. *Journal of the National Cancer Institute, 91*(15), 1310–1316.

Brekelmans, C. T. M., Seynaeve, C., Bartels, C. C. M., et al.

(2001). Effectiveness of breast cancer surveillance in BRCA1/2 gene mutation carriers and women with high familial risk. *Journal of Clinical Oncology, 19*(4), 924–930

Butchko, H. H., Stargel, W. W., Comer, C. P. et al. (2002). Aspartame: review of safety. *Regulatory Toxicology and Pharmacology Journal, 35*(2 Pt 2), S1–S93

Duckworth, L. T., Frank-Stromborg, M., Oleckno, W. A., Duffy, P., & Burns, K. (2002). Relationship of perception of radon as a health risk and willingness to engage in radon testing and mitigation. *Oncology Nursing Forum, 29*(7), 1099–1107.

Inskip, P. D., Tarone, R. E., Hatch, E. E., et al. (2001). Cellular telephone use and brain tumors. *New England Journal of Medicine, 344*(2), 79–86.

Li, S., Hursting, S. D., Davis, B. J., et al. (2003). Environmental exposure, DNA methylation, and gene regulation: lessons from diethylstilbestrol-induced cancers [review]. *Annals of New York Academy of Science, 983*(1), 161–169.

Martin, A. M., & Weber, B. L. (2000). Genetic and hormonal risk factors in breast cancer. *Journal of the National Cancer Institute, 92*(14), 1126–1135.

National Cancer Institute. (2003). *Fluoridated water*. National Cancer Institute's Cancer Facts website. Retrieved April 2, 2004, from http://cis.nci.nih.gov/fact/3_15.htm.

National Centers for Health Statistics. (2001). Leading causes of death. Retrieved April 2, 2004, from www.cdc.gov/nchs/data/nvsr/nvsr49/nvsr49_11.pdf.

Palli, D., Russo, A., Sajeva, C., et al (2000). Dietary and familial determinants of 10-year survival among patients with gastric carcinoma. *Cancer, 89,* 1205–1213.

Richardson, M. A., Sanders, T., Palmer, J. L., Greisinger, A., & Singletary, S. E. (2000). Complementary/alternative medicine use in a comprehensive cancer center and the implications for oncology. *Journal of Clinical Oncology, 18*(13), 2505–2514.

Thomas, C. (2003). Common sense about food and cancer. *Cancerpage.com.* Retrieved May 27, 2003, from www.cancerpage.com/cancernews/cancernews2081.htm.

Trichopoulos, D., & Adami, H. O. (2001). Cellular telephones and brain tumors. *New England Journal of Medicine, 344*(2), 133–134.

Turchetti, D., Cortesi, L., Federico, M., Romagnoli, R., & Silingardi, V. (2002). Hereditary risk of breast cancer: not only BRCA. *Journal of Experimental Clinical Cancer Research, 21*(3 Suppl), 17–21.

Walker, L., & Covinsky, K. E. (2001). Cancer screening in elderly patients: A framework for individualized decision making. *Journal of the American Medical Association, 285,* 2750–2765.

Ward, M. H., Mark, S. D., Cantor, K. P., Weisenburger, D. D., Correa-Villasenor, A., et al. (2000). Non-Hodgkin's lymphoma and nitrate in drinking water. *Journal of Epidemiology and Community Health, 54*(10), 772–723

Warren, H.G., Prevatt, A. A., Daly, K. A., & Antonelli, P. J. (2003). Cellular telephone use and risk of intratemporal facial nerve tumor. *Laryngoscope, 13*(4), 663–667.

● Recommended Readings

American Cancer Society. (2000). *American Cancer Society's Guide to Complementary and Alternative Cancer Methods.* Atlanta, GA: American Cancer Society.

Centers for Disease Control and Prevention. (1999). Achievements in public health, 1900–1999: fluoridation of drinking water to prevent dental caries. *Morbidity and Mortality Weekly Report, 48*(41)933–940.

Devita, V. T., Hellman, S., & Rosenberg, S. A. (2001). *Cancer: Principles and Practices of Oncology* (6th ed.). Philadelphia: Lippincott Williams & Wilkins.

Eisenberg, D. M., Davis, R. B., Ettner, S. L., et al. (2000). Trends in alternative medicine use in the United States, 1990–1997. *Journal of the American Medical Association, 280*(18), 1569–1675.

Gates, R. A., & Fink, R. M. (2001). *Oncology nursing secrets.* Philadelphia: Lippincott Williams & Wilkins.

Jacobs, J. (1997). Unproven alternative methods of cancer treatment. In: DeVita, Hellman, Rosenberg (Eds.). *Cancer: Principles and practice of oncology* (5th ed., pp. 2993–3001). Philadelphia: Lippincott-Raven Publishers.

Kao, G. D., & Devine, P. (2000). Use of complementary health practices by prostate carcinoma patients undergoing radiation therapy. *Cancer, 88*(3), 615–619.

Love, S. M., & Lindsey, K. (2000). *Dr. Susan Love's breast book.* Perseus Publishing.

McGinn, K. A., & Haylock, P. J. (2003). *Women's cancers: How to prevent them, how to treat them, how to beat them.* Alameda, CA: Hunter House.

Otto, S. E. (2001). *Oncology nursing.* St. Louis: Mosby.

Sparber, A., Bauer, L., Curt, G., et al. (2000). Use of complementary medicine by adult patients participating in cancer clinical trials. *Oncology Nursing Forum, 27*(4), 623–630.

Walsh, P. C., & Worthington, J. F. (2002). *Dr Patrick Walsh's guide to surviving prostate cancer.* New York: Warner Books.

Wilkes, G. M., Ingwersen, K., & Barton-Burke, M. (2003). *Oncology nursing drug handbook.* New York: Jones and Bartlett Publishers.

Conditions Affecting Mood and Cognition

■ Chapter Outline

Aging and mental health
  Myths
  Incidence of mental health problems
Promoting mental health
  Good lifelong mental health practices
  Principles of care
  Common problems confronting the
    elderly
Selected conditions
  Delirium
  Dementia
    Alzheimer's disease
    Other dementias
    Caring for persons with dementia
  Depression
  Suicide
  Anxiety
  Alcohol abuse
  Paranoia
  Hypochondriasis
Nursing considerations
  Monitoring medications
  Promoting a positive self-concept
  Managing behavioral problems

■ Learning Objectives

After reading this chapter, you should be able to:

- describe the realities of mental health and illness in late life

- list measures that enhance mental health for older adults

- differentiate delirium from dementia

- identify factors that cause delirium

- describe the progression of symptoms of dementia

- list causes of dementia

- outline nursing actions for the patient with Alzheimer's disease

- describe the symptoms and care of the older person with depression

- identify indications of suicidal thoughts

- describe interventions to reduce anxiety

- discuss the scope and signs of alcohol abuse in the elderly

- list reasons for hypochondriasis
- identify factors to consider in monitoring psychotropic medications
- describe factors that promote a positive self-concept
- identify nursing actions to manage disruptive behavior

Mental health indicates a capacity to cope effectively with and manage life's stresses in an effort to achieve a state of emotional homeostasis. Older people have an advantage over other age groups in that they probably have had more experience with coping, problem solving, and managing crises by virtue of the years they have lived. Most older persons have few delusions regarding what they are or what they are going to be. They know where they have been, what they have accomplished, and who they really are. Immigrating to a new country, watching loved ones die from epidemics, fighting in world wars, and surviving the Great Depression may be among the numerous stresses that today's elderly have faced and overcome. Such experiences have provided them with unique strength that should not be underestimated. This is not to imply that psychiatric illness is not a problem among the older population. More people than ever are reaching old age; many bring to their later years the mental health problems they have possessed throughout their lifetimes. The many losses and challenges of old age may exceed the physical, emotional, and social resources of some persons and promote mental illness. By promoting mental health, detecting problems early (Display 34-1, Nursing Diagnosis Table 34-1), and minimizing the impact of existing psychiatric problems, nurses can help older people achieve optimal satisfaction and function.

✔ **Point to Ponder**
What does mental health mean to you?

Aging and Mental Health

Many myths prevail regarding mental health and the elderly. For instance, many people still believe that loss of mental functioning, senility, or mental incompetence is a natural part of old age. Stereotypes about personality in later life propagate through descriptions of elders being childlike, rigid, or cantankerous. Frequently, these misconceptions are so widely accepted that when pathological signs are demonstrated by an older person, it is considered normal and no attempt is made to intervene. Nurses can play a significant role in ensuring that the myths and realities of mental health in old age are understood.

Cognitive function in later life is highly individualized, based on personal resources, health status, and the unique experiences of the individual's life. The incidence of mental illness is higher among the old than among the young. A significant number of elderly in the community and in nursing homes have symptoms of serious mental health problems. Nearly 10% of the older population has a problem with alcoholism, and nearly one fourth of all suicides are committed by persons aged 65 years and older (Knauer, 2003). Between 4% and 5% of the elderly are victims of Alzheimer's disease, and scientists project a dramatic increase in prevalence unless new ways to prevent and treat the disease are discovered (National Institutes of Health, 2003). Depression increases in prevalence and intensity with age (Charney, Reynolds, & Lewis, 2003). Multiple losses, altered sensory function, and alterations, discomforts, and demands associated with illnesses that the elderly frequently encounter set the stage for a variety of mental health problems.

> **KEY CONCEPT**
> Cognitive function among elders is highly individualized based on their health status, experiences, and personal resources.

Promoting Mental Health

Mental health in old age implies a satisfaction and interest in life. This can be displayed in a variety of ways, ranging from silent reflection to zealous activity. The quiet individual who stays at home does not necessarily have less mental capacity or mental health than the person who is actively involved in every possible community program. There is no single profile for mental health; thus, attempts to assess an older

D I S P L A Y   3 4 - 1

Assessment of Mental Health

Every comprehensive assessment includes an evaluation of mental status. Because patients may be anxious, embarrassed, or insulted by having their mental status reviewed, an explanation of the importance of and the reasons for it can prove useful. The evaluation should be approached in a matter-of-fact manner, not in an apologetic or intimidating one, with reassurance that this evaluation is part of every patient's assessment. Making the patient comfortable and establishing rapport before the assessment can reduce some of the barriers to an effective examination.

General Observations

Assessment of mental status actually begins the moment the nurse meets the patient. The initial observation can yield insight into mental health, and as such, attention should be paid to the following indicators:

Grooming and dress: Is clothing appropriate for the season, clean and presentable, appropriately worn? Is the patient clean? Is the hair clean and combed? Are makeup and accessories excessive or bizarre?

Posture: Does the patient appear stooped and fearful? Is body alignment normal?

Movement: Are tongue rolling, twitching, tremors, or hand wringing present? Are movements hyperactive or hypoactive?

Facial expression: Is it masklike or overly dramatic? Are there indications of pain, fear, or anger?

Level of consciousness. Does the patient drift into sleep and need to be aroused (ie, lethargic)? Does the patient offer only incomplete or slow responses and need repeated arousal (ie, stuporous)? Are painful stimuli the only thing the patient responds to (ie, semiconscious)? Is there no response, even to painful stimuli (ie, unconscious)?

While the nurse observes the patient, general conversation can aid in evaluating mental status. The nurse can note the tone of voice, rate of speech, ability to articulate, use of unusual words or combinations of words, and appropriateness of speech. Mood also can be evaluated during this time.

Interview

Through effective questioning, much can be revealed about the patient's mental health.

Direct questions can be asked to unveil specific problems, such as the following:

"How do you feel about yourself? Would you say others would say you are a good or bad person?"

"Do you have many friends? How do you get along with people?"

"Do you feel that anyone is trying to harm you? Who? Why?"

"Are you moody? Do you quickly go from laughing to crying or from being happy to sad?"

"Do you have trouble falling asleep or staying asleep? How much sleep do you get? Do you use any drug or alcohol to become sleepy?"

"How is your appetite? How does your appetite and eating pattern change when you are sad or worried?"

"Do you ever have feelings of being nervous, such as palpitations, hyperventilating, or restlessness?"

"Are there any particular problems in your life or anything you are concerned about now?"

"Do you see or hear things that other people do not? Have you ever heard voices? If so, how do you feel about them?"

"Does life bring you pleasure? Do you look forward to each day?"

"Have you ever thought about suicide? If so, what were those ideas like? How would you do it?"

"Do you feel you are losing any of your mental abilities? If so, describe how."

"Have you ever been hospitalized or had treatment for mental problems? Has any member of your family?"

Listen carefully to the answers and how they are given. It is important to pick up nonverbal clues.

(Continued)

DISPLAY 34-1 (Continued)

Cognitive Testing

A variety of reliable, validated tools can be used in assessing mental function, such as the Short Portable Mental Status Questionnaire (Pfeiffer, 1975), the Philadelphia Geriatric Center Mental Status Questionnaire (Fishback, 1977), Mini-Mental Status (Folstein et al. 1975), Symptoms Check List 90 (Derogatis et al., 1974),

General Health Questionnaire (Goldberg, 1972), OARS (Duke University, 1978), and, specifically for depression, the Zung Self-Rating Depression Scale (Zung, 1965). Most mental status evaluation tools test orientation, memory and retention, the ability to follow commands, judgment, and basic calculation and reasoning. Even without the use of a tool, the nurse can assess basic cognitive function in the following ways.

Orientation: Ask the patient his or her name, where he or she is, the date, time, and season.

Memory and retention: At the beginning of the assessment, ask the patient to remember three objects (eg, watch, telephone, boat). First ask the patient to recall the items immediately after being told; then, after asking several other questions, ask for recall of the three items again; near the end of the assessment, ask what the three items were one last time.

Three-stage command: Ask the patient to perform three simple tasks (eg, "Pick up the pencil, touch it to your head, and hand it to me.").

Judgment: Present a situation that requires basic problem solving and reasoning (eg, "What is meant by the statement 'A bird in the hand is worth two in the bush'?").

Calculation: Ask the patient to count backwards from 100 by increments of 5; if this is difficult, ask the patient to count backward from 20 by increments of 2. Simple arithmetic problems may be asked also, if they are within the realm of the patient's educational experience.

Whenever cognitive function is tested, the unique experiences, educational level, and cultural background of the patient must be considered, as must the role of sensory deficits, health problems, and the stress associated with being examined.

Persons with Alzheimer's disease or other cognitive deficits may become overwhelmed by the assessment and react with anger, tears, or withdrawal. This is referred to as a catastrophic reaction. The assessment may need to be discontinued temporarily and the patient reassured and comforted.

Physical Examination

Physical health problems are often at the root of many cognitive disturbances; as such, it is essential that a complete physical examination supplement the mental status evaluation. A complete review of medications being used is crucial. In addition, a variety of laboratory tests may be conducted, including the following:

- complete blood count
- serum electrolytes
- serologic test for syphilis
- blood urea nitrogen
- blood glucose
- bilirubin
- blood vitamin level
- sedimentation rate
- urinalysis

Depending on the problem suspected, cerebrospinal fluid may be tested and a variety of diagnostic procedures performed, including electroencephalography, computed tomography, magnetic resonance imaging, and positron emission tomography scan. The mental status evaluation often presents only a snapshot of the individual. Cerebral blood flow, body temperature, blood glucose, fluid and electrolyte balance, and the stress to which the patient is subjected can change from one day to the next and cause different levels of mental function to occur. Repeated assessments may be necessary to obtain an accurate evaluation of the patient's mental status.

Nursing Diagnosis

ND **TABLE 34-1** ● *Nursing Diagnoses Related to Mental Health Problems*

Causes or Contributing Factors	Nursing Diagnosis
Depression, lack of motivation, sensory overload, fatigue, medications	Activity Intolerance
Threat to self-concept, losses	Anxiety
Psychomotor slowing, medications, inactivity, lack of recognition of need to defecate	Constipation
Anxiety, medications, stress	Diarrhea
Hyperactivity, sensory overload, suicidal attempt	Pain
Impaired cerebral function, anxiety, suspiciousness	Impaired Verbal Communication
Stress, altered body function, low self-esteem, dependency, sensory overload, loss of significant other	Ineffective Coping
Patient dependency; history of poor family relationships	Disabled Family Coping
Physical, mental, or social limitations	Deficient Diversional Activity
New or misperceived environment, losses	Fear
Loss of body part, function, role, significant other	Anticipatory Grieving
Cognitive impairment, lack of motivation, misperceptions	Ineffective Health Maintenance
Cognitive impairment, misperceptions, lack of motivation	Impaired Home Maintenance
Medications, inactivity, inability to protect self	Risk for Infection
Cognitive impairment, fatigue, medications, suicidal attempt	Risk for Injury
Medications, fatigue	Impaired Physical Mobility
Cognitive impairment, lack of motivation or capacity, suicidal desires	Noncompliance
Depression, anxiety, stress, paranoia, cognitive impairment, suicidal attempt	Impaired Nutrition: Less Than Body Requirements
Depression, anxiety, cognitive impairment, inactivity, suicidal attempt	Impaired Nutrition: More Than Body Requirements
Paranoia, depression, disability, stress	Powerlessness
Cognitive impairment, lack of motivation, knowledge, skill	Self-Care Deficit
Altered body image or function, losses, ageism	Body Image Disturbance
Cognitive impairment, medications, paranoia, sensory deficits, isolation, stress	Sensory–Perceptual Alterations
Depression, anxiety, paranoia, guilt, stress, altered self-concept, medications	Sexual Dysfunction
Cognitive impairment (inability to protect self), malnutrition	Impaired Skin Integrity
Anxiety, paranoia, depression, confusion, medications	Disturbed Sleep Pattern
Altered body part or function, cognitive impairment, anxiety, depression, misperceptions, paranoia, hypochondriasis	Impaired Social Interaction
Anxiety, depression, paranoia, cognitive impairment	Social Isolation
Cognitive impairment, fear, depression, anxiety, stress, isolation	Disturbed Thought Processes
Cognitive impairment, anxiety, depression, medications	Impaired Urinary Elimination
Cognitive impairment, paranoia, stress, misperceptions, fear, suicidal attempt	Risk for Other-Directed Violence

individual's mental status based on any given stereotype must be avoided (Fig. 34-1).

Good mental health practices throughout an individual's lifetime promote good mental health in later life. To preserve mental health, people need to maintain the activities and interests that they find satisfying. They need opportunities to sense their value as a member of society and to have their self-worth reinforced. Security through the provision of adequate income, safe housing, the means to meet basic human needs, and support and assistance through stressful situations will promote mental health. Connection with others is also an aspect of mental health. Finally, a basic ingredient in the preservation and promotion of mental health that cannot be overstated is the importance of optimum physical health.

> 🔑 **KEY CONCEPT**
> Good mental health practices throughout the life
> span promote good mental health in old age.

Nurses must recognize that there are times in everyone's life when disturbances occur and alter the capacity to manage stress. The same principles guiding the care of physical health problems can be applied to the care of persons with mental health problems. The following are actions related to those principles that can be used in care.

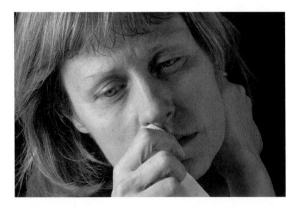

FIGURE 34-1

Astute assessment of behavior and cognitive function aids in differentiating symptoms of psychiatric illness from normal reactions to life events.

Strengthen the individual's capacity to manage the condition: improvement of physical health, good nutrition, increased knowledge, meaningful activity, income supplements, and socialization

Eliminate or minimize the limitations imposed by the condition: providing consistency in care, not fostering hallucinations, reality orientation, correction of physical problems, and modifying the environment to compensate for deficits

Act for or do for the individual only when absolutely necessary: selecting an adequate diet, assisting with bathing, managing finances, and coordinating activities for the patient

Mental health conditions must be seen in the perspective of the patient's total world. The elderly confront many problems that challenge their emotional homeostasis, such as the following:

Illness: acceptance, related self-care demands, pain, altered function or body image

Death: friends, family, significant support person

Retirement: loss of status, role, income, sense of purpose

Increased vulnerability: crime, illness, disability, abuse

Social isolation: lack of transportation, funds, health, friends

Sensory deficits: decrease in or loss of function of hearing, vision, taste, smell, and touch

Greater awareness of own mortality: increased number of deaths among peers

Increased risk of institutionalization, dependency: loss of self-care capabilities to varying degrees

With these factors in mind, some of the symptoms displayed may be revealed to be normal reactions to the circumstances at hand. Before labeling the patient with a psychiatric diagnosis, there should be an attempt to explore such factors in the patient's behavior and to address the cause of the problem rather than its effects alone.

Selected Conditions

DELIRIUM

A variety of conditions can impair cerebral circulation and cause disturbances in cognitive function (Display

34-2). The onset of symptoms tends to be rapid and can include disturbed intellectual function; disorientation of time and place but usually not of identity; altered attention span; worsened memory; labile mood; meaningless chatter; poor judgment; and altered level of consciousness, including hypervigilance, mild drowsiness, and semicomatose status. Disturbances in sleep-wake cycles can occur; in fact, restlessness and sleep disturbances may be early clues. The patient may be suspicious, have personality changes, and experience illusions more often than delusions. Physical signs, such as shortness of breath, fatigue, and slower psychomotor activities, may accompany behavioral changes.

KEY CONCEPT
Delirium alters level of consciousness, whereas dementia does not.

Nurses can play a significant role by detecting signs of confusion promptly. A good history and assessment of mental status on initial contact can provide the baseline data with which changes can be compared. Any change in behavior or cognitive pattern warrants an evaluation. There is the risk that delirium may not be recognized if persons unfamiliar with the patient assume that poor cognition is normal

for him or her. Likewise, persons with dementia can develop delirium as a response to an acute condition but be undiagnosed because changes are not understood or identified.

Delirium is reversible in most circumstances, and prompt care, treating this condition as a medical emergency, can prevent permanent damage. Treatment depends on the cause (eg, stabilizing blood glucose, correcting dehydration, or discontinuing a medication). Treating the symptoms rather than the cause or accepting the symptoms as normal and failing to obtain treatment can result not only in worsened mental status but also in the continuation of a physical condition that could be life threatening.

During the initial acute stage, maintaining stability and minimizing stimulation are primary goals. Consistency in care is important; thus, the patient benefits from interaction with only a limited number of people. Control environmental temperature, noise, and traffic flow. Avoid bright lights, but provide ample lighting to enable the patient to adequately visualize the environment. Ensure that the patient does not harm himself or herself or others and that physical care needs are met. Regardless of the level of intellectual function or consciousness, it is important to speak to the patient and offer explanations of activities or procedures being done. Families may need considerable support during this time and realistic

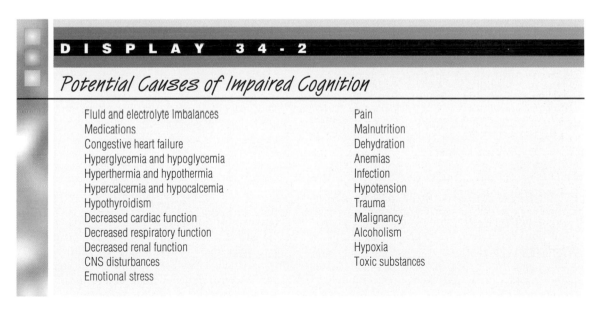

DISPLAY 34 - 2

Potential Causes of Impaired Cognition

Fluid and electrolyte Imbalances	Pain
Medications	Malnutrition
Congestive heart failure	Dehydration
Hyperglycemia and hypoglycemia	Anemias
Hyperthermia and hypothermia	Infection
Hypercalcemia and hypocalcemia	Hypotension
Hypothyroidism	Trauma
Decreased cardiac function	Malignancy
Decreased respiratory function	Alcoholism
Decreased renal function	Hypoxia
CNS disturbances	Toxic substances
Emotional stress	

explanations to alleviate their anxieties (eg, "No, he does not have Alzheimer's disease. His confusion occurred because the level of glucose, or sugar, in his blood dropped too low. He'll be better as soon as the level is brought back to normal.").

DEMENTIA

Alzheimer's Disease

It is estimated that 4 million older adults suffer some form of dementia. Alzheimer's disease is the most common cause of dementia in older adults; in fact, the likelihood of developing Alzheimer's disease doubles every 5 years after the age of 60 (Kochanek, Smith, & Andersen, 2001; National Institute on Aging, 2002, p. 6).

Alzheimer's disease is characterized by the following changes in the brain:

- *The presence of neuritic plaques, which contain deposits of beta-amyloid protein (excess amounts of this are found in persons with Alzheimer's disease and Down syndrome).* Beta-amyloid protein is a fragment of amyloid precursor protein that helps the neurons grow and repair. The beta-amyloid fragments clump together into plaques that impair the function of nerve cells in the brain. It is unclear at this point if the plaques are a cause or by-product of the disease.
- *Neurofibrillary tangles in the cortex.* Microtubules, structures within healthy neurons, normally are stabilized by a special protein called tau. In Alzheimer's disease, tau is changed and begins to pair with other threads of tau that become tangled. This causes the microtubules to disintegrate and collapse the neuron's transport system.

These changes lead to a loss or degeneration of neurons and synapses, especially within the neocortex and hippocampus. Interestingly, the cause-and-effect relationship between these brain changes and Alzheimer's disease is unclear at present.

There are changes in neurotransmitter systems associated with Alzheimer's disease, including reductions in serotonin receptors, serotonin uptake into platelets, production of acetylcholine in the areas of the brain in which plaque and tangles are found, acetylcholinesterase (which breaks down acetylcholine), and choline acetyltransferase. (Cholinesterase inhibitors

and nicotinic, muscarinic, and cholinergic agonists are among the neurotransmitter-affecting drugs used in the treatment of Alzheimer's to compensate for the neurotransmitter changes.)

Possible Causes

Although environmental factors play a role, genetic factors do increase the risk for Alzheimer's disease. Studies have revealed several generations of Alzheimer's disease patients occurring in the same family. Chromosomal abnormalities have been identified. A strong argument for the genetic formulation of the disease stems from its connection with Down syndrome. An extra chromosome 21 exists in persons with Down syndrome; not only do people with Down syndrome begin to develop symptoms of dementia after age 35, but also the prevalence of Alzheimer's disease is higher in families with Down syndrome, and vice versa (Isacson et al., 2002; Prasher et al., 2003). An altered chromosome 21 causes an abnormal amyloid precursor protein to be produced. Chromosomes 14 and 1 also have been found to have mutations within families who have a high prevalence of Alzheimer's disease; these mutations cause abnormal proteins to be produced. If only one of these mutated genes is inherited from a parent with Alzheimer's disease, a person has a 50-50 chance of developing the disease (National Institute on Aging, 2002, p. 33).

> ✔ **Point to Ponder**
>
> *Would you want to know if you had a genetic predisposition toward Alzheimer's disease? What difference could this make in your life?*

There is some investigation into the role of free radicals in the development of Alzheimer's disease. Free radicals are molecules that can build up in neurons, resulting in damage (called oxidative damage). Substances are blocked from flowing in and out of the cell leading to brain damage. Some studies suggest that a diet rich in antioxidants may offer protection (National Institute on Aging, 2002, p. 36).

Higher than normal levels of aluminum and mercury have been found in the brain cells of Alzheimer's disease patients, causing some speculation regarding the role of environmental toxins in the disease. However, the results are inconclusive as to their role in the development of Alzheimer's disease. Low zinc levels are present in persons with Alzheimer's disease, although it is not certain if this is a cause or result of the disease.

There has been some speculation about a slow-acting virus causing the neurofibrillary tangles in the brain, but no conclusive evidence exists at present to support this theory. At present, no one theory can explain this complex disease.

Symptoms

The symptoms of this progressive, degenerative disease develop gradually and progress at different rates among affected individuals. The Global Deterioration Scale/Functional Assessment Staging (GDS/FAST) offers a means of staging Alzheimer's disease (Fig. 34-2) (Auer & Reisberg, 1997). Although staging of the disease can help predict its general course and anticipate plans for care, it must be appreciated that many factors affect the progression of the disease and that there will be individual variation.

Early in the disease, the patient may be aware of changes in intellectual ability and become depressed or anxious or attempt to compensate by writing down information, structuring routines, and simplifying responsibilities. It may take some time for symptoms to be detected, even by those close to the patient.

> **KEY CONCEPT**
> The greatest risk for suicide for a person with dementia is in the early stage of the disease when the individual is aware of the changes experienced.

Other Dementias

In addition to Alzheimer's disease, dementia may be caused by a variety of pathologies:

Vascular dementia. This form of dementia results from small cerebral infarctions. Damage to brain tissue can be diffuse or localized, the onset is more rapid, and the disease progresses more predictably than Alzheimer's disease. It is associated with risk factors such as smoking, hyper-

tension, hyperlipidemia, inactivity, and a history of stroke or cardiovascular disease.

Frontotemporal dementia. Rather than neurofibrillary tangles and plaques, this form of dementia is characterized by neuronal atrophy affecting the frontal lobes of the brain. A unique characteristic of this type of dementia is the appearance of behavioral rather than cognitive abnormalities in the early stage. Also, rather than poor memory, early cognitive changes can include impairments in abstract thinking and speech and language skills. Pick's disease is the most common form of frontotemporal dementia.

Lewy body dementia, also known as *cortical Lewy body disease,* is associated with subcortical pathology and the presence of Lewy body substance in the cerebral cortex. The similarity in the brain matter of both Alzheimer's and Lewy body dementias causes some gerontologists to view Lewy body dementia as a type of Alzheimer's disease.

Creutzfeldt-Jacob disease is an extremely rare brain disorder that causes dementia. This dementia has a rapid onset and progression and is characterized by severe neurological impairment that accompanies the dementia. It is believed that this disease can be transmitted through a slow virus; a familial tendency toward the disease is possible. The pathological process displays destruction of neurons in the cerebral cortex, overgrowth of glia, abnormal cellular structure of the cortex, hypertrophy and proliferation of astrocytes, and a spongelike appearance of the cerebral cortex. Symptoms are more varied than with Alzheimer's disease and include psychotic behavior, heightened emotional lability, memory impairment, loss of muscular function, muscle spasms, seizures, and visual disturbances. The disease progresses rapidly, and death typically occurs within 1 year of diagnosis.

Wernicke encephalopathy and *Parkinson's disease* are responsible for a small percentage of dementias. Many persons with AIDS will develop dementia in the final phase of the disease. Trauma and toxins are among the other causes of this problem.

Symptoms similar to those associated with Alzheimer's disease can present with other forms of dementia. The ability of other dementias' symptoms

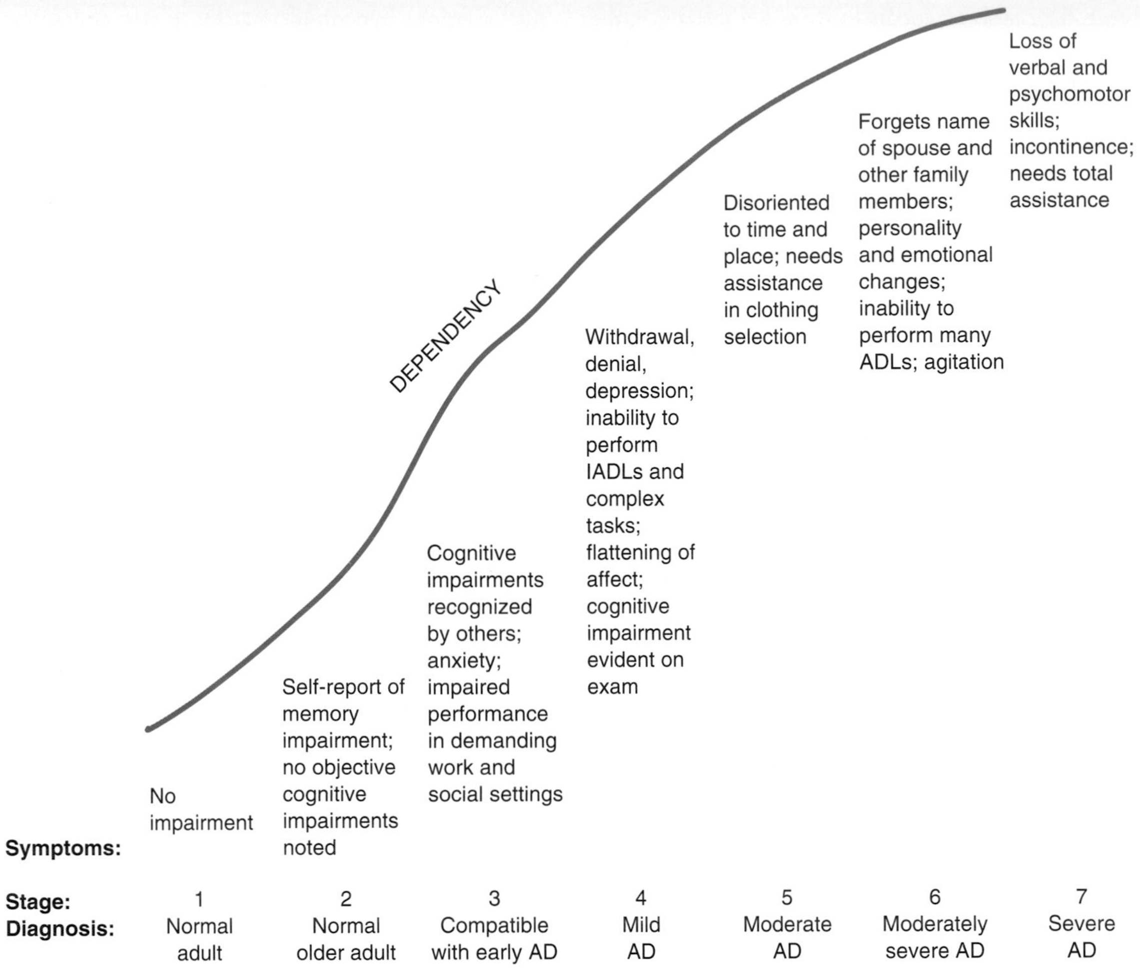

FIGURE 34-2

Stages of Alzheimer's disease. (Based on Reisberg, B., Ferris, S.H., & de Leon, M.J. [1982]. The global deterioration scale for assessment of primary dementia. *American Journal of Psychiatry, 139,* 1136–1139; and Auer, S., & Reisberg, B. [1997]. The GDS/FAST Staging System. *International Psychogeriatrics, 9* [Suppl. 1], 167–171.)

to mimic symptoms commonly associated with Alzheimer's disease reinforces the importance of comprehensive evaluation of causes of dementia symptoms. Without a comprehensive evaluation to identify or exclude other causes of dementia, the label of Alzheimer's disease cannot be accurately given to a dementia.

In addition to the history of symptoms from the patient and family members or significant others, di-

agnosis is aided by brain scans that can reveal changes in the brain's structure that are consistent with the disease, neuropsychological testing that evaluates cognitive functioning, and laboratory tests and neurological examinations.

Although currently there is no treatment to prevent or cure Alzheimer's disease, clinical trials are being conducted by the National Institutes of Health and private industry in hopes of finding a means to improve function and slow the progress of the disease. There has been interest in estrogen's role in enhancing cognitive function, with speculation that estrogen has a role in protecting postmenopausal women from developing Alzheimer's disease or other age-related cognitive decline; however, research has produced conflicting results as the women's Health Initiative Memory Study demonstrated an increased risk for dementia in postmenopausal women in women taking estrogen with progestin (Shumaker et al., 2003). Antioxidants, antiinflammatory agents, supplements (folic acid and vitamins B_6, and B_{12}), gene therapy that adds a nerve growth factor to the aging brain, and the development of a vaccine are among the other areas being investigated in clinical trials (National Institute on Aging, 2002, p. 44).

Because acetylcholine falls sharply in people with Alzheimer's disease, medications that stop or slow the enzyme (acetylcholinesterase) that breaks down acetylcholine have been developed to help people with Alzheimer's disease; these drugs include donepezil (Aricept), rivastigmine (Exelon), and galanthamine (Reminyl).

> **KEY CONCEPT**
> Other diseases can mimic Alzheimer's disease; therefore, a comprehensive evaluation is essential to rule out other possible causes of dementia before the diagnosis of Alzheimer's disease is made.

Caring for Persons With Dementia

The irreversible nature of dementia and its progressive deteriorating course can have devastating effects on affected individuals and their families. A majority of the care required by persons with dementia falls within the scope of nursing practice. One of the foremost considerations is the safety of these patients. Their poor judgment and misperceptions can lead to serious behavioral problems and mishaps. A safe, structured environment is essential. The persons and components of the environment should be consistent (Fig. 34-3). Items to trigger memory are useful to include, such as photographs of the patient or a consistently used symbol (eg, flower or triangle) on the bedroom door or personal possessions. Noise, activity,

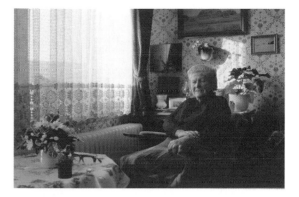

FIGURE 34-3

Familiar objects, a stable environment, and consistency of caregivers can reduce some of the behavioral problems associated with dementias.

and lighting levels can overstimulate the patient and further decrease function; thus, they need to be controlled. This is particularly useful in preventing and managing sundowner syndrome (Display 34-3). Cleaning solutions, pesticides, medications, and nonedible items that could be ingested accidentally must be stored in locked cabinets. Coverings should be applied to unused sockets, electrical outlets, fans, motors, and other items into which fingers may be poked. Matches and lighters should not be accessible; if the patient smokes, it must be under close supervision. Windows and doors can be protected with Plexiglas, and nonremovable screens can be installed to avoid falls from windows. Wandering is common among patients with dementia; rather than restrain or restrict them, it is more advantageous to provide a safe area in which they can wander. Protective gates can be installed to prevent patients from wandering away; alarms and bells on doors can signal when they are attempting to exit. With the great risk of patients wandering away and not being able to give their names or residence when found, it is beneficial to have identification bracelets on them at all times and a recent photograph available.

Various therapies and activities can be offered to the patient with dementia, depending on the patient's level of function. Occupational therapy and expressive therapies can benefit those with early dementia. Various degrees of reality orientation, ranging from daily groups to reminding the patient who he or she

D I S P L A Y   3 4 - 3

Sundowner Syndrome

Individuals with cognitive impairments may experience a nocturnal confusion, named sundowner syndrome due to its presentation "after the sun goes down." Some of the factors that increase the risk of this condition include unfamiliar environment (eg, recent admission to a facility), disturbed sleep patterns (eg, from sleep apnea), use of restraints, excess sensory stimulation, sensory deprivation, or change in circadian rhythms.

Nurses can prevent and manage sundowner syndrome by:

- placing familiar objects in the person's room
- providing physical activity in the afternoon to help the person expend energy
- adjusting lighting in the environment to prevent the room from becoming dark in the evening
- keeping a nightlight on throughout the night
- having frequent contact with the person to offer reassurance and orientation
- using touch to provide human contact and calm the person
- assuring the environmental temperature is within a comfortable range for the person
- controlling noise and traffic flow in the evening
- assuring the person's basic needs are met (eg, adequate fluids, toileting, dry clothing)

is during every interaction, can be used. Even the most regressed patient can maintain contact and derive stimulation through activities, such as listening to music and touching various objects. Being touched is also a pleasurable and stimulating experience.

The physical care needs of patients with dementia are at risk of being overlooked. These individuals may not complain that they are hungry, so no one notices that they have consumed less than one quarter of the food served; they cannot remember to drink water, so they become dehydrated; they fight their bath so strongly that they are left unbathed; and pressure ulcers on their buttocks go unnoticed. These patients need close observation and careful attention to their physical needs. Consideration must be given to the fact that they may be unable to communicate their needs and discomforts; a subtle change in behavior or function, a facial grimace, or repeated touching of a body part may give clues that a problem exists. This reinforces the importance of consistency in caregivers because they will be familiar with a patient's unique behaviors and more quickly recognize a deviation from that individual's norm.

A variety of alternative medical therapies are being used to treat Alzheimer's disease and other forms of dementia. Nutritional supplements that have been used include vitamins B_6, B_{12}, C, and E; folic acid; zinc; and selenium. The herb ginkgo biloba has been shown to improve circulation and mental function in several clinical trials (Howes, Pery, Houghton, 2003; Oken, Storzbach, & Kaye, 2000); caution is needed, however, because ginkgo biloba can increase the risk of intraocular hemorrhage and subdural hematoma when taken for an extended period of time or when an anticoagulant drug is being taken concurrently. Dong quai, ginseng, and ho-shou-wu also are used (Howes et al., 2003). Chinese medicine, in addition to herbs and nutrition, uses a form of therapeutic exercise called qigong; it is believed that oxygenation to the brain improves by the breathing exercises and visualization used in qigong exercises.

As patients regress, their dignity, personal worth, freedom, and individuality may be jeopardized. Loved ones may view the demented family member as a stranger living inside the body that once housed the person they knew. Staff see another dependent or total-care patient before them with no sense of that person's unique life history. Viewed less and less as a normal human being or as the same person that has been known, the person with dementia may be treated in a dehumanizing manner. Special attention must be paid to maintaining and promoting the following qualities:

Individuality. The personal history and uniqueness of the patient should be learned and incorporated into caregiving activities.

Independence. Even if it takes three times longer to guide patients through dressing than it would take to dress them, they should be afforded every opportunity for self-care.

Freedom. As major freedoms become limited, minor choices and control become especially important. Nurses must be careful that, in the name of efficiency and safety, such severe restrictions to freedom are not imposed that the quality of life becomes minimal.

Dignity. To become angry or laugh at the behaviors of a demented person is no less cruel than reacting in a similar fashion to a stroke victim who falls during ambulation. These patients should be afforded the respect given to any adult, including attractive clothing, good grooming, adult hairstyles, use of their name, privacy, and confidentiality.

Connection. Persons with dementia continue to be valued human beings who are members of families, communities, and the universe. Interaction and connection with other people and nature show recognition and respect for the spiritual beings that live within the altered bodies and minds.

Assistance and support to the families of patients are integral parts of nursing persons with dementia. The physical, emotional, and socioeconomic burden of caring for a cognitively impaired relative can be immense. It should not be assumed that family members understand basic care techniques. Basic, specific care techniques need to be reviewed, including lifting, bathing, and managing inappropriate behaviors. Families should be prepared for the guilt, frustration, anger, depression, and other feelings that normally accompany this responsibility. Helping them plan respite, network with support groups, and obtain counseling may be beneficial. Most states now have chapters of the Alzheimer's Association to which families can be referred (see Resources listing).

Display 34-4 describes the care of a person with Alzheimer's disease.

> 🔑 **KEY CONCEPT**
> It cannot be assumed that family members understand feeding, bathing, lifting, and other basic caregiving skills.

DEPRESSION

Depression is the most frequent problem that psychiatrists treat in the elderly, and although major depression declines with age, minor depression increases in incidence with age. Various estimates have placed the prevalence of depression at 15% to 25% in community-based elders and as many as 25% in older adults who are residents of long-term care facilities, with another 20% to 30% of institutional residents displaying symptoms of depression although not diagnosed with clinical depression (National Mental Health Association, 2003).

Although depressive episodes may have been a lifelong problem for some individuals, it is not uncommon for depression to be a new problem in old age. This is not surprising when one considers the adjustments and losses the elderly face, such as the independence of one's children; the reality of retirement; significant changes or losses of roles; reduced income restricting the pursuit of satisfying leisure activities and limiting the ability to meet basic needs; decreasing efficiency of the body; a changing self-image; the death of family members and friends, reinforcing the reality of one's own shrinking life span; and overt and covert messages from society that one's worth is inversely proportional to one's age. In addition, drugs can cause or aggravate depression (Display 34-5).

Depression is a complex syndrome and is demonstrated in a variety of ways in older persons. The most common manifestations of this problem are the vegetative symptoms, which include insomnia, fatigue, anorexia, weight loss, constipation, and decreased interest in sex. Depressed persons may express self-deprecation, guilt, apathy, remorse, hopelessness, helplessness, and feelings of being burdens. They may have problems with their personal relationships and social interactions and lose interest in people. Changes

DISPLAY 34-4

Case Study

A home health nurse is making an initial home visit to evaluate 69-year-old Mr. Stebbins, who has Alzheimer's disease, and assist his wife in developing effective caregiving plans. Mr. Stebbins was diagnosed approximately 1 year earlier as a result of an evaluation initiated by the university where he taught. University sources stated the Mr. Stebbins was behaving inappropriately: entering other professors' classrooms and beginning to lecture, forgetting to be present for classes and meetings, failing to bathe or change his clothes for days, addressing his class in an incoherent manner, and asking coworkers for assistance in operating office equipment that he had used for years without difficulty. After observing Mr. Stebbins' condition progressively worsen over time, the dean of the university telephoned Mrs. Stebbins to discuss the situation. Mrs. Stebbins claims that she noticed that her husband was acting unusually (forgetting names and appointments, bouncing checks, arguing for no reason, making unkind comments to friends, confusing days off with work days) but thought this could be related to "getting older" and job stress. When the dean spoke with her, Mrs. Stebbins realized that a serious problem might exist and accompanied her husband for an evaluation, the result of which was the establishment of a diagnosis of Alzheimer's disease. Mr. Stebbins retired immediately from the university and has been with his wife for 24 hours each day since. Mrs. Stebbins offered no complaints until this past month, when she repeatedly called the physician to discuss the new problems of incontinence, eating difficulties, and wandering that Mr. Stebbins was exhibiting. These new problems have devastated Mrs. Stebbins; she looks fatigued and claims to be eating and sleeping poorly. She firmly states that she "will never consider placing her husband in an institution" and that she'll take care of him at home "if it kills her."

Based on the brief information available, the nurse could develop the following care plan:

Nursing Diagnosis

Self-care deficit: feeding related to altered cognition

Goals

The patient:

maintains weight within ideal range
is free from signs of malnutrition

Actions

■ Weigh patient to establish baseline weight and advise wife to weigh patient weekly and report weight loss of 5 pounds or more.
■ Review with patient and wife patient's food likes and dislikes; assist wife in planning meals that incorporate patient's preferences; consult with dietitian as necessary.
■ Advise wife to provide nutritious snacks, finger foods and soft/pureed foods for patient.
■ Discourage patient's eating of nuts, hard candy, popcorn, or other foods that could easily be aspirated.
■ Suggest that patient eat in the same location (preferably a room with minimal distractions) at consistent times daily.
■ Instruct wife to guide patient through meals by placing appropriate utensil in his hand, giving him one-stage instructions, and praising good eating habits.
■ Discuss with wife referral to Meals on Wheels or similar service in community.

Desired Outcomes

The patient:

maintains weight within ideal range
is free from signs of malnutrition

Nursing Diagnosis

Self-care deficit: toileting and altered urinary elimination: incontinence related to altered cognition

Goals

The patient:

establishes toileting routine to prevent incontinence (if possible)

(Continued)

is free from complications associated with incontinence

Actions

- Assess urinary elimination pattern and attempt to determine whether incontinence is result of altered cognition or another problem; refer for evaluation if indicated.
- Assist wife in identifying length of time between voiding episodes and develop plan to toilet patient half an hour prior to anticipated voiding time.
- Ensure that bathroom is easily accessible; arrange to obtain commode chair and urinal if necessary.
- Reinforce proper cleansing technique and skin care to prevent irritation.
- Suggest clothing that is easy for patient to remove for toileting; replacement of pants' buttons and zippers with Velcro.
- Supply with information regarding urine containment products and availability in community.

Desired Outcomes

The patient:

reduces incontinent episodes through habit training
is free from complications associated with incontinence

Nursing Diagnosis

Risk for injury due to wandering, poor judgment secondary to altered cognition

Goal

The patient is free from injury

Actions

- Inspect home with wife for potential safety hazards and make appropriate recommendations.
- Ensure that home is equipped with smoke alarm and fire extinguisher.
- Recommend preventive measures, such as storing chemicals, medications, and other potentially

hazardous substances in locked cabinet, setting hot water heater temperature below 120°F, alarming doors to signal patient's wandering from home, keeping environment well lighted and clutter free, capping electrical outlets, locking and securing windows, keeping spare key with neighbor. Assist in locating stores to purchase safety equipment.
- Instruct wife to administer medications for patient.
- Assure patient wears stable shoes, safe clothing.
- Advise wife to have current photograph of patient readily available in the event he becomes lost and must be located by persons unfamiliar with him.
- Supply with information on obtaining identification bracelet for patient.

Desired Outcome

The patient is free from injury

Nursing Diagnosis

Disturbed sleep pattern related to dementia

Goals

The patient:

sleeps 5 to 7 hours at night
takes one nap during the day
is free from fatigue, insomnia, and other sleep/rest disturbances

Actions

- Recommend that wife maintain a record of patient's sleep and nap times to assess patterns.
- Advise wife to adhere to simple, consistent bed-time routine, provide soft lighting and music as this facilitates sleep, prevent patient from excess daytime napping, encourage early evening exercise.

Desired Outcomes

The patient:

sleeps 5 to 7 hours each night
is free from signs of fatigue

(Continued)

D I S P L A Y 3 4 - 4 (C o n t i n u e d)

Nursing Diagnosis

Impaired verbal communication and disturbed thought processes related to Alzheimer's disease

Goals

The patient:

is oriented to person, place, and time (to maximum extent possible)
effectively communicates needs

Actions

- Instruct wife in helpful communication techniques, such as:
  using calm relaxed manner of communication
  approaching patient from the front and getting his attention before speaking
  using basic language
  giving one instruction or comment at a time
  avoiding overstimulating or overloading patient
  allowing ample time for patient to respond
  identifying terms used by patient to describe needs or items
  using distractions when patient becomes upset
- Encourage wife to keep patient oriented, place clocks and calendars in rooms used by patient.
- Help wife to identify and avoid aspects of environment that could promote misperceptions, such as shadows cast by light, radios playing in empty rooms.

Desired Outcomes

The patient:

is oriented to person, place and time
effectively communicates needs

Nursing Diagnosis

Interrupted family processes and caregiver role strain related to altered roles and function of patient and demands of caregiving

Goals

The family:

is free from adverse effects from patient's illness
develops effective means of coping with patient's condition

Actions

- Assess wife's reactions to patient's condition, impact on her roles and functions; identify her risks and needs.
- Discuss realities of disease and patient's prognosis with wife.
- Identify other family resources or significant others who can offer support and assistance to wife.
- Refer family to local chapter of Alzheimer's Disease and Related Disorders Association, counseling services, and other support services.
- Assist in locating respite care; recommend adult day care program for patient.
- Discuss potential for nursing home placement; listen to wife's concerns; clarify misconceptions and offer facts.
- Assist wife in identifying her own needs and developing plans for her own life as husband's condition declines.
- Allow and encourage expression of feelings; offer support.

Desired Outcomes

The family:

is free from adverse effects from patient's illness
develops effective means of coping with patient's illness

---

in sleep and psychomotor activity patterns can be evident. Hygienic practices may be neglected. Physical complaints of headache, indigestion, and other problems often surface. Altered cognition may be present, caused by malnutrition or other effects of the depression. The symptoms of depression can mimic those of dementia; thus, careful assessment is crucial to avoid misdiagnosis. However, a decline in intellect and personality is usually indicative of dementia, not depression. Depression can occur in the early stage of dementia as the patient becomes aware of declining intellectual abilities.

DISPLAY 34-5

Drugs That Can Cause Depression

Antihypertensives and cardiac drugs; β blockers, digoxin, procainamide, guanethidine, clonidine, reserpine, methyldopa, spironolactone

Hormones: corticotropin, corticosteroids, estrogens

Central nervous system (CNS) depressants, anti-anxiety agents, psychotropics: alcohol, haloperidol, flurazepam, barbiturates, benzodiazepines

Others: cimetidine, L-dopa, ranitidine, asparaginase, tamoxifen

KEY CONCEPT
Some older adults who are depressed demonstrate cognitive deficits secondary to the effects of depression.

This pseudodementia can delay or prevent the underlying depression from being recognized and treated.

The relationship of life events to the depression is essential to explore during the assessment; the approach for a person depressed from the effects of a drug obviously will differ from that for a person who has just become widowed. The underlying problem should be addressed. Although depressions do tend to last longer in the elderly, prompt treatment can hasten recovery. Treatment should not be withheld because it is associated with a serious or terminal illness; alleviating the depression may help the individual cope more effectively and be in a better position to manage other health problems.

Psychotherapy and antidepressants (Display 34-6) can alleviate many depressions to varying degrees. Electroconvulsive therapy has been shown to be effective in patients who have serious depressions that have been unresponsive to other therapies. Some herbs have been known to have antidepressant effects; these include St. John's wort (this herb can cause photosensitivity and should not be used with an antidepressant medication), gotu kola, ginseng, skullcap, and lavender; these herbs require close monitoring when used due to the possibility of adverse effects (Boehnlein & Oakley, 2002; National Health Information, 2003). Acupressure, acupuncture, guided imagery, and light therapy, in conjunction with psychotherapy, can also prove helpful. Good basic health practices, including proper nutrition and regular exercise, can also have a positive effect on mood. Display 34-7 describes other helpful measures.

SUICIDE

Suicide is a real and serious risk among depressed persons. The suicide rate increases with age and is highest among older white men. Twenty-five percent of all suicides are elderly individuals. All suicide threats from the elderly should be taken seriously. In addition to recognizing obvious suicide attempts, nurses must learn to recognize those that are more subtle but equally destructive.

KEY CONCEPT
All suicide threats from the elderly should be taken seriously.

Medication misuse, either in the form of overdoses or omission of dosages, may be a suicidal gesture. Self-starvation is another sign and can occur even in an institutional setting if staff members are not attentive to monitoring intake and nutritional status. Engaging in activities that oppose a therapeutic need or threaten a medical problem (eg, ignoring dietary restrictions or refusing a particular therapy) may indicate a desire to die. Walking through a dangerous area, driving while intoxicated, and subjecting oneself to other risks can also be signals of suicidal

DISPLAY 34-6

Antidepressants

Selective Serotonin Reuptake Inhibitors (SSRIs)

Fluvoxamine (Luvox)
Fluoxetine (Prozac)
Paroxetine (Paxil)
Sertraline (Zoloft)

Cyclic Compounds

Amitriptyline HCl (Elavil, Amitril)
Amoxapine (Ascendin)
Desipramine HCl (Norpramine, Pertofrane)
Doxepin HCl (Adapin, Sinequan)
Imipramine pamoate (Trofanil)
Maprotiline (Ludiomil)
Nortriptyline HCl (Aventyl, Pamelor)

Monoamine Oxidase Inhibitors (MAOIs)

Phenelzine (Nardil)
Tranyllcypromine (Parnate)

Lithium Carbonate

Lithium (Eskalith, Lithonate)

Nursing Guidelines

■ Dosages for elders should begin at about one-half that recommended for the general adult population.

■ Sedation commonly occurs during the initial few days of treatment; take precautions to reduce the risk for falls.

■ At least 1 month of therapy is needed before therapeutic effects will be noted; advise and support the patient during this period.

■ Bedtime administration is preferable with antidepressants that produce a sedative effect.

■ Prepare patients for side effects, including dry mouth, diaphoresis, urinary retention, indigestion, constipation, hypotension, blurred vision, drowsiness, increased appetite, weight gain, photosensitivity, fluctuating blood glucose levels. Assist patient in preventing complications secondary to side effects.

■ Be alert to anticholinergic symptoms, particularly when cyclic compounds are used.

■ Ensure that elders and their caregivers understand dosage, intended effects, and adverse reactions to the drugs. Instruct about drug–drug, and drug–food interactions, eg,
antidepressants can increase the effects of anticoagulants, atropine-like drugs, antihistamines, sedatives, tranquilizers, narcotics, and levodopa
antidepressants can decrease the effects of clonidine, phenytoin, and some antihypertensives
alcohol and thiazide diuretics can increase the effects of antidepressants

---

desires. Suicidal risk can further be assessed by asking the patient about recent losses, lifestyle changes, new or worsening health problems, new symptoms of depression, changes in or a limited support system, and a family history of suicide.

The suicidal elderly need close observation, careful protection, and prompt therapy. Treatment of the underlying depression should be supported. The environment should be made safe by removing items that could be used for self-harm. Nurses need to convey a willingness to listen to and discuss thoughts and feelings about suicide. Being able to reach out for help by

expressing their suicidal thoughts to nursing staff may prevent patients from taking actions to end their lives.

ANXIETY

Adjustments to physical, emotional, and socioeconomic limitations in old age and the new problems that frequently are encountered due to aging add to the variety of causes for anxiety. Anxiety reactions, not uncommon in older persons, can be manifested in various ways, including somatic complaints, rigidity in thinking and behavior, insomnia, fatigue, hos-

---

DISPLAY 34-7

Basic Goals in Caring for Depressed Patients

Help the patient develop a positive self-concept. It must be emphasized that, although the situation may be bad, the person is not. Opportunities for success, regardless of how minor, should be provided, and new goals should be formed.

Encourage the expression of feelings. Anger, guilt, frustration, and other feelings should be vented. Nurses should afford time to listen and guide patients through these feelings. In addition to verbalization, feelings can be expressed through writing.

Statements such as "Don't worry, things will get better" or "Don't talk that way; you have a lot to be thankful for" offer little benefit to depressed persons.

Ensure that physical needs are met. Good nutrition, activity, sleep, and regular bowel movements are among the factors that enhance a healthy physical state, which in turn strengthen the patient's capacities to work through depression. Physical-care problems must be aggressively addressed.

Offer hope. While being realistic regarding the individual situation, nurses can, by words and deeds, convey their belief that the future will have meaning and that the patient's life is of value.

---

tility, restlessness, chain smoking, pacing, fantasizing, confusion, and increased dependency. An increase in blood pressure, pulse, respirations, psychomotor activity, and frequency of voiding may occur. Appetite may increase or decrease. Anxious individuals often handle their clothing, jewelry, or utensils excessively, become intensively involved with a minor task (eg, folding a piece of linen), and have difficulty concentrating on the activity at hand.

Treatment of anxiety depends on its cause. Nurses should probe into the patient's history for recent changes or new stresses (eg, rent increase, increased neighborhood crime, divorce of child). The consumption of caffeine, alcohol, nicotine, and over-the-counter drugs should be reviewed for possible causes. Interventions specific to the underlying cause should be planned. In addition to drugs, interventions such as biofeedback, guided imagery, and relaxation therapy can prove helpful. Anxious persons need their lives to be simplified and stable, with few unpredictable occurrences. Environmental stimuli must be controlled. Basic nursing interventions that could prove beneficial include the following:

- allow adequate time for conversations, procedures, and other activities
- prepare the individual for all anticipated activities

- provide thorough, honest, and basic explanations
- control the number and variety of persons with whom the patient must interact
- adhere to routines
- keep and use familiar objects
- prevent overstimulation of the senses by reducing noise, using soft lights, and maintaining a stable room temperature

✔ Point to Ponder

What types of situations cause you to become depressed or anxious? What implications does this have for your senior years?

ALCOHOL ABUSE

Abuse of, dependency on, or addiction to alcohol affects the elderly but often is a problem that goes unnoticed. More than 60% of elders consume alcohol, with 13% of men and 2% of women reporting heavy use (Knauer, 2003). Alcoholism can seriously threaten the physical, emotional, and social health of elders; therefore, it is important that gerontological nurses recognize this problem and help patients seek appropriate treatment.

A majority of older adults who are alcoholic are chronic alcohol abusers who have used it heavily throughout their lives. A significant number of chronic abusers die before reaching old age, contributing to a decreased incidence of alcoholism with age. The other type of older alcoholic is the one who begins abusing alcohol in late life because of situational factors (eg, retirement, widowhood, or poor health status).

Many health care professionals possess the same stereotype of alcoholics as the general public, believing alcoholics to be sloppy, "skid row bum" type of people. Consequently, even professionals may fail to detect alcohol abuse in the retired professional who drinks at the country club daily or the frail widow who begins sipping brandy at midmorning. Nurses must keep an open mind and recognize that alcoholics come in many forms.

> **KEY CONCEPT**
> Alcoholics come in many forms and often do not fit the stereotypical profile.

Alcohol abuse can be manifested in a variety of ways, some of which may be subtle or easy to confuse with other disorders (Display 34-8). Symptoms can develop secondary to complications from alcoholism, such as cirrhosis, hepatitis, and chronic infections (related to suppressed immune system). These signs should be noted during an assessment and trigger questions regarding the patient's drinking pattern.

Display 34-9 describes the criteria for a definitive diagnosis of alcoholism.

Ongoing supervision of the older alcoholic's health status can help identify and, in some cases, correct complications early. Chronic alcoholism can cause magnesium deficiencies, gastritis, pancreatitis, and polyneuropathy. Cardiac disorders can result from alcoholism and can be displayed by hypertension, irregular heart beat, and heart failure due to cardiomyopathy. Cognition can be impaired by a loss of brain cells and enlargement of the ventricles.

In caring for the patient who has an alcohol problem, the long-term goal is sobriety; this can be achieved only if the patient acknowledges the problem and takes responsibility for doing something about it. Family involvement can be significant to the success of the treatment plan because outcomes can be negatively affected by loved ones denying or enabling the drinking problem.

Alcoholism treatment programs designed specifically for older adults are rare, and it is likely that traditional program staff are unfamiliar with the unique characteristics and needs of the older alcoholic. Gerontological nurses must ensure that the needs of the older alcoholic are competently addressed. For example, benzodiazepines, commonly used for detoxification, can cause toxicity in older people at the same dosage levels that are prescribed for younger adults. Dosage adjustments are necessary, as is close monitoring for complications.

Alcoholics Anonymous (see the Resources at the end of the chapter) is a free program for recovery, available

---

DISPLAY 34-8

Possible Indications of Alcohol Abuse

Drinking alcohol to calm nerves or improve mood	Irritability
Gulping or rapidly consuming alcoholic beverages	Depression
Memory blackouts	Mood swings
Malnutrition	Lack of motivation or energy
Confusion	Injuries, falls
Social isolation and withdrawal	Insomnia
Disrupted relationships	GI distress
Arrests for minor offenses	Clumsiness
Anxiety	

D I S P L A Y   3 4 - 9

Criteria for Diagnosing Alcoholism

- Drinks a fifth of whiskey a day or its equivalent in wine or beer (for a 180-pound person)
- Alcoholic blackouts
- Blood alcohol level greater than 150 mg/100 mL
- Withdrawal syndrome: hallucinations, convulsions, gross tremors, delirium tremens (DTs)
- Continued drinking despite medical advice or problems caused by drinking (U.S. Department of Health and Human Services, National Institute on Alcohol Abuse and Alcoholism)

---

in most communities, which provides counseling and opportunities for alcohol-free socialization for the older alcoholic. Supplying patients with locations, meeting times, and encouragement to attend meetings can be significant to helping them get on the treatment path.

PARANOIA

Paranoid states frequently occur in older persons, which is not surprising considering the following:

- sensory losses, so common in later life, easily cause the environment to be misperceived
- illness, disability, living alone, and a limited budget promote insecurity
- ageism within society sends a message of the undesirability of the old
- older people are frequent victims of crime and unscrupulous practices

The initial consideration in working with paranoid older individuals is to explore mechanisms that could reduce insecurity and misperception. Corrective lenses, hearing aids, supplemental income, new housing, and a stable environment are potential interventions. Psychotherapy and medications can be used when improvement is not achieved through other interventions. Nurses should ensure that these patients do not become withdrawn from the rest of the world because of self-imposed isolation.

Not to be overlooked is the impact of the paranoid state on general health and well-being. Nutritional status can be threatened if the patient refuses to eat, believing his or her food to be poisoned; sleep deprivation can result if there is suspicion that a stranger is

in the house; and health problems may not be diagnosed if the person believes the doctor is an enemy. Honest, basic explanations and approaches to dealing with paranoid misperceptions are beneficial; at no time should delusions be supported.

HYPOCHONDRIASIS

Hypochondriasis may be a problem of older individuals. Although it is commonly associated with depression, for some elderly it may be an attention-getting mechanism. Often, health professionals reinforce this behavior by reacting to physical complaints promptly but not reinforcing periods of good function and health. Staff members may not respond to a request to sit down and talk with a patient, but they give undivided attention when that same person expresses physical discomfort. Some older people find hypochondriasis an effective means of controlling a spouse or children. Older people may use it as a means of socialization; if they do not have travels, professions, or interests they can share with others, they can count on their peers having similar ailments, which can serve as the common ground for conversation.

 KEY CONCEPT
Health care professionals may promote hypochondriatic behavior by investing more time and interest reviewing the complaints of the older person than in discussing interests and normal life activities.

Regardless of how unfounded they seem, complaints must be evaluated for their validity before assuming that they are part of hypochondriasis. Even the complaints of a known hypochondriac deserve evaluation, particularly if a new set of complaints emerges. It is beneficial to help these people find alternatives to their obsession with their bodily functions. Spending time in nonillness-related conversation can demonstrate that one can receive attention without resorting to physical complaints. Family members need to understand the dynamics of this problem so that they can reinforce positive behaviors and not be manipulated. Telling these patients that nothing is wrong is of little help; the underlying reason for this reaction must be addressed.

Nursing Considerations

MONITORING MEDICATIONS

Medications used to treat psychiatric disorders can bring significant improvement to patients, but they can also have profound adverse effects on older adults. Some of the adverse effects of these medications can lead to anorexia, constipation, falls, incontinence, anemia, lethargy, sleep disturbances, and confusion. The lowest possible dosage should be used, and any reactions should be observed closely. It may be useful to initiate a checklist for problem identification, as shown in Table 34-1, to track the impact of medications on behavior and function. Of course, drugs complement and do not substitute for other forms of treatment.

> **KEY CONCEPT**
> Drugs should be viewed as an adjunct to rather than as a substitute for other forms of treatment.

PROMOTING A POSITIVE SELF-CONCEPT

The importance of promoting a positive self-concept in all older adults cannot be overemphasized. All people need to feel that their lives have had meaning and that there is hope. A sense of meaninglessness and hopelessness threatens mental health and minimizes the pleasures that the last segment of life can bring. Nurses should take a sincere interest in the lives and accomplishments of their elderly patients. It must be remembered that the disabled or frail person who now presents to the nurse may once have demonstrated the courage to venture from a native country to America, risked his life to save fellow soldiers in a war, scrubbed floors at night to support a family during the Great Depression, or developed a successful business from scratch. Struggles and accomplishments exist in every life and can be recognized to help promote self-esteem. Activities such as life-review discussions, taping oral histories, and compiling a scrapbook of life events not only help older adults feel a sense of worth about the lives they have lived but also provide a sense of history and legacy for younger generations. In addition to the past, the present and future should hold meaning for the elderly, and this can be promoted by helping patients participate in relevant activities, engage in meaningful social interactions, have opportunities to do for others, exercise the maximal amount of control possible over their lives, maintain religious and cultural practices, and be respected as individuals.

MANAGING BEHAVIORAL PROBLEMS

Behavioral problems are actions that are annoying, disruptive, harmful, or generally deviate from the norm and that tend to be recurrent in nature, such as physical or verbal abuse, resistance to care, repetitive actions, wandering, restlessness, suspiciousness, and inappropriate sexual behavior and undressing. These problems can occur in persons with altered cognitive status who are incapable of thinking rationally and making good judgments. Any type of illness that lowers the patient's ability to cope with changes and stress can also contribute to these problems. Medications, environmental factors, a loss of independence, and insufficient activity can cause problematic behaviors as well.

Assessing the cause of the behavior is the first step in assisting the patient who displays behavioral problems. Factors associated with the behavior should be closely observed and documented and include the following information:

- time of onset
- where it occurred
- environmental conditions
- persons present

| TABLE 34-1 ● *Checklist for Documenting Drugs and Behavior* | | | | | | | | | | | | | | | | | | | | | | | | |

Date	AM 12	1	2	3	4	5	6	7	8	9	10	11	PM 12	1	2	3	4	5	6	7	8	9	10	11
Medications:																								
Disoriented regarding: Self																								
Others																								
Place																								
Day																								
Time																								
Forgetful of: Today's events																								
Past events																								
Inappropriate: Speech																								
Behavior																								
Hallucinations																								
Wandering																								
ADL deficits: Feeding																								
Bathing																								
Dressing																								
Toileting																								
Mobility																								
Incontinence, urinary																								
Pulse																								
Blood pressure																								
Bowel movement																								
Sleeping/napping																								
Other symptoms:																								

Food Intake	100%	75%	50%	25%	0%	Comments
Breakfast						
Lunch						
Dinner						
Snacks						

Use back to describe specific problems or changes

- activities that preceded
- pattern of behavior
- signs and symptoms present
- outcome
- measures that helped or worsened behavior

It is beneficial to correct the underlying cause of the problem whenever possible. Likewise, factors that precipitate the behavioral problem should be avoided (eg, if it is identified that the patient becomes agitated when seated in a busy hallway, try to avoid seating the patient in this area). Staff or care-givers can prevent behavioral problems by identifying signs and symptoms that precipitate the behaviors and intervening in a timely manner. Environmental considerations that can decrease behavioral problems include maintaining a room temperature between 70°F (21°C) and 75°F (24°C), avoiding wall coverings and linens that have busy patterns, limiting traffic flow, controlling noise, preventing dramatic transitions from daylight to nighttime darkness, and installing safety devices for monitoring, such as alarms on doors and video cameras. Table 34-2 reviews some of the major behaviors, their causes, and related nursing interventions.

Critical Thinking Exercises

1. Discuss factors associated with aging in America that contribute to mental illness in late life.
2. Describe situations that an older patient could experience during a hospitalization for surgery that could cause delirium.
3. Discuss the impact of an older adult's diagnosis of Alzheimer's disease on the spouse, adult children, and grandchildren.
4. Why could dementia be confused with delirium or depression?
5. Why is alcoholism sometimes missed in the elderly?
6. Describe questions and observations that could be used in an interview to uncover mental health problems.
7. Describe reasons for an older adult being suspicious other than a paranoid disorder.

Web Connect

Access an online booklet prepared by the Alzheimer's Association that provides an overview of Alzheimer's disease and current research at http://www.alzheimers.org/unravel.html.

● Resources

Al-Anon Family Group Headquarters (local chapters available)
1600 Corporate Landing Parkway
Virginia Beach, VA 23454
888-4AL-ANON
www.al-anon-alateen.org

Alcoholics Anonymous (local chapters available)
Grand Central Station
P.O. Box 459
New York, NY 10163
(212) 683-3900
www.alcoholics-anonymous.org

Alzheimer's Association
919 N. Michigan Avenue, Suite 1000
Chicago, IL 60611
(800) 272-3900

www.alz.org (local chapters available)

Alzheimer's Disease Education and Referral (ADEAR) Center
P.O. Box 8250
Silver Spring, MD 20907
(800) 438-4380
www.alzheimers.org

Anxiety Disorders Association of America
6000 Executive Boulevard
Suite 513
Rockville, MD 20852
(301) 231-9350
www.aada.org

National Mental Health Association
1021 Prince Street
Alexandria, VA 22314
(800) 969-6642
www.nmha.org

TABLE 34-2 ● *Understanding and Managing Common Behavioral Problems*

Behavior	Possible Causes	Nursing Actions
Violent/physically abusive (eg, hitting, kicking, biting others)	Dementia Paranoia Misinterpretation of actions of others Anger Feeling powerless Anxiety Fatigue	Avoid putting person in situations that trigger behaviors Recognize warning signs (eg, cursing, pacing) Get help to protect self and others Address in calm, quiet manner Distract Move person to area away from others
Verbally abusive (eg, insulting, accusing, threatening)	Dementia Feeling powerless Anger	Avoid arguing, reasoning, reacting to comments Distract with activities Reinforce positive behaviors Allow maximum decision-making and participation
Resisting care	Dementia Misinterpretation of actions, objects, environment Depression	Prepare for activities Break activities into single, simple steps Use alternatives if possible (eg, sponge bath instead of tub bath) Monitor hygiene, nutritional status, intake and output, elimination
Undressing inappropriately	Dementia Soiled clothing Irritation from clothing Feeling too warm	Ensure clothing is clean, dry; replace as necessary Examine clothing for irritation, poor fit Inspect skin for irritation Redress Use clothing that is difficult to unfasten Offer positive reinforcement when person remains dressed
Repetitive actions	Dementia Agitation Anxiety Boredom	Ignore Distract with other activities Replace with a more acceptable repetitive activity (eg, folding laundry, stacking papers)
Wandering	Dementia Boredom Restlessness Anxiety	Schedule times for supervised walking Provide activities Safeguard environment (eg, alarm doors, install door locks that require punching in code to open, ensure window screens cannot be removed) Ensure person is wearing some form of identification Familiarize person with environment; orient
Night wandering, restlessness	Dementia Excess daytime sleeping Misinterpretation of environment Sundowner syndrome Medications (eg, sedatives, hypnotics, diuretics, laxatives)	Provide daytime activities Provide late day exercise Toilet before bed time Keep night light on in bedroom and bathroom Reassure and orient when person awakens Safeguard environment
Inappropriate sexual behavior	Dementia, leading to poor judgment, loss of inhibition Misinterpretation of actions and messages from others	Relocate person to private area Distract with other activities Set limits and remind of acceptable behaviors Review medications for those that can cause reduced inhibitions (eg, antianxiety agents) or that increase libido (eg, L-dopa) Provide acceptable means of touch, human contact
Suspiciousness	Paranoid state Dementia Suspicious personality Medications (eg, anticholinergics, L-dopa, tolbutamide)	Assess cause Don't react to behavior; depersonalize Protect from harm Provide explanations; prepare for activities, changes Afford maximum decision-making Do not try to explain to person that suspicions are unfounded or wrong; this will not be helpful

(Eliopoulos, C. [1991]. Common behavior problems. *Long-Term Care Educator 2*[5], 5.)

National Clearinghouse for Alcohol and Drug Information
11426-28 Rockville Pike, Suite 200
Rockville, MD 20852
(800) 729-6686
www.health.org

National Depressive and Manic-Depressive Association
730 North Franklin
Suite 501
Chicago, IL 60610
(800) 826-3632
www.ndmda.org

Respite Programs for Caregivers of Alzheimer's Disease Patients (Hotline)
(800) 648-COPE

●**References**

Auer, S., & Reisberg, B. (1997). The GDS/FAST staging system. *International Psychogeriatrics, 9*(Suppl 1), 167–171.

Boehnlein, B., & Oakley, L. D. (2002). Implications of self-administered St. John's wort for depression symptom management. *Journal of the American Academy of Nurse Practitioners, 14*(10), 443–448.

Charney, D. S., Reynolds, C. F., & Lewis, L. (2003). Depression and Bipolar Support Alliance consensus statement on the unmet needs in diagnosis and treatment of mood disorders in late life. *Archives of General Psychiatry, 60*(7), 664–672.

Derogatis, R. S., Lipma, K., Rickels, E. H., Uhlenbath, E. H., & Covi, L. (1974). The Hopkins symptom checklist: A measure of primary symptom dimensions. *Pharmacopsychiatry, 7,* 79.

Duke University Center for the Study of Aging. (1978). *Multidimensional functional assessment: The OARS methodology.* Durham, NC: Duke University.

Fishback, D. B. (1977). Mental status questionnaire for organic brain syndrome, with a new visual counting test. *Journal of the American Geriatric Society, 25,* 167.

Folstein, M. F., Folstein, S., & McHugh, P. R. (1975). Mini-mental state: A practical method for grading the cognitive state of patients for the clinician. *Journal of Psychiatry Research, 12,* 189.

Goldberg, D. (1972). *The detection of psychiatric illness by questionnaire.* London: Oxford University Press.

Howes, M. J., Perry, N. S., & Houghton, P. J. (2003). Plants with traditional uses and activities, relevant to the management of Alzheimer's disease and other cognitive disorders. *Phytotherapy Research, 17*(1), 1–18.

Isacson, O., Seo, H., Lin, L., et al. (2002). Alzheimer's disease and Down's syndrome: Roles of APP, trophic factors and ACh. *Trends in Neuroscience, 25*(2), 79–84.

Knauer, C. (2003). Geriatric alcohol abuse: A national epidemic. *Geriatric Nursing 24*(3), 152–154.

Kochanek, K. D., Smith, B. L., & Andersen, R. N. (2001). *Deaths: Preliminary data for 1999. National Vital Statistics Reports,* Vol. 49, No. 3. Hyattsville, MD: National Center for Health Statistics.

National Health Information. (2003). St. John's wort in depression: A new meta-analysis. *Alternative Medicine Research Report, 2*(1), 1–5.

National Institute on Aging. (2002). *Alzheimer's disease: Unraveling the mystery.* Publication No. 02-3782, Rockville, MD: National Institutes of Health.

National Institutes of Health. (2003). New prevalence study suggests dramatically rising numbers of people with Alzheimer's disease. *National Institutes of Health Press Release,* August 13, 2003. Retrieved August 23, 2003, from www.nia.nih.gov/news/pr/2003/0820.htm.

National Mental Health Association. (2003). *Depression and older Americans.* Retrieved May 30, 2003, from www.nmha.org/ccd./support/factsheet.older.cfm.

Oken, B. S., Storzbach, D. M., & Kaye, J. A. (2000). The efficacy of Ginkgo biloba on cognitive function in Alzheimer disease. In P. B. Fortanarosa (Ed.). *Alternative medicine: An objective assessment* (pp. 332–339). Chicago: American Medical Association.

Pfeiffer, E. (1975). A short portable mental status questionnaire for the assessment of organic brain deficit in elderly patients. *Journal of the American Geriatric Society, 23*(10), 433.

Prasher, V., Cumella, S., Natarajan, K., et al, (2003). Magnetic resonance imaging, Down's syndrome and Alzheimer's disease: research and clinical implications. *Journal of Intellectual Disabilities Research, 47*(Pt 2), 90–100.

Shumaker, S. A., Legault, C., Rapp, S. R., et al. (2003). Estrogen plus progestin and the incidence of dementia and mild cognitive impairment in postmenopausal women. The Women's Health Initiative Memory Study: A randomized controlled trial. *Journal of the American Medical Association, 289*(20), 2651.

Zung, W. W. K. (1965). A self-rating depression scale. *Archives of General Psychiatry, 12,* 63.

●**Recommended Readings**

Algase, D. L. (1999). Wandering: Dementia-compromised behavior. *Journal of Gerontological Nursing, 25*(9), 10–16.

Allen, L. A. (1999). Treating agitation without drugs. *American Journal of Nursing, 99*(4), 36–42.

Antai-Otang, D.(2003). Suicide: Life span considerations. *Nursing Clinics of North America, 38*(1), 137–150

Blixen, C. E. (1998). Aging and mental health care. *Journal of Gerontological Nursing, 14*(11), 11.

Buettner, L. L. (1998). A team approach to dynamic programming on the special care unit. *Journal of Gerontological Nursing, 24*(1), 23–30.

Buettner, L., & Kolanowski, A. (2003). Practice guidelines for recreation therapy in the care of people with dementia. *Geriatric Nursing, 24*(1), 18–25.

Burgener, S. C., & Dickerson-Putnam, J. (1999). Assessing patients in the early stages of irreversible dementia: The relevance of patient perspectives. *Journal of Gerontological Nursing, 25*(2), 33–41.

Cacchione, P. Z., Culp, K., Laing, J., & Tripp-Reimer, T. (2003). Clinical profile of acute confusion in the long-term care setting. *Clinical Nursing Research, 12*(2), 145–158.

Carey, M. (2003). Entering Donald's world. Creative interventions in Alzheimer's. *Journal of Christian Nursing, 20*(1), 9–12.

Clark, M. E., Lipe, A. W., & Bilbrey, M. (1998). Use of music to decrease aggressive behaviors in people with dementia. *Journal of Gerontological Nursing, 24*(7), 10–17.

Clavel, D. S. (1999). Vocalizations among cognitively impaired elders: What is your patient trying to tell you? *Geriatric Nursing, 20*(2), 90–93.

Colling, K. B. (1999). Passive behaviors in dementia: Clinical application of the need-driven dementia-compromised behavior model. *Journal of Gerontological Nursing, 25*(9), 27–32.

Connell, C. M., & Gibson, G. D. (1997). Racial, ethnic, and cultural differences in dementia caregiving: Review and analysis. *The Gerontologist, 37,* 355–364.

Davis, K. M., & Matthew, E. (1998). Pharmacologic management of depression in the elderly. *The Nurse Practitioner, 23*(6), 16, 18, 26.

Denney, A. (1997). Quiet music: An intervention for mealtime agitation? *Journal of Gerontological Nursing, 23*(7), 16–23.

Donovan, C., & Dupuis, M. (2000). Specialized care unit: Family and staff's perceptions of significant elements. *Geriatric Nursing, 21*(1), 30–33.

Fick, D., & Foreman, M. (2000). Consequences of not recognizing delirium superimposed on dementia in hospitalized elderly individuals. *Journal of Gerontological Nursing, 26*(1), 30–39.

Futrell, M., Melillo, K. D., & Tang, J. H. (2002). Evidence-based protocol: Wandering. *Journal of Gerontological Nursing, 28*(11):14–22.

Gray-Vickrey, P. (2002). Advances in Alzheimer's disease. *Nursing, 32*(11 Pt 1), 64.

Guse, L., Inglis, J., Chicoine, J., Leche, G., Stadnyk, L.,

& Whitbread, L. (2000). Life albums in long-term care: Residents, family, and staff perceptions. *Geriatric Nursing, 21*(1), 34–37.

Hultsch, D. F. (1998). *Memory change in the aged.* New York: Cambridge University Press.

Kaempf, G., O'Donnell, C., & Oslin, D. W. (1999). The BRENDA model: A psychosocial addiction model to identify and treat alcohol disorders in elders. *Geriatric Nursing, 20*(6), 302–304.

Kaas, M. J., & Lewis, M. L. (1999). Cognitive behavior group therapy for residents in assisted-living facilities. *Journal of Psychosocial Nursing and Mental Health Services, 37*(10), 9–15.

Kelley, L. S., Specht, J. K. P., & Maas, M. L. (2000). Family involvement in care for individuals with dementia protocol. *Journal of Gerontological Nursing, 26*(2), 13–21.

Kurlowicz, L., & Wallace, M. (1999). Mini-mental state examination: Try this. *Journal of Gerontological Nursing, 25*(5), 8–9.

Larrimore, K.L. (2003). Alzheimer disease support group characteristics: A comparison of caregivers. *Geriatric Nursing, 24*(1), 32–35.

Lilly, M. L., Richards, B. S., & Buckwalter, K. C. (2003). Friends and social support in dementia caregiving: Assessment and intervention. *Journal of Gerontological Nursing, 29*(1), 29–36.

Lim, Y. M. (2003). Nursing intervention for grooming of elders with mild cognitive impairments in Korea. *Geriatric Nursing, 24*(1), 11–17.

Long, C. O., & Dougherty, J. (2003). What's new in Alzheimer's disease? *Home Healthcare Nurse, 21*(1), 8–14

Mathiasen, P., & LaVert, S. (1998). *Late life depression.* New York: Dell Publishers.

McAiney, C. A. (1998). The development of the empowered aide model: An intervention for long-term care staff who care for Alzheimer's residents. *Journal of Gerontological Nursing, 24*(1), 17–22.

McGee, E. M. (2000). Alcoholics Anonymous and nursing: Lessons in holism and spiritual care. *Journal of Holistic Nursing, 18*(1), 11–26.

McKhann, G., & Albert, M. (2002). *Keeping your brain young: The complete guide to physical and emotional health and longevity.* Hoboken, NJ: John Wiley and Sons.

Moore, S. L., Metcalf, B., & Schow, E. (2000). Aging and meaning in life: Examining the concept. *Geriatric Nursing, 21*(1), 27–29.

Nissenboim, S., & Vroman, C. (1998). *The positive interactions program of activities for people with Alzheimer's disease.* Baltimore: Health Professions Press.

Onega, L. L., & Abraham, I. L. (1998). Differentiated nursing assessment of depressive symptoms in community-dwelling elders. *Nursing Clinics of North America, 33*(3), 407–416.

Ostwald, S. K., Hepburn, K. W., & burns, T. (2003). Training family caregivers of patients with dementia: A structured workshop approach. *Journal of Gerontological Nursing, 29*(1), 37–44.

Petersen, R. (Ed.). (2002). *Mayo Clinic on Alzheimer's disease.* Rochester, MN: Mayo Clinic Health Information.

Poveda, A. M. (2003). An anthropological perspective of Alzheimer disease. *Geriatric Nursing, 24*(1), 26–31.

Resnick, B. (2003). Dementia, delirium, and depression in older adults. *Advance for Providers of Post-Acute Care, January/February,* 49–52.

Restak, R. (2001). *The secret life of the brain.* Washington, DC: Joseph Henry Press.

Rinaldi, P., Mecocci, P., Benedetti, C., et al. (2003). Validation of the five-item geriatric depression scale in elderly subjects in three different settings. *Journal of the American Geriatric Society, 51*(5), 694–698.

Robie, D., Edgemon-Hill, E. J., Phelps, B., Schmitz, C., & Laughlin, J. A. (1999). Suicide prevention protocol. *American Journal of Nursing, 99*(12), 53–63.

Rowe, M., & Alfred, D. (1999). The effectiveness of slow-stroke massage in diffusing agitated behaviors in individuals with Alzheimer's disease. *Journal of Gerontological Nursing, 25*(6), 22–34.

Ryden, M. B., Pearson, V., Kaas, M. J., Hanscom, J., Lee, H., Krichbaum, K., Wang, J. J., & Snyder, M. (1999). Nursing interventions for depression in newly admitted nursing home residents. *Journal of Gerontological Nursing, 25*(3), 20–29.

Salvatore, T. (2000). Elder suicide: A preventable tragedy. *CARING Magazine, 19*(3), 34–37.

Smyer, M. A., & Qualls, S. H. (1999). *Aging and mental health.* Malden, MA: Blackwell Publishers.

Snowden, D. (2001). *Aging with grace: What the nun study teaches us about leading longer, healthier, and more meaningful lives.* New York: Random House.

Stewart, D. E. (2003). Physical symptoms of depression: Unmet needs in special populations. *Journal of Clinical Psychiatry, 64*(Suppl 7), 12–16.

Thimis, A. (1995). An alternative for Alzheimer's residents. *Provider, 21*(6), 41–43.

Tsang, H. W., Mok, C. K., Au Yeung, Y. T., & Chan, S. Y. (2003). The effect of Qigong on general and psychosocial health of elderly with chronic physical illnesses: A randomized clinical trial. *International Journal of Geriatric Psychiatry, 18*(5), 441–449

U.S. Preventive Services Task Force. (2002). Screening for depression: Recommendations and rationale. *American Journal of Nursing, 102*(7), 77–80.

Wallace, M. (1999). Creutzfeldt-Jakob disease: Assessment and management update. *Journal of Gerontological Nursing, 25*(10), 17–24.

Warner, M. L. (1998). *The complete guide to Alzheimer's-proofing your home.* West Lafayette, IN: Purdue University Press.

Whall, A. L., & Hoes-Gurevich, M. L. (1999). Missed depression in elderly individuals: Why is this a problem? *Journal of Gerontological Nursing, 25*(6), 44–46.

Winters, S. (2003). Alzheimer disease from a child's perspective. *Geriatric Nursing, 24*(1), 36–39.

Wolf, T. P. (2003). Building a caring client relationship and creating a quilt. A parallel and metaphorical process. *Journal of Holistic Nursing, 21*(1), 81–87.

Yen, P. K. (2003). Maintaining cognitive function with diet. *Geriatric Nursing, 24*(1), 62–63.

Zarit, S. H., & Zarit, J. M. (1998). *Mental disorders in older adults: Fundamentals of assessment and treatment.* New York: Guilford Press.

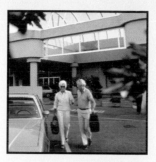

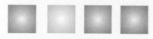

Gerontological Care Issues

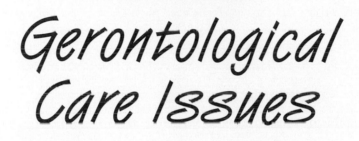

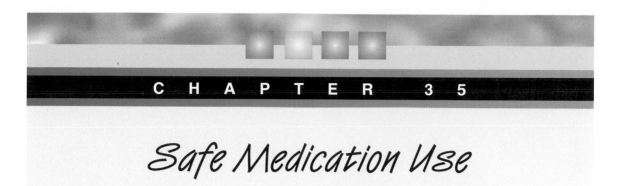

C H A P T E R 3 5

Safe Medication Use

■ *Learning Objectives*

After reading this chapter, you should be able to:

• describe the unique aspects of drug pharmacokinetics and pharmacodynamics in the aged

• list measures to promote safe drug use

• describe alternatives to medications

Drugs Consumed by the Older Population

The high prevalence of health conditions in the older population causes this group to use a large number and variety of medications. Although they account for approximately 13% of the total population, elders consume slightly more than one third of all prescription drugs and spend billions annually on medications (Center for Medicare Education, 2002) (Fig. 35-1). A majority of the elderly use at least one drug regularly, with the more typical situation involving the use of several drugs daily. Researchers have found that the number of drugs used by elders increases with age (Kaufman et al., 2002). The most commonly used drugs by the older population include:

• cardiovascular agents
• antihypertensives
• analgesics
• antiarthritic agents
• sedatives
• tranquilizers
• laxatives
• antacids

The drugs on this list can cause adverse effects (eg, confusion, dizziness, falls, fluid and electrolyte imbalances) that threaten the elderly's quality of life. Furthermore, when taken together, some of these drugs can interact and cause serious adverse effects (Table 35-1).

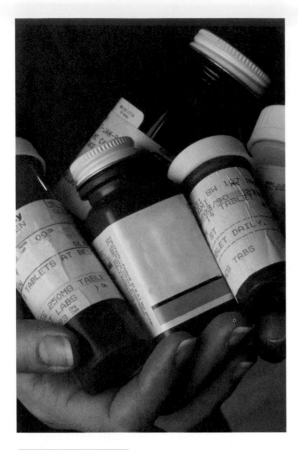

FIGURE 35-1

The high prevalence of drugs consumed by the elderly and the complexity of drug dynamics in old age require gerontological nurses to evaluate regularly the continued need, appropriateness of dosage, and intended and adverse effects of every drug given to older individuals.

Point to Ponder

How often do you rely on medications to curb appetite, promote sleep, stimulate bowel elimination, or manage a headache or some other symptom? Why do you choose to use medications rather than address the underlying cause or use a natural means to correct the problem? How can you change this?

Response of Older Adults to Drugs

In addition to the type and volume of drugs used by the older population, age-related differences in pharmacokinetics and pharmacodynamics heighten the risks associated with drug therapy in this age group. *Pharmacokinetics* refers to the absorption, distribution, metabolism, and excretion of drugs; *pharmacodynamics* refers to the biologic and therapeutic effects of drugs at the site of action or on the target organ. Drugs behave differently in older adults than in younger adults and require careful dosage adjustment and monitoring. To minimize the risks associated with drug therapy and ensure that medications do not create more problems than they solve, close supervision and adherence to sound principles of safe drug use are essential in gerontological nursing.

> **KEY CONCEPT**
> The risk of adverse drug reactions is high in older adults because of age-related differences in pharmacokinetics and pharmacodynamics.

Pharmacokinetics

ABSORPTION

Generally, older people have fewer problems in the area of drug absorption than with distribution, metabolism, and excretion of drugs. A variety of factors can alter the absorption of drugs, such as:

- *Age-related changes:* Decreased intracellular fluid, increased gastric pH, decreased gastric blood flow and motility, reduced cardiac output and circulation, and slower metabolism can slow drug absorption.
- *Route of administration:* Drugs given intramuscularly, subcutaneously, orally, or rectally are not absorbed as efficiently as drugs that are inhaled, applied topically, or instilled intravenously.
- *Concentration and solubility of drug:* Drugs that are highly soluble (eg, aqueous solutions) and in higher concentrations are absorbed with greater speed than less soluble and concentrated drugs.

TABLE 35-1 ● *Interactions Among Popular Drug Groups*

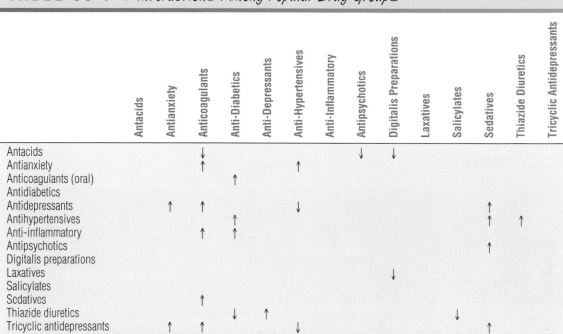

	Antacids	Antianxiety	Anticoagulants	Anti-Diabetics	Anti-Depressants	Anti-Hypertensives	Anti-Inflammatory	Antipsychotics	Digitalis Preparations	Laxatives	Salicylates	Sedatives	Thiazide Diuretics	Tricyclic Antidepressants
Antacids			↓					↓	↓					
Antianxiety			↑			↑								
Anticoagulants (oral)				↑										
Antidiabetics														
Antidepressants	↑	↑				↓						↑		
Antihypertensives				↑								↑	↑	
Anti-inflammatory			↑	↑										
Antipsychotics												↑		
Digitalis preparations														
Laxatives									↓					
Salicylates														
Sedatives			↑											
Thiazide diuretics				↓	↑									
Tricyclic antidepressants		↑	↑			↓					↓	↑		

Arrows indicate the effect of drugs listed in the left-hand column on those listed across the top. (Adapted from Eliopoulos, C. [1990]. Safe drug use in the elderly. In Eliopoulos, C. [Ed.]. *Caring for the elderly in diverse care settings.* Philadelphia: J.B. Lippincott.)

● *Diseases and symptoms:* Conditions such as diabetes mellitus and hypokalemia can increase the absorption of drugs, whereas pain and mucosal edema will slow absorption.

Although nurses can do little to improve many of the underlying factors responsible for altered drug absorption, they can use measures to maximize the absorption of drugs. Exercise will stimulate circulation and should be encouraged. Properly used heat and massage likewise will increase blood flow at the absorption site. Preventing fluid volume deficit, hypothermia, and hypotension is beneficial in facilitating absorption. Preparations that neutralize gastric secretions should be avoided if a low gastric pH is required for drug absorption. Drug–drug and drug–food interactions should be monitored (Table 35-2). With the increasing use of herbal remedies, drug-herb interactions also must be reviewed (Table 35-3). Consideration should be given to using the most effective administration route for the drug.

DISTRIBUTION

Although it is difficult to predict with certainty how drug distribution will differ among older adults, changes in circulation, membrane permeability, body temperature, and tissue structure can modify this process. For example, adipose tissue increases compared to lean body mass in the elderly and occurs to a greater extent in women; drugs stored in adipose tissue (ie, lipid-soluble drugs) will have increased tissue concentrations, decreased plasma concentrations, and a longer duration in the body. Decreased cardiac output can raise the plasma levels of drugs while reducing their deposition in reservoirs; this is particularly apparent with water-soluble drugs. Reduced serum albumin levels can be problematic if several protein-bound drugs are consumed and compete for the same protein molecules; the unbound drug concentrations will rise and the effectiveness of the drugs will be threatened. Highly protein-bound drugs that may compete at protein-binding sites and displace each other include acetazo-

TABLE 35-2 ● *Examples of Food and Drug Interactions*

Drug	Potential Interactions
Acetaminophen	Accumulation to toxic level if more than 500 mg vitamin C supplements are ingested daily
Allopurinol	Impairs iron absorption leading to iron deficiency anemia
	Combined with alcohol or simple carbohydrates can increase blood uric acid level
Aluminum antacids	Depletes phosphate and calcium
	Decreases absorption of vitamins A, C, and D, and magnesium, thiamine, folacin, and iron
Antihistamines	Ingestion of large amounts of alkaline foods (eg, milk, cream, almonds, alcohol) can prolong action
Aspirin	Can cause iron deficiency anemia as a result of gastrointestinal bleeding
	Causes vitamin C deficiency (12+ aspirin tablets daily)
	Causes thiamine deficiency
Calcium carbonate antacids	Cause deficiencies of phosphate, folacin, iron, thiamine
Calcium supplements	Combined with large doses of vitamin D can cause hypercalcemia
	Absorption decreased by foods rich in oxalate (eg, spinach, rhubarb, celery, peanuts), phytic acid (eg, oatmeal and other grain cereals), phosphorous (chocolate, dried beans, dried fruit, peanut butter)
Chlorpromazine HCl	Large amounts of alkaline foods can delay excretion
	Can increase blood cholesterol
Cimetidine	Reduces iron absorption
Clonidine HCl	Effectiveness reduced by tyramine-rich foods (eg, chicken and beef livers, bananas, sour cream, meat tenderizers, salami, yeast, chocolate)
	Can cause sodium and fluid retention
Colchicine	Effectiveness decreased by caffeine
	Some herbal teas contain phenylbutazone, which can increase blood uric acid and decrease effectiveness of antigout drugs
Dicumarol	Effectiveness reduced by foods rich in vitamin K (eg, cabbage, broccoli, asparagus, spinach, turnip greens)
Digitalis	Can cause deficiencies of thiamine, magnesium, and zinc
	Calcium supplements increase risk of toxicity
Estrogen	Hastens breakdown of vitamin C
Ferrous supplements	Absorption decreased by antacids, increased by vitamin C
Furosemide	Increases excretion of calcium, magnesium, potassium, and zinc
Hydralazine	Can cause vitamin B_6 deficiency
Levodopa	Effectiveness reduced by high-protein diet
	Can cause deficiencies of potassium, folacin, and vitamins B_6 and B_{12}
Magnesium antacids	Can deplete phosphate and calcium
Magnesium-based laxatives	30 ml contains nearly four times the average daily intake of magnesium; toxicity can result
Mineral oil	Decrease absorption of vitamins A, D, and K
Phenobarbital	Increases breakdown of vitamins D and K
	Impairs absorption of vitamins B_6 and B_{12} and folic acid
Phenylbutazone	Inhibits absorption of iodine
Phenytoin	Increases breakdown of vitamins D and K
	Reduces absorption of folacin
Potassium supplements	Absorption decreased by dairy products
	Impairs absorption of vitamin B_{12}
Probenecid	Effectiveness decreased by coffee, tea, or cola
Spironolactone	Increases excretion of calcium
	Decreases excretion of potassium leading to potassium toxicity
Theophylline	Effectiveness reduced by high-carbohydrate diet
Thiazides	Increases excretion of calcium, potassium, magnesium, zinc
	Can decrease blood glucose level
Thioridazine	Excretion delayed by high-alkaline diet
Warfarin	Effectiveness reduced by large amounts of vitamin K in diet

(From Eliopoulos, C. [1990]. Safe drug use in the elderly. In Eliopoulos, C. [Ed]. *Caring for the elderly in diverse care settings*. Philadelphia: J.B. Lippincott.)

TABLE 35-3 ● *Potential Adverse Effects of Selected Herbs*
Aloe: allergic dermatitis; increases effects of cardiac glycosides; increases potassium loss when taken with corticosteroids or thiazide diuretics
Angelica: rash when the person is exposed to sunlight
Balm: interferes with thyroid-stimulating hormone
Barberry: drastic reductions in blood pressure, heart rate, and respirations with large doses
Bayberry: edema, elevation of blood pressure; contraindicated in persons with history of cancer
Black cohosh: depression of cardiac function leading to bradycardia and hypotension; estrogen-like properties can cause abnormal coagulation and liver dysfunction
Bloodroot: bradycardia, arrhythmia, impaired vision, thirst
Cascara sagrada: severe intestinal cramps
Celery: hypokalemia with long-term use
Chaparral: liver damage
Coltsfoot: liver toxicity, fever
Comfrey: liver toxicity
Dandelion: hypokalemia with long-term use
Ephedra (ma huang): elevation of blood pressure and heart rate, insomnia, dizziness, anxiety
Feverfew: interference with coagulation; when taken orally can cause mouth ulcers, loss of taste sensation, swelling of oral cavity; increases anticoagulation effects of aspirin and warfarin sodium
Garlic: anticoagulation effect, hypotension, increases effects of antidiabetic agents
Ginkgo biloba: anticoagulation effect, irritability, restlessness, insomnia, nausea, vomiting, diarrhea; increases effects of anticoagulants
Ginseng: elevation of blood pressure, insomnia
Goldenseal: vasoconstriction
Hawthorne: dramatic reductions in blood pressure
Hops: drowsiness, increased effects of sedatives and tranquilizers
Licorice: edema, hypertension, hypokalemia, and hypernatremia with long-term use
Mistletoe: bradycardia; potentially fatal
Parsely: hypokalemia with long-term use
Red clover: estrogen-like effects, contraindicated in persons with estrogen-dependent cancer
Rhubarb: severe abdominal cramps, diarrhea
Senna: can increase effects of digoxin
St. John's wort: acts as monoamine oxidase inhibitor; hypertension, photosensitivity, nausea, vomiting

lamide, amitriptyline, cefazolin, chlordiazepoxide, chlorpromazine, cloxacillin, digitoxin, furosemide, hydralazine, nortriptyline, phenylbutazone, phenytoin, propranolol, rifampin, salicylates, spironolactone, sulfisoxazole, and warfarin. When monitoring the blood levels of medications, it is also important to evaluate the serum albumin level. For instance, raising the dosage of phenytoin because the blood level is low can lead to toxicity if the serum albumin also is low.

KEY CONCEPT
When several are taken concurrently, protein-bound drugs may not achieve desired results because of ineffective binding to reduced protein molecules.

Conditions such as dehydration and hypoalbuminemia decrease drug distribution and result in higher drug levels in the plasma. When these conditions exist, lower dosage levels may be necessary.

METABOLISM, DETOXIFICATION, AND EXCRETION

The renal system is primarily responsible for the body's excretory functions, and among its activities is the excretion of drugs. Drugs follow a path through the kidneys similar to that of most constituents of urine. After systemic circulation, the drug filters through the walls of glomerular capillaries into the Bowman capsule. The drug continues down the tubule, where substances beneficial to the body will be reabsorbed into the bloodstream through proximal convoluted tubules and where waste substances excreted through the urine flow into the pelvis of the kidney. Capillaries surrounding the tubules reabsorb the filtered blood and join to form the renal vein. It is estimated that to promote this filtration process almost 10 times more blood circulates through the kidneys than through similarly sized body organs. The reduced efficiency of body organs with advanced age affects the kidneys as well, complicating drug excretion in the elderly. Nephron units are decreased in number, and many of the remaining ones can be nonfunctional in older individuals. The glomerular filtration rate and tubular reabsorption are reduced. Decreasing cardiac function contributes to the almost 50% reduction in blood flow to the kidneys. The implications of reduced kidney efficiency are important. Drugs are not as quickly filtered from the bloodstream and are present in the body longer. The biological half-life, or the time necessary for half of the drug to be excreted, can increase as much as 40% and increase the risk for adverse drug reactions. Drugs that have a likelihood of accumulating because of an increased biological half-life include antibiotics, barbiturates, cimetidine, digoxin, and salicylate.

🔑 **KEY CONCEPT**
The extended biological half-life of drugs in older adults increases the risk of adverse reactions.

The liver also has many important functions that influence drug detoxification and excretion. Carbohydrate metabolism in the liver converts glucose into glycogen and releases it into the bloodstream when needed. Protein metabolism in the parenchymal cells of the liver is responsible for the loss of the amine groups from amino acids, which aid in the formation of new plasma proteins, such as prothrombin and fibrinogen, as well as in the conversion of some poisonous nitrogenous by-products into nontoxic substances such as vitamin B_{12}. Also important is the liver's formation of bile, which breaks down fats through enzymatic action and removes substances such as bilirubin from the blood. The liver decreases in size and function with age, and hepatic blood flow declines by 45% between the ages of 25 and 65 years. This could affect the distribution of some drugs, such as antibiotics, cimetidine, chlordiazepoxide, digoxin, lithium, meperidine, nortriptyline, and quinidine.

Certain enzymes may not be secreted, which interferes with the metabolism of drugs that require enzymatic activity. Most important, the detoxification and conjugation of drugs may be significantly reduced, so that the drug stays in the bloodstream longer. Some evidence indicates larger drug concentrations at administration sites in older persons.

Conditions such as dehydration, hyperthermia, immobility, and liver disease can decrease the metabolism of drugs. As a consequence, drugs can accumulate to toxic levels and cause serious adverse reactions. Careful monitoring is essential. Along this line, the extended biological half-life of many of the drugs consumed by the elderly warrants close evaluation of drug clearance. Estimated creatinine clearance must be calculated based on the age, weight, and serum creatinine level of the individual because serum creatinine levels alone may not reflect a reduced creatinine clearance level.

Pharmacodynamics

Information on pharmacodynamics in the older population is limited but will grow as increased research is done in this area. At this point, some of the known differences in older adults' responses to drugs include increased myocardial sensitivity to anesthesias and increased central nervous system receptor sensitivity to narcotics, alcohol, and bromides.

ADVERSE REACTIONS

The risk of adverse reactions to drugs is so high in the elderly that some geropharmacologists suggest that any symptom in an older adult be suspected as being related to a drug until proved otherwise (Patel, 2003). The following are some general factors to remember in regard to adverse reactions.

- The signs and symptoms of an adverse reaction to a given drug may differ in older persons.
- A prolonged time may be required for an adverse reaction to become apparent in older adults.
- An adverse reaction to a drug may be demonstrated even after the drug has been discontinued.
- Adverse reactions to a drug that has been used over a long period without problems can develop suddenly.

Varying degrees of mental dysfunction often are early symptoms of adverse reactions to commonly prescribed medications for the elderly, such as codeine, digitalis, methyldopa, phenobarbital, L-dopa, Valium, and various diuretics. Any medication that can promote hypoglycemia, acidosis, fluid and electrolyte imbalances, temperature elevations, increased intracranial pressure, and reduced cerebral circulation also can produce mental disturbances. Even the most subtle changes in mental status could be linked to a medication and should be reviewed with a physician. The elderly easily may become victims of drug-induced mental illness. Unfortunately, mental and behavioral dysfunction in the elderly is sometimes treated symptomatically (ie, with medications but without full exploration of the etiology). This will not correct a drug-related problem and can predispose the individual to additional complications from the new drug.

> **KEY CONCEPT**
> Gerontological nurses should ensure that drug-induced cognitive and behavioral problems are not treated with additional drugs.

Promoting the Safe Use of Drugs

The scope of drug use and significant adverse reactions that can result necessitate that gerontological nurses ensure drugs are used selectively and cautiously. Nurses should review all prescription and nonprescription medications used by patients and ask themselves these questions.

Why is the drug ordered?

Consider whether the drug is really needed. Perhaps warm milk and a back rub could eliminate the need for the sedative; maybe the patient had a bowel movement this morning and now does not need the laxative. Perhaps the medication is prescribed because it has been prescribed for years and no one has considered its discontinuation.

Is the smallest possible dosage ordered?

The elderly usually require lower dosages of most medications because of the delayed time for excretion of the substance. Larger dosages increase the risk of adverse reactions.

Is the patient allergic to the drug?

Sometimes the physician may overlook a known allergy, or perhaps the patient neglected to share an allergy problem with the physician. The nurse may be aware of a patient's sensitivities to certain drugs. Consideration must also be given to new signs that could indicate a reaction to a drug that has been used for a long period without trouble.

Can this drug interact with other drugs, herbs, or nutritional supplements that are being used?

It is useful to review resource material to identify potential interactions—they are too numerous for anyone to commit to memory!

Are there any special instructions accompanying the drug's administration?

Some drugs should be given on an empty stomach, others with a meal. Certain times of the day may be better for drugs to be given than others.

Is the most effective route of administration being used?

A person who cannot swallow a large tablet may do better with a liquid form. Suppositories that are expelled because of ineffective melting or oral drugs that are vomited obviously will not have the therapeutic effect of the drug given in a different manner.

Nurses must go through a mental checklist of these questions when administering medications and teach older persons who are responsible for their own medication administration, as well as their caregivers, to do the same.

> **KEY CONCEPT**
> Regular review of a drug's ongoing necessity and effectiveness is essential.

The most common way to administer drugs is orally. Oral medications in the form of tablets, capsules, liquids, powders, elixirs, spirits, emulsions, mixtures, and magmas are used either for their direct action on the mucous membrane of the digestive tract (eg, antacids) or for their systemic effects (eg, antibiotics and tranquilizers). Although administration is simple, certain problems can interfere with the process. Dry mucous membranes of the oral cavity, common in older individuals, can prevent capsules and tablets from being swallowed. If they are then expelled from the mouth, there is no therapeutic value; if they dissolve in the mouth, they can irritate the mucous membrane. Proper oral hygiene, ample fluids for assistance with swallowing and mobility, proper positioning, and examining the oral cavity after administration will ensure that the patient receives the full benefit of the medicine during its travel through the gastrointestinal system. Some elderly people may not even be aware that a tablet is stuck to the roof of their dentures or under their tongue.

KEY CONCEPT
To ensure that oral medications achieve full benefit, encourage good oral hygiene, ample fluids, and proper positioning to facilitate swallowing.

Because enteric-coated and sustained-release tablets should not be crushed, the nurse should consult with a physician for an alternative form of the drug if a tablet is too large to be swallowed. As a rule, capsules are not to be broken open and mixed. Medications are put into capsule form so that unpleasant tastes will be masked or the coating will dissolve when it comes into contact with specific gastrointestinal secretions. Some vitamin, mineral, and electrolyte preparations are bitter, and even more so for older persons, whose taste buds for sweetness are lost long before those for sourness and bitterness. Combining the medication with foods and drinks such as applesauce and juices can make them more palatable and prevent gastric irritation, although there may be a problem if the full amount of medicated food is not ingested. Individuals should be informed that the food or drink they are ingesting contains a medication. Oral hygiene after the administration of oral drugs will prevent an unpleasant aftertaste.

Drugs prescribed in suppository form for local or systemic action are inserted into various body cavities and act by melting from body heat or dissolving in body fluids. Because circulation to the lower bowel and vagina is decreased and the body temperature is lower in many older individuals, a prolonged period may be required for the suppository to melt. If no alternative route can be used and the suppository form must be given, a special effort must be made to ensure that the suppository is not expelled.

KEY CONCEPT
Lower body temperature and decreased circulation to the lower bowel and vagina can prolong the time required for suppositories to melt.

Intramuscular and subcutaneous administration of drugs is necessary when immediate results are sought or when other routes are not able to be used, either because of the nature of the drug or the status of the individual. The upper, outer quadrant of the buttocks is the best site for intramuscular injections. Frequently, the older person will bleed or ooze after the injection because of decreased tissue elasticity; a small pressure bandage may be helpful. Alternating the injection site will help to reduce discomfort. Medication should not be injected into an immobile limb because the inactivity of the limb will reduce the rate of absorption. A person receiving frequent injections should be checked for signs of infection at the injection site; reduced subcutaneous sensation in older persons or absence of sensation, as that experienced with a stroke, may prevent the person from being aware of a complication at the injection site.

Occasionally, intravenous administration of drugs is essential. In addition to observing the effects of the medication, the nurse needs to be alert to the amount of fluid in which the drug is administered. Declining cardiac and renal function make the elderly more susceptible not only to dehydration but also to overhydration. Signs of circulatory overload must be closely monitored, including elevated blood pressure, increased respirations, coughing, shortness of breath, and symptoms associated with pulmonary edema. Intake and output balance, body weight, and specific gravity are useful to monitor. Of course, patients should be observed for complications associated with intravenous therapy in any age group, for example, infiltration, air embolism, thrombophlebitis, and pyrogenic reactions. Decreased sensation may mask any of these potential complications, emphasizing the necessity for close nursing observation.

KEY CONCEPT
The elderly are at risk for circulatory overload during intravenous drug therapy; close monitoring is essential.

Because so many elderly people are responsible for self-medication, nurses should promote self-care capacity in this area. An assessment of a patient's risk for medication errors should be done (Display 35-1) and interventions planned to minimize those risks. A detailed description, both verbal and written, should be given to the elderly and their caregivers, outlining the drug's name, dosage schedule, route of administration, action, special precautions, incompatible foods or drugs, and adverse reactions. A color-coded dosage schedule can be developed to assist persons who have visual deficits or who are illiterate. Medication labels with large print and caps that can be easily removed by weak or arthritic hands should be provided. During every patient-nurse visit, the patient's medication schedule should be reviewed and new symptoms explored. A variety of potential medication errors can be prevented or corrected by close monitoring. Some of the classic self-medication errors include incorrect dosage, noncompliance arising from misunderstanding, discontinuation or unnecessary continuation of drugs without medical advice, and the use of medications prescribed for previous illnesses. Display 35-2 describes guidelines to use in teaching elders about safe drug use.

Alternatives to Drugs

Older adults have many health conditions for which drugs can prove helpful. On the other hand, drugs can produce serious adverse effects that can result in greater threats to elders than their primary health condition. It is crucial that drugs be used cautiously and that the benefits and risks of drugs be weighed to ensure they are resulting in more good than harm.

Sometimes lifestyle changes can improve conditions and eliminate the need for medications. These can include diet modifications, regular exercise, effective stress management techniques, and regular schedules for sleep, rest, and elimination.

Alternative and complementary therapies provide new avenues for treating health conditions. These therapies have grown in acceptance and popularity among consumers and can offer effective and safe approaches to managing health conditions. Often, alternative therapies can replace the need for drugs or enable lower dosages of drugs to be used. It is crucial for nurses to be aware of the uses, limitations, precautions, and possible adverse reactions associated with alternative therapies so that they can help elders be informed consumers. (**Visit the Connection website to learn about some useful alternative therapies.**)

✔ **Point to Ponder**
How can you envision using alternative and complementary therapies as substitutes for or adjuncts to drug therapy in your practice? What obstacles could you face in attempting to integrate these therapies into your practice and what could you do to overcome them?

DISPLAY 35-1

Risk Factors for Medication Errors

Use of multiple medications	Lack of knowledge regarding medications
Cognitive impairment	Limited finances
Visual deficits	Illiteracy
Hearing deficits	Lack of support system
Arthritic or weak hands	History of inappropriate self-medication
History of noncompliance with medical care	Presence of expired or borrowed medications in home

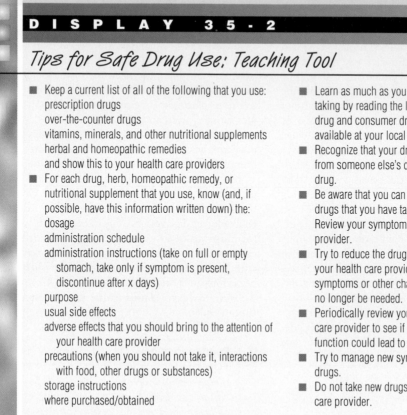

DISPLAY 35-2

Tips for Safe Drug Use: Teaching Tool

- Keep a current list of all of the following that you use:
  prescription drugs
  over-the-counter drugs
  vitamins, minerals, and other nutritional supplements
  herbal and homeopathic remedies
  and show this to your health care providers
- For each drug, herb, homeopathic remedy, or nutritional supplement that you use, know (and, if possible, have this information written down) the:
  dosage
  administration schedule
  administration instructions (take on full or empty stomach, take only if symptom is present, discontinue after x days)
  purpose
  usual side effects
  adverse effects that you should bring to the attention of your health care provider
  precautions (when you should not take it, interactions with food, other drugs or substances)
  storage instructions
  where purchased/obtained

- Learn as much as you can about the drugs you are taking by reading the literature that comes with the drug and consumer drug reference books that are available at your local library or bookstore.
- Recognize that your drug dosage may be different from someone else's dosage who is taking the same drug.
- Be aware that you can develop adverse effects to drugs that you have taken for years without problems. Review your symptoms with your health care provider.
- Try to reduce the drugs you are using. Discuss with your health care provider improvements in your symptoms or other changes that could cause a drug to no longer be needed.
- Periodically review your drug dosages with your health care provider to see if any changes in your body's function could lead to reduced dosages.
- Try to manage new symptoms naturally rather than with drugs.
- Do not take new drugs without consulting your health care provider.

Critical Thinking Exercises

1. List age-related changes that affect the way in which drugs behave in older persons.
2. What key points would you include in a program to educate senior citizens about safe drug use?
3. What interventions could you employ to aid an older adult who has poor memory to safely administer medications?
4. Review the major drug groups and identify those that address problems that could potentially be managed with nonpharmacologic means.

Web Connect

Review consumer safety tips for buying medications through the internet by visiting www.fda.gov and clicking *Buying Medications and Medical Products Online.*

● References

Center for Medicare Education. (2002). Prescription drug coverage for people with Medicare. *Issue Brief. Center for Medicare Education, 3*(9), 1.

Kaufman, D. W., Kelly, J. P., Rosenberg, L., Anderson, T. E., et al. (2002). Recent patterns of medication use in the ambulatory adult population of the United States: The Slone survey. *Journal of the American Medical Association, 287*(3), 337–344.

Patel, R. B. (2003). Polypharmacy and the elderly. *Journal of Infusion Nursing, 26*(3), 166–169.

● Recommended Readings

Allen, L. B. (1998). Treating agitation without drugs. *American Journal of Nursing, 99*(4), 36–41.

Avorn, J., & Gurwitz, J. H. (1997). Principles of pharmacology. In C. K. Cassel, H. J. Cohen, E. B. Larson, et al. (Eds.), *Geriatric medicine* (3rd ed., pp. 55–70). New York: Springer.

Bretherton, A., Day, L., & Lewis, G. (2003). Polypharmacy and older people. *Nursing Times, 99*(17), 54–55.

Eliopoulos, C. (1999). *Integrating alternative and conventional therapies: Holistic care of chronic conditions.* St. Louis: Mosby.

Facts and Comparisons and American Nurses Association. (1996). *Nurses drug facts. Reference set 1996.* St. Louis: Author.

George, C. F. (1998). *Drug therapy in old age.* Chichester, NY: Wiley.

Horowitz, S. (1999). Migraine: Magnets and other non-drug treatments. *Alternative and Complementary Therapies, 5*(3), 124–129.

Logue, R. M. (2002). Self-medication and the elderly: How technology can help. *American Journal of Nursing, 102*(7), 51–56.

Medical Economics Company. (1998). *PDR for herbal medicines.* Montvale, NJ: Author.

Miller, C. A. (2000). Advising older adults about pain remedies. *Geriatric Nursing, 21*(1), 55.

Miller, C. A. (2002). The connection between drugs and falls in elders. *Geriatric Nursing, 23*(2), 171–172.

Miller, C. A. (2002). Cardiovascular drugs: Reason for promise and vigilance. *Geriatric Nursing, 23*(3), 171–172.

Roberts, J. (Ed.). (1996). *Handbook of pharmacology of aging* (2nd ed.). Boca Raton, FL: CRC Press.

Schuurmans, M. J, Duursma, S. A., Shortridge-Baggett, L. M., et al. (2003). Elderly patients with a hip fracture: The risk for delirium. *Applied Nursing Research, 16*(2), 75–84.

Semla, T. P., & Beizer, J. L. (1997). *Guide to preferred drugs in long-term care: A comparative formulary for geriatric specialists.* Hudson, OH: Lexi-Comp.

Spellbring, A. M., & Ryan, J. W. (2003). Medication administration by unlicensed caregivers: A model program. *Journal of Gerontological Nursing, 29*(6), 48–56.

Tabloski, P. A., Cooke, K. M., & Thoman, E. B. (1998). A procedure for withdrawal of sleep medication in elderly women who have been long term users. *Journal of Gerontological Nursing, 24*(9), 20–27.

Turkoski, B. B. (1998). Medication timing for the elderly: The impact of biorhythms on effectiveness. *Geriatric Nursing, 19*(4), 146–151.

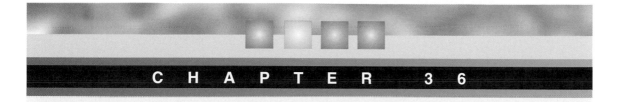

Living in Harmony With Chronic Conditions

■ Learning Objectives

After reading this chapter, you should be able to:

- discuss the scope of chronic conditions among the older population
- differentiate between healing and curing
- list chronic care goals
- outline components of assessment of chronic care needs
- discuss approaches to maximize the benefits of conventional treatments
- identify alternative therapies that could benefit chronically ill persons
- discuss institutional care of the chronically ill

*I*llness is not an easy situation to accept. Even a common cold disrupts our lives and makes us uncomfortable, irritable, and unmotivated to work and play. When sick, the basic activities of daily living can become a chore; our appearance may be the least of our worries; and our lives may revolve around the medications, treatments, and doctor's visits that

479

will make us feel better. Fortunately, for most people, illness is an unusual and temporary event; we recover and return to life as usual.

Some illnesses, however, will accompany people for the remainder of their lives—chronic conditions. Potentially every aspect of one's life can be affected by chronic conditions. The success to which a chronic condition is managed can make the difference between a satisfying lifestyle, in which control of the illness is but one routine component, and a life controlled by the demands of the illness.

> **KEY CONCEPT**
> The manner in which a chronic condition is managed can make the difference between a high-quality, satisfying life and one in which the person is prisoner to the illness.

Chronic Conditions and the Elderly

Medical technology has helped many people survive illnesses that once would have killed them; greater numbers of people are reaching old age, in which the incidence of chronic disease is higher. Thus, it should be no surprise that more than 80% of the elderly possess at least one chronic disease. Chapter 1, Table 1-11, lists the rates of chronic illness for various age groups and shows the profound increase in the rate of most chronic illnesses with age. From that list, the major chronic problems for the elderly can be derived (Display 36-1) and the following facts surface:

- Nearly half of older adults suffer from arthritis.
- More than one third have hypertension.
- Nearly one third have a hearing impairment.
- More than one fourth have a heart condition.
- More than one eighth have a visual impairment.
- Nearly another one eighth have a deformity or orthopedic impairment.
- Almost 10% have diabetes.
- Approximately 1 in 12 are affected by hemorrhoids and varicose veins.

These are profound numbers, particularly considering the impact of these diseases on the individual elderly person who is affected. When some of the potential nursing diagnoses that can be associated with these chronic conditions are considered (Table 36-1), the disruption to physical, emotional, and social well-being can be realized fully.

> **KEY CONCEPT**
> Most of the chronic conditions that are common in the elderly can significantly affect the quality of daily life.

Healing Versus Curing

Because chronic diseases cannot be cured, it would be inappropriate to direct care activities in a curative direction. Rather, healing is of the utmost importance. *Healing* implies the mobilization of the body, mind, and spirit to control symptoms, promote a sense of well-being, and enhance the quality of life. The person

---

DISPLAY 36-1

Major Chronic Conditions of Older Adults

Arthritis	Hypertension
Hearing impairment	Heart condition
Cataracts	Chronic sinusitis
Visual impairment	Deformity or orthopedic impairment
Hernia (abdominal cavity)	Diabetes
Varicose veins	Hemorrhoids

TABLE 36-1 ● *Potential Nursing Diagnoses Associated With Twelve Major Chronic Problems of the Elderly*

	Arthritis	Hypertension	Hearing Impairment	Heart Condition	Cataracts	Chronic Sinusitis	Visual Impairment	Deformities, Orthopedic Impairment	Hernia	Diabetes	Varicose Veins	Hemorrhoids
Activity Intolerance	✓	✓		✓	✓			✓	✓	✓	✓	✓
Anxiety	✓	✓	✓	✓	✓	✓	✓	✓	✓	✓	✓	✓
Constipation									✓		✓	
Decreased Cardiac Output												
Impaired Verbal Communication				✓								
Ineffective Coping	✓	✓	✓	✓	✓	✓	✓	✓	✓	✓	✓	✓
Disabled Family Coping	✓	✓	✓	✓	✓		✓	✓	✓		✓	✓
Deficient Diversional Activity	✓	✓	✓	✓	✓	✓	✓	✓	✓		✓	✓
Interrupted Family Processes	✓	✓	✓	✓	✓	✓	✓	✓	✓		✓	✓
Fear	✓	✓	✓	✓	✓	✓	✓	✓			✓	✓
Deficient Fluid Volume								✓				
Excess Fluid Volume					✓							
Grieving												
Ineffective Health Maintenance	✓	✓	✓	✓	✓	✓	✓	✓			✓	✓
Impaired Home Maintenance	✓	✓	✓	✓	✓	✓	✓	✓			✓	✓
Risk for Infection				✓		✓			✓	✓	✓	✓
Risk for Injury	✓	✓	✓	✓	✓	✓	✓					
Knowledge Deficit	✓	✓	✓	✓	✓	✓	✓	✓	✓	✓		✓
Impaired Physical Mobility	✓	✓		✓	✓		✓	✓	✓		✓	
Noncompliance	✓	✓	✓	✓	✓	✓	✓	✓	✓	✓	✓	✓
Imbalanced Nutrition: Less Than Body Requirements	✓			✓	✓	✓	✓	✓	✓			
Imbalanced Nutrition: More Than Body Requirements	✓	✓		✓	✓					✓		
Impaired Oral Mucous Membrane										✓		
Pain	✓	✓		✓		✓		✓	✓		✓	✓
Powerlessness	✓		✓	✓			✓	✓				
Ineffective Breathing Pattern				✓		✓		✓				
Self Care Deficit	✓	✓	✓	✓	✓	✓	✓	✓		✓	✓	✓
Disturbed Body Image	✓	✓	✓	✓	✓	✓	✓	✓		✓	✓	✓
Disturbed Sensory Perception	✓		✓				✓	✓				
Ineffective Sexuality Patterns	✓	✓		✓				✓		✓		
Impaired Skin Integrity				✓				✓		✓	✓	✓
Disturbed Sleep Pattern	✓	✓		✓		✓		✓	✓	✓	✓	✓
Impaired Social Interaction	✓	✓	✓	✓	✓	✓	✓	✓		✓		
Social Isolation	✓	✓	✓	✓	✓		✓	✓				
Spiritual Distress												
Disturbed Thought Processes		✓	✓	✓			✓			✓		
Ineffective Tissue Perfusion				✓								
Impaired Urinary Elimination				✓						✓		

with a chronic condition can learn to live effectively with the disease and develop a sense of inner peace and harmony through the recognition that he or she is defined by more than the physical body. The nurse serves a healing role in facilitating this process and guiding individuals with chronic conditions to achieve their maximum potential and highest attainable quality of life. Rather than administer care and treatments *for* or *to* patients, the nurse stimulates patients' self-healing capabilities by:

- creating a therapeutic human and physical environment
- educating
- empowering
- reinforcing, affirming, and validating
- removing barriers to self-care and self-awareness

> **KEY CONCEPT**
> Healing implies the mobilization of the body, mind, and spirit to control symptoms, promote a sense of well-being, and enhance the quality of life.

Chronic Care Goals

Most health professionals were educated in the acute care model, in which care activities focus on diagnosis, treatment, and cure of illness. Nursing actions were based on interventions that would cure patients, and success was judged on how quickly and totally patients were able to recover.

Chronic conditions are an entirely different situation. Patients will not recover from their disease; care measures focus on helping patients effectively live in harmony with, rather than cure, the condition. Professionals who seek success through the number of patients who recover will be frustrated and disappointed when working with persons who have chronic conditions; they must reorient themselves to a new set of care goals (Display 36-2). The following goals are appropriate to chronic care:

Maintain or improve self-care capacity. Chronic conditions often place additional demands on people. They may need to eat special diets, modify their activities, administer medications, perform treatments, or learn to use assistive devices or equipment. A variety of measures may be required for these demands to be met, and nurses may need to assist patients in increasing their abilities to engage in these measures. Actions toward achieving this goal include education about the disease and its management, stabilization and improvement of health status, promotion of interest and motivation for self-care, use of assistive devices, and provision of periodic assistance with care.

Manage the condition effectively. Individuals need to be knowledgeable about their conditions and related care. Skills may need to be mastered, such as injecting medications, changing dressings, or applying prostheses. However, motivation is essential to mobilize knowledge and skills in effective self-care, so assessing motivational factors and planning and implementing strategies to enhance motivation are crucial aspects.

Boost the body's healing abilities. The body's tremendous potential to fight disease and heal naturally is often underestimated. Helping patients mobi-

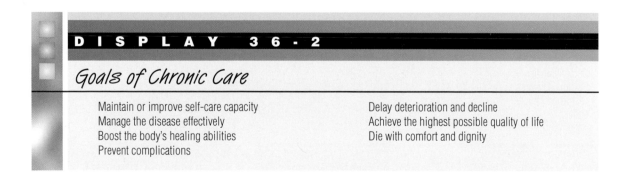

DISPLAY 36-2

Goals of Chronic Care

Maintain or improve self-care capacity	Delay deterioration and decline
Manage the disease effectively	Achieve the highest possible quality of life
Boost the body's healing abilities	Die with comfort and dignity
Prevent complications	

lize natural resources is an important nursing function. Stress management, guided imagery, exercise, immune-boosting nutrients, and biofeedback are among the strategies that can be used to promote self-healing.

Prevent complications. Chronic diseases and conventional treatments used to manage them can increase the risk for infections, injuries, and other complications. Potential risks should be identified and actively prevented, recognizing that risks change over time. Complications must be prevented because they risk weakening self-care capacity, increasing disability, and hastening decline. Whether a patient with diabetes lives an active life or becomes a blind amputee is largely determined by the extent to which treatment plans are followed and complications are actively prevented.

Delay deterioration and decline. By their nature, chronic conditions often will progressively worsen. For example, a person with Alzheimer's disease will demonstrate a progressive decline in status even if highly effective care is provided. However, preventive practices can influence whether that individual is ambulatory or bedbound at the end of a period. A conscious effort must be made to reinforce the importance of preventive care measures and identify problems early.

Achieve the highest possible quality of life. Sitting in bed attached to an oxygen tank may keep the body functioning but offers little stimulation to the mind and spirit. Consideration should be given to helping patients participate in activities that bring pleasure, stimulation, and reward. The extent to which recreational, social, spiritual, emotional, sexual, and family needs are met should be assessed, and assistance provided to fulfill those needs (eg, introduction to new hobbies, counseling for alternate positions for intercourse, provision of transportation by specially equipped vehicles, arrangements for home visits by clergy). A positive self-concept needs to be promoted. It is important for health professionals to periodically evaluate the extent to which treatment of the condition promotes or prohibits a satisfying lifestyle.

Die with comfort and dignity. As health status declines and patients face their final days of life, they will need increasing physical and psychosocial support. Pain relief, preservation of energy, provision of comfort, and assistance in meeting basic needs become crucial. Nurses also must be sensitive to the importance of listening and talking to dying persons, anticipating their needs, and, most importantly, instilling a feeling that the nurse can be depended on for support through this period.

The goals of chronic care are such that success and progress must be measured differently. A deterioration of a patient from ambulatory to wheelchair status can be judged a success if, without nursing intervention, that patient may have become bedridden or died. Likewise, a physically and an emotionally comfortable death that left positive memories for the patient's family can be a significant accomplishment. These determinants of success are different from those of acute care but are no less important.

> **KEY CONCEPT**
> Successes in chronic care are measured differently from those in acute care.

Assessing Chronic Care Needs

There is a great deal of difference in the self-care capacities of persons who have chronic conditions. There will also be variation in the self-care capacity of the same individual at different times throughout the course of the illness. Keen assessment and reassessment are thus necessary. The individual's capacity to fulfill each of the health-related requirements should be reviewed, as well as the person's capacity to meet the demands imposed by illness (eg, medication administration, dressings, and special exercises). From this, deficits in fulfilling care needs can be determined.

A majority of people with chronic conditions will be managing their conditions in a community setting, most likely with family support or involvement; therefore, assessment must consider not only the capacity of the individual to fulfill the care demands but also the capacity of the family to assist and cope with caregiving. For instance, a man with diabetes and severe arthritis in his hands may not be able to manipulate a syringe for his insulin injections, but his wife may be able to give him injections; thus, he does not have a deficit in this area. Likewise, a victim of Alzheimer's disease may not be able to protect herself from safety hazards, but if she lives with a daughter who supervises her activities, this patient may not have a deficit in her ability to protect herself. Within this framework, *the family is the patient,* and the capacities and limitations of the total family unit must be evaluated. Remember that family is not limited to relatives but can include a variety of significant others.

Nurses cannot assume, however, that the presence of family members guarantees compensation for the patient's care deficits. Sometimes the caregivers may not have the physical, mental, or emotional abilities to meet the patient's care needs. For instance, the patient's caregiver daughter may be a frail older adult herself. Likewise, the family may not want to provide care because of the imposition on their lifestyle or their feelings toward the patient. These factors must be considered before care is delegated to family members.

Once identified, care needs should be reviewed with the patient and family members. This not only helps to validate data but also promotes understanding by all parties involved about what the care needs actually are. Methods of meeting care needs should be identified jointly (eg, the daughter will assist with bathing, the son will provide transportation to the clinic for monthly visits, the daughter-in-law will call twice daily to remind the patient to take medications). The family should be informed of the services available in their community to supplement their efforts. In fairness to the family, the costs and limitations of community services must be included in this discussion.

Setting goals is important in helping patients and their families understand the realistic direction of care. For instance, a long-term goal of restoring ambulation sets a different tone from a goal of preventing complications as function deteriorates. Acceptance of long-term goals may require acceptance of the realities of the condition, which is not an easy task for patients and their families. It may take time and considerable nursing support for families to come to the understanding that the patient's physical or mental status will decline over time. This is not to suggest that hope should be destroyed, but rather that it be tempered with a realistic sense of what the future may hold. Short-term goals offer a means of evaluating ongoing efforts and serve as benchmarks in care; these

goals can be set on a daily, weekly, or monthly basis, depending on the situation.

> **KEY CONCEPT**
> The patient and family caregivers should validate care plan priorities and goals.

Finally, written care plans are beneficial to patients and their families. Having the plans in writing avoids discrepancies between perceptions and reality. It also prevents directions from being forgotten and ensures that anyone who participates in the patient's care will have the same understanding.

> **Point to Ponder**
> *How would your life change if you learned that you had a chronic condition that would progressively worsen? What would you do differently? From where and whom would you draw emotional and spiritual support?*

Maximizing Function

With similar diagnoses and care requirements, one individual may remain an active participant in society, enjoying a high quality of life, whereas another may become a homebound prisoner to the disease. The difference can depend on how the person approaches and manages care activities.

SELECTING AN APPROPRIATE PHYSICIAN

Because chronic conditions demand long-term medical supervision, selection of a physician becomes a significant issue for the patient. The patient should have contact with a specialist who is knowledgeable about state-of-the-art practices related to the condition. The nurse may assist the patient by providing the names of specialists for the patient to consider. In addition to qualifications and expertise in the field, the patient should feel at ease with the physician; a good chemistry between physician and patient will allow the patient to ask questions freely, discuss concerns, and report problems. Some factors that promote a positive physician–patient relationship include:

- accessibility of the physician
- sufficient time allocation for office visits and telephone consultations
- comfortable and patient-appropriate communication style
- respect for patient's involvement and decision-making
- consideration of needs of entire family unit
- openness to alternative and complementary therapies
- attitude of hope and optimism

> **KEY CONCEPT**
> In addition to expertise in treating the specific condition, the physician should have a style with which the patient is comfortable because the relationship will be a long-term one.

Patients have a responsibility to use their health care provider's time effectively. Patients can be advised to prepare for office visits by writing down questions, symptoms, and concerns and to maintain their own records of laboratory tests, vital signs, and other relevant medical data.

USING A CHRONIC CARE COACH

Anyone who has attempted a weight-reduction diet or exercise program appreciates the benefits of having a friend with whom the experience can be shared. Likewise, the person who must face life adjustments every day for the rest of his or her life can benefit from a buddy or coach who can provide support and assistance. The chronic care coach can be a spouse, child, friend, or someone with a similar condition who cares about and has regular contact with the patient. The coach may accompany the patient to diagnostic tests or routine office visits and check on the patient's status routinely. Feedback and positive reinforcement can be provided by the coach, as can a listening ear when the patient has "slipped off" the treatment regimen or regressed (Display 36-3). Also, the coach can help the patient stay current about the disease by clipping articles from magazines and sharing information gained through media features. Gerontological nurses can advise and support persons who function as

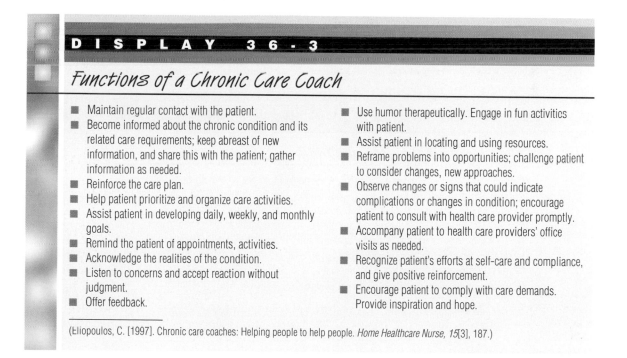

DISPLAY 36-3

Functions of a Chronic Care Coach

- Maintain regular contact with the patient.
- Become informed about the chronic condition and its related care requirements; keep abreast of new information, and share this with the patient; gather information as needed.
- Reinforce the care plan.
- Help patient prioritize and organize care activities.
- Assist patient in developing daily, weekly, and monthly goals.
- Remind the patient of appointments, activities.
- Acknowledge the realities of the condition.
- Listen to concerns and accept reaction without judgment.
- Offer feedback.

- Use humor therapeutically. Engage in fun activities with patient.
- Assist patient in locating and using resources.
- Reframe problems into opportunities; challenge patient to consider changes, new approaches.
- Observe changes or signs that could indicate complications or changes in condition; encourage patient to consult with health care provider promptly.
- Accompany patient to health care providers' office visits as needed.
- Recognize patient's efforts at self-care and compliance, and give positive reinforcement.
- Encourage patient to comply with care demands. Provide inspiration and hope.

(Eliopoulos, C. [1997]. Chronic care coaches: Helping people to help people. *Home Healthcare Nurse, 15*[3], 187.)

chronic care coaches to elders by outlining some of the basic steps of this process (Display 36-4).

> **KEY CONCEPT**
> A chronic care coach provides support, encouragement, reinforcement, assistance, and feedback.

INCREASING KNOWLEDGE

An informed patient is well equipped to manage the chronic condition successfully and prevent complications. Also, knowledge helps empower the patient. Various organizations for virtually every health condition can provide useful educational materials, often free of charge (see the Resources lists throughout this book). Most newspapers carry regular health columns that provide current information on health conditions and treatments. Local libraries not only possess a wealth of information on their shelves but also can assist people with literature searches. Also, ever-increasing numbers of individuals use the Internet to learn about new information and share knowledge. (If patients do not own a computer, they often can use ones provided at public libraries.) Patients should be encouraged to obtain as much information as they can and to maintain a file on their condition.

LOCATING A SUPPORT GROUP

Support groups can be important for persons with chronic illnesses; they provide the opportunity not only for obtaining valuable information but also in gaining perspectives from those living with similar situations. Patients may be more willing to ask questions and express concerns with their peers than with health care professionals. Most support groups can be located through local telephone directories or the information and referral services of the local agency on aging; national headquarters of organizations also can direct patients to local chapters.

MAKING SMART LIFESTYLE CHOICES

Patients with lifelong health conditions need to commit to smart lifestyle choices to maximize their health and quality of life. Such activities include:

* compliance with the prescribed treatment plan
* sound dietary practices
* regular exercise
* stress management
* assertiveness in protecting one's own needs

DISPLAY 36-4

Steps in Chronic Care Coaching

Contact: Schedule regular telephone or face-to-face contact to check on the patient's status.
Observe: Be attentive to comments, mood, body language, energy, general status, presence of symptoms, compliance.
Affirm: Reinforce care plan and actions, recognize patient's efforts and accomplishments.
Clarify: Ask questions, validate observations, correct misconceptions, reinforce information.
Help: Offer assistance when self-care capacity is diminished; locate and negotiate resources.
Inspire: Encourage patient to comply with care plan, build on positive experiences and accomplishments; offer hope.
Nurture: Provide education, information, support.
Guide: Assist in setting realistic goals, developing plans, prioritizing, seeking resources.

(Eliopoulos, C. [1997]. Chronic care coaches: Helping people to help people. *Home Healthcare Nurse, 15*[3], 188.)

- development of a healing attitude and mind-set to live positively with the illness

USING COMPLEMENTARY AND ALTERNATIVE THERAPIES

Growing numbers of Americans use complementary and alternative therapies for health promotion and illness management, and increasing evidence of the effectiveness of these measures is available. Such therapies use the body's capacity to heal itself and place the patient in charge of the healing process. Display 36-5 lists some of the alternative therapies that can be used to complement conventional therapies. In some cases, complementary and alternative therapies can replace conventional treatments, as when an analgesic is replaced by the use of therapeutic touch or guided imagery. The fact that complementary and alternative therapies have not been widely used in this country in the past does not mean that they are ineffective; people in other countries have used some of these measures successfully for centuries. Furthermore, the scarcity of research supporting the use of some of these therapies does not mean that they are useless. (Consider that researchers stand a better chance of obtaining funds for well-understood conventional therapies than for less familiar alternatives, pharmaceutical companies are not going to invest large sums of money testing herbal remedies that cannot be patented for their exclusive use, and most medical researchers have been educated in a system that perpetuates the use of conventional practices.) This is not to say that there are not charlatans eager to take advantage of people who have chronic conditions. The nurse plays a significant role in helping the patient evaluate the validity of complementary and alternative therapies and use only sound, safe practices. Patients should be encouraged to discuss these therapies with their physicians and other health care providers. (In some circumstances, patients may need to provide literature about complementary and alternative therapies to their providers to educate them about these practices!) Ideally, patients should be able to use the best of both complementary/alternative and conventional health care practices.

> **KEY CONCEPT**
> Many individuals can benefit from using a combination of conventional and complementary and alternative health practices for the care of their conditions.

DISPLAY 36-5

Alternative Therapies for Chronically Ill People

Acupressure	Light therapy
Acupuncture	Meditation
Aromatherapy	Naturopathic medicine
Ayurvedic medicine	Nutritional supplements
Biofeedback	Osteopathy
Chiropathy	Progressive relaxation
Guided imagery	Qigong
Herbal medicine	Sound therapy
Homeopathy	T'ai chi
Hydrotherapy	Therapeutic touch
Hypnotherapy	Yoga

Following the Course of Chronic Care

Anyone who has dieted can appreciate the difficulty of sustaining the initial weight-loss behaviors (eg, food restrictions, exercise) on a long-term basis without regular reinforcement and support. The same is true for the new behaviors associated with managing a chronic condition. Persons with chronic conditions cannot be given their instructions for care, discharged, and forgotten. They will need periodic contact and reevaluation of their capacity, resources, and motivation to manage their conditions.

A variety of factors can change patients' abilities to manage their illnesses. The status of the illness may change, placing more or different demands on the patient. The status of the patient may change, reducing self-care ability. The status of the caregiver may change, limiting the degree to which the patient's deficits can be compensated. All the factors affecting the patient's ongoing care must be evaluated regularly.

DEFENSE MECHANISMS AND IMPLICATIONS

The lifestyle changes, frustrations, and losses commonly experienced by persons who must live with chronic conditions may cause certain reactions to emerge that could disrupt the flow of care. These reactions are defense mechanisms, used when the situation at hand may be too much for the patient to cope with, and include:

Denial: making statements or taking actions that are not consistent with the realities of the illness (eg, abandoning a special diet, discontinuing medications independently, committing to responsibilities that cannot be fulfilled)

Anger: acting in a hostile manner, having violent outbursts

Depression: making statements regarding the hopelessness of a situation, refusing to engage in self-care activities, withdrawing, questioning the purpose of life

Regression: becoming increasingly dependent unnecessarily, abandoning self-care behaviors

These and other reactions are indications that the patient's ego strength is threatened and that extra support is needed. Rather than reacting to the patient's behavior, caregivers need to understand its origin and help the patient work through it (eg, by providing an opportunity to vent frustrations and offering respite from the routines of care by doing for the patient until he or she feels psychologically able to resume self-care).

IMPACT OF ONGOING CARE ON THE FAMILY

In the home management of a chronic illness, the entire family is the patient; therefore, in evaluating care, the impact on the total family must be considered. The patient with Alzheimer's disease may be well groomed, well nourished, and free from complications; looking at the patient in isolation, an evaluation could be made that her home care has been successful. However, the patient's status may have been achieved at great cost to the entire family. For example, her husband may have had to forfeit his job to care for her during the day; her daughter's family life may have been disrupted because she needs to sleep at her parents' home to assist her father in controlling her mother's night wandering; the son's plans to expand his business may have been postponed because he began subsidizing his parents' income. Some sacrifices and compromises are common when family members assume caregiver roles, but serious disruption to their health or their lives should not result. Families may be so embroiled in the situation that they are unable to see the full impact that the caregiving situation is having on their own lives. Sometimes they feel that they must be a "bad" spouse or child to feel that the patient's care is a burden. Nurses can assist by helping family members realistically evaluate their caregiving responsibilities and identify when other caregiving options should be considered. For instance, the family may sense that it is in the patient's best interest to enter a nursing home, but they need the health care professional to introduce the suggestion and help them through the process of making this difficult decision.

KEY CONCEPT
In chronic care, the entire family is the patient.

Point to Ponder
What would you do if a parent, spouse, or child needed considerable care? How much care could you realistically provide, and what resources would you have available?

INSTITUTIONAL CARE

Although only 5% of the older population is in a nursing home or other institutional setting at any given time, nearly one half of all older women and one third of all older men will spend some time in a long-term care facility during their lives (American Association of Homes and Services for the Aging, 2003). Most families seek institutional care after having attempted caregiving of their elder relative at home, not as a first choice. By the time they seek such assistance, their physical, emotional, and socioeconomic resources can be significantly depleted, and they may require special support and assistance from nurses. (Chapter 39 discusses the care of individuals who are in long-term care facilities.)

Effective chronic care is not an easy nursing challenge. It requires knowledge and skills related to the management of multiple medical problems, skilled assessment and planning, individualized promotion of self-care capacity, monitoring of family health, and a variety of other demands. The patient's comfort, independence, and quality of life are largely influenced by the type of services rendered; in chronic care, most of those services will fall within the scope of nursing. Perhaps this type of care, more than any other, provides an opportunity for nursing to demonstrate its facets of independent practice and full leadership potential.

Critical Thinking Exercises

1. Discuss the way in which your life would be affected if you developed a chronic disease. What additional issues exist for an older adult faced with this same situation?
2. Mr. Arni is a 72-year-old widower with multiple chronic conditions, including hypertension, arthritis, emphysema, and diet-controlled diabetes mellitus. He is employed part-time as a salesman and enjoys his work; however, he is complaining that his antihypertensive medication is making him "tired" and that he is impatient with having to forfeit "all the good food when joining his clients for lunch" to comply with his special diet. Furthermore, he has recently established a relationship with a middle-aged woman and is experiencing some impotency that he attributes to his antihypertensive medication. He asks, "What is the point of living a long life if you aren't enjoying it?"

   What nursing diagnoses are evident and what could be done to assist Mr. Arni?
3. Describe factors that cause most nurses and physicians to be ill-informed of or resistant to alternative therapies.
4. Identify measures that could help empower an older adult who has a chronic illness.
5. Review the major chronic illnesses affecting the older population and identify the threats to the quality of life that could be associated with each.

Web Connect

Be directed to a wide range of support groups by visiting www.supportpath.com.

● Reference

American Association of Homes and Services for the Aging. (2003). *Nursing Home Statistics.* Retrieved August 5, 2003, from www.aahsa.org/public/backgrd1.htm.

● Recommended Readings

Acton, G. J., & Miller, E. W. (2003). Spirituality in caregivers of family members with dementia. *Journal of Holistic Nursing, 21*(2), 117–130.

Arras, J. D. (Ed.). (1995). *Bringing the hospital home: Ethical and social implications of high-tech home care.* Baltimore, MD: Johns Hopkins University Press.

Astor, B. (1998). *Baby boomers guide to caring for aging parents.* New York: Macmillan.

Baird, C. L. (2003). Holding on. Self-caring with osteoarthritis. *Journal of Gerontological Nursing, 29*(6), 32–39.

Baldwin, K., & Shaul, M. (2001). When your patient can no longer live independently: A guide to supporting the patient and family. *Journal of Gerontological Nursing, 27*(11), 10–18.

Benet, A. (1996). A portrait of chronic illness: Inspecting the canvas, reframing the issues. *American Behavioral Sciences, 39*(6), 767–777.

Berman, B. M., & Anderson, R. W. (1994). Improving health care through the evaluation and integration of complementary medicine. *Complementary Therapies in Medicine, 2,* 217–220.

Calkins, E. (1999). *New ways to care for older people: Building systems based on evidence.* New York: Springer.

Clark, C. C. (2003). *American Holistic Nurses' Association guide to common chronic conditions.* Hoboken, NJ: John Wiley and Sons.

Eason, L. R. (2003). Concepts in health promotion: Perceived self-efficacy and barriers in older adults. *Journal of Gerontological Nursing, 29*(5), 11–19.

Eliopoulos, C. (1997). Chronic care coaches. *Home Healthcare Nursing, 15*(3), 185–188.

Eliopoulos, C. (1999). *Integrating conventional and alternative therapies: Holistic care for chronic conditions.* St. Louis: Mosby.

Eliopoulos, C. (2003). *Nursing administration manual for long-term care facilities* (6th ed.). Glen Arm, MD: Health Education Network.

Evans, L. K., Yurkow, J., & Siegler, E. L. (1995). The CARE program: A nurse-managed collaborative outpatient program to improve function of frail older people. *Journal of the American Geriatrics Society, 43*(10), 1155–1160.

Hagen, B. (2001). Nursing home placement: Factors affecting caregivers' decisions to place family members with dementia. *Journal of Gerontological Nursing, 27*(2), 44–53.

Hayes, J. M. (1999). Respite for caregivers: A community-based model in a rural setting. *Journal of Gerontological Nursing, 25*(1), 22–26.

Hughes, E. M. (1995). Creating functional environments for elder care facilities. *Geriatric Nursing, 16*(4), 1727–1736.

Keller, V., & Baker, L. (2000). Communicate with care. *RN, 63*(1), 32–33.

Kelley, L. S., Specht, J. K., & Maas, M. L. (2000). Family involvement in care for individuals with dementia protocol. *Journal of Gerontological Nursing, 26*(2), 13–21.

Krechting, J. L., & Koper, V. E. (1995). *Interdisciplinary care plans for long-term care.* Gaithersburg, MD: Aspen.

Larrimore, K. L. (2003). Alzheimer disease support group characteristics: A comparison of caregivers. *Geriatric Nursing, 24*(1), 32–35.

Levin, N. J. (1997). *How to care for your parents: A practical guide to eldercare.* New York: Norton.

Lewis, M., Hepburn, K., Corcoran-Perry, S., Narayan, S., & Lally, R. M. (1999). Options, outcomes, values, likelihoods. Decision-making guide for patients and their families. *Journal of Gerontological Nursing, 25*(12), 19–25.

Lilly, M. L., Richards, B. S., & Buckwalter, K. C. (2003). Friends and social support in dementia caregiving: Assessment and intervention. *Journal of Gerontological Nursing, 29*(1), 29–36.

Lubkin, I. M. (1995). *Chronic illness: Impact and interventions* (3rd ed.). Boston: Jones and Bartlett.

McCall, J. B. (1999). *Grief education for caregivers of the elderly.* New York: Haworth Pastoral Press.

McCullough, L. B., & Wilson, N. L. (1995). *Long-term care decisions: Ethical and conceptual dimensions.* Baltimore, MD: Johns Hopkins University Press.

Meyer, M. M., & Derr, P. (1998). *The comfort of home: An illustrated step-by-step guide for caregivers.* Portland, OR: CareTrust Publications LLC.

Moore, S. L., Metcalf, B., & Schow, E. (2000). Aging and meaning in life: Examining the concept. *Geriatric Nursing, 21*(1), 27–29.

Morse, S., & Robbins, D. Q. (1998). *Moving mom and dad: Why, where, how, and when to help your parents relocate* (2nd ed.). Berkeley, CA: Lanier Publishing International.

National Family Caregivers Association. (1996). *The resourceful caregiver: Helping caregivers help themselves.* St. Louis: Mosby Lifeline.

Resnick, B., & Simpson, M. (2003). Restorative care nursing activities: Pilot testing self-efficacy and outcome expectation measures. *Geriatric Nursing, 24*(2), 82–88.

Ruppert, R. A. (1996). Caring for the lay caregiver. *American Journal of Nursing, 96*(3), 40–45.

Schomp, V. (1997). *The aging parent handbook.* New York: Harper Paperbacks.

Stocker, S. (1996). Six tips for caring for aging parents. *American Journal of Nursing, 96*(9), 32–33.

Tsuji, I., Whalen, S., & Finucane, T. E. (1995). Predictors of nursing home placement in community-based long-term care. *Journal of the American Geriatrics Society, 43*(7), 761–766.

Turner, D. C. (1996). The role of culture in chronic illness. *American Behavioral Sciences, 39*(6), 717–729.

Williamson, A. T., Fletcher, P. C., & Dawson, K. A. (2003). Complementary and alternative medicine: Use in an older population. *Journal of Gerontological Nursing, 29*(5), 20–28.

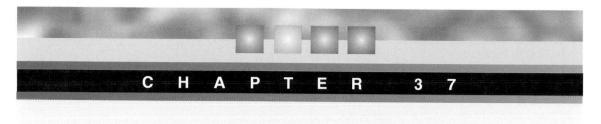

Rehabilitative Care

■ Learning Objectives

After reading this chapter, you should be able to:

- discuss the challenges of living with a disability
- describe the principles of rehabilitative nursing
- list components of the assessment of activities of daily living and instrumental activities of daily living
- identify positions for proper body alignment
- describe types of range-of-motion exercises
- list considerations in the proper use of mobility aids
- outline components of bowel and bladder training programs
- describe measures to promote mental function
- identify resources to assist in patients' rehabilitation

The prevalence of chronic conditions, frailty, and disability among the elderly is significant. Many older persons must learn to live with limited mobility, pain, impaired communication, and multiple risks to their safety and well-being. As increasing numbers of people achieve old age, surviving once-fatal conditions but with residual disabilities, the prevalence of disability among elders will rise. The emphasis on saving lives must be balanced with an emphasis on preserving the quality of the lives that have been saved. The advantages of modern technology in diagnosing and treating disease and improving life expectancy may be minimized if older adults must live with disabilities that result in discomfort, dependency, and distress.

> ### Point to Ponder
> *Advances in health care technology have enabled people to be saved from serious illnesses, although in some cases they are left with significantly limited function and discomfort. Would you want every effort made to save your life regardless of the consequences? Why or why not?*

Functional status, rather than diagnoses, provides direction to rehabilitative needs. Among the elderly, functional status varies widely. Some elders actively hold down jobs and regularly provide volunteer service, others are able to perform activities of daily living (ADLs) if some assistance is provided, and a portion are so severely impaired that total care is required. Furthermore, functional status can change within an individual from time to time, depending on factors such as control of symptoms, progression of the disease, and mood.

Frailty is a particular challenge to elders that must be considered in rehabilitative care. A person is considered frail if he or she has at least three of the following symptoms (Fried et al., 2001):

- unplanned weight loss (10 or more pounds in the past year)
- slow walking speed
- low grip strength
- fatigue, poor endurance
- low levels of activity

Elders who meet the criteria for frail are at high risk for falls, disability, hospitalization, nursing home placement, and death. Positive health practices and effective management of health conditions are beneficial in helping older adults to avoid becoming frail. Early recognition and intervention for symptoms of frailty (eg, correcting weight loss, assisting with muscle strengthening exercises) can prevent or delay some of the frailty elders experience. This emphasizes the usefulness of reviewing symptoms of frailty during nursing assessments of older adults.

Although it differs from handicap and impairment (Display 37-1), the term disability will be used throughout this chapter to discuss rehabilitative needs.

Living With Disability

An accident or a stroke may bring sudden disability to a previously independent, functional adult, or perhaps a chronic condition progressively worsens and its disabling impact is more acutely realized. What-

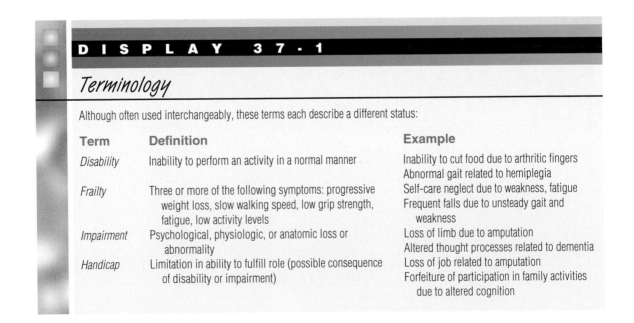

DISPLAY 37-1

Terminology

Although often used interchangeably, these terms each describe a different status:

Term	Definition	Example
Disability	Inability to perform an activity in a normal manner	Inability to cut food due to arthritic fingers Abnormal gait related to hemiplegia
Frailty	Three or more of the following symptoms: progressive weight loss, slow walking speed, low grip strength, fatigue, low activity levels	Self-care neglect due to weakness, fatigue Frequent falls due to unsteady gait and weakness
Impairment	Psychological, physiologic, or anatomic loss or abnormality	Loss of limb due to amputation Altered thought processes related to dementia
Handicap	Limitation in ability to fulfill role (possible consequence of disability or impairment)	Loss of job related to amputation Forfeiture of participation in family activities due to altered cognition

ever the circumstances, few of us are prepared to deal with disability. It is difficult to accept in ourselves and our loved ones. Relationships, roles, and responsibilities are disrupted; disfigurement and dysfunction alter body image and self-concept. Losses and limitations cause a new vulnerability to emerge and make death seem more real and close. Concern arises over potential physical and emotional pain, and frustration occurs in wanting to eliminate the cause of the problem and knowing we cannot. Disability can be an extremely difficult and devastating mountain to climb.

Point to Ponder

What examples have you seen within your own family of differences in the way people respond to health challenges?

IMPORTANCE OF ATTITUDE AND COPING CAPACITY

The severity of the disability can be less important to rehabilitation efforts than the attitude and coping capacity of disabled patients and their families. Someone with a mild cardiac problem may confine himself to his home, become preoccupied with his illness, and demand to be waited on, whereas a patient with hemiplegia could return to independent living in his modified apartment, find a job, and cultivate new friends and interests. Previous attitudes, personality, and lifestyle have a strong influence on reactions to disability. A person who has always felt that life has dealt her a bad hand could view a disability as the last straw and give up all hope. On the other hand, an optimistic person who has approached problems as new challenges to overcome may be determined not to allow a disability to control her life. Individuals who relish independence and refuse to let illness slow their lifestyles will respond to disability differently from those who use real or exaggerated ills for other gains. The family's response to the disabled person will also influence that person's reactions. Families that reinforce sick role behaviors and insist on doing everything for the disabled person can cripple him physically and psychologically, whereas families that promote self-care and treat the disabled person as a responsible family member can help him to feel like a normal, useful human being.

KEY CONCEPT

Previous attitudes, personality, experiences, and lifestyle influence reactions to a disability.

LOSSES ACCOMPANYING DISABILITY

Many losses may accompany disability, such as the loss of function, role, income, status, independence, or perhaps a body part. Disabled persons mourn these losses, often demonstrating the same reactions experienced during the stages of dying. They may deny their disabilities by making unrealistic plans and not complying with their care plans. They may have angry outbursts and become impatient with those who are trying to help them. They may shop for medical advice that will offer them a more optimistic outlook or invest their hopes in any faith healer they can find. On one day they may optimistically state that their disability has given them a new perspective on life, yet the very next day they tearfully question what they have to live for. These reactions can fluctuate; it is the rare individual who accepts a disability without some periods of regret or resentment.

KEY CONCEPT

Disability can be accompanied by many losses, including function, role, income, status, independence, and anatomic structure.

Rehabilitative Nursing

Most of the disabilities that older adults have cannot be eliminated or, in many cases, significantly improved. Damaged lungs, amputations, diseased heart muscle, partial blindness, presbycusis, and deformed joints may accompany patients for the remainder of their lives. Often these chronic disabilities receive the least intervention; reimbursement and aggressive attention are given to restore the function of someone who has suffered a stroke or fracture, but those with "no rehabilitation potential" often are overlooked in their need to maintain function and prevent further decline.

Rehabilitation must be defined broadly in geriatric care. It may be regarded as those efforts that help individuals gain ways to improve their functional capacity so that they can better cope, be maximally independent, have a sense of well-being, and enjoy a satisfying life. The principles guiding gerontological nursing care are of particular significance in rehabilitation and include the following actions:

- increase self-care capacity
- eliminate or minimize self-care limitations
- act for or do for when the person is unable to take action for himself or herself

---

KEY CONCEPT
Improving the functional capacity of older adults can promote a sense of well-being and a higher quality of life.

Efforts to increase self-care capacity could include building the patient's arm muscles to enable better transfer to and propelling of a wheelchair or teaching the patient how to inject insulin with the use of only one hand. Relieving pain and having a ramp installed for easier wheelchair mobility are efforts that minimize or eliminate limitations. Obtaining a new prescription from the pharmacy and performing range-of-motion exercises demonstrate ways in which nurses act for or do for the patient. Whenever nurses act or do for patients, they need to question what could be done to enable patients to perform this act independently. Patients will always be dependent on others for some activities, but for other actions patients can assume responsibility with sufficient education, time allocation, encouragement, and assistive devices. The following information should be remembered in rehabilitative nursing.

- Know the unique capacities and limitations of the individual. Assess the patient's self-care capacity, mental status, level of motivation, and family support.
- Emphasize function rather than dysfunction, capabilities rather than disabilities.
- Provide time and flexibility. At times, institutional routines (eg, having all baths completed by 9 AM, collecting all food trays 45 minutes after delivery) cause caregivers to do tasks for patients so that they may be completed efficiently. Staff desires for effi-

ciency and orderliness should never supersede the patient's need for independence.

- Recognize and praise accomplishments. Seemingly minor acts, such as combing hair or wheeling themselves to the hallway, can be the result of tremendous effort and determination on the part of disabled persons.
- Do not equate physical disability with mental disability. Treat disabled persons as mature, intelligent adults.
- Prevent complications. Recognize potential risks (eg, skin breakdown, social isolation, depression) and actively prevent them.
- Demonstrate hope, optimism, and a sense of humor. It is difficult for disabled persons to feel positive about rehabilitation if their caregivers appear discouraged or disinterested.
- Keep in mind that rehabilitation is a highly individualized process, requiring a multidisciplinary team effort for optimal results.

Assessing Functional Capacity

Determining individual levels of independence in meeting the activities of daily living (ADLs) and instrumental activities of daily living (IADL) is essential to understanding the rehabilitation needs of the patient. An assessment of ADLs explores the skills the patient possesses to meet basic requirements such as eating, washing, dressing, toileting, and moving. Assessment of IADL examines those skills beyond the basics that enable the individual to function independently in the community, such as the ability to prepare meals, shop, use a telephone, safely use medications, clean, travel in the community, and manage finances. Persons can be totally independent, partially independent, or dependent in their ability to perform these activities (Table 37-1).

KEY CONCEPT
Instrumental activities of daily living (IADL) include functions that enable a person to manage in the community, such as preparing meals, shopping, using a telephone, self-administering medications, managing finances, and traveling in the community.

TABLE 37-1 ● *Assessing Capacity to Perform Activities of Daily Living*

Total Independence	Partial Independence	Dependence
Eating		
Uses all utensils	Needs tray set up	Needs to be fed
Cuts meats	Cannot cut foods or butter bread	
Butters bread	Needs encouragement, reminders to eat	
Drinks from cup or glass		
Hygiene		
Transfers in or out of tub or shower	Reaches some body parts to cleanse	Needs complete bathing assistance
Reaches and bathes all body parts	Unable to brush teeth, dentures	
Brushes teeth or dentures	Unable to turn faucets or flush toilet	
Brushes or combs hair	Needs assistance transferring in or out of	
Cleanses self after toileting	tub or shower	
Turns faucets, flushes toilet	Needs assistance to comb or brush hair	
	Must have basin brought	
	Needs reminders, encouragement to bathe	
Dressing		
Selects appropriate garments	Needs assistance with some garments,	Needs to be fully dressed
Puts on all clothing	zippers, buttons, snaps	
Slips on shoes, socks, stockings	Unable to select appropriate garments	
Ties shoelaces	Needs encouragement, reminders to dress	
Able to manage zippers, buttons, snaps		
Continence		
Continent of bladder and bowels	Incontinent less than once daily	Total incontinent
Toileting		
Uses bedpan or toilet without assistance	Needs to be taken to toilet or have bedpan	Needs assistance getting on or
Able to reach or transfer to and from	brought or taken	off bedpan or commode
bedpan or toilet	Needs encouragement or reminders to toilet	Unable to use bedpan or commode
Manages ostomy or catheter	Needs assistance with ostomy or catheter care	Unable to perform ostomy or
independently		catheter care
Mobility		
Ambulates with no assistance	Ambulates with assistance	Bedbound
Turns corners	Climbs stairs with assistance	Needs to be pushed in wheelchair
Climb stairs	Transfers with assistance	Unable to transfer
Sits or lifts from chair and bed	Propels wheelchair but needs to be assisted	Unable to climb stairs
Uses wheelchair, cane, walker with	in and out	Wanders away if not supervised
no assistance	Wanders in limited area	

When a deficit in ADL capacity exists, its specific cause must be identified so that appropriate interventions can be planned. For example, a person who is partially dependent in bathing because he needs to have a basin of water brought to him will have different nursing requirements than one who forgets what he is doing as he bathes and needs to be reminded of the next action to take.

Proper Positioning

Correct body alignment facilitates optimal respiration, circulation, and comfort and prevents complications such as contractures and pressure ulcers. When patients are unable to position their bodies independently, nurses must be attentive to keeping their bodies properly aligned. Figure 37-1 demonstrates proper alignment in various positions.

🔑 **KEY CONCEPT**
Correct body alignment facilitates the optimal function of major systems, promotes comfort, and prevents complications.

Range-of-Motion Exercises

Exercise is an essential component of the health maintenance and promotion plan of every adult and is particularly significant for the elderly. Exercise has many benefits, including the promotion of joint motion

and muscle strength, stimulation of circulation, maintenance of functional capacity, and prevention of contractures and other complications. Exercises can be done in the following degrees:

- *active*—independently by patients
- *active assistive*—with assistance to the patient
- *passive*—with no active involvement of the patient

During the assessment, all joints should be put through a full range of motion to determine the degree of movement possible actively, with active assistance, and passively. The most significant concern is the degree to which range of motion is sufficient to participate in ADL.

Patients should be encouraged to put all joints through a full range of motion at least once daily. Figure 37-2 demonstrates basic range-of-motion exercises

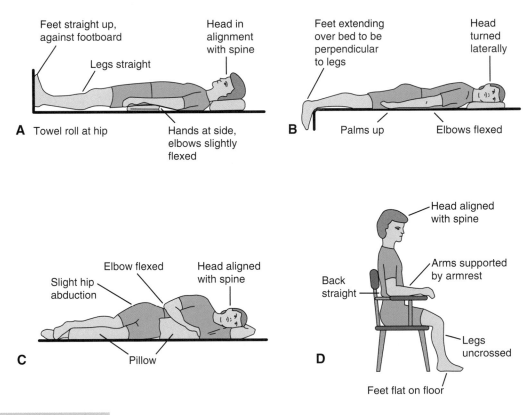

FIGURE 37-1

(**A**) Supine position. (**B**) Prone position. (**C**) Lateral position. (**D**) Chair position.

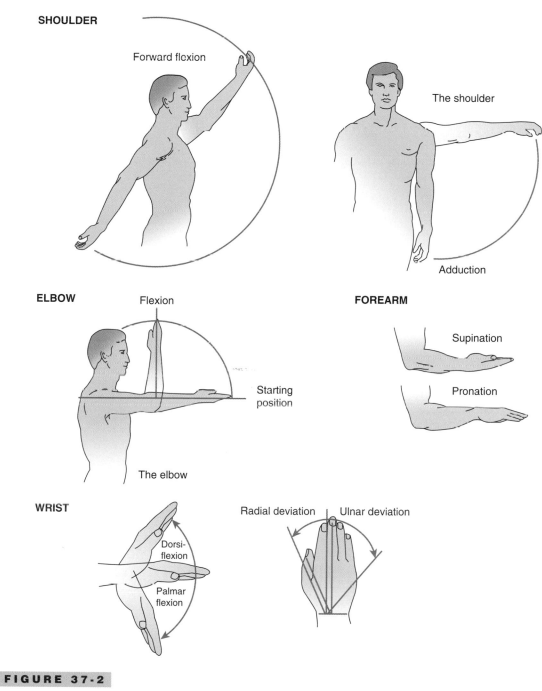

SHOULDER

Forward flexion

The shoulder

Adduction

ELBOW

Flexion

Starting position

The elbow

FOREARM

Supination

Pronation

WRIST

Dorsi-flexion

Palmar flexion

Radial deviation   Ulnar deviation

FIGURE 37-2

Range-of-motion exercises.

HIP

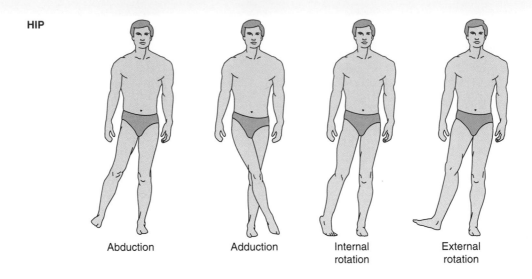

Abduction Adduction Internal rotation External rotation

KNEE

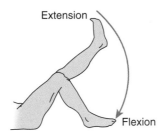

Extension

Flexion

CERVICAL SPINE

 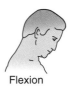

Neutral Flexion Extension

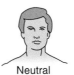

Neutral Rotation

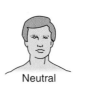 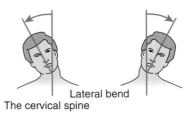

Neutral Lateral bend
The cervical spine

FIGURE 37-2

Range-of-motion exercises. (*continued*)

THUMB

Adduction

Abduction

Opposition

FINGERS

Adduction

Abduction

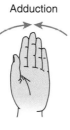

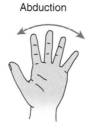

Extension

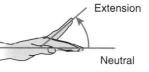

Neutral

ANKLE

Dorsiflexion

Plantar flexion

Eversion

Inversion

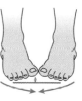

TOES

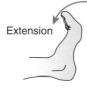

Extension

Flexion

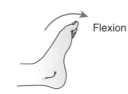

Adduction

Abduction

FIGURE 37-2

Range-of-motion exercises. (*continued*)

that should be incorporated into the older adult's daily activities. When nurses need to assist patients with these exercises, they should remember the following points. First, offer support below and above the joint being exercised. Next, move the joint slowly and smoothly, exercising it at least three times. Third, do not force the joint past the point of resistance or pain. Next, record joint mobility. Display 37-2 lists some of the terms used in describing joint motion. Table 37-2 offers a tool that can be used to document the patient's range of motion.

With any exercise program, caution must be taken to ensure that the physical activity does not overexert the older patient. Some of the signs that would warrant stopping an exercise include the development of:

- a resting heart rate greater than or equal to 100 beats/minute
- an exercise heart rate greater than or equal to 35% above the resting heart rate
- increase or decrease in systolic blood pressure by 20 mm Hg
- angina
- dyspnea, pallor, cyanosis
- dizziness, poor coordination
- diaphoresis
- acute confusion, restlessness

Mobility Aids

Wheelchairs, canes, and walkers can make the difference between older persons living a full life or being confined to their immediate environments. Mobility aids can enable patients to independently fulfill their universal needs and enhance functional capacity. If misused, however, these aids can present significant safety risks; thus, nurses must ensure that these pieces of equipment are used properly.

> **KEY CONCEPT**
> Inappropriately used canes, walkers, and wheelchairs can subject the older adult to falls and other injuries.

The first principle in using mobility aids is to use them only when necessary. Using a wheelchair because it is quicker or easier can result in unnecessary dependency and decline of functional capacity. The true need for the aid must be evaluated. If a mobility aid is deemed necessary, it must be individually selected according to the certain criteria.

- Canes are used to provide a wider base of support and should not be used for bearing weight.
- Walkers offer a broader base of support than canes and can be used for weight-bearing.
- Wheelchairs provide mobility for persons unable to ambulate because of various disabilities, such as paralysis or severe cardiac disease.

These aids are individually fitted based on the patient's size, need, and capacities. Patients should be fully instructed in their proper use. Physical therapists are excellent resources for sizing and instructing patients for cane, walker, or wheelchair use. Figure 37-3 depicts some of the considerations involved in using these aids.

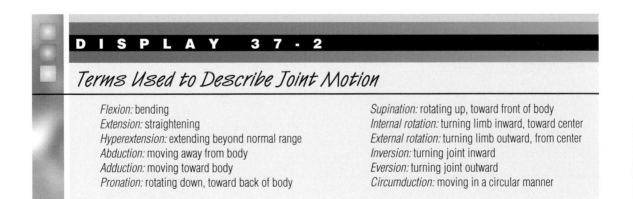

DISPLAY 37-2

Terms Used to Describe Joint Motion

Flexion: bending
Extension: straightening
Hyperextension: extending beyond normal range
Abduction: moving away from body
Adduction: moving toward body
Pronation: rotating down, toward back of body

Supination: rotating up, toward front of body
Internal rotation: turning limb inward, toward center
External rotation: turning limb outward, from center
Inversion: turning joint inward
Eversion: turning joint outward
Circumduction: moving in a circular manner

TABLE 37-2 ● *Tool for Assessing Range of Motion*

Joint	Normal Range	Patient's Range
Shoulder	Flexion 160°	
	Extension 50°	
Elbow	Flexion 160°	
	Extension from 160° to 0°	
Wrist	Flexion 90°	
	Extension 70°	
	Abduction 55°	
	Adduction 20°	
Hip	Flexion (bent knee) 120°	
	Flexion (straight knee) 90°	
	Abduction 45°	
	Adduction 45°	
Knee	Flexion 120°	
Neck	Extension 55°	
	Flexion 45°	
	Lateral bending 40°	
	Rotation 70°	
Ankle	Dorsiflexion 20°	
	Plantar flexion 45°	
	Inversion 30°	
	Eversion 20°	
Great toe	Distal phalange:	
	Flexion 50°	
	Proximal phalange:	
	Flexion 35°	
	Extension 80°	
Finger	Proximal phalange:	
	Flexion 90°	
	Extension 30°	
	Middle phalange:	
	Flexion 120°	
	Distal phalange:	
	Flexion 80°	
Thumb	Proximal phalange:	
	Flexion 70°	
	Distal phalange:	
	Flexion 90°	

(Eliopoulos, C. [1991]. Range of motion exercises. *Long-Term Care Educator, 2*[9], 3.)

Bowel and Bladder Training

Incontinence can have a profound impact on a person's general health and well-being. Skin breakdown can result from the moisture and irritation to which the skin is subjected. Urine or feces on the floor can cause falls. Soiled, odorous clothing can lead to embarrassment and social isolation. Infections, fractures, depression, altered self-concept, anorexia, and other problems can stem from poor bladder and bowel control.

The physical and mental capacity of the patient to achieve continence must be evaluated before a training program is begun. Some patients may not have the functional capacity to control their elimination despite good intentions; to initiate a training program

Cane

Depending on the disability, various canes may be recommended:

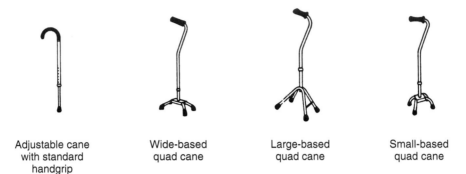

| Adjustable cane with standard handgrip | Wide-based quad cane | Large-based quad cane | Small-based quad cane |

Canes should be individually fitted, usually based on the distance from the greater trochanter to a distance 6 inches from the side of the patient's foot.

The cane is used on the *unaffected* side and is advanced when the affected limb advances.

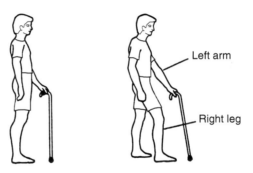

Left arm

Right leg

For example, if the right leg is affected, the cane is held in the left hand. The cane is advanced with the advance of the right leg.

Walker

A variety of walkers can be used to provide support and stability during ambulation.

 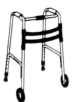 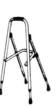 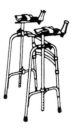

| Regular walker | Walker with wheels | Walker-cane | Walker with forearm attachments |

FIGURE 37-3

Proper use of mobility aids.

Walkers are sized by the measurement from the patient's trochanter to the floor. The hands are placed on the sides of the walker, with the elbows slightly flexed.

During ambulation, the walker is advanced, and then the patient steps.

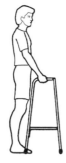

Person standing with walker	Walker advanced	Person advancing to walker

Appropriate use of the walker for transfer activities is

When lowering to seat: back walker to seat

When lifting from seat: push on arms of seat to a standing position; walker should not be used to pull to a standing position.

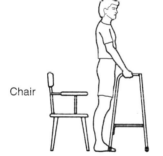

Chair

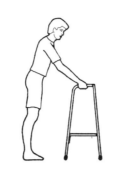

Hand should be on chair arm as person is lifting

Walker

Wheelchair

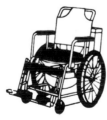

A wheelchair should be individually fitted to the patient. The seat should be slightly larger than the patient's width to prevent pressure and friction; the patient's arm should be able to reach the wheels easily; footrests should be adjusted to support the patient's foot in a flat position.

Removable or fold-down armrests facilitate transfer.

Wheelchairs should be checked routinely for ease of wheeling, function of brakes, jagged edges, tears in upholstery, and broken or missing hardware.

FIGURE 37-3

Proper use of mobility aids. (*continued*)

with them would be unrealistic and frustrating. If the patient has the capacity to be continent, training should begin as early as possible (Displays 37-3 and 37-4). Consistency is a crucial factor in training programs; the gains of the day shift in keeping the patient continent are lost if the evening and night shifts do not toilet the patient at the appropriate intervals. Success should be recognized and praised; patients should not be chastised for accidents, but the reasons for the incontinent episodes should be discussed with them. Encouraging patients to wear street clothes promotes a positive self-image and normality and often discourages regression. Accurate documentation can assist in determining the effectiveness of the plan.

KEY CONCEPT

Consistency and adherence to the toileting schedule by all caregivers on all shifts is essential to bladder and bowel retraining programs.

Maintaining and Promoting Mental Function

The functioning of muscles and joints is only one aspect of rehabilitation. Equally important are efforts to

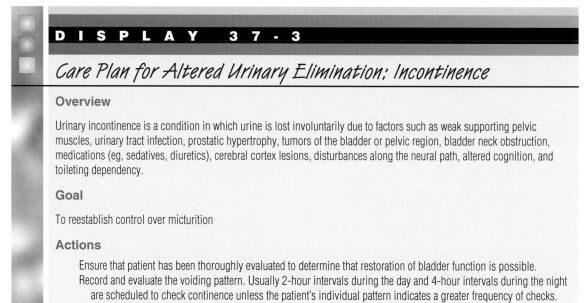

DISPLAY 37-3

Care Plan for Altered Urinary Elimination: Incontinence

Overview

Urinary incontinence is a condition in which urine is lost involuntarily due to factors such as weak supporting pelvic muscles, urinary tract infection, prostatic hypertrophy, tumors of the bladder or pelvic region, bladder neck obstruction, medications (eg, sedatives, diuretics), cerebral cortex lesions, disturbances along the neural path, altered cognition, and toileting dependency.

Goal

To reestablish control over micturition

Actions

Ensure that patient has been thoroughly evaluated to determine that restoration of bladder function is possible.
Record and evaluate the voiding pattern. Usually 2-hour intervals during the day and 4-hour intervals during the night are scheduled to check continence unless the patient's individual pattern indicates a greater frequency of checks.
Half an hour before anticipated voiding time, having the patient drink a glass of water.
Tell the patient to make a conscious effort not to void.
Sit patient on commode at scheduled time.
Have patient rock back and forth or prop feet on stool to increase intra-abdominal pressure.
Instruct patient to massage over bladder area.
Encourage voiding by running water.
Record results.
Reinforce desired behaviors. Give positive feedback for successes. When incontinent episodes do occur the patient should not be chastised, nor should the incident be ignored; instead, discuss the causes for the incontinence with the patient and establish goals for improvement.
As continence improves, the interval between voiding times can be increased.
It is essential that the schedule be rigidly followed.

DISPLAY 37-4

Care Plan for Altered Bowel Elimination: Incontinence

Overview

Bowel incontinence refers to the inability to voluntarily control the passage of stool. It can result from decreased anal muscle tone, disturbances in the neural enervation of the rectum, loss of cortical control, rectal prolapse, diarrhea, constipation with overflow related to impaction, or altered cognition.

Goal

To control bowel elimination

Actions

Record and evaluate patient's bowel elimination pattern.
Establish consistent time to toilet based on pattern.
Position patient in best physiologic position for bowel movement: sitting with normal posture.
Have patient lean forward or prop feet on stool to increase intra-abdominal pressure.
Instruct patient to bear down and attempt to defecate.
Record results; ensure that patient does not develop fecal impaction.
If necessary, stimulate anorectal reflex with glycerin suppository 30 to 45 minutes before scheduled bowel movement.
Supplement toilet activities with exercise and good fluid and roughage intake.

restore, maintain, and promote mental function. In institutional settings where the contact patients have with staff mainly revolves around illness-related issues, or in their own homes where they may be socially isolated, healthy mental stimulation may be sorely lacking. Like any other function, mental function can deteriorate if not exercised; thus, all rehabilitative efforts include the promotion of mental activity.

IMPORTANCE OF INDIVIDUALIZATION

Mental stimulation is a highly individualized process, based on the unique intellectual and educational level of the patient. Some people enjoy reading the classics; others are barely interested in reading the local newspaper. Some people thrive on large social events, whereas others could spend days alone solving a crossword puzzle. Some people want to make things happen; others derive pleasure from watching them happen. This diversity, present in all age groups, reinforces the need to gear mental activities to the unique capacities and interests of the individual.

KEY CONCEPT
Like younger adults, older individuals show variation in activities that bring them intellectual stimulation and enjoyment.

METHODS

Patients can take part in a wide range of intellectual, recreational, and social activities. Some activities have specific therapeutic aims, one of which is *reminiscence*. Since Butler and Lewis first described reminiscence, or life review (Butler & Lewis, 1982), studies have supported the value of this process as a means of validating existence, resolving past conflicts, and finding meaning in remaining life (Hsieh & Wang, 2003). Nurses can guide patients in reminiscing through individual or group means. Often, patients can supply meaningful themes for reminiscence. For example, a patient may comment, "Kids today have it a lot easier than I did when I was young," which could lead the nurse to explore the patient's youth and feelings associated with that period of his or her life. Knowing something of the patient's personal history can help nurses find relevant topics for reminiscence, such as the patient's immigration to America, development of a business, or efforts to assist the country during war time. As the patient discusses the topic, questions can be asked and comments made to encourage greater exploration. If the patient begins to ramble aimlessly, he or she can be redirected to the topic by comments such as, "Yes, you've mentioned that before . . . I can tell it was important to you. Now tell me what happened after that." Themes can be selected for group reminiscing, including playing old records and asking participants what their lives were like when those records were popular, showing old photographs and asking participants what memories arise, and asking them to describe the important pieces of history they have witnessed. Perhaps the most important skill for nurses to use in reminiscing activities is listening.

Patients with moderate-to-severe memory loss, confusion, or disorientation demand therapeutic efforts to keep them mentally integrated with the world around them. For these patients, *reality orientation* is an effective tool. Reality orientation frequently is assumed to be special group sessions that review day, date, weather, next meal, and next holiday. Actually, reality orientation encompasses much more; it is a total approach to keeping the patient oriented. Every nurse-patient contact can enhance orientation. For example, when passing medications, the nurse can state, "Hello, Mr. Richards. I'm Nurse Jones with

your medicine. How are you on this sunny Tuesday? It's very warm for March 10th, isn't it?" This simple exchange adds no more time to the act of administering the medications but provides helpful orientation. Misinformation and misperceptions of the patient should be clarified simply, for instance: "No, your son will not be visiting today. He comes on Sunday and today is Wednesday." Chastising or becoming frustrated with the patient for not remembering serves no therapeutic value. Clocks, calendars, holiday theme decorations, and reality boards enhance, but do not substitute for, staff interactions. Consistency is crucial to promoting orientation; it makes little sense for the day shift to reinforce to the patient that she is in a nursing home while the evening shift agrees with the patient's claim that she is on her grandfather's farm.

Resources for Rehabilitative Needs

Every community has its unique resources for persons with rehabilitative needs; such resources provide education, support, and various forms of assistance to the disabled and their caregivers. Social workers, physical therapists, occupational therapists, speech and hearing therapists, and rehabilitation and vocational counselors are among the professionals who can offer guidance in locating appropriate resources. Local libraries, health departments, and information and referral services for the elderly can also provide valuable assistance.

Critical Thinking Exercises

1. Discuss the way in which a disability can progress to a handicap and measures that can be taken to avoid this.
2. Consider the way in which your average routine would be altered if you possessed a disability. What resources could you use?
3. Describe the way in which prejudices and misinformed attitudes regarding disabilities can affect disabled persons.
4. Identify ways to assist persons in your community who have aphasia, blindness, bilateral amputation, and alcoholism.

Web Connect

Download clinical guidelines for a variety of rehabilitation issues from the website of the Paralyzed Veterans of American website at www.pva.org/NEWPVASITE/publications/consortpubs.htm.

● Resources

Alcoholism

Alcoholics Anonymous
P.O. Box 459
Grand Central Station
New York, NY 10017
(212) 686-1100
www.alcoholics-anonymous.org

National Clearinghouse for Alcohol and Drug Information
11426-28 Rockville Pike
Suite 200
Rockville, MD 20852
(800) 729-6686
www.health.org

Alzheimer's Disease

Alzheimer's Disease and Related Disorders Association, Inc.
919 North Michigan Avenue
Suite 1000
Chicago, IL 60601
(800) 272-3900
www.alz.org

Amputations

National Amputation Foundation
40 Church Street
Malvern NY 11565
(516) 887-3600
www.nationalamputation.org

Arthritis

Arthritis Foundation
1314 Spring Street NW
Atlanta, GA 30309
(800) 283-7800
www.arthritis.org

Asthma

Asthma and Allergy Foundation of America
1125 15th Street NW
Suite 502
Washington, DC 20005
(800) 7-ASTHMA
www.aafa.org

Asthma Hotline
(800) 222-LUNG

Cancer

American Cancer Society
1599 Clifton Road NE
Atlanta, GA 30329
(800) 227-2345
www.cancer.org

National Cancer Institute
Office of Cancer Communications
Building 31, Room 10A18
Bethesda, MD 20205
(800) 492-6600
www.nci.gov

Diabetes

American Diabetes Association
1660 Duke Street
Alexandria, VA 22314
(800) 232-3472
www.diabctcs.org

Diabetes Education Center
4959 Excelsior Boulevard
Minneapolis, MN 55416
(612) 927-3393
www.lilly.com/diabetes/diabetes_education.html

Head Injuries

National Head Injury Foundation
1776 Massachusetts Avenue NW #100
Washington, DC 20036
800-444-6443
www-nmcp.med.navy.mil/Neurology/dzchi.asp

The Brain Injury Association Inc.
105 North Alfred Street
Alexandria, VA 22314
703-236-6000
www.biausa.org

Hearing Impairments

American Humane Association
Hearing Dog Program
1500 West Tufts Avenue
Englewood, CO 80110
(303) 762-0342
(Local SPCAs operate Hearing Dog Programs)

Independent Living Aids
200 Robbins Lane
Jericho, NY 11753
(800) 537-2118
www.independentliving.com

National Institute of Neurological and Communicative Disorders
9000 Rockville Pike
Bethesda, MD 20892
(202) 496-4000
www.nidcd.nih.gov

National Association for the Deaf
814 Thayer Avenue
Silver Spring, MD 20910
(301) 587-1788
www.nad.org

Self-Help for Hard of Hearing People
P.O. Box 34889
Washington, DC 20034
www.shhh.org

Heart Disease

American Heart Association
7320 Greenville Avenue
Dallas, TX 75231
(800) 242-8721
www.amhrt.org

The Mended Hearts
7320 Greenville Avenue
Dallas, TX 55231
(214) 750-5442
www.mendedhearts.org

Lung Disease

American Lung Association
1740 Broadway
New York, NY 10019
(800) 586-4872
www.lungusa.org

Emphysema Anonymous
726 N. Highland Avenue
Clearwater, FL 34615
(818) 391-9977

National Heart, Lung, and Blood Institute
Information Center
PO Box 30105
Bethesda, MD 20824-0105
(301) 592-8573
www.nhlbi.nih.gov

Mental Illness

Alzheimer's Disease and Related Disorders Association, Inc.
919 North Michigan Avenue
Suite 1000
Chicago, IL 60601
(800) 272-3900
www.alz.org

Anxiety Disorders Association of America
8730 Georgia Avenue, Suite 600
Silver Spring, MD 20910
(240) 485-1001
www.adaa.org

National Alliance for the Mentally Ill
2107 Wilson Blvd. Suite 300
Arlington, VA 22201
(800) 950-6264
www.nami.org

National Foundation for Depressive Illness
PO Box 2257
New York, NY 10116
(800) 239-1265
www.depression.org
Neurologic Diseases

American Parkinson's Disease Association
1250 Hylan Boulevard
Suite 4B
Staten Island, NY 10305
(800) 223-2732
www.apdaparkinson.org/

Epilepsy Foundation of America
4351 Garden City Drive
Landover, MD 20785
(301) 459-3700
www.epilepsyfoundation.org

Myasthenia Gravis Foundation
5841 Cedar Lake Road
Suite 204
Minneapolis, MN 55416
(800) 541-5454
www.mysathenia.org

National Huntington's Disease Association
158 West 29th Street, 7th floor
New York, NY 10001
(800) 345-HDSA
www.hdsa.org

National Multiple Sclerosis Society
733 Third Avenue

New York, NY 10017
(800) 344-4867
www.nmss.org

National Stroke Association
8480 East Orchard Road
Suite 1000
Englewood, CO 80111
(800) STROKES
www.stroke.org

Ostomies

United Ostomy Association
19772 MacArthur Blvd.
Suite 200
Irvine, CA 92612
(800) 826-0826
www.uoa.org

Spinal Cord Disorders

National Spinal Cord Injury Foundation
369 Elliot Street
Newton Upper Falls, MA 02164
(617) 964-0521
www.spinalcord.org

Paralyzed Veterans of America
4350 East-West Highway
Suite 900
Washington, DC 20014
(301) 652-2135
www.pva.org

Visual Impairments

American Foundation for the Blind
15 West 16th Street
New York, NY 10011
(212) 620-2000
www.afb.org

Blinded Veterans Association
1735 DeSales Street, NW
Washington, DC 20036
(202) 347-4010
www.bva.org

Guide Dogs for the Blind
P.O. Box 1200
San Rafael, CA 94902
(415) 479-4000
www.guidedogs.com

Guiding Eyes for the Blind
250 East Hartsdale Avenue
Hartsdale, NY 10530
(914) 723-2223
www.guiding-eyes.org

Leader Dogs for the Blind
1039 South Rochester Road
Rochester, MN 48063
(313) 651-9011
www.leaderdog.org

National Association for the Visually Handicapped
305 East 24th Street
New York, NY 10010
(212) 899-3141
www.navh.org

National Braille Association
3 Townline Circle
Rochester, NY 14623
(716) 427-8260
http://members.aol.com/nbaoffice

National Eye Institute
Building 31, Room 6A-32
Bethesda, MD 20205
(301) 496-5248
www.nei.nih.gov

National Library Service for the Blind and Physically Handicapped
Library of Congress
1291 Taylor Street, NW
Washington, DC 20542
(202) 287-5100
lcweb.loc.gov/nls

Recordings for the Blind
215 East 58th Street
New York, NY 10022
(212) 751-0860
www.rfbd.org

General

Disabled American Veterans
P.O. Box 14301
Cincinnati, OH 45214
(606) 441-7300
www.dav.org

National Rehabilitation Information Center
Catholic University of America
4407 8th Street, NE
Washington, DC 20017
(202) 635-5822

Sister Kenny Institute
800 East 28th St.
Minneapolis, MN 55407
(612) 863-4400
www.allina.com/ahs/ski.nsf

● References

Butler, R. N., & Lewis, M. I. (1982). *Aging and mental health* (p. 58). St. Louis: Mosby.

Fried, L. P., Tangen, C. M., Walston, J., Newman, A. B., Hirsch, C., Gottdiener, J., et al. (2001). Frailty of older adults: Evidence for a phenotype. *Journals of Gerontology: Biological Sciences and Medical Sciences, 56A*(3), M146–M156.

Hsieh, H. F., & Wang, J. J. (2003). Effect of reminiscence therapy on depression in older adults: A systematic review. *International Journal of Nursing Studies, 40*(4), 335–345.

● Recommended Readings

Baird, C. L. (2003). Holding on: Self-caring with osteoarthritis. *Journal of Gerontological Nursing, 29*(6), 32–39.

Cohen, H., Feussner, J., Weinberger, M., Carnes, M., Hamdy, R., Hsieh, F., et al. (2002). A controlled trial of inpatient and outpatient geriatric evaluation and management. *New England Journal of Medicine, 346*(12), 905–912.

Diwan, S., Ivy, C., Merino, D., & Brower, T. (2001). Assessing the need for intensive case management in long-term care. *The Gerontologist, 41*(5), 680–686.

Eliopoulos, C. (1999). *Integrating alternative and conventional therapies: Holistic care of chronic conditions.* St. Louis: Mosby.

Eliopoulos, C. (2003). Holistic nursing, In. Leskowitz, E. *Complementary and alternative medicine in rehabilitation.* St. Louis, MO: Churchill Livingstone, pp. 275–283.

Hart, B., Birkas, J., Lachmann, M., & Saunders, L. (2002). Promoting positive outcomes for elderly persons in the hospital: Prevention and risk factor modification. *AACN Clinical Issues, 13*(1), 22–33.

Hoeman, S. P. (2002). *Rehabilitation nursing: Process and application* (3rd ed.). St. Louis: Mosby.

Hughes, E. M. (1995). Creating functional environments for elder care facilities. *Geriatric Nursing, 16*(4), 172–176.

Kelly, M. (1995). Consequences of visual impairment on leisure activities of the elderly. *Geriatric Nursing, 16*(6), 273–275.

Lai, S. C., & Cohen, M. N. (1999). Promoting lifestyle changes. *American Journal of Nursing, 99*(4), 63–67.

Lewis, M., Hepburn, K., Corcoran-Perry, S., Narayan, S., & Lally, R. M. (1999). Options, outcomes, values, likelihoods. Decision-making guide for patients and their families. *Journal of Gerontological Nursing, 25*(12), 19–25.

Lohrmann, C., Dijkstra, A., & Dassesn, T. (2003). The care dependency scale: An assessment instrument for elderly patients in German hospitals. *Geriatric Nursing, 24*(1), 40–43.

Lord, S. R., Ward, J. A., Williams, P., & Strudwick, M. (1995). The effect of a 12-month exercise trial on balance, strength, and falls in older women. *Journal of the American Geriatrics Society, 43*(8), 1198–1206.

Lunney, J. R., Lynn, J., Foley, D. J., Lipson, S., & Guralnik, J. M. (2003). Patterns of functional decline at the end of life. *Journal of the American Medical Association, 289*(18), 2387–2392.

McMurtry, C. T., & Rosenthal, A. (1995). Predictors of 2-year mortality among older male veterans on a geriatric rehabilitation unit. *Journal of the American Geriatrics Society, 43*(10), 1123–1126.

Moore, S. L., Metcalf, B., & Schow, E. (2000). Aging and meaning in life: Examining the concept. *Geriatric Nursing, 21*(1), 27–28.

Ostwald, S. K., Hepburn, K. W., & Burns, T. (2003). Training family caregivers of patients with dementia: A structured workshop approach. *Journal of Gerontological Nursing, 29*(1), 37–44.

O'Sullivan, S. B., & Schmitz, T. J. (2001). Physical rehabilitation: Assessment and treatment. Philadelphia: F.A. Davis.

Resnick, B., & Fleishell, A. (2002). Developing a restorative care program. *American Journal of Nursing, 102*(7), 91–97.

Resnick, B., & Simpson, M. (2003). Restorative care nursing activities: Pilot testing self-efficacy and outcome expectation measures. *Geriatric Nursing, 24*(2), 82–89.

Skelton, D. A., Young, A., Grieg, C. A., & Malbut, K. E. (1995). Effects of resistance training on strength, power, and selected functional abilities of women aged 75 and older. *Journal of the American Geriatrics Society, 43*(10), 1081–1087.

Stokes, S. A., & Gordon, S.E. (2003). Common stressors experienced by the well elderly. Clinical implications. *Journal of Gerontological Nursing, 29*(5), 38–46.

Walsh, C. (1995). Managing a head injury program. *Provider 21*(6), 35–38.

Young, H. (May 31, 2003). Challenges and solutions for care of frail older adults. *Online Journal of Issues in Nursing, 8*(2), manuscript 4. Retrieved April 2, 2004, from www.nursingworld.org/ojin/topic21/tpc21_4.htm.

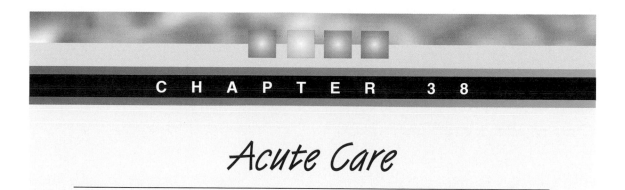

Acute Care

■ Learning Objectives

After reading this chapter, you should be
able to:

- list measures to minimize risks faced
  by acutely ill older adults
- describe risks and precautions for older
  patients undergoing surgery
- discuss common geriatric emergencies
  and related nursing actions
- identify measures to reduce the risk of
  infection
- discuss the importance of early
  discharge planning
- describe factors that influence
  postdischarge outcomes

Risks Associated With Hospitalization

Today's acute care hospitals play a significant role
in geriatric care. The elderly have a high rate of hospitalization as compared with other age groups,
with one quarter of all inpatient hospital days used
by persons over 75 years of age (U.S. Census Bureau, 2002). Furthermore, the elderly are significant consumers of outpatient hospital services.
Acute care settings definitely are in the geriatric care
business!

Many older adults who have lived independently
in their homes prior to admission to the hospital are
not discharged with the same level of function;
some are transferred to a long-term care facility. Although the decline in status can be attributed to the

513

effects of aging on the older adult's ability to withstand the stress of an acute condition, the elderly are at high risk for iatrogenic complications and nosocomial infections. Nurses should anticipate and minimize the common risks faced by the acutely ill elderly in an effort to promote optimal functional independence (Display 38-1). Some useful measures include:

- careful assessment to identify problems and risks
- early discharge planning
- encouragement of independence

DISPLAY 38-1

Potential Risks of Older Adults During Hospitalization

Risk	Contributing/ Causative Factors	Risk	Contributing/ Causative Factors
Delirium	New environment	Incontinence	Diuresis
	Sensory deprivation		Sedation
	Inaccessible eyeglasses, hearing aid		Weakness
	Altered cognition or level of consciousness		Inaccessible commode, bedpan
	Excess stimuli		Indwelling catheterization
	Adverse drug reactions		Lack of assistance
	Physiologic disturbance	Constipation	Age-related changes to GI system
Falls	Dizziness		Effects of medications
	Orthostatic hypotension		Effects of surgery
	Weakness, fatigue		Dietary modifications
	Unfamiliar environment		Reduced activity
	Altered cognition or level of consciousness		Poor positioning during defecation
	Presence of equipment, supplies		Inaccessible commode, bedpan
	Chemical or physical restraints		Lack of toileting assistance
	Failure to use bed rails	Loss of functional independence	Stereotypical expectations by staff
	Effects of medications		Unnecessary restrictions
	Lack of assistance		Insufficient time for self-care
Pressure ulcers	Age-related changes to skin		Knowledge deficit
	Immobilization		Immobility
	Shearing forces		Development of complications
	Sedation		Failure to ambulate, mobilize early
	Pain		
	Weakness		
	Debilitating condition		
	Lack of assistance		
Dehydration	Age-related decrease in thirst sensation		
	Sedation		
	Nausea, vomiting		
	Altered cognition or level of consciousness		
	Inaccessible fluids		
	Lack of assistance		

- close monitoring of medications and assurance that age-adjusted dosages are used
- reminders and assistance to patient with frequent repositioning, coughing, deep breathing, toileting
- early identification and correction of complications, recognizing that atypical signs and symptoms may be present
- avoidance of urinary catheterization if possible
- strict adherence to aseptic techniques and infection control practices
- close monitoring of intake and output, vital signs, mental status, and skin status
- environmental modifications to accommodate older patients' needs (eg, room temperature of 75°F, noise control, use of nightlights, avoidance of glare)
- use of bed rails
- assistance, as necessary, with activities of daily living
- patient and family education
- orientation as necessary
- referral to resources to promote self-care ability and independence

> **Point to Ponder**
> *What do you perceive are the positive and negative aspects of caring for elders in an acute hospital setting?*

Surgical Care

Improved surgical procedures and the increasing number of persons living to old age account for the fact that nurses now are caring for many more surgical patients of advanced age. Also, people are no longer denied the benefit of surgery based on their age alone. Surgical intervention has provided many older people not only with more years to their lives but also with more functional years. Successful surgical management of an older person's health problems depends on the nurse's understanding of the age-related factors that alter normal surgical procedures.

> **KEY CONCEPT**
> Surgical intervention not only adds years to an older adult's life but also improves the quality and functional independence of those added years.

SPECIAL RISKS

In general, older adults have a smaller margin of physiologic reserve and are less able to compensate for and adapt to physiologic changes. Infection, hemorrhage, anemia, blood pressure changes, and fluid and electrolyte imbalances are more problematic in the elderly (Fig. 38-1). Unfortunately, inelasticity of blood vessels, malnourishment, increased susceptibility to infection, and reduced cardiac, respiratory, and renal reserves cause complications to occur more frequently in the elderly, especially during emergency or complicated surgical procedures. By strengthening their capacities preoperatively, maintaining these capacities postoperatively, and being alert to early signs of complications, the nurse can help reduce the risk of surgical problems (Nursing Diagnosis Table 38-1).

PREOPERATIVE PROCEDURES

The gerontological nurse must be sensitive to the fears that many older patients have concerning surgery.

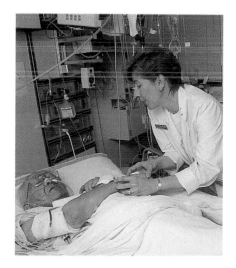

FIGURE 38-1

The hospitalized older adult requires nursing interventions to prevent complications and to promote a return to wellness. (Craven, R.F., & Hirnle, C.J..(2003). *Fundamentals of nursing: Human health and function* [4th ed., p. 201]. Philadelphia: Lippincott Williams & Wilkins.)

Throughout their lifetimes, today's elders may have witnessed severe disability or death in older persons having surgery, and they may worry about similar outcomes from their operation. Patients need to understand the increased success of surgical procedures through the following advances:

- better diagnostic tools facilitating earlier diagnosis and treatment
- improved therapeutic measures, including surgical techniques and antibiotics
- increased knowledge concerning the unique characteristics of older adults

In addition to reassurance, patients and their families should be taught what to expect before, during, and after the operative procedure, including the following information:

- preoperative preparation—scrubs, medications, nothing to eat by mouth (NPO)
- types of reactions to anesthesia
- length of the surgery and a brief description of it
- routine recovery room procedures
- expected pain and its management
- turning, coughing, and deep-breathing exercises
- rationale for and frequency of dressing changes,

Nursing Diagnosis

ND **TABLE 38-1** ● *Nursing Diagnoses Related to Surgical Interventions*

Causes or Contributing Factors	Nursing Diagnosis
Altered oxygen transport, pain	Activity Intolerance
Fear of death or disability, pain, lack of knowledge	Anxiety
Anesthesia, immobility, actual or perceived pain, analgesics	Constipation
Shock, fluid and electrolyte imbalances, sepsis, anesthesia	Decreased Cardiac Output
Diagnostic tests, positioning, tissue trauma, immobility	Pain
Decreased cerebral blood flow, endotracheal intubation, pain, anesthesia, central nervous system depressants	Impaired Verbal Communication
Concern about loss of body function or part, death, outcome of surgery	Fear
Shock, infection, excessive wound drainage, NPO status, electrolyte imbalance, blood loss	Deficient Fluid Volume
Excessive or rapid IV infusion, venous pooling/stasis	Excess Fluid Volume
IV therapy, intubation, break in aseptic technique, catheterization	Risk for Infection
Altered cerebral function, pain	Risk for Injury
Lack of knowledge of surgical procedure, expected outcome, risks, postoperative care	Deficient Knowledge
Pain, weakness, altered cognition, restrictions	Impaired Physical Mobility
Anorexia, nausea, vomiting, pain, inability to feed self	Imbalanced Nutrition: Less Than Body Requirements
Trauma from endotracheal tube, NPO status, mouth breathing, inadequate oral hygiene	Impaired Oral Mucous Membrane
Inability to help self, lack of knowledge	Powerlessness
Anesthesia, narcotics, immobility, pain, secretions	Impaired Gas Exchange
Immobility, weakness, restrictions from IV apparatus	Self-Care Deficit
Change in body function or part, pain, dependency	Body Image Disturbance
Immobility, pressure from operating table, edema, dehydration	Impaired Skin Integrity
Immobility, anxiety, pain, new environment, drugs	Disturbed Sleep Pattern
Anesthesia, drugs, confusion, dehydration, indwelling catheter	Impaired Urinary Elimination

suctioning, oxygen, catheters, and other anticipated procedures

Explanations given by the nurse should also be communicated to others responsible for care through documentation in the patient's record. The nurse identifies concerns, questions, and fears during assessment and preoperative preparation and makes the physician aware of these findings.

The nurse also reviews with the physician the medications the patient is receiving to determine those that must be continued throughout the hospitalization. The patient's routine medications may need to be administered despite NPO restrictions. For instance, sudden interruption of steroid therapy can cause cardiovascular collapse. The nurse may learn that the patient has been taking antihypertensive, tranquilizing, or other medications before hospitalization. Occasionally, patients forget or are reluctant to tell the physician about these drugs. Because cardiac and pulmonary functions can be altered by certain drugs, it is important to make sure this information is communicated to the physician. Likewise, the physician needs to know about herbal medications that the patient may be using as some of these (such as ginseng and gingko biloba) can affect clotting.

Nurses should ensure that basic preoperative screening has been completed, including the following:

- analysis of blood samples: creatinine clearance, glucose, electrolytes, complete blood counts, total plasma proteins, arterial blood gases, cardiac enzymes, lymphocyte count, serum albumin, hemoglobin, hematocrit, total iron-binding capacity, transferrin
- chest x-ray
- electrocardiogram (ECG)
- pulmonary function testing: for obese individuals and those with a history of smoking or pulmonary disease
- nutritional assessment: height, weight, midarm circumference, triceps skin-fold, diet history
- mental status

Because of the direct nature of the care they provide, nurses may be the only health care professionals to recognize certain problems. For example, they may discover loose teeth, which can become dislodged and aspirated during the surgical procedure, causing un-

necessary complications. Such a problem should be brought to the physician's attention to ensure preoperative dental correction.

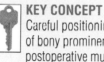

KEY CONCEPT

Before the patient undergoes surgery, nurses should examine the individual for loose teeth, which can become dislodged and aspirated during surgical procedures.

Another precaution during surgery preparation if prolonged surgery is anticipated is to pad the bony prominences of older patients to protect them from lying on a hard operating room table and subsequently acquiring pressure ulcers or experiencing muscle and bone discomfort following surgery.

KEY CONCEPT

Careful positioning of the patient and padding of bony prominences can reduce some of the postoperative muscle and bone soreness that the elderly may experience with prolonged surgery.

Infection control must be at the forefront of the nurse's mind during the entire hospitalization and begins early during the preoperative preparation. Promoting a good nutritional state and correcting existing infections are important preoperative considerations. To further reduce the risk of infection, three preoperative bathings—in the morning and at bedtime on the day before surgery and on the morning of surgery, using an antiseptic—are recommended, as is performing preoperative shaving as close to the time of surgery as possible. Although it is the physician's legal responsibility, nurses can ensure that the patient's informed consent has been obtained preoperatively.

OPERATIVE AND POSTOPERATIVE PROCEDURES

Anesthesia must be considered carefully. Because anesthesia produces depression of the already compromised functions of the cardiovascular and respiratory systems of the older patient, it must be carefully selected. Close monitoring by the anesthesiologist during surgery can detect and prevent difficulties in the patient's vital functions. Prolonged surgery for the older patient is discouraged. Rough, frequent handling of the tissue during surgery usually is avoided because this stimulates reflex activity, increasing the demand for anesthesia. If inhaled agents are used for anesthesia, the nurse should be aware that the patient may remain anesthetized for a longer time because of the slower elimination of these agents; turning and deep breathing will facilitate faster elimination of inhaled agents.

Hypothermia is one of the major complications older adults face intraoperatively and postoperatively. Factors that contribute to this problem include the lower normal body temperatures possessed by many older persons, the cool temperature of operating rooms, and the use of medications that slow metabolism. The cool environment and shivering that may result can increase cardiac output and ventilation and deprive the heart and brain of necessary oxygen; however, shivering occurs less frequently in the elderly. Furthermore, the slowing of metabolism that occurs with hypothermia delays awakening and the return of reflexes. Close monitoring of body temperature is essential. Some hypothermia may be preventable with proper warming measures; research has demonstrated that forced-air warming during the intraoperative and early postoperative periods resulted in higher core temperatures and a lower incidence of hypothermia (Grossman, Bautista, & Sullivan, 2002).

> **KEY CONCEPT**
> Hypothermia is a major intraoperative and postoperative risk to older patients.

Frequent, close postoperative observation and monitoring are extremely important. The decreased ability of the elderly to manage stress reinforces the need to detect and treat symptoms of shock and hemorrhage promptly. Although not fully conscious after surgery, the older person may demonstrate restlessness as the primary symptom of hypoxia. It is important that this restlessness not be mistaken for pain; administration of a narcotic could deplete the body's oxygen supply even more. Prophylactic administration of oxygen may be a beneficial component of the postoperative therapy. Blood loss should be accurately measured and, if excessive, promptly corrected. Frequent checking of urinary output can help reveal the onset of serious complications. Finally, fluid and electrolyte imbalances can be avoided and detected through strict recording of intake and output. Output should include drainage, bleeding, vomitus, and all other sources of fluid loss.

> **KEY CONCEPT**
> Postoperative restlessness could indicate hypoxia, not pain; inappropriate administration of a narcotic analgesic could further deplete the body's oxygen supply.

Because the older patient has a greater risk of developing infections, strict attention must be paid to caring for wounds and changing dressings. A good nutritional status is beneficial to tissue healing and should be encouraged. To conserve the patient's energy and provide comfort, relief of pain is essential. Maintaining regular bowel and bladder elimination, keeping joints mobile, and helping the patient achieve a comfortable position can aid in pain control. If medications are used for pain relief, attention should be given to the reduced activity that may result and to the prevention of the ill effects of such immobilization. The nurse should also be aware that positioning on the hard operating room table and pulling and moving of the unconscious patient may cause muscle and bone soreness for several days postoperatively. Finally, it is vital to observe the patient for respiratory depression if narcotic analgesics are administered.

Older patients are particularly subject to several postoperative complications. Respiratory complications include pneumonia, pulmonary emboli, and atelectasis; with atelectasis there may be decreased lung sounds and a low-grade fever, although the chest x-ray may not show the condition. Atelectasis increases the risk for the development of pneumonia. If pneumonia develops in an elder, it is more problematic than it would be for a younger adult and requires a longer recovery period. Cardiovascular complications include embolus, thrombus, myocardial infarction, and arrhythmias. Cerebrovascular accident and coronary occlusion occur, but they are less common than other complications. Reduced activity and lowered resistance can cause pressure ulcers to develop easily. Drug-induced renal failure is not uncommon; drugs that commonly cause this complication include cimetidine, digoxin, aminoglycosides, cephalosporins, ampicillin, and neuromuscular-blocking agents. Postoperative older patients, particularly those with hip repair, tend to have a higher incidence of delirium than the general adult population. Paralytic ileus, accompanied by fever, dehydration, abdominal tenderness, and distention, is an additional postoperative complication that the aged may experience. Table 38-1 lists other complications.

The nurse is in a key position to help the older patient achieve the maximal benefit from surgery. The most sophisticated surgical procedure in the world performed by the most skillful surgeon is of little value if poor rehabilitative care causes disability or death from avoidable complications. To combine the principles and practices of surgical nursing with the unique characteristic of the older patient is an immense challenge to the gerontological nurse. However, to see the increased capacity and more meaningful life many elders derive from the benefits of surgery is an immense satisfaction.

Emergencies

Emergencies in older persons are particularly problematic. First, they occur frequently because of the age-related changes that lower resistance and make the body more susceptible to injury and illness. Second, they often present an atypical picture that complicates diagnosis. Next, they can be more difficult to treat or stabilize because of the elderly's altered response to treatment. Finally, they carry a greater risk of causing serious complications and death. By recognizing emergency situations and intervening promptly, nurses can spare considerable discomfort and disability to older patients and, in many situations, save their lives.

Regardless of the type of emergency, the following basic goals guide nursing actions:

- maintain life functions
- prevent and treat shock

- control bleeding
- prevent complications
- keep the patient physically and psychologically comfortable
- observe and record signs, treatments, and responses
- assess for causative factors

Whenever there is a question regarding whether a true emergency exists, nurses should err on the side of safety. It is far better to obtain an x-ray or ECG that results in a negative finding than to believe it would be an unnecessary bother or expense and have the patient suffer from a delayed diagnosis.

🔑 **KEY CONCEPT**
When an emergency condition is suspected, it is better to err on the safe side and obtain diagnostic tests rather than risk delaying the diagnosis.

Display 38-2 highlights some of the emergency conditions that may be encountered with older adults and related nursing measures. (**Visit the Connection website to learn about other problems that can present as emergency situations or require prompt action.**)

Infection Control

Infections are common acute conditions that demand prompt attention. A variety of factors can be responsible for the high risk for infection in the elderly (Display 38-3).

Not only do infections develop more easily in the elderly, but they also are more difficult to identify early because of altered symptomatology. That is, the atypical presentation of symptoms can complicate early identification and correction. For example, lower body temperature can cause fever to appear atypically; reduced cough efficiency can prohibit the productive cough that can give a clue to a respiratory infection; and anorexia, fatigue, and altered cognition can be ascribed to other health problems or "old age." Gerontological nurses should suspect an infection when any abrupt, unexplained change in physical or mental function is detected.

TABLE 38-1 ● *Common Complicating Conditions in Elderly Surgical Patients*

Complicating Condition	Medical-Surgical Factors	Aging Processes	Nursing Interventions
Fluid and electrolyte imbalance	Blood, fluid losses during surgery, cool operating room, fluids evaporate from tissues, surgery and anesthesia stimulate ADH and aldosterone, overhydration with IV infusion	Decreased renal function—nephron loss, GFR, decreased renal blood flow and creatinine clearance; decreased cardiopulmonary function	Careful monitoring of intake and output, assessment of skin turgor—over sternum or forehead, assess for signs of hypervolemia and hypovolemia, determine urinary status, note nonmeasured fluid losses such as diaphoresis, assess for sacral edema, correct imbalances with isotonic IV infusions and electrolytes
Malnutrition	NPO for test preparations, decreased intake post-operatively, psycho-social influences, operative site, stress of surgery increases nutritional needs	Decreased secretion, motility, and absorption; decreased basal metabolic rate; loss of taste buds; loss of appetite; reduced absorption of iron, B_{12}, calcium; sensory losses	Preoperative nutritional assessment, monitor weight, fluid balance, food intake and laboratory values, preoperative nutritional preparation, calorie and protein increases postoperatively, hyperalimentation if indicated, use of nutritional support team, maintain positive nitrogen balance postoperatively; vitamin/mineral supplements
Pneumonia, atelectasis	Heavy smokers with cough, obesity, bronchitis, chronic pulmonary disease, thoracic or upper abdominal surgery, anesthesia and pain medication reduce functional residual capacity, lung expansion and gas exchange	Reduced bronchopulmonary movement, decreased pulmonary function—tidal volume, loss of protective airway reflexes	*Preoperatively*—cease smoking for 1 week, weight reduction, pulmonary function testing; if bronchitis present, give antibiotics, expectorants and bronchodilators, teach pulmonary maneuvers; cough (tongue extended to loosen secretions), deep breathing, incentive spirometer *Postoperatively*—position change hourly, monitor blood gases, off ventilator as soon as possible, continue pulmonary maneuver; O_2 to ensure adequate oxygenation, early ambulation, chest physiotherapy
Pressure ulcers	Malnutrition; chronic disease (eg, diabetes, CHF, PVD); length of time on OR table	Moisture loss, thinning epidermis, capillary loss in dermis, loss of sensory receptors, loss of subcutaneous fat	Frequent turning, correct positioning, pressure relieving devices, avoidance of shearing forces, early movement and ambulation, good skin hygiene, lotions, gentle massage, nutritional supplements, increase fluid intake, high-protein, high-calorie diet *(continued)*

TABLE 38-1 ● *Common Complicating Conditions in Elderly Surgical Patients (Continued)*

Complicating Condition	Medical-Surgical Factors	Aging Processes	Nursing Interventions
Wound dehiscence, wound evisceration	Malnutrition; large, sudden weight loss	Delayed immune response, delayed wound healing—slowing of inflammatory response, mitosis, cell proliferation, abnormal collagen formation causing poor tensile strength in wound, decreased muscle strength	1–3 weeks preoperative nutritional preparation, hyperalimentation, vitamin supplements, strict aseptic wound care, encourage rest—slow wave sleep aids wound healing, inspiratory breathing exercises, coughing only if secretions present, prevent/reduce vomiting; discharge teaching, proper wound care and observation for complications, diet instructions
Incidental hypothermia	Cold operating rooms, room temperature infusions, exposure of skin for draping and preparation, exposure of peritoneum/pleura during surgery, peripheral vasodilation	Impaired thermoregulatory mechanisms, decreased cardiopulmonary reserves, impaired ability to increase basal metabolic rate	Temperature monitoring in OR, careful cardiac monitoring, hyperthermia blanket, warm top blankets after incision closure, warm IV fluids, transfer from OR quickly, thermal top blankets in RR, transfer blankets with patient to surgical unit
Joint stiffness, contractures	Presence of degenerative joint disease, osteoporosis, reduced mobility during preoperative preparation, immobility during surgery, pain limiting motion in postoperative period	Decreased muscle strength and wasting, decreased bone mass, ossification of cartilage in joints, flexion of joints, stooped posture, slowed movement, gait changes	Assess prior functioning level, leg exercises preoperatively, early ambulation, proper positioning and movement in bed, active/passive range of motion, encourage active movement by patient
Acute confusional states, delirium	Type of anesthesia, penetration of blood-brain barrier by certain drugs, presence of preexisting depression or dementia, environmental factors, number of medications taken, hypoxemia, psychosocial factors	Loss of neurons, brain atrophy, decreased cerebral blood flow and oxygen consumption, decreased renal function, slowed clearance of drugs from system, sensory losses, decreased cardiopulmonary reserves	*Preoperatively*—baseline assessment of mental status and emotional state, psychological support, allow time for questions and verbalization of fears, provide pastoral care if desired, correct electrolyte imbalances, anemia *Postoperatively*—monitor level of consciousness, avoid restraints, provide calm environment, avoid use of indwelling catheters, orient to environment, progressive mobility, small doses of haloperidol (Haldol) if organic causes, reassurance from all staff, need special attention if have hearing loss, monitor electrolytes and fluid balance, ensure adequate oxygenation *(continued)*

TABLE 38-1 ● *Common Complicating Conditions in Elderly Surgical Patients (Continued)*

Complicating Condition	Medical-Surgical Factors	Aging Processes	Nursing Interventions
Cardiac failure	Existing cardiac disease, hypertension, anesthesia effects on blood pressure, stress of surgery increases metabolic needs and increases workload on heart	Decreased cardiac output, altered O_2 transport, fatty accumulations in heart valves, atherosclerosis of vessels, widening pulse pressure	*Preoperatively*—risk assessment, correct, treat existing conditions; low dosage heparinization; improved nutritional status will improve cardiac function. *Postoperatively*—continuous CVP monitoring; assess JVD and breath sounds hourly; continuous ECG monitoring; close observation of vital signs, level of consciousness and urinary output, maintain infusion rates; check intake and output; observe peripheral circulation, color; maintain cardiovascular functions; careful, early mobilization, rest periods

ADH, antidiuretic hormone; CHF, congestive heart failure; CVP, central venous pressure; ECG, electrocardiogram; GFR, glomerular-filtration rate; IV, intravenous; JVD, jugular vein distention; NPO, nothing by mouth; OR, operating room; PVD, pulmonary vascular disease; RR, recovery room. (From Palmer, M. A. [1990]. Care of the older surgical patient. In Eliopoulos, C. [Ed.], *Caring for the elderly in diverse care settings.* Philadelphia: J.B. Lippincott.)

🔑 KEY CONCEPT
An infection should be suspected when there is an abrupt change in the physical or mental status of the older adult.

The most common infection in the elderly is urinary tract infection (UTI). In the elderly, signs of UTI could include confusion, incontinence, vague abdominal pain, anorexia, nausea, and vomiting. Patients with diabetes may experience a loss of glycemic control. Diagnosis can be confirmed by laboratory tests.

Bacterial pneumonia is the leading cause of infection-related death in older adults. As with other infectious processes, symptoms can be atypical and include confusion, lethargy, and anorexia, in addition to the typical signs associated with pneumonia in any age group. Serum and blood testing are done to confirm the diagnosis.

Careful attention must be paid to infection prevention in older adults. Measures that assist in this effort include:

- promoting good hydration and nutritional status
- monitoring vital signs, mental status, and general health status
- maintaining intact skin and mucous membrane
- avoiding immobility
- ensuring pneumococcal and influenza vaccines have been administered (unless contraindicated)
- maintaining a clean environment
- restricting contact with persons who have infections or suspected infections
- storing foods properly
- preventing injuries
- adhering to infection-control practices

A variety of vitamins and herbs have been promoted for the prevention and management of infections. Vitamin C and vitamin A supplements are recommended, as is the elimination of refined sugar from the diet. The herbs echinacea, goldenseal, and garlic can prevent and treat infections; in small doses, they are believed to boost resistance to infection, and in larger doses, they may fight pathogens. Siberian ginseng can protect the body from the hazardous effects of stress and boost resistance to infection. Patients

DISPLAY 38-2

Selected Emergencies

Acute Confusion/Delirium

Clinical manifestations: rapid decline in cognitive function, disturbed intellectual function, disorientation to time and place, diminished attention span, poorer memory, labile mood, meaningless chatter, poor judgment, altered level of consciousness, restlessness, insomnia, personality changes, suspiciousness

Goal: identify and correct causative factor.

Assess for changes in physical health, stresses, lifestyle changes, medications taken, dietary intake, other problems.

Obtain blood samples for evaluation.

Monitor vital signs, intake and output, and behaviors.

Support treatment plan, for example, electrolyte replacement, medication change, and fever control.

Goal: protect from injury and complications.

Supervise activities closely.

Remove hazardous substances, medications, and machinery from patient's immediate environment.

Ensure adequate nutritional intake, toileting, and hygiene.

Goal: reduce confusion.

Limit number of staff who provide care. Offer consistency of approach.

Maintain stable, calm environment. Avoid bright lights, excessive noise, and extreme room temperatures.

Offer orienting statements, such as "Mr. Jones, you are in the hospital. It is Tuesday evening. Your wife is at your side."

Clarify misconceptions.

Note: a thorough evaluation is crucial when confusion exists. This problem can result from a wide range of disturbances such as hypoglycemia, hypercalcemia, malnutrition, infection, trauma, and drug reactions.

Dehydration

Clinical manifestations: concentrated urine, decreased or excessive urine output, weight loss, output exceeds intake, increased pulse rate, increased temperature, decreased skin turgor, dry-coated tongue, dry skin and mucous membrane, weakness, lethargy, confusion, nausea, anorexia; thirst may or may not be present.

Goal: restore lost fluids.

Obtain blood sample for analysis of electrolytes.

Force fluids unless contraindicated. Administer intravenous solutions as ordered.

Monitor and record intake and output, weight, and vital signs.

Goal: minimize or eliminate causative factors. Assess for possible causes (eg, insufficient intake, fever, vomiting, diarrhea, wound drainage).

Correct underlying cause.

Monitor and encourage good fluid intake.

Note: the reduction in intracellular fluid that occurs with age contributes to less total body fluids; thus, any fluid loss is more significant in older adults. Unless there is a medical need for restriction, fluid intake should range between 2000 and 3000 mL daily. Special factors that can lead to dehydration should be assessed in older patients, such as diminished thirst sensations, disabilities that restrict independent fluid intake, altered mental status, and desires to minimize frequency and nocturia.

Falls

Clinical manifestations: patient found on floor or reports falling

Goal: evaluate and treat injury sustained from fall.

Do not move patient until status is evaluated.

Request x-ray if fracture is suspected.

Control bleeding.

Relieve patient's anxiety.

Assess vital signs, mental status, and functional capacity. Note signs and symptoms (eg, incontinence, tremors, weakness).

Review events preceding fall (eg, position change, medication administration, pain, dizziness).

(Continued)

DISPLAY 38-2 (Continued)

Observe and monitor patient's status for the next 24 hours.

Goal: prevent future falls.

Assess and correct factors contributing to falls (eg, gait disturbances, poor vision, confusion, improper use of assistive device, medications, environmental hazards).

Teach patient how to fall safely (eg, protect head and face, do not move until checked).

Teach patient how to reduce risk of falls.

Wear safe shoes; avoid long robes.

Sit on edge of bed for a few minutes before rising.

Use rails, particularly in tubs and stairways.

Walk only in well-lighted areas.

Eliminate clutter and loose rugs from environment.

Note: an older person who falls once is at great risk of falling again; thus, active prevention is necessary. Falls are the second leading cause of accidental death; the morbidity and mortality associated with falls increase with age.

Myocardial Infarction

Clinical manifestations: acute confusion/delirium, dyspnea, reduced blood pressure, pale skin, weakness; chest pain may or may not be present

Goal: aid in prompt diagnosis.

Identify signs early. Signs may be missed or attributed to other problems.

Even with the slightest suspicion that a myocardial infarction exists, proceed with a diagnostic evaluation.

Obtain an ECG and blood specimen—sedimentation rate will be elevated.

Monitor vital signs.

Goal: reduce cardiovascular stress.

Support prescribed treatment. Administer antiarrhythmics.

Provide oxygen. Monitor blood gases. Observe for signs of carbon dioxide retention.

Support limbs.

Control stress.

Relieve pain and anxiety.

Goal: prevent and promptly identify complications.

Perform range-of-motion exercises. Ensure frequent change of position.

Monitor intake and output. Anuria can develop; straining due to constipation can produce strain on heart. Evaluate response to medications. Note adverse reactions, for example, bleeding, bradycardia, hypokalemia.

Observe for signs of congestive heart failure (eg, dyspnea, cough, rhonchi, rales).

Observe for signs of shock (eg, drop in blood pressure, increased pulse, cool moist skin, decreased urine output, restlessness).

---

should be advised to consult with their health care providers before using an alternative therapy.

Please consult with Chap. 23 for a more complete discussion of infections.

Discharge Planning

Hospitalized older adults require early and competent discharge planning to prevent complications, reduce the risk of rehospitalization, and minimize stress to themselves and their caregivers. Effective discharge planning is particularly significant in this era of ab-

breviated hospital stays that cause patients to leave the hospital in sicker, more debilitated states.

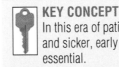

KEY CONCEPT
In this era of patients being discharged sooner and sicker, early discharge planning is essential.

Many factors can influence postdischarge outcomes of hospitalized elderly, such as:

- patients' perceptions of health status and prognosis
- number and complexity of medical conditions

DISPLAY 38-3

Factors Contributing to the High Risk for Infection in Older Adults

Age-related changes

- altered antigen–antibody response
- decreased respiratory activity
- reduced ability to expel secretions from lungs
- weaker bladder muscles facilitating urinary retention
- prostatic hypertrophy
- increased alkalinity of vaginal secretions

- increased fragility of skin and mucous membrane
  High prevalence of chronic disease
  Immobility
  Greater likelihood of malnutrition, urinary catheter use, invasive procedures, hospitalization, institutionalization

- prior history of self-care practices
- family or social support and resources

The patient's needs after discharge should be assessed and anticipated as early as possible so the individual and the caregivers can be adequately educated, referrals made, and home preparation done by the time the patient leaves the hospital. Some acute care settings use an interdisciplinary geriatric team that consults with staff and develops discharge plans. A gerontological nurse specialist in the acute care setting may also perform this activity.

The needs of the family or significant others who provide support and caregiving assistance should not be overlooked in the discharge planning efforts. The plan must be one that works for all parties involved, not just the patient, to be fully successful. (A more complete discussion of caregiving is provided in Chap. 40.)

Critical Thinking Exercises

1. A new gerontological nurse specialist on an inpatient surgical unit has been given the task of implementing nursing interventions to help reduce the elderly's risk of complications during their hospitalization. What protocols, staff development activities, and other actions could this nursing specialist consider?
2. Eighty-two-year-old Mrs. Hanks is brought to the emergency department by her daughter, with whom she lives. Mrs. Hanks had been ambulatory and able to perform all self-care activities until 6 days ago, when she became increasingly confused and weak; she has also lost weight and begun to experience urinary incontinence. She is diagnosed with bacterial pneumonia, and admission to the hospital is planned.
   Based on the information provided:
   What risks does Mrs. Hanks face during her hospitalization and what can be done to minimize them?
   What plans would you make to assist her daughter in caregiving activities after Mrs. Hanks' discharge?
3. Develop an outline of concepts you would review in teaching community-based elderly measures to prevent infection.
4. What prejudices or misinformed views could jeopardize the health and well-being of acutely ill older people?

Web Connect

Learn what the American Society of Laser Medicine and Surgery has to say about specialty laser surgery use by visiting its website at www.aslms.org/health/intro.html.

● References

Grossman, S., Bautista, C., & Sullivan, L. (2002).Using evidence-based practice to develop a protocol for postoperative surgical intensive care unit patients. *Dimensions of Critical Care Nursing, 21*(5), 206–214.

U.S. Census Bureau. (2002). Hospital discharges and days of care: 1995 and 2000. Washington, DC: *Statistical Abstract of the U.S. 2002.* Table No. 159.

● Recommended Readings

Alternative Update. (1995). Aromatherapy massage and cardiac surgery. *Nursing Times, 91*(43), 52.

Arras, J. D. (1995). *Bringing the hospital home: Ethical and social implications of high-tech home care.* Baltimore, MD: Johns Hopkins University Press.

Cook, L. (1999). The value of lab values. *American Journal of Nursing, 99*(5), 66–70.

Day, N., Musallam, K., & Wells, M. (1999). Observed behaviors of patients with probable Alzheimer's disease who are hospitalized for diagnostic tests. *Journal of Gerontological Nursing, 25*(11), 35–39.

Duthie, E. H., & Katz, P. R. (1998). *Practice of geriatrics* (3rd ed.). Philadelphia: Saunders.

Fick, D., & Foreman, M. (2000). Consequences of not recognizing delirium superimposed on dementia in hospitalized elderly individuals. *Journal of Gerontological Nursing, 26*(1), 30–39.

Fleming, A. W. (2001). Trauma in the elderly. *Clinical Geriatrics, 9*(3), 52–54.

Fulmer, T. T., Foreman, M. D., Walker, M., & Montgomery, K. S. (Eds.). (2001). *Critical care nursing of the elderly* (2nd ed.). New York: Springer Publishing.

Hamilton, L. (1995). A nursing-driven program to preserve and restore functional ability in hospitalized elderly patients. *Journal of Nursing Administration, 25*(4), 30–37.

Hazzard, W. R. (1999). *Principles of geriatric medicine and geriatrics* (4th ed.). New York: McGraw-Hill.

Horan, M. A., & Little, R. A. (1998). *Injury in the aging.* New York: Cambridge University Press.

Huckstadt, A. A. (2002). The experience of hospitalized elderly patients. *Journal of Gerontological Nursing, 28*(9), 24–29.

Jacelon, C. S. (1999). Preventing cascade iatrogenesis in hospitalized elders: An important role for nurses. *Journal of Gerontological Nursing, 25*(1), 27–33.

Kaufman, D. L. (1997). *Injuries and illness in the elderly.* St. Louis: Mosby.

Kelly, M. (1995). Surgery, anesthesia, and the geriatric patient. *Geriatric Nursing, 16*(5), 213–216.

Kresevic, D. M., & Mezey, M. (1997). Assessment of function: Critically important to acute care of elders. *Geriatric Nursing, 18*(5), 209–215.

McMahon, M. M. (2003). Emergency: ED triage. *American Journal of Nursing, 103*(3), 61–68.

Milisen, K., Foreman, M., Wouters, B., et al. (2002). Documentation of delirium in elderly patients with hip fracture. *Journal of Gerontological Nursing, 28*(11), 23–29.

Netting, F. E., & Williams, F. G. (1999). *Enhancing primary care of elderly people.* New York: Barland Publishers.

Rapp, C. G., Mentes, J. C., & Titler, M. G. (2001). Acute confusion/delirium protocol. *Journal of Gerontological Nursing, 25*(4), 21–33.

Robbins, L. M., & Courts, N. F. (1997). Care of the traumatized older adult. *Geriatric Nursing, 18*(5), 209–215.

Rogers, P. D., & Bocchino, N. L. (1999). Restraint-free care: Is it possible? *American Journal of Nursing, 99*(10), 26–34.

Schafer, S., & Sampsei, D. (1989). 33-day laceration stay. *Geriatric Nursing 10*(3), 124.

Siegler, E. L., Hyer, K., Fulmer, T., & Mezey, M. (1998). *Geriatric interdisciplinary team training.* New York: Springer.

Sullivan-Marx, E. M. (2001). Achieving restraint-free care of acutely confused older adults. *Journal of Gerontological Nursing, 27*(4), 56–61.

Szirony, T. A. (1999). Infection with HIV in the elderly population. *Journal of Gerontological Nursing, 25*(10), 25–31.

Williams, M. E. (1999). *The American Geriatrics Society's complete guide to aging and health* (pp. 63–67). New York: Harmony Books.

Yarnold, B. D. (1999). Hip fracture: Caring for a fragile population. *American Journal of Nursing, 99*(2), 36–41.

Young, D. M., & Mentes, J. C. (1999). Acute pain management protocol. *Journal of Gerontological Nursing, 25*(6), 10–21.

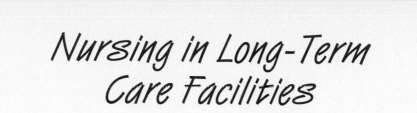

Nursing in Long-Term Care Facilities

■ Chapter Outline

Development of long-term institutional care
Before the 20th century
During the 20th century
Lessons to be learned from history
Facility residents
Facility standards
Nursing responsibilities
A new model of long-term care
Hierarchy of residents' needs
Hygiene
Holism
Healing
Assumptions of the new model

■ Learning Objectives

After reading this chapter, you should be able to:

- describe the development of long-term institutional care
- discuss the problems resulting from the lack of a unique model for long-term care
- identify major categories of standards described in regulations
- list various roles of nurses in long-term care facilities
- describe hygiene, holism, and healing needs of facility residents

The long-term care facility, which had been regarded as a low-status area for nursing practice, is emerging as a complex and dynamic clinical setting. Increasingly, such facilities are caring for a more medically complex population than ever before; many of these facilities are establishing subacute care units that provide ventilator care, hyperalimentation, and other services that were once confined to hospital settings. Consumers are more informed of the standards of good nursing home care and have higher expectations of providers than previously. Also, to many nurses who have become frustrated with the caregiving limitations of abbreviated hospital stays and fragmented care, such facilities offer an opportunity to establish long-term relationships and use nursing's healing arts.

Although the number of facilities providing long-term care has declined since the implementation of tougher standards, the number of residents who are served in long-term care facilities has grown along

TABLE 39-1 ● *Number of Nursing Facilities and Nursing Facility Residents*

Year	Nursing Facilities	Residents (in thousands)
1940	1,200	25
1960	9,582	290
1970	22,004	1,076
1980	30,111	1,396
1990	14,744	1,558
2002	16,886	1,795

Source: U.S. Census Bureau. (2002). Nursing homes: Selected characteristics, Table No. 168. Washington, DC: *Statistical Abstract of the U.S.*

with the growth of the older population (Table 39-1). Nearly one half of all older women and one third of all older men will spend some time in a long-term care facility during their lives (American Association of Homes and Services for the Aging, 2003).

Development of Long-Term Institutional Care

The many positive aspects of geriatric nursing in long-term care facilities are often overshadowed by an uncomplimentary image of this care setting, influenced by a history laden with scandals and the media's readiness to highlight the abuses and substandard conditions demonstrated by a small minority. This is compounded by reimbursement policies that significantly limit the ability to provide high-quality care. Reviewing the manner in which nursing home care developed helps one understand some of the reasons for the current challenges nurses face in working in this setting and avoiding similar problems in the future.

BEFORE THE 20TH CENTURY

Institutions to care for persons who were mentally ill, developmentally disabled, aged, orphaned, poor, or suffering from a contagious disease were common in most European countries by the end of the 17th century. Typically, all of these individuals were housed together, often with criminals and with limited funds

and low public interest in these populations, care was custodial at best.

In the United States, any type of inpatient care, acute or long-term, was scarce until the 19th century because it was expected that respectable people would be cared for at home, by private help or family. Philadelphia's Pennsylvania Hospital and the New York Hospital were the only hospitals in existence at the beginning of the 1800s.

The number of hospitals soon began to increase, but they discouraged long-term stays by poor persons with chronic conditions. The growing need for long-term institutional care was realized, and communities responded by developing almshouses, the primary source of institutional care in the 19th century. In small communities, the local almshouse placed all patients in a single building, sometimes segregating the very ill ones on separate wards so that they could receive some medical attention. The larger communities that had more people in need of institutional care were more likely to house people by category in separate wards; there were wards for "the destitute, the orphaned, the marginally criminal, and the permanently incapacitated . . . " (Rosenberg, 1987). During this period, a variety of terms were used to describe institutions that provided long-term care, including almshouse, hospital, asylum, home for the incurable, and chronic disease hospital. Typically, these facilities were located outside the main community to minimize the contact average citizens would have with these persons who were "different."

In this era, before the time of government reimbursement for long-term care, funding for these institutions came from limited public funds and charities. With limited resources, care was basic at best. Supplies were grossly inadequate, nurses tore up threadbare sheets to serve as bandages, some residents slept on the floor because of overcrowded conditions, and food was so inadequate that many residents developed recurrent cases of scurvy. Furthermore, theft, drunkenness, and sex between residents and their caregivers were common occurrences (Lawrence, 1905). Residents who were able were expected to work in the institution. Many recovered residents with no better option in the community remained in the institution and received room, board, and a very small salary in exchange for caring for residents, cooking, and cleaning. Physicians (who at that time usually were of society's elite) found these institutions unappealing and unstimulating, attitudes that most likely had a ripple effect on other caregiving professionals.

The promotion of a high quality of care, residents' rights, and rehabilitation were foreign concepts to these early long-term care facilities. The primary concern of the managers of these early institutions was running an efficient operation; this was done through the establishment of rules and routines that offered residents minimal autonomy and individuality of care. During this era, sociologist Erving Goffman offered a profile of these facilities, which he labeled "total institutions," when he described them as being characterized by the following (Goffman, 1961):

- all activities conducted in the same manner, in the same place
- all individuals treated in the same manner and required to comply with the same activities and schedules
- strict, inflexible schedule of activities
- numerous and heavily enforced rules
- activities that furthered the aims of the institution more than serving the needs of its residents

This approach to care, which viewed residents as inmates rather than as unique individuals in need of assistance, in combination with the isolation of residents from mainstream society, led to an erosion of their identities, development of maladaptive behaviors, apathy, inactivity, and stereotypical behaviors—in other words, institutionalized behaviors.

KEY CONCEPT
The many rules and routines that were implemented to keep the poorly funded early institutions operating efficiently resulted in residents developing abnormal behaviors.

DURING THE 20TH CENTURY

By the early 1900s, public and charitable institutions began to replace almshouses. Residents lived in institutions dedicated to their specific population, for example, orphanages, homes for the aged, mental hospitals, prisons, and chronic disease hospitals. However, funding was scarce, so care improved little. The public viewed long-term care institutions as a dreaded last resort.

It is significant to note that there was no careful assessment of the special needs of persons in need of long-term institutional care. There was no strategic planning and no thought given to the differences between facilities housing frail, dependent individuals for an extended period and other types of institutions. There was neither a model of long-term care nor a set of standards describing the unique care expectations for this special population. Instead, facilities providing long-term care modeled themselves after hospitals, prisons, and other institutions of the period. Patterning themselves after institutions that served very different populations for very different purposes was like trying to fit a square peg into a round hole; the absence of a clear model of long-term institutional care laid a weak foundation that affected the growth of this clinical setting.

KEY CONCEPT
Long-term care facilities were fashioned after prisons, hospitals, and other institutions rather than on a model based on the unique needs of the population served.

In 1935, the enactment of Social Security provided a means for many elders to seek alternatives to the public and charitable institutions that carried a highly negative public image. Older adults now had private funds to purchase services. In response, small facilities began to develop, offering room, board, and some personal care. Some of these facilities were operated by nurses or persons who called themselves nurses; thus the term "nursing home" became popularized. As the public's demand for nursing homes was realized, entrepreneurs and health and social service agencies became interested in constructing facilities. In 1946, the government contributed to nursing home growth by granting funds to help construct these facilities through the Hill-Burton Hospital Survey and Construction Act. As the name implies, the act's original intent was to assist in the construction of hospitals; therefore, the physical plant standards attached to the funding reflected characteristics desirable in an acute hospital setting. Indeed, despite the significant difference between hospitals and nursing homes, there were no separate standards for nursing homes. Consequently, nursing homes constructed during this time were replicas of hospitals and, unfortunately, hospitals provided the model for nursing home design for many years thereafter. Nursing homes modeled hospitals not only in their architectural features but also in their style of operation. White linens and uniforms, rigid schedules, passive residents, strict visitation policies, and restriction of pets were among the similarities.

The infusion of government funds through the Hill-Burton Act stimulated nursing home growth, but not nearly as much as the availability of reimbursement through Medicaid and Medicare. In the 1960s,the impact of the growing elder population was being realized. This population was beginning to exercise its political power by requesting increased and improved health care services. Hospitals were frustrated with the growing numbers of older patients filling their beds for extended periods of time who needed nursing home care but lacked the ability to privately pay for this service. Nursing homes were eager for government reimbursement. These pressures resulted in provisions for nursing home reimbursement through Medicare and Medicaid.

As a result of the enactment of Medicare and Medicaid, between 1960 and 1970 the number of nursing homes more than doubled and the number of residents served in this setting more than tripled (see Table 39-1). Unfortunately, instead of being owned and operated by clinicians like nurses who understood the unique needs of a geriatric population, most nursing home owners and operators were business-oriented individuals with minimal experience and understanding of nursing care. Federal standards (regulations) were very minimal, and monitoring and enforcement systems were lax. This situation led to deplorable conditions in some nursing homes. The media's investigation and exposure of these conditions led to a public outcry for stricter government regulation and a stigma that continues to cloud long-term care facilities.

> ✔ **Point to Ponder**
>
> *What perceptions of nursing homes have you heard family, friends, and other health care professionals express? How has this affected your thoughts about employment in this setting?*

The seriousness of nursing home conditions and resulting public outrage caused the Department of Health and Human Services to commission the Institute of Medicine (IOM) to study long-term care facilities and recommend changes. The IOM study reported widespread problems with the quality of care and recommended strengthening nursing home regulations (Institute of Medicine, 1986). In response, highly stringent nursing home regulations were developed under legislation known as the Omnibus Budget Reconciliation Act of 1987 (OBRA '87). OBRA required the following:

- use of a standardized assessment tool called the Minimum Data Set (MDS)
- timely development of a written care plan
- reduction in the use of restraints and psychotropic drugs
- increase in staffing
- protection of residents' rights
- training for nursing assistants

Furthermore, enforcement provisions were tougher; deficient nursing homes could receive sanctions that included termination of Medicare and Medicaid reimbursement. Interestingly, as regulations became more stringent, the number of nursing homes declined.

> 🔑 **KEY CONCEPT**
> OBRA '87 brought about the most profound changes in nursing home care that have ever been witnessed.

Conditions in nursing homes, now referred to as nursing facilities, have improved. Licensed staff must be on duty around the clock, nursing assistants must complete a certification process, the use of chemical and physical restraints has declined, and documentation has improved. However, problems do remain. Issues such as insufficient staffing and high staff turnover and conditions such as pressure ulcers, dehydration, and malnutrition continue to plague this care setting.

LESSONS TO BE LEARNED FROM HISTORY

There are lessons for gerontological nurses in this history.

A vision and a clear model are important founda-tions. The lack of a vision for long-term care and a clear model contributed to disorganization and confusion regarding the purpose, function, and standards for nursing homes. The facilities attempted to replicate the style of hospitals and other institutions rather than design systems and operations that were tailored to their unique population and services.

When nursing fails to exercise leadership, nonnurses will determine nursing practice. The essence of long-term care is *nursing care;* therefore, who bet-ter than nurses to define nursing facility care? Un-fortunately, nurses took a reactive, passive role and allowed persons with minimal understanding of caregiving to dictate nursing practice.

When nursing does not attempt to correct problems in the health care system, others will, and public per-ception will be that nurses are part of the problem. When conditions in long-term care facilities reached scandalous proportions, it was not the nursing community who was outraged and de-manded change, but the public. Nurses who worked in nursing homes witnessed and com-plained of substandard conditions but took no organized public action to effect change. Nurses who did not work in nursing homes often were critical of the conditions that caused them to stay away from this practice setting, yet they also did nothing to improve the situation. When they are not part of the solution, nurses create the perception that they are part of the problem.

Entrepreneurial thinking can benefit nursing and pa-tients. In the era of rapid nursing home growth, many entrepreneurs saw the opportunity to reap considerable financial gains by owning and op-erating long-term care facilities; many did be-come millionaires as a result. These business-people were not necessarily brighter, richer, or harder working than nurses, but they were more apt to see opportunities and take risks. By not being entrepreneurs and owning and operating nursing homes themselves, nurses not only missed the opportunity to benefit financially but also—and more importantly—were not in posi-tions of power from which they could influence the quality of care, staffing levels, salaries, and other critical aspects of nursing home care.

These lessons should have meaning for nurses and students today, as they observe financial professionals making decisions that determine clinical practice, work in settings in which staffing and services are be-low acceptable standards, and see new services and agencies develop in response to income potential rather than need.

> ✔ **Point to Ponder**
> *What would you do if you worked in a setting in which care was substandard?*

Facility Residents

People who seek long-term care are those who are func-tionally dependent on a long-term basis as a result of physical or mental impairment. It is the *level of func-tion,* therefore, not the medical diagnosis, that influ-ences the need for long-term care. Typically, residents of nursing facilities have dependencies in their ability to fulfill activities of daily living; most are incontinent and many are cognitively impaired. A majority of long-term care facilities' residents are older adults, with the average age being 85 years (National Center for Health Statistics, 2002). (Fifty-five percent of nursing facility residents are elders, 42% are adults under age 65, and 3% are children.) At any given time, only 5% of all eld-ers reside in a long-term care facility, although as men-tioned, a higher percentage will need nursing home care at some point in their lives (American Association of Homes and Services for the Aging, 2002).

For most of these residents, nursing home place-ment was not the first or most desirable choice. In many situations, family members tried to assist in caregiving but found that caregiving needs exceeded the family's capacities. By the time the decision to seek nursing fa-cility care is made, many families are physically, emo-tionally, and financially drained, adding to whatever guilt, depression, and frustration they feel about the sit-uation. Often, a crisis triggers the need for placement in a long-term care facility, placing families in the posi-tion of having to seek and decide on a facility under less than ideal circumstances. An important function of the gerontological nurse is to help residents and their fam-ilies as they face the challenges of selecting and adjust-ing to a nursing facility (Displays 39-1 and 39-2).

DISPLAY 39-1

Factors to Consider When Selecting a Nursing Facility

Cost

- daily rate
- type of health insurance accepted
- out-of-pocket costs necessary to supplement health insurance
- services covered and excluded in daily rate
- charge for services not covered in daily rate
- policy regarding care of resident when reimbursement limits are reached

Philosophy of Care

- custodial versus restorative/rehabilitative
- promotion of independence and individuality
- encouragement of residents and families to be active participants in care

Administration

- organizational structure
- ownership
- accessibility and availability of administrator, director of nursing, medical director, deparment heads
- existence of regularly scheduled meetings between administration and residents and families

Special Services

- availability of podiatry, speech therapy, occupational therapy, physical therapy, transportation, beauty/barber shop
- cost for special services
- conditions and arrangements for transfer to hospital

Staff

- number of caregivers available on typical shift
- ratio of RNs, LPNs, nursing assistants to residents
- number of supervisory staff on duty on typical shift
- frequency and type of inservice education offered to staff
- appearance, image portrayed by staff
- quality of staff–resident interactions
- courtesy, helpfulness of staff

Residents

- cleanliness, grooming, general appearance
- type of clothing worn (pajamas, street clothes, clean, wrinkled)
- activity level
- ease of interaction with staff and other residents

Physical Facility

- cleanliness, attractiveness, fresh-smelling
- ease of use for disabled and frail
- lighting
- noise control
- safe areas for walking
- general fire and safety precautions
- proximity of bathrooms, dining rooms, activity rooms, nursing stations, and exits to residents' rooms
- visibility of residents to staff
- outdoor areas for residents' use

Meals

- meal schedule
- type of food served
- attractiveness, temperature of food served
- availability of staff to assist residents at mealtime
- location where residents dine (eg, bedroom, communal dining hall)
- availability of dietitian or nutritionist for consultation
- range of special diets
- ability to have meal substitutions, ethnic preferences

Activities

- posted activity schedule
- range and frequency of activities
- ability of families and visitors to participate in activities with residents
- existence of resident council
- mechanisms for residents to have input into planning and evaluation of activities

(Continued)

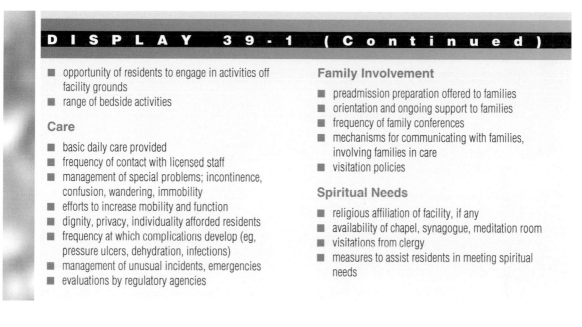

DISPLAY 39-1 (Continued)

- opportunity of residents to engage in activities off facility grounds
- range of bedside activities

Care

- basic daily care provided
- frequency of contact with licensed staff
- management of special problems; incontinence, confusion, wandering, immobility
- efforts to increase mobility and function
- dignity, privacy, individuality afforded residents
- frequency at which complications develop (eg, pressure ulcers, dehydration, infections)
- management of unusual incidents, emergencies
- evaluations by regulatory agencies

Family Involvement

- preadmission preparation offered to families
- orientation and ongoing support to families
- frequency of family conferences
- mechanisms for communicating with families, involving families in care
- visitation policies

Spiritual Needs

- religious affiliation of facility, if any
- availability of chapel, synagogue, meditation room
- visitations from clergy
- measures to assist residents in meeting spiritual needs

Facility Standards

Most long-term care facilities are concerned with complying with regulations. Regulations describe minimal standards that a long-term care facility must meet in order to comply with the law and qualify for reimbursement (Display 39-3). It must be emphasized that these standards are the *minimum* ones that must be fulfilled for facilities to comply with the law and be licensed and certified.

States can add to the basic federal regulations and create higher standards that facilities are obliged to meet. Also, the Joint Commission for the Accreditation of Healthcare Organizations offers higher standards that facilities can voluntarily choose to follow. It is crucial for nurses working in this setting to be familiar with the regulations pertaining to nursing facilities in their specific states.

Nursing Responsibilities

As mentioned earlier, OBRA '87 placed new demands on nursing facilities for competent resident assessment, care planning, quality assurance, and protection of residents' rights. The increased demands and com-

plexities of long-term care facilities necessitate that highly competent nurses be employed in this setting.

Unlicensed nursing personnel currently deliver most care in the nursing facility setting. This imposes greater demands on licensed staff; not only must nurses oversee the status of residents, but they also must monitor the competency and performance of unlicensed caregivers. Staff education, role modeling, good supervision, coaching, performance evaluation, and correction of performance problems become responsibilities of most long-term care nurses that are superimposed on their major clinical and administrative duties.

Gerontological nurses have increasing opportunities for role variety in the nursing facility. They can fill administrative and management roles as director of nursing, supervisor, unit nurse coordinator, or charge nurse. They can fill specialized roles, such as staff development director, quality assurance coordinator, infection control coordinator, geropsychiatric nurse specialist, or rehabilitative nurse. Of course, nurses can also be direct care providers to residents.

Nurses influence the quality of care provided to residents in a variety of ways. Admission assessments and the completion of the MDS assessment tool are coordinated by a registered nurse, and most of the entries on the MDS rely on nursing assessment. Problems identified on the MDS trigger care planning

DISPLAY 39·2

Measures to Help Families With Nursing Facility Admission of a Relative

Prior to Admission

- Encourage the family to visit the facility and allocate a block of uninterrupted time to spend with them. Review basic information about the facility and its routines without overloading. Introduce the family to the director of nursing, medical director, administrator and other key personnel.

- Ask for information about the resident that will enable staff to understand the resident's unique history, needs, and preferences. Demonstrate an interest in the resident as an individual.

- Accompany the family to a private area and offer them an opportunity to express their concerns and feelings. Communicate to them that it is normal for families to feel guilty, angry, and depressed at having a loved one enter a long-term care facility; assure them that these feelings will improve in time. Advise them that it is not unusual for the resident initially to be angry at them, beg to go home, or reject them; assure them that as the resident adjusts to the facility, these reactions usually diminish.

- Describe the rights and responsibilities of families within the facility.

- Provide written description of facts communicated verbally.

At Admission

- Attempt to have a staff member who has met the family prior to admission meet the family and accompany them through the admission process.

- Inform family members of the location of cafeteria, vending machines, and rest rooms. If possible, order a snack or lunch tray for family members so that they may share the resident's first meal time in the facility.

- Arrange for staff who will be caring for the resident to introduce themselves to the family. It is beneficial for staff to write their names on a paper that the family can consult for future reference.

- Introduce the family to another resident's family member, and encourage them to develop a "buddy

system." Often families can provide significant support to each other and make visitations more pleasurable.

- Advise the family of the anticipated sequence of events for the resident (eg, the resident will be examined by the physician this afternoon, attend a group activity this evening, visit physical therapy tomorrow morning). Inform the family of the dates and times for care planning conferences and other events in which they are invited to participate.

- Encourage the family to go home at a reasonable time. Reinforce to them that the admission process is tiring to both them and the resident and that both could benefit from some rest. Express understanding that they and the resident may have many uncomfortable feelings at this time, but that these feelings normally improve with time.

During Visitations

- Encourage the family to be actively involved in care planning and care activities. Instruct family members on care activities that they can perform, such as feeding, back rubs, range-of-motion exercises, and grooming.

- Suggest activities that the family can share with the resident during visits (eg, card games, bringing in a pet, compiling a photo album, reading, puzzles, decorating a bulletin board). If possible, take the resident to an activity room or outdoors for the visit, and encourage the family to take the resident off the premises for short periods.

- Encourage touch between the family and the resident.

- Offer and respect privacy during visits.

In General

- Be courteous and patient. Remember that having a relative in a health care facility is difficult and can cause various reactions that can be displaced to staff.

- Call the family when there is a change in status or an incident involving the resident.

- Listen to and investigate complaints. Encourage families to discuss problems and concerns with unit-level staff.

- Invite the family's participation in care planning and delivery to the fullest extent possible.

(Eliopoulos, C. [1990]. Understanding and supporting families. *Long-Term Care Educator, 1*[5], 6.)

D I S P L A Y   3 9 - 3

Regulations Related to Nursing Facilities

- Resident rights
- Admission, transfer, and discharge rights
- Resident behavior and facility practices
- Quality of life
- Nursing services
- Dietary services
- Physician services

- Specialized rehabilitation services
- Dental services
- Pharmacy services
- Infection control
- Physical environment
- Administration

activity. (**Visit the Connection website to access the current MDS.**) The written care plan guides nursing actions; staff are held accountable by regulatory agencies for ensuring that care plans are accurate and followed. Nurses ensure that nursing assistants provide care appropriately and monitor residents to evaluate the effectiveness of care and to recognize changes in status. Display 39-4 lists some of the major responsibilities of nurses in this setting.

KEY CONCEPT
The Minimum Data Set (MDS) is a standardized assessment tool that must be completed on admission, whenever there is a change in the resident's status, and annually.

Unlike many other clinical settings, the average long-term care facility does not have physicians and other professionals on site at all times. Although this places a greater burden on nurses for assessment and management of problems, it does offer the opportunity for nurses to function independently and use a wide range of knowledge and skills. Independent nursing practice and the ability to develop long-term relationships with residents and their families are among the exciting features of nursing in this setting.

A New Model of Long-Term Care

As this chapter's discussion about the development of long-term care reflected, nursing facilities emerged without a clearly defined model. Rather than a tapestry

D I S P L A Y   3 9 - 4

Major Responsibilities of Gerontological Nurses in Long-Term Care Facilities

Assist residents and their families in the selection of and adjustment to the facility.

Assess and develop an individualized care plan based on assessment data.

Monitor residents' health status.

Recommend and use rehabilitative and restorative care techniques when possible.

Evaluate the effectiveness and appropriateness of care.

Identify changes in residents' conditions and take appropriate action.

Communicate and coordinate care with the interdisciplinary team.

Protect and advocate for residents' rights.

Promote a high quality of life for residents.

Ensure and promote the competency of nursing staff.

of a wide range of therapeutic interventions that enable persons relying on others for long-term assistance to achieve optimum physical, psychosocial, and spiritual health and well-being, nursing facilities are more like a patchwork quilt of poorly fitted fragments of traditional medical care loosely held together by weak threads of regulations and institutional rules.

Because most resident needs and care activities in long-term care facilities fall within the realm of nursing, nurses are the logical professionals to define the model of long-term care. Recognizing the limitations of the medical model in long-term care facilities, the themes of the new model could be holism and healing. Figure 39-1 offers a hierarchy of residents' needs that can help nurses and nurses-to-be envision this new model and challenge them to consider a design for long-term care services that exceeds the minimum requirements. The levels of needs shown are the following:

Hygiene. The most basic needs include physiologic needs, assurance of safety of the human and physical environment, treatment of medical conditions, and restoration and/or stabilization of physical and mental health. Basic survival depends on the fulfillment of these needs; however, having these needs met does not ensure a satisfying, fulfilling life.

Holism. At this level, psychological, social, and spiritual aspects are considered. To attain harmony and balance among mind, body, and spirit, individuals need to exercise individual rights, assume responsibility for self-care to the fullest extent possible, prevent avoidable declines and dysfunction, and experience a dynamic relationship with the community inside and outside the facility.

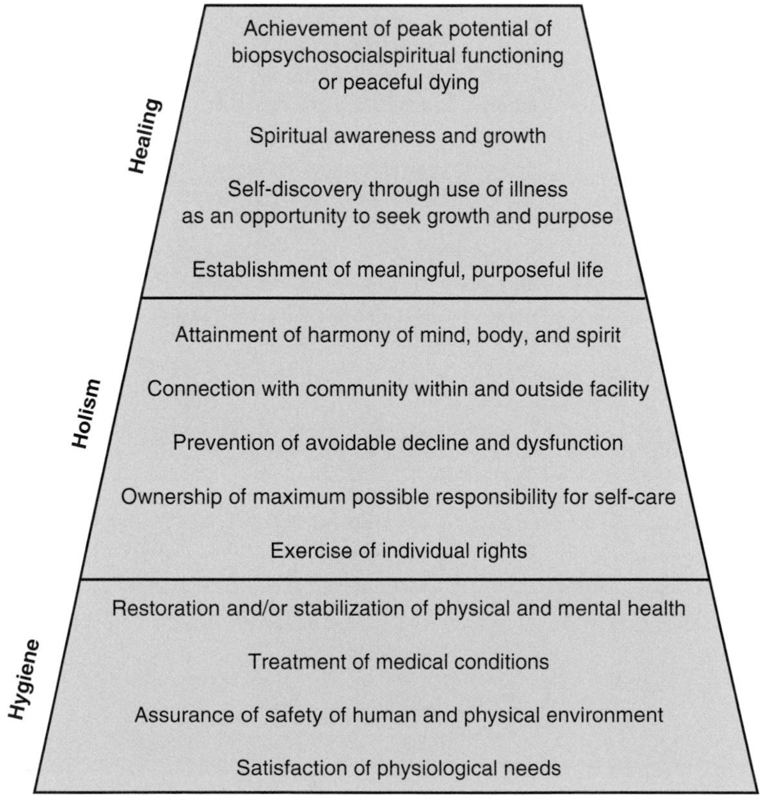

Healing
- Achievement of peak potential of biopsychosocialspiritual functioning or peaceful dying
- Spiritual awareness and growth
- Self-discovery through use of illness as an opportunity to seek growth and purpose
- Establishment of meaningful, purposeful life

Holism
- Attainment of harmony of mind, body, and spirit
- Connection with community within and outside facility
- Prevention of avoidable decline and dysfunction
- Ownership of maximum possible responsibility for self-care
- Exercise of individual rights

Hygiene
- Restoration and/or stabilization of physical and mental health
- Treatment of medical conditions
- Assurance of safety of human and physical environment
- Satisfaction of physiological needs

FIGURE 39-1

Hierarchy of nursing facility residents' needs. (Eliopoulos, C. [1998]. *Transforming nursing homes into healing centers: A holistic model for long-term care.* Glen Arm, MD: Health Education Network.)

Healing. The fulfillment of hygiene and holism needs provides the foundation for healing to occur. Healing does not imply cure but, rather, establishing a meaningful and purposeful life, using illness as an opportunity for self-discovery, deepening spiritual awareness and growth, and transcending the physical being.

Woven within this model of holism and healing are the following assumptions (Eliopoulos, 1998):

- Psychological, social, and spiritual well-being are of equal and sometimes greater importance than physical well-being.
- Medical supervision and treatment are only one component of the overall needs of residents.
- Many of the needs resulting from chronic conditions can be effectively and safely met with the use of alternative and complementary therapies.

- Caregivers' presence and interactions affect health, healing, and the quality of nursing facility life.
- The physical environment can be used as a therapeutic tool.
- The nursing facility is an integral and active member of the community at large.

Gerontological nurses must reclaim nursing's healing role and cast a new vision for long-term care that can enable residents of nursing facilities to experience the highest possible quality of life for the remaining time in their lives.

> ✔ **Point to Ponder**
>
> *If you could design a long-term care facility that promoted holism and healing, what would it look like?*

Critical Thinking Exercises

1. Consider the expectations baby boomers will have when they use long-term care facilities in the future and outline the environmental features, services, and operations that will accommodate them.
2. Imagine that you are a director of nursing in a long-term care facility and describe:
   - activities that could be planned to encourage the local community to become involved in facility activities
   - services the facility could offer persons living in the neighboring community
   - programs and services that could be provided for families of residents
3. Describe actions nurses can take to improve long-term care facilities.

Web Connect

The National Association of Directors of Nursing in Long-Term Care (NADONA/LTC) publishes a journal, provides legislative representation, grants scholarships, and offers other benefits to promote long-term care nursing; learn more by visiting its website at www.NADONA.org.

● **Resources**

American Association of Homes and Services for the Aging
2519 Connecticut Avenue, NW
Washington, DC 20008
(202) 783-2242
www.aasha.org

American Health Care Association
1201 L Street, NW
Washington, DC 20005
(202) 833-2050
www.ahca.org

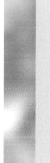

American Nurses Association, Inc.
Council on Nursing Home Nurses
600 Maryland Avenue, SW
Suite 100 West
Washington, DC 20024
(800) 274-4262
www.nursingworld.org

National Association of Directors of Nursing Administration in Long-Term Care
10999 Reed Hartman Highway
Suite 234
Cincinnati, OH 45242
(800) 222-0539
www.NADONA.org

National Citizens Coalition for Nursing Home Reform
1424 16th Street, NW
Washington, DC 20036
(202) 339-2275
www.nccnhr.org

National Gerontological Nursing Association
7250 Parkway Drive
Suite 510
Hanover, MD 21076
(800) 723-0560
www.nursingcenter.com/people/nrsorgs/ngna

● References

American Association of Homes and Services for the Aging. (2003). *Nursing Home Statistics.* Retrieved August 25, 2003, from www.aahsa.org/public/backgrd1.htm.

Eliopoulos, C. (1998). *Transforming nursing homes into healing centers: A holistic model for long-term care.* Glen Arm, MD: Health Education Network.

Goffman, E. (1961). *Asylums.* Garden City, NY: Anchor Books.

Institute of Medicine, Committee on Implications of For-Profit Enterprise in Health Care. (1986). Profits and health care: An introduction to the issues. In B.H. Gray (Ed.). *For-profit enterprise in health care* (pp. 3–18). Washington, DC: National Academy Press.

Lawrence, C. (1905). *History of the Philadelphia almshouses and hospitals.* Privately printed.

National Center for Health Statistics. (2002). Nursing home residents 65 years of age and over according to functional status and age, sex, and race. Retrieved June 20, 2003, from www.cdc.gov/nchs/data/hus/tables/2002/02hus111pdf.

Rosenberg, C. E. (1987). *The care of strangers: The rise of America's hospital system.* New York: Basic Books.

● Recommended Readings

Barba, B. E. (2002). Nursing home environments. *Journal of Gerontological Nursing, 28*(3), 5–6.

Barba, B. E., Tesh, A. S., & Courts, N. F. (2002). Promoting thriving in nursing homes: The Eden Alternative. *Journal of Gerontological Nursing, 28*(3), 7–13.

Buettner, L. L. Therapeutic recreation in the nursing home: Reinventing a good thing. *Journal of Gerontological Nursing, 27*(5), 8–13.

Coleman, M., Looney, S., O'Brien, J., et al. (2002). The Eden Alternative: Findings after one year of implementation. *Journal of Gerontology Medical Sciences, 57A*(7), M422–M427.

Davidson, K. M. (2003). Evidence-based protocol: Family bereavement support before and after the death of a nursing home resident. *Journal of Gerontological Nursing, 29*(1), 10–18.

Donovan, C., & Dupuis, M. (2000). Specialized care unit: Family and staff's perceptions of significant elements. *Geriatric Nursing, 21*(1), 30–33.

Eliopoulos, C. (1999). *Integrating alternative and conventional therapies: Holistic care for chronic conditions.* St. Louis: Mosby.

Eliopoulos, C. (2003). *Nursing administration of long-term care facilities* (6th ed.). Glen Arm, MD: Health Education Network.

Eliopoulos, C., & Seiler, K. (2003). *Staff development handbook for long-term care facilities* (6th ed.). Glen Arm, MD: Health Education Network.

Forbes, S. (2001). This is heaven's waiting room? End of life in one nursing home. *Journal of Gerontological Nursing, 27*(11), 37–45.

Gladstone, J., & Wexler, E. (2000). A family perspective of family/staff interaction in long-term care facilities. *Geriatric Nursing, 21*(1), 16–19.

Guse, L., Inglis, J., Chicoine, J., Leche, G., Stadnyk, L., & Whitbread, L. (2000). Life albums in long-term care: Residents, family, and staff perceptions. *Geriatric Nursing, 21*(1), 34–37.

Hagen, B. (2001). Nursing home placement: Factors affecting caregivers' decisions to place family members with dementia. *Journal of Gerontological Nursing, 27*(2), 44–53.

Henderson, M. L., Hanson, L. C., & Kimberly, S. R. (2003). *Improving nursing home care of the dying. A training manual for nursing home staff.* New York: Springer Publishing Company.

Horgas, A. L., & Dunn, K. (2001). Pain in nursing home residents: Comparison of residents' self-report and nursing assistants' perceptions. *Journal of Gerontological Nursing, 27*(3), 44–53.

Iwasiw, C., Goldenberg, D., Bol, N., & MacMaster, E. (2003). Resident and family perspectives: The first year in a long-term care facility. *Journal of Gerontological Nursing, 29*(1), 45–54.

Lindgren, C. L., & Murphy, A. M. (2002). Nurses' and family members' perceptions of nursing home residents' needs. *Journal of Gerontological Nursing, 28*(8), 45–53.

Logue, R. M. (2003). Maintaining family connectedness in long-term care: An advanced practice approach to family-centered nursing homes. *Journal of Gerontological Nursing, 29*(6), 24–31.

MacLean, D., & MacIntosh, R. (1998). Health and disease in organizations. *Journal of Alternative and Complementary Medicine, 4,* 185–188.

McGilton, K. S. (2002). Enhancing relationships between care providers and residents in long-term care: Designing a model of care. *Journal of Gerontological Nursing, 28*(12), 13–21.

Muder, R. R., Brennen, C., & Swenson, D. L. (1996). Pneumonia in the long-term care facility. *Archives of Internal Medicine, 156,* 2365–2370.

Mullins, L. C., & Hartley, T. M. (2002). Residents' autonomy: Nursing home personnel's perceptions. *Journal of Gerontological Nursing, 28*(2), 35–44.

National Committee to Preserve Social Security and Medicare. (April 1997). Nurse staffing in nursing homes: Viewpoint. *Legislative Agenda for the 105th Congress.*

Pattillo, M. (2002). Assessing the gifts, talents, and skills of nursing home residents. *Geriatric Nursing, 23*(1), 48–50.

Pearson, A., Fitzgerald, M., & Nay, R. (2003). Mealtimes in nursing homes: The role of nursing staff. *Journal of Gerontological Nursing, 29*(6), 40–47.

Rice, V. H. (1997). Ethical issues relative to autonomy and personal control in independent and cognitively impaired elders. *Nursing Outlook, 45,* 27–34.

Shearer, N. B. C. (2002). Loss of power within the nursing home. *Journal of Gerontological Nursing, 28*(11), 54–56.

Thomas, W. H. (1996). *Life worth living: How someone you love can still enjoy life in a nursing home. The Eden Alternative in action.* Acton, MA: VanderWyk & Burham.

Yaffe, K., Fox, P., Newcomer, R., Sands, L., Lindquist, et al. (2002). Patient and caregiver characteristics and nursing home placement in patients with dementia. *Journal of the American Medical Association, 287*(16), 2090–2097.

Yeaworth, R. C. (2002). Long-term care and insurance. *Journal of Gerontological Nursing, 28*(11), 45–51.

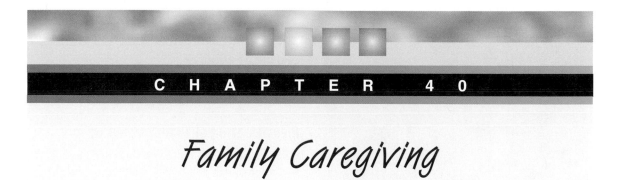

CHAPTER 40

Family Caregiving

■ Learning Objectives

After reading this chapter, you should be able to:

- list the various structures and functions of families

- discuss various roles that family members can assume

- describe classic family relationships

- identify risks to caregivers and ways to reduce them

- identify signs of elder abuse

- discuss interventions to reduce family dysfunction

Aging is a family affair. Whether it is the retiree's concern about living and supporting his family on a pension, a middle-aged daughter's decision to accept her mother into her household, or a sister's attempt to care for her dying brother at home, the impact of one individual's aging process has a ripple effect on the entire family unit (Fig. 40-1). This impact is also felt when older members of the family require assistance with daily needs and care. Families are absorbing more complex responsibilities for caregiving for longer periods of time than ever before, and with growing numbers of people reaching the old-old years and the trend toward maintaining very ill older individuals in the home setting, the burdens faced by family caregivers will grow. Nurses need to understand the various structures, roles, and relationships that exist among families so that they can be effective when working with the older adults and their caregivers.

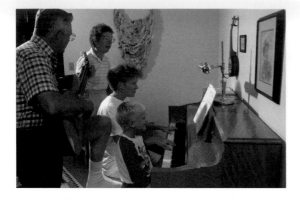

FIGURE 40-1

Aging is a family affair.

KEY CONCEPT

Greater numbers of families are providing more complex care for their older members for longer periods of time than ever before.

Various Family Compositions

Almost every individual is part of a family unit, although that family may not reflect the stereotypical nuclear family. In fact, one may find among the elderly a diversity of family structures, including:

- couples (married, unmarried, heterosexual, homosexual)
- couples with children (heterosexual, homosexual, married, unmarried)
- parent and child or children
- siblings
- groups of unrelated individuals
- multigenerations

When interviewing older adults, it is important to explore all persons who are "significant others" to an individual and fulfill a family role, regardless of whether they are unrelated or reside in different households. For example, a widow can have a friend with whom she shares a close emotional tie or a cousin in a neighboring community who provides assistance and support.

KEY CONCEPT

Caregivers can be significant others, not just family.

IDENTIFICATION OF FAMILY MEMBERS

One can identify family members by looking for those individuals who fulfill family functions. In aging families, family functions are somewhat modified to address the special needs of the elderly and focus on the following:

- ensuring fulfillment of physical needs
- providing emotional support and comfort
- maintaining connections with family and community
- instilling a sense of meaning to life
- managing crises

Asking older adults the following questions can also facilitate the identification of significant persons who perform family functions for them.

- Who checks on them regularly?
- Who shops with or for them?
- Who escorts them to the clinic or physician?
- Who assists with or manages their problems?
- Who takes care of them when they are ill?
- Who helps them make decisions?
- Who do they seek for emotional support?

All persons fulfilling significant family functions should be included in the care plan of older adults.

Family Roles

Frequently, family members assume certain roles as a result of their socialization process and family needs and expectations. Possible roles include the following:

Decision-maker: the person who is granted or assumes responsibility for making important decisions or is called on in times of crisis; may not be geographically close or involved in daily activities but consulted for problem solving

Caregiver: the person who provides direct services, looks after, or assists with personal care and home management of another member

Deviant: the "problem child" who has strayed from family norms; may be used to fulfill family need for scapegoat or provide sense of purpose for family members who "rescue" or compensate for this individual

Dependent: an individual who depends on the other members of the family for economic or caregiving assistance

Victim: a person who forfeits his or her legitimate rights and may be physically, emotionally, socially, or economically abused by the family

> ✔ **Point to Ponder**
> *What are the dynamics within your own extended family? What different roles and functions do various members fulfill?*

The impact of these roles should be explored when assessing the family unit. Nurses must be sensitive to the fact that certain "negative" roles may not have the adverse effects on the family unit that would be anticipated; likewise, "positive" roles may not be welcomed by the family. For example, the middle-aged son who drifts from town to town, regularly contacting his elderly parents for funds to pay off his latest indulgences, may not be representative of a responsible, mature adult, but he may bring excitement and a sense of being needed to his parents' lives, thereby bringing them some rewards. On the other hand, his financially secure, responsible brother who takes care of his parents' affairs may be less liked because of his dullness and practicality.

> 🔑 **KEY CONCEPT**
> Even seemingly negative roles can be fostered by and meet certain needs of the family.

Family Dynamics

The dynamics among family members can have positive or negative effects on the elderly. In assessing the family unit it is useful to explore the following issues:

How family members feel about each other. Do they love but not like, admire, respect, or enjoy each other? How do they express affection?

The manner of communication. Do they share daily events or have contact only on holidays? Is their style of interaction parent-child or adult-adult?

Their attitudes, values, and beliefs. Do they feel that the young should take care of the old or that children owe their parents nothing? What are their expectations of family members, friends, and society?

Links with organizations and the community. How involved are they with persons external to the family unit? Is the family similar to others in the community?

As discussed in Chap. 1, the majority of older people are not abandoned by their children; most do enjoy regular contact with them. Nevertheless, lifestyles, housing, and societal expectations are not conducive to healthy parents and their adult children living together. Most elderly people want to live in their own residences, if possible, and the majority do. The arrangement of generations living under separate roofs but within a 30-minute trip of each other is generally the most satisfactory. It is understood that parents and children will provide assistance and share a household if an unusual circumstance arises.

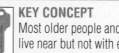

> 🔑 **KEY CONCEPT**
> Most older people and their families prefer to live near but not with each other.

More than 9 of 10 elders are grandparents. Grandparenting can be a positive experience for older adults because they obtain enjoyment, affection, and a sense of purpose from caring for their grandchildren without the 24-hour stress of child-rearing responsibilities. Grandchildren can provide new interests and meaning to life. In turn, grandchildren usually receive the benefit of unconditional love and attention. As grandchildren grow into adulthood, their involvement with grandparents often lessens, but a strong bond continues to exist.

Next to that between parent and child, the relationship between siblings is stronger than any other relationship. The typical pattern is for siblings to drift apart during young and middle adulthood but then reestablish strong ties in later life. Siblings can provide socialization, emotional support, and financial and household assistance. Usually, earlier conflicts and differences become insignificant as siblings develop mutually supportive relationships in later life.

Elderly couples have a low rate of divorce, although it is increasing. Rocky marriages often stabilize in later life as the couple faces a new interdependency. Elderly spouses look to each other for security, support, and safety in an imperfect world. After years of experiencing and reinforcing one another's behaviors, the couple can understand, anticipate, and complement one another's actions. Spouses look after the care and welfare of their mates and derive security in having someone available to care about them.

Relationships in old age are affected by the forms of relationships experienced throughout life. Parents who ignored or abused their children early in life may produce children who want nothing to do with them in adulthood. Siblings who have unresolved anger over favoritism displayed by their parents may express their feelings by refusing to assist when the favored child is in need. Couples who never shared intimacy and friendship may exist in separate worlds under the same roof. Nurturing relationships during every stage of life are an investment in having meaningful, supportive relationships in later life.

> **KEY CONCEPT**
> Children who feel their parents were insensitive to their needs throughout their lives may be reluctant caregivers to these parents in old age.

Scope of Family Caregiving

Most of the home care of older persons is provided by family members, not formal agencies. It is estimated that more than 10 million people are involved in parent care, approximately half of whom provide care on a regular basis. More than half of the elderly's caregivers are wives; the next largest group of caregivers is daughters and daughters-in-law. Indeed, today the average woman will spend more time providing care

for her parents than for her children; often, responsibilities for care of their parents and children are faced by these women concurrently, causing them to be named the "sandwich generation." One in 60 full-time workers are caregivers, and 1 in 12 are potential caregivers.

> **KEY CONCEPT**
> Most of the home care of elders is provided by family members, not formal agencies.

Families provide many types of assistance to their older members (Display 40-1). Often, the provision of assistance is a subtle, gradual process. For example, a daughter may begin by telephoning her mother after the mother has returned from a physician's visit and inquiring about medication changes. As time progresses, the daughter may accompany her mother to the physician's office, discuss the medications directly with the physician, and telephone her mother to monitor the response to the drugs. Eventually, the daughter may need to lift her mother in and out of the car, push her into the physician's office in a wheelchair, undress her for the examination, and administer the medications to her on a regular basis.

> ✔ **Point to Ponder**
> *If you suddenly faced the situation of having to provide care to a parent or older relative, how would your life change and how would you manage the added responsibilities?*

Protecting the Health of Patient and Caregiver

A family is a strong chain of human experience that bonds its members through life's challenges and joys; however, that chain is only as strong as its weakest link. Effective gerontological nursing recognizes that the health of all family members must be maintained and promoted.

Maintaining older persons' independence facilitates normality in family relationships. Having to live with or be cared for by family members can threaten

DISPLAY 40-1

Types of Assistance Families Provide to Their Older Members

Maintaining and cleaning the home	Cooking and providing meals
Managing finances	Reminding to take medications, keep appointments,
Shopping	and take actions
Transporting	Monitoring and administering medications
Providing opportunities for socialization	Performing treatments
Advising	Supervising
Explaining	Protecting
Troubleshooting	Bathing and dressing
Reassuring	Feeding
Accompanying to physician's office and hospital	Toileting
Negotiating services	

the status and roles of older persons and cause anger, resentment, and other feelings to develop (see Nursing Diagnosis Highlight). Sound health practices to prevent disease and disability are crucial to maintaining self-care ability and independence. If illness occurs, aggressive attention should be paid to avoiding complications and restoring the affected person to a healthy state. Interventions such as environmental modifications, financial aid, home-delivered meals, assistance with chores, transportation for the handicapped, telephone reassurance, or a home companion can supplement deficits and strengthen the elderly's reserves for independent living.

KEY CONCEPT
Caregivers of older persons frequently are senior citizens themselves.

If the caregiver is a spouse or sibling, chances are that he or she is an elderly person as well. Even the children of the elderly person can be aged themselves. The physical, emotional, and social health of the caregivers must be evaluated periodically to ensure that they are competent to provide the required services and are not jeopardizing themselves in the process.

Provisions must be made for what gerontological nurses refer to as their TLC:

T—training in care techniques, safe medication use, recognition of abnormalities, and available resources

L—leaving the care situation periodically to obtain respite and relaxation and maintain their normal living needs

C—caring for themselves via adequate sleep, rest, exercise, nutrition, socialization, solitude, support, financial aid, stress reduction, and health management

Gerontological nurses should review the TLC needs of caregivers during every contact to ensure their continued effectiveness.

KEY CONCEPT
Caregivers need TLC: training, leave, and care for self.

A particularly vulnerable group of caregivers is middle-aged daughters who are a likely caregiver group. After years of sacrificing and struggling with childrearing, they are beginning to taste some freedom

NURSING DIAGNOSIS HIGHLIGHT

ALTERED FAMILY PROCESSES

Overview

An alteration in family processes exists when the family's normal functions are altered. When this problem is present, the family may be unable to meet the physical, emotional, socioeconomic, or spiritual needs of its members, may deal with stress ineffectively, may communicate ineffectively or inappropriately, and may refuse to seek or accept help from others. They may be fearful, guarded, or suspicious when visited or interviewed.

Causative or Contributing Factors

Illness or injury of family member, change in dependency level of member, change in role or function of family member, addition or loss of family member, relocation, reduced income, added expenses, social or sexual deviance by family member, break in religious or cultural practices by family members

Goal

The family will demonstrate support and assistance to members in their fulfillment of physical, emotional, and socioeconomic needs; the family will seek and accept assistance from external sources as appropriate.

Interventions

- Collect a comprehensive family history that includes profile of family (include significant oth-

ers who fill family functions as family members); age, health, and residence of members; roles and responsibilities of each member; typical patterns of communication, problem-solving, and crisis management; recent changes in composition of the family and members' roles, responsibilities, and health statuses; new burdens; and the family's assessment of problem.
- Identify factors related to family dysfunction and plan appropriate interventions such as family therapy, financial aid, family conference, visiting nurse, or clergy visit.
- Facilitate open, honest communication among family members; assist in planning family conferences, promoting discussion by all members, developing realistic goals and plans, and allocating responsibility; provide privacy for family.
- When a member is receiving health services, explain care activities and expected outcomes, prepare for changes, and involve the family in care to the maximum extent possible.
- Provide caregiver education and support; help caregivers identify community resources; and emphasize the importance of respite for caregivers.
- Make the family aware of support and self-help groups that can assist them, such as Alzheimer's Disease and Related Disorders Association, American Cancer Society, Alcoholics Anonymous, and American Diabetes Association.

as their children gain independence and begin to leave home. They are concerned for their children's success and well-being and experience ambivalence over the less intense parental role. Ever-increasing numbers of them are in the workforce, perhaps resuming delayed careers. Some may be coping with spouses who are experiencing midlife crises, having mixed feelings about their marriage, or reacting to undesirable changes in their physical appearance. They are clouded with the

"superwoman" myth and desperately try to be the supportive parent, understanding wife, exciting lover, interesting friend, and aspiring employee. In short, they are overwhelmed. At this point in life, the final straw may be dependent parents and their demands. These daughters feel that they certainly cannot deprive their parents, trust their care to strangers, or institutionalize them. However, what will this mean to their careers, income, marital relationships, friendships, leisure pursuits, and energy? As a growing number of middle-aged women confront this dilemma, special nursing intervention is warranted. Display 40-2 describes some ways in which nurses can aid family caregivers.

Family Dysfunction

Many factors can threaten the healthy functioning of the family unit; the gerontological nurse must be skilled in identifying such problems and providing interventions for them (see the Nursing Diagnosis Highlight). Family dysfunction occurs in many forms, ranging from an older parent's domination and manipulation of an adult child, to incestuous relationships. A lifelong history of dysfunction may exist, or the dysfunction may be a recent problem, associated with a wide range of factors (eg, divorce, loss of income, increased dependency of elder, illness of caregiver). Families experiencing dysfunction may be:

- less able to fulfill the physical, emotional, socioeconomic, and spiritual needs of their members
- rigid in roles, responsibilities, and opinions
- unable or unwilling to obtain and use help from others
- composed of members with psychopathology or behavioral disorders
- inexperienced or ineffective at managing crises
- ineffective or inappropriate with their communication and behavior (including learned violence patterns)

ELDER ABUSE

One form of dysfunction that has gained increased visibility in recent years is elder abuse. It is estimated as many as 1.2 million older adults are abused annually in the United States, primarily by a close family member (Fulmer, 2003). The profile of the older adult at greatest risk for abuse is a disabled woman, older than 75

DISPLAY 40-2

Nursing Strategies to Assist Family Caregivers

Guide the family to view the situation realistically. Perhaps a leave of absence rather than resignation from a job is warranted to assist a parent or spouse through convalescence. Perhaps the needs are such that a lay caregiver (eg., family member) will not be able to care for them adequately. Often an objective outsider can guide the family in viewing the real situation and understanding the extent of care needs.

Provide information that can assist in anticipating needs. Caregivers need to be guided in exploring the various scenarios that can arise and developing plans before a crisis occurs. Encourage the expression of feelings. Raised with an abundance of "shoulds" and "oughts" regarding the treatment of older persons, families need to know that the guilt, anger, resentment, and depression they feel are neither uncommon nor bad.

Assess and monitor the impact of the caregiving on the total family unit. Although caregivers may feel they alone are assuming responsibility for care, they need to examine the effects on the total family unit. How will their children's tuition be paid if they quit their jobs to care for a parent? Will someone have to forfeit a bedroom if the relative moves in? What is the relationship of the spouse with the in-laws? Who will help lift grandma into the tub? Will the family be able to take vacations and entertain at home? Is someone available to relieve them if they want to go out for a special occasion?

Introduce and promote a review of care options. Often family members believe that care must be one of two extremes: institutionalization or total care provided solely by the caregiver. Although these are options, other possibilities exist within these extremes, including home health aides, live-in companions, geriatric day care, or shared family care in which the elder lives at specific times with various relatives, or relatives spend designated days at the elder's home. Caregivers also should be aided in identifying their limitations and the need for institutional care when necessary. See Chapter 37 for more information about services for the elderly and their caregivers.

years of age, who lives with a relative and is physically, socially, or financially dependent on others. It is important to remember that abuse occurs in all sorts of families, regardless of social, financial, or ethnic background, and can present in many forms, including:

- inflicting pain or injury
- withholding food, money, medications, or care
- confinement, physical or chemical (drug) restraint
- theft or intentional mismanagement of assets
- sexual abuse

Not only is the actual commission of any of the above abuse, but also the threat of committing the act is considered abuse.

KEY CONCEPT
Both the actual commission of a harmful act and the threat of committing it are considered abuse.

The older adult may be reluctant to report or admit to abuse. Subtle clues of abuse include malnutrition, failure to thrive, injuries, oversedation, and depression. Nurses must manage this situation tactfully. Once abuse is detected, the nurse needs to assess the degree of immediate danger and take appropriate actions. Abused persons must have assurances that their plight will not be worsened by making the abuse public; they may prefer being verbally threatened or having their money taken to the alternative of living in an institution or foster home.

The family needs empathy, not judgment, from the nurse. Although some individuals are consciously malicious and abusive for their own gain, most abusers are distressed persons who find themselves in stressful caregiving situations and have lost their ability to cope effectively. Abuse can also be associated with a family pattern of violence, emotional or cognitive dysfunction of the abused or abuser, a history of dependency of the abuser on the victim, or retaliation for a history of earlier abuse. A good family history can be helpful in gaining insight into the family dynamics that could contribute to abuse.

Abuse may be stopped and family health salvaged by helping the family find effective ways to manage its situation, such as counseling or respite care. The nurse must consider that caregiving burdens often increase over time; therefore, ongoing interventions are necessary to prevent future abuse after the immediate episode has been resolved.

Rewards of Caregiving

A caring, interested family is one of the most valuable resources an individual can possess in old age. In turn, the love and richness of experience offered by older persons adds a unique depth and meaning to the family. Caregiving experiences provide opportunities for relatives to learn more about each other as individuals and to obtain gratification in the young giving something back to the aged who may have sacrificed for them. Gerontological nurses must view older adults in the perspective of their family units and structure care to enhance the functional capacity of all family members.

KEY CONCEPT
A caring and interested family is one of the most valuable assets possessed in old age.

Critical Thinking Exercises

1. Describe the potential changes the average family would face if they suddenly had to provide care for an older relative.

2. Mary Kant is a 45-year-old single parent who is the sole wage earner for herself and her three teenage children. Several years ago, when Ms. Kant's father was diagnosed with dementia, she arranged to have him move into an apartment in the same complex in which her apartment is located. His condition has since deteriorated, and he is now incontinent and unable to eat or dress without assistance; he has also started fires in his apartment and has been found wandering around the complex grounds at all hours of the night. Ms. Kant has decided to take her father into her three-bedroom apartment. Ms. Kant's 2 daughters share one bedroom, her son has his own room, and she has one bedroom for herself; therefore, she has moved her father into her son's room, much to her son's resentment. In fact, her son states that he cannot stand the urine odor and noise made by his grandfather, so he has begun sleeping on the living room sofa and staying at friends' homes whenever possible. Ms. Kant's father's pension is not sufficient to pay the additional cost for a larger apartment because of the expense of his medication and incontinence care supplies.

   Between the stress and her father's nighttime activity, Ms. Kant is unable to obtain adequate rest and has been late for and "nodding off" at work as a result. Her employer knows of her situation but states that Ms. Kant's job could be in jeopardy if she is unable to perform her duties and be dependable. Although Ms. Kant's children understand that their grandfather has no one else to care for him, they are angry at how this situation has disrupted their lives: they no longer feel comfortable bringing friends home, they forfeit social activities to help with their grandfather's care, and they have less money to spend. Together, the children confront Ms. Kant and suggest that their grandfather be placed in a nursing home. Ms. Kant becomes upset and responds, "How can you even suggest putting your own flesh and blood in a place like that? If it kills me, I'll never put your grandfather in a nursing home."

   In regard to this situation:

   Describe the actual and potential problems associated with caring for Ms. Kant's father.

   Discuss the impact of this situation on each family member.

   Describe approaches that could be used to introduce Ms. Kant to other caregiving options, including nursing home care of her father.

   Develop a care plan to assist this family.

3. Discuss satisfactions and benefits family members can derive from caring for older relatives.

4. Identify resources in your community to assist families with caregiving.

Web Connect

Find resources and statistics related to eldercare by visiting the Elderweb website at www.elderweb.com.

● Resources

Clearinghouse on Abuse and Neglect of the Elderly
College of Human Resources
University of Delaware
Newark, DE 19716
(302) 831-3525
www.elderabusecenter.org

National Center on Elder Abuse
810 First Street, NE
Suite 500
Washington, DC 20002
(202) 682-2470
www.gwjapan.com/NCEA

National Council on Family Relations
3989 Central Avenue, NE
Suite 550
Minneapolis, MN 55420
(612) 781-9331
www.ncfr.com

National Eldercare Locator
1112 16th Street, NW
Suite 100
Washington, DC 20036
(800) 677-1116
www.eldercare.gov

● Reference

Fulmer, T. (2003). Elder abuse and neglect assessment. *Journal of Gerontological Nursing, 29*(6), 4.

● Recommended Readings

Acton, G. J., & Miller, E. W. (2003). Spirituality in caregivers of family members with dementia. *Journal of Holistic Nursing, 21*(2), 117–130.

Astor, B. (1998). *Baby boomers guide to caring for aging parents.* New York: Macmillan.

Backer, J. (1995). Perceived stressors of financially secure, community-residing older women. *Geriatric Nursing, 16*(4), 155–159.

Baumhover, L. A., & Beall, S. C. (Eds.). (1996). *Abuse, neglect, and exploitation of older persons: Strategies for assessment and intervention.* Baltimore, MD: Health Professionals Press.

Brandl, B., & Raymond, J. (1997). Unrecognized elder abuse victims: Older abused women. *Journal of Case Management, 6*(2), 62–68.

Brandt, A. L. (1998). *Caregivers' reprieve: A guide to emo-*
tional survival when you're caring for someone you love. San Luis Obispo, CA: Impact Publishers.

Brownell, P. J. (1998). *Family crimes against the elderly: Elder abuse and the criminal justice system.* New York: Garland Publications.

Conlin, M. M. (1995). Silent suffering: A case of elder abuse and neglect. *Journal of the American Geriatrics Society, 43*(8), 1303–1308.

Courts, N. F., Barba, B. E., & Tesh, A. (2001). Family caregivers' attitudes toward aging, caregiving, and nursing home placement. *Journal of Gerontological Nursing, 27*(8), 44–52.

Davidhizar, R., Bechtel, G. A., & Woodring, B. C. (2000). The changing role of grandparenthood. *Journal of Gerontological Nursing, 26*(1), 24–29.

Eliopoulos, C. (1997). Chronic care coaches. *Home Healthcare Nursing, 15*(3), 185–188.

Eliopoulos, C. (1999). *Integrating conventional and alternative therapies: Holistic care for chronic conditions.* St. Louis: Mosby.

Farran, C. J. (2001). Family caregiver intervention research: Where have we been? Where are we going? *Journal of Gerontological Nursing, 27*(7), 38–45.

Gladstone, J., & Wexler, E. (2000). A family perspective of family/staff interaction in long-term care facilities. *Geriatric Nursing, 21*(1), 16–19.

Grollman, E. A., & Grollman, S. H. (1997). *Your aging parents: Reflections for caregivers.* Boston: Beacon Press.

Hostel, M. O., & Curry, L. C. (1999). Elder abuse revisited. *Journal of Gerontological Nursing, 25*(7), 10–18.

Kelley, L. S., & Specht, J. K. P. (2000). Family involvement in care for individuals with dementia protocol. *Journal of Gerontological Nursing, 26*(2), 13–21.

Larrimore, K. L. (2003). Alzheimer disease support group characteristics: A comparison of caregivers. *Geriatric Nursing, 24*(1), 32–35.

Levin, N. J. (1997). *How to care for your parents: A practical guide to eldercare.* New York: Norton.

Li, H. (2002). Family caregivers preferences in caring for their hospitalized elderly relatives. *Geriatric Nursing, 23*(2), 204–207.

Li, Y. (1999). The graying of American and Chinese societies: Young adults' attitudes toward the care of their elderly parents. *Geriatric Nursing, 20*(1), 45–47.

Lilly, M. L., Richards, B. S., & Buckwater, K. C. (2003). Friends and social support in dementia caregiving: Assessment and intervention. *Journal of Gerontological Nursing, 29*(1), 29–36.

Logue, R. M. (2003). Maintaining family connectedness in long-term care: An advanced practice approach to family-centered nursing homes. *Journal of Gerontological Nursing, 29*(6), 24–31.

Lubkin, I. M. (1995). *Chronic illness: Impact and interventions* (3rd ed.). Boston: Jones & Bartlett.

Luggen, A. S., & Rini, A. G. (1995). Assessment of social networks and isolation in community-based elderly men and women. *Geriatric Nursing, 16*(4), 179–181.

Manion, P. S., & Rantz, M. J. (1995). Relocation stress syndrome: A comprehensive plan for long-term care admissions. *Geriatric Nursing, 16*(3), 108–112.

McCall, J. B. (1999). *Grief education for caregivers of the elderly.* New York: Haworth Pastoral Press.

McCullough, L. B., & Wilson, N. L. (1995). *Long-term care decisions: Ethical and conceptual dimensions.* Baltimore, MD: Johns Hopkins University Press.

Meyer, M. M., & Derr, P. (1998). *The comfort of home: An illustrated step-by-step guide for caregivers.* Portland, OR: CareTrust Publications LLC.

Moore, S. L., Metcalf, B., & Schow, E. (2000). Aging and meaning in life: Examining the concept. *Geriatric Nursing, 21*(1), 27–29.

Morse, S., & Robbins, D. Q. (1998). *Moving mom and dad: Why, where, how, and when to help your parents relocate* (2nd ed.). Berkeley, CA: Lanier Publishing International.

National Family Caregivers Association. (1996). *The resourceful caregiver: Helping caregivers help themselves.* St. Louis: Mosby Lifeline.

Ostwald, S. K., Hepburn, K. W., & Burns, T. (2003). Training family caregivers of patients with dementia: A structured workshop approach. *Journal of Gerontological Nursing, 29*(1), 37–44.

Penhale, B., & Kingston, P. (1995). Elder abuse: Recognizing and dealing with abuse of older people. *Nursing Times, 91*(42), 27–28.

Ruppert, R. A. (1996). Caring for the lay caregiver. *American Journal of Nursing, 96*(3), 40–45.

Schomp, V. (1997). *The aging parent handbook.* New York: Harper Paperbacks.

Stocker, S. (1996). Six tips for caring for aging parents. *American Journal of Nursing, 96*(9), 32–33.

Stokes, S. A., & Gordon, S. E. (2003). Common stressors experienced by the well elderly: Clinical implications. *Journal of Gerontological Nursing, 29*(5), 38–46.

Tsuji, I., Whalen, S., & Finucane, T. E. (1995). Predictors of nursing home placement in community-based long-term care. *Journal of the American Geriatrics Society, 43*(7), 761–766.

Turner, D. C. (1996). The role of culture in chronic illness. *American Behavioral Sciences, 39*(6), 717–729.

Winters, S. (2003). Alzheimer disease from a child's perspective. *Geriatric Nursing, 24*(1), 36–39.

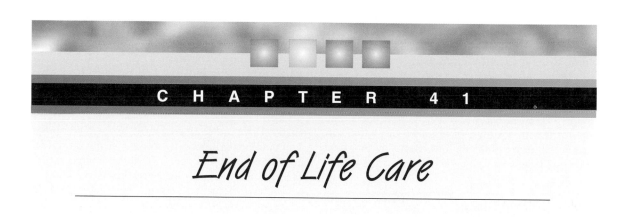

CHAPTER 41

End of Life Care

■ *Learning Objectives*

After reading this chapter, you should be able to:

- discuss the difficulty people have in facing death
- describe the coping mechanisms people use in facing death and related nursing interventions
- list physical care needs of dying individuals and related nursing interventions
- discuss ways in which nurses can support family and friends of dying individuals

eath is an inevitable, unequivocal, and universal experience, common to all. Despite the reality that it touches every person's life at one time or another, death is difficult for many individuals to face—perhaps the most difficult and painful reality of all. Although a certainty, the cessation of life is often dealt with in terms of fury and fear. Humans can be very reluctant to accept their mortality.

Gerontological nurses commonly face the reality of death because more than 80% of all who die are elderly. It is not only the event of death that gerontological nurses must learn to deal with but also the entire dying process—the complexity of experiences that dying individuals, their family, their friends, and all others involved with them go through. Working with those who undergo this complicated process requires a blend of sensitivity, insight, and knowledge about the complex topic of death so that nurses can diagnose nursing problems and effectively intervene (Nursing Diagnosis Table 41-1).

Definitions of Death

REFLECTIONS IN LITERATURE

The final termination of life, the cessation of all vital functions, the act or fact of dying—these are definitions the dictionary offers concerning death—attempts at succinct explanations of this complex experience. But we are often reluctant to accept such simple descriptions. For example, the world of literature contains many eloquent words on the topic of death:

Do not go gentle into that good night,
Old age should burn and rave at close of day
Rage, rage against the dying of the light.
Dylan Thomas

Each person is born to one possession which outvalues all the others—his last breath.
Mark Twain

Death is fortunate for the child,
bitter to the youth,
too late to the old.
Publilius Syrus

A man can die but once:
We owe God a death.
Shakespeare, Henry IV

CLINICAL DEFINITIONS

Dramatic or amusing, the descriptions of death offered in literature have done little to enhance our knowledge of its true meaning. Current scientific literature does not provide much more in the way of specific definitions of death. The United Nations Vital Statistics definition says that death is the permanent disappearance of every vital sign. However, terms such as brain death (the death of brain cells determined by a flat electroencephalogram [EEG]), somatic death (determined by the absence of cardiac and pulmonary functions), and molecular death (determined by the cessation of cellular function) confuse the issue. The controversy lies in deciding at which level of death a person is considered dead. In some situations, an individual with a flat EEG still has cardiac and respiratory functions; could this individual be considered dead? In other situations, individuals with flat EEGs and no cardiopulmonary functions still have living cells that permit their organs to be transplanted; are individuals really dead if they possess living cells? The answers to these questions are not simple. Much current thought and investigation are focused on the need for a single criterion in the determination of death.

Family Experience With Mortality in the Past

At one time, most births and deaths occurred in the home. In multigenerational family living, older persons were part of the household and could be naturally observed as they grew old and died. Personal involvement with births and the dying process was common. Viewed as natural processes, these events were managed by familiar faces in familiar surroundings. Intimate encounters with the beginning and end of life were rich experiences that provided insights and helped foster understanding of these realities. Perhaps the family felt a certain comfort and closeness by being with and doing for the person whose life was about to begin or end. And who can determine the benefit to the infant or the dying individual of being comforted and cared for by close loved ones?

A high mortality rate also made experiences with the dying process more common in the past (Fig. 41-1). Not only were living conditions poor, health care facilities inadequate, disease control techniques limited, and technologies to fight and control nature's elements unheard of, but also there were fewer numbers of hospitals and other institutions in which people could die.

Nursing Diagnosis

ND TABLE 41-1 ● *Nursing Diagnoses Related to Death and Dying*

Causes or Contributing Factors	Nursing Diagnosis
Depression, fatigue, pain, treatments, immobility	Activity Intolerance
Separation from loved one, loss of body function or part, realization of impending death, concern about treatment prior to and at death	Anxiety
Narcotics, immobility, diet, stress	Constipation
Stress, antibiotics, tube feedings, cancer, fecal impaction	Diarrhea
Congestive heart failure, cardiogenic shock, anemia, fluid and electrolyte imbalances, drugs, stress	Decreased Cardiac Output
Cancer, diagnostic tests, poor positioning, overactivity	Pain
Pain, drugs, fatigue	Impaired Verbal Communication
Changes in body integrity, separation from loved one, ineffective family coping, helplessness, powerlessness	Ineffective Coping
Impending death of loved one, lack of knowledge or support	Disabled Family Coping
Hospitalization, treatment demands, depression	Deficit Diversional Activity
Loss of family member, changes in roles, care costs	Interrupted Family Processes
Treatments, pain, death	Fear
Shock, fever, infection, anorexia, inability to drink independently, depression	Deficient Fluid Volume
Loss of body function or part, pain, separation from family	Chronic Sorrow
Cancer, renal failure, treatments, immobility, lowered resistance, drugs (eg, antibiotics, steroids), malnutrition	Risk for Infection
Altered ability to protect self, pain, drugs, fatigue	Risk for Injury
Diagnostic tests, treatments, drugs, pain management	Knowledge Deficit
Weakness, pain, bed rest	Impaired Physical Mobility
Denial, lack of knowledge, impaired functional capacity	Noncompliance
Anorexia, depression, pain, treatments, nausea, vomiting	Imbalanced Nutrition: Less Than Body Requirements
Cancer, infection, drugs, malnutrition, dehydration, mouth breathing, poor hygiene	Impaired Oral Mucous Membrane
Dependency, disability, institutional constraints, inability to reverse condition	Powerlessness
Thick secretions, pain, anxiety, drugs, immobility, decreased lung elasticity and activity, mouth breathing	Ineffective Breathing Pattern
Pain, weakness, disability	Self-Care Deficit
Loss of body function or part, institutionalization, pain	Body Image Disturbance
Metabolic alterations, pain, immobility, isolation, drugs	Disturbed Sensory Perception
Separation from partner, pain, fatigue, depression, drugs, treatments, hospitalization	Sexual Dysfunction
Immobility, infections, edema, dehydration, emaciation	Impaired Skin Integrity
Immobility, pain, anxiety, depression, drugs, new environment	Disturbed Sleep Pattern
Loss of body function or part, depression, anxiety	Impaired Social Interaction
Hospitalization, disability, deformity, discomfort of others	Social Isolation
Loss of body function or part, barriers imposed by treatments or hospitalization, feelings toward dying process	Spiritual Distress
Depression, anxiety, fear, isolation	Disturbed Thought Processes

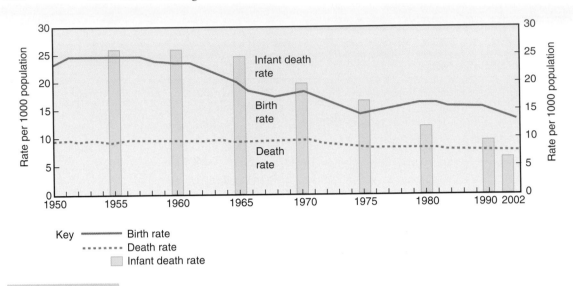

FIGURE 41·1

Changes in birth and death rates from 1950 to 2002. (Modified from U.S. Bureau of the Census [2002]. *Statistical abstract of the United States* [122nd ed.]. Washington, D.C.: U.S. Government Printing Office.)

Family Experience With Mortality in the Present

As Figure 41-1 indicates, the mortality rate has decreased over the years. Health and medical care are now easily available and accessible, and new medications and therapeutic interventions increase the possibility of surviving an illness. Sophisticated and widespread lifesaving technologies and improved standards of living have also lowered the number of deaths in the population.

The declining mortality rate is one of several factors that have limited our experience with the dying process. Another factor is that our more mobile nuclear families are frequently composed of young members, with older parents and grandparents living in different households, often in different parts of the country. The funeral of the older family members may be the only part of the dying process shared by other age groups. Furthermore, older people in the family or community will most likely not die in their familiar home environment. With a majority of deaths occurring in an institutional or hospital setting, rarely do family and friends remain with the individual or witness the dying process.

> **KEY CONCEPT**
> With fewer people dying at earlier ages than in the past and most deaths occurring in hospitals or nursing homes, most people have minimal direct involvement with dying individuals.

The separation of individuals from their loved ones and familiar surroundings during the dying process seems discomforting, stressful, and unjust. How inhumane to remove dying persons from intimate involvement with their support systems at the time of their greatest need for support. As our direct experiences with dying and death are lessened, death becomes a more impersonal and unusual event. Its reality is difficult to internalize; it is held at arm's distance.

Perhaps this explains why many persons have difficulty accepting their own mortality. Avoiding discussions about death and not making a will or other plans related to one's own death are clues to the lack of internalization of one's mortality. Although the topic of death can be confronted on an intellectual level, it is often this internalization of life's finiteness that remains difficult.

NURSES' ATTITUDES TOWARD DEATH

To assist the dying and their families effectively, nurses should analyze their own attitudes toward death. Denying their own mortality or feeling angry about it, nurses may tend to avoid dying persons, discourage their efforts to deal realistically with their death, or instill false hopes in them and their families. The difficult process of confronting and realizing one's own mortality need not be viewed as depressing by the nurse; it can provide a fuller appreciation of life and the impetus for making the most of every living day. Nurses who understand their own mortality are more comfortable helping individuals through the dying process.

KEY CONCEPT
An examination of one's own feelings and attitudes about death can be therapeutic to the nurse personally, as well as helpful in the care of dying patients.

Supporting the Dying Individual

For a long time, nurses were more prepared to deal with the care of a dead body than with the dynamics involved with the dying process. Not only was open discussion of an individual's impending death rare, but also it was typical for the dying person to be moved to a separate and often isolated location during the last few hours of life. If the family was present, they were frequently left alone with the dying person, without benefit of a professional's support. Rather than planning for additional staff support for the dying person and the family, nurses were concerned with whether a patient would live until their next shift and require postmortem care. When death did occur, the body was removed from the unit in secrecy so that other patients would be unaware of the event. Nurses were discouraged from showing emotion when a patient died. A detached objectivity was promoted as part of nursing the dying patient.

Nursing now offers a more humanistic approach to caring for the dying patient. Emphasis on meeting the total needs of the patient in a holistic manner has stimulated greater concern for the psychosocial/spiritual care of the dying. In addition, there is now recognition that family and significant others play a vital role in the dying process and must be considered by the nurse. Knowledge has increased in the field of thanatology (ie, the study of death and dying), and more nurses are exposed to this body of knowledge. Hospice care has developed into a specialty (Display 41-1). The nursing profession has come to realize that professionalism does not preclude human emotions in the nurse–patient relationship. These factors have contributed to increased nursing involvement with the dying individual.

Because the dying process is unique for every human being, individualized nursing intervention is required. Patients' previous experiences with death, religious and spiritual beliefs, philosophy of life, age, and health status are among the multitude of complex ingredients affecting the dying process. The nurse must carefully assess the particular experiences, attitudes, beliefs, and values that all individuals bring to their dying process. Only through this assessment can the most therapeutic and individualized support be given to the dying person.

KEY CONCEPT
Patients' reactions to dying are influenced by previous experiences with death, age, health status, philosophy of life, and religious, spiritual, and cultural beliefs.

STAGES OF DYING AND RELATED NURSING INTERVENTIONS

Although the dying process is a unique journey for each individual, common reactions that have been observed to occur provide a basis for generalizations. After several years of experiences with dying patients, Elisabeth Kübler-Ross developed a conceptual framework outlining the coping mechanisms of dying in terms of five stages that has now become classic

---

DISPLAY 41-1

Hospice

Hospice is a way of caring for the terminally ill and their families. It aids in adding quality and meaning into the remaining period of life. Although most hospice care is provided in the home, these services are required to be provided in nursing home settings also. The first hospice program was St. Christopher's Hospice in London. In 1974, the first hospice in the United States began at Hospice, Inc., in New Haven, Connecticut. The National Hospice Organization has developed standards for hospice care to guide local hospice programs; however, individuality and autonomy of each program are encouraged. Hospice care uses interdisciplinary efforts to address physical, emotional, and spiritual needs, including:

- pain relief
- symptom control
- coordinated home care and institutional care
- bereavement follow-up and counseling

For more information, contact the National Hospice Organization, 1901 North Fort Meyer Drive, Suite 402, Arlington, VA 22209, (703) 243-5900. Hospice referral line: (800) 659-8898

(Kübler-Ross, 1969). It behooves the nurse to be familiar with these stages and to understand the most therapeutic nursing interventions during each stage. Not all dying persons will progress through these stages in an orderly sequence. Neither will every dying person experience all of these stages. However, an awareness of Kübler-Ross' conceptual framework can help the nurse support dying individuals as they demonstrate complex reactions to death. A brief description of these stages, along with pertinent nursing considerations, follows.

Denial

On becoming aware of their impending death, most individuals initially react by denying the reality of the situation. "It isn't true" and "There must be some mistake" are among the comments reflective of this denial. Patients sometimes "shop" for a physician who will suggest a different diagnosis or invest in healers and fads that promise a more favorable outcome. Denial serves several useful purposes for the dying person. It is a shock absorber after learning the difficult news that one has a terminal condition, it provides an opportunity for people to test the certainty of this information, and it allows people time to internalize the information and mobilize their defenses.

 KEY CONCEPT
Denial can serve as a shock absorber to afford time for the dying person to mobilize emotional energy to confront the reality of the situation.

Although the need is strongest early on, dying persons may use denial at various times throughout their illness. They may fluctuate between wanting to discuss their impending death and denying its reality. Although such a contradiction may be confusing, the nurse must be sensitive to the person's need for defenses while also being ready to participate in discussions on death when the person needs to do so. The nurse should try to accept the dying person's use of defenses rather than focus on the conflicting messages. An individual's life philosophy, unique coping mechanisms, and knowledge of the condition determine when denial will be replaced by less radical defense mechanisms. Perhaps the most important nursing action during this stage is to accept the dying individual's reactions and to provide an open door for honest dialogue.

Anger

The stage of denial is gradually replaced, and the "No, not me" reaction is substituted for one of "Why me?"

This second stage, anger, is often extremely difficult for individuals surrounding the dying person because they are frequently the victims of displaced anger. In this stage, the dying person expresses the feeling that nothing is right. Nurses don't answer the call light soon enough; the food tastes awful; the doctors don't know what they are doing; and visitors either stay too long or not long enough. Seen through the eyes of the dying person, such anger is understandable. Why wouldn't people resent not having what they want when they want it when they won't be wanting it very much longer? Why wouldn't they be envious of those who will enjoy a future they will never see? Their unfulfilled desires and the unfinished business of their life may cause outrage. Perhaps their complaints and demands are used to remind those around them that they are still living beings.

During this time, the family may feel guilt, embarrassment, grief, or anger as a result of the dying person's anger. They may not understand why their intentions are misunderstood or their actions unappreciated. It is not unusual for them to question whether they are doing things correctly. The nurse should help the family gain insight into the individual's behavior, which can relieve their discomfort and, thus, create a more beneficial environment for the dying person. If the family can come to realize that the person is reacting to impending death and not to them personally, it may facilitate a more supportive relationship.

The nurse should also guard against responding to the dying person's anger as a personal affront. The best nursing efforts may receive criticism for not being good enough; cheerful overtures may be received with scorn; the call light goes on the minute the nurse leaves the room. It is important that the nurse assess such behavior and understand that it may reflect the anger of the second stage of the dying process. Instead of responding to the anger, the nurse should be accepting, implying to the dying person that it is fine to vent these feelings. Anticipating needs, remembering favorite things, and maintaining a pleasant attitude can counterbalance the anticipated losses that are becoming more apparent to the dying individual. It may be useful for nurses to discuss their feelings about the patient's anger with an objective colleague who can serve as a sounding board so that the nurse-patient relationship continues to be therapeutic.

Bargaining

After recognizing that neither denial nor anger changes the reality of impending death, dying persons may attempt to negotiate a postponement of the inevitable. They may agree to be a better Christian if God lets them live through one more Christmas; they may promise to help themselves more if the physician initiates aggressive therapy to prolong life; they may promise anything in return for an extension of life. Most bargains are made with God and usually kept a secret. Sometimes such agreements are shared with members of the clergy. The nurse should be aware that dying persons may feel disappointed at not having their bargain honored or guilty over the fact that, having gained time, they want an additional extension of life even though they agreed that the request would be their last. It is important that these often covert feelings be explored with the dying person.

Depression

When a patient is hospitalized with increasing frequency and experiences declining functional capacity and more symptoms, the reality of the dying process is emphasized. The older patient may already have had many losses and experienced depression. Not only may lifetime savings, pleasurable pastimes, and a normal lifestyle be gone, but also bodily functions and even bodily parts may be lost. Understandably, all this leads to depression. Unlike other forms of depression, however, the depression of the dying person may not benefit from encouragement and reassurances. Urging dying persons to cheer up and look at the sunny side of things implies that they should not contemplate their impending death. It is unrealistic to believe that dying people should not be deeply saddened by the most significant loss of all—their life.

The depression of the dying person is usually a silent one. It is important for the nurse to understand that cheerful words may be far less meaningful to dying individuals than holding their hand or silently sitting with them (Fig. 41-2). Being with the dying person who openly or silently contemplates the future is a significant nursing action during this stage. Finally, an interest in prayer and a desire for visits from clergy are commonly seen during this stage. The nurse should be particularly sensitive to the dying person's

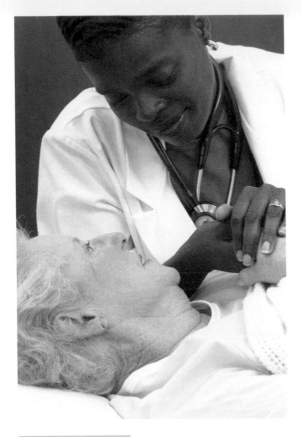

FIGURE 41-2

Touching, comforting, and being near the dying individual are significant nursing actions.

religious needs and facilitate the clergy–patient relationship in every way possible.

The nurse may need to help the family understand this depression, explaining that their efforts to cheer the dying person can hinder the patient's emotional preparation rather than enhance it. The family may require reassurance for the helplessness they feel at this time. The nurse may emphasize that this type of depression is necessary for the individual to be able to approach death in a stage of acceptance and peace.

> **KEY CONCEPT**
> Family members may experience feelings of helplessness when faced with the dying person's depression.

Acceptance

For many dying persons, a time comes when struggling ends and relief ensues. It is as though a final rest is being taken to gain the strength for a long journey. This acceptance should not be mistaken for a happy state; it implies that the individual has come to terms with death and has found a sense of peace. During this stage, patients may benefit more from nonverbal than verbal communication. It is important that their silence and withdrawal not result in isolation from human contact. Touching, comforting, and being near the person are valuable nursing actions. An effort to simplify the environment may be required as the dying person's circle of interests gradually shrinks. It is not unusual for the family to need a great deal of assistance in learning to understand and support their loved one during this stage.

Significantly, hope commonly permeates all stages of the dying process. Hope can be used as a temporary but necessary form of denial, as a rationalization for enduring unpleasant therapies, and as a source of motivation. It may provide a sense of having a special mission to comfort an individual through the last days. A realistic confrontation of impending death does not negate the presence of hope.

> **KEY CONCEPT**
> Hope permeates all stages of the dying process.

PHYSICAL CARE NEEDS

Pain

Concern regarding the degree of pain that will be experienced and its management may be a considerable source of distress for dying individuals; nurses can reduce distress for patients by supplying them with realistic information regarding pain. Patients with cancer are more likely to experience severe pain than persons dying from other causes, and even among terminally ill cancer patients, pain can be managed effectively.

Gerontological nurses must be aware that patients will perceive and express pain differently based on their cultural background, medical diagnosis, emotional state, cognitive function, and other factors. Complaints of pain or discomfort, nausea, irritability, restlessness, and anxiety are common indicators of pain; however, the absence of such expressions of pain does not mean it does not exist. Some patients may not overtly express their pain; in these individuals, signs such as sleep disturbances, reduced activity, diaphoresis, pallor, poor appetite, grimacing, and withdrawal may provide clues to the presence of pain. In some circumstances, confusion can be associated with pain.

Pain must be regularly reassessed because it can increase or decrease over time. Patients should be encouraged to report their pain in a timely manner and openly discuss their concerns about pain. It can be useful for patients to rate their pain on a scale of 0 to 10 (0 being no pain and 10 the most severe pain); nursing staff can record patients' self-appraisal of pain along with other factors on a flow sheet.

For the dying patient, the goal of pain management is to prevent pain from occurring rather than re-

sponding to it after it occurs. Pain prevention not only helps patients avoid discomfort but also ultimately reduces the amount of analgesics they use. After the pattern of pain has been assessed, a schedule for the administration of analgesics can be developed. The type of analgesic used will depend on the intensity of the pain, ranging from aspirin or acetaminophen for mild pain to codeine or oxycodone for moderate pain to morphine or hydromorphone for severe pain. Meperidine and pentazocine are contraindicated for pain control in the elderly because of their high incidence of adverse effects, particularly psychosis, at relatively low dosages. Nurses should note and patients should be instructed to report indications of ineffectiveness of analgesics or their schedule of administration, overdosage, and adverse reactions (Display 41-2).

DISPLAY 41·2

Pain Management for the Dying Patient

Mr. Lugio is a terminally ill nursing home resident who is suffering from pain secondary to metastasis of his lung cancer to his spine. His pain has been managed with a nonsteroid anti-inflammatory drug that he receives PRN, but nursing staff feel that the drug may be ineffective because Mr. Lugio is seen grimacing with pain periodically throughout the day. A review of his medication administration record reveals that he sometimes asks for his pain medication at 6- to 8-hour intervals, although he is able to have the drug every 4 hours. The nurses observe that he complains of pain more frequently during the week than on weekends when his family visits.

Nursing staff could consider the following in helping to achieve improved pain control for Mr. Lugio:

■ Assess the pattern and severity of pain. Provide Mr. Lugio with a chart to record his pain. Instruct him to rate his pain on a scale of 0 to 10, in which 0 indicates no pain and 10 indicates severe pain. Analyze the pattern.

■ Recommend that Mr. Lugio take his analgesic on a regular basis rather than sporadically. Rather than change the type or dosage of analgesic at this time, determine if a regular schedule of administration could improve pain control. Often, regularly scheduled doses can maintain an analgesic level that prevents pain and provides greater relief. If regularly scheduled doses prove ineffective, a change in dosage or the type of analgesic can be considered.

■ Assess Mr. Lugio's understanding of analgesic use. He should understand that addiction or "overuse" of the analgesic is not a primary concern and encouraged to inform nursing staff of the need for pain relief when necessary.

■ Consider the impact of psychological factors on his physical pain. The worsening of his pain when his family is not present could be related to anxiety, boredom, or other psychosocial factors. Psychosocial discomfort can intensify or exacerbate physical discomfort. Mr. Lugio may benefit from a listening ear, counseling, diversional activities, or more frequent visits from his family.

■ Use nonpharmacologic pain relief measures. Back rubs, therapeutic touch, guided imagery, relaxation exercises, and counseling could prove effective in managing pain. Trained practitioners could provide acupressure, acupuncture, and hypnosis. These measures should be reviewed with the physician.

KEY CONCEPT
For the dying patient, the goal of pain management is to prevent pain from developing rather than treating it once it occurs.

Alternatives to medications should be included in the pain-control program of dying patients. Such measures include guided imagery, hypnosis, relaxation exercises, massage, acupressure, acupuncture, therapeutic touch, diversion, and the application of heat or cold. Even if these measures cannot substitute for medications, they could reduce the amount of drugs used or potentiate the drugs' effects.

Respiratory Distress

Respiratory distress is a common problem in dying patients. In addition to the physical discomfort resulting from dyspnea, patients can experience tremendous psychological distress associated with the fear, anxiety, and helplessness that results from the thought of suffocating. The causes of respiratory distress can range from pleural effusion to deteriorating blood gas levels. Interventions such as elevating the head of the bed and administering oxygen can prove beneficial. Atropine or furosemide may be administered to reduce bronchial secretions; narcotics may be used for their ability to control respiratory symptoms by blunting the medullary response.

Constipation

Reduced food and fluid intake, inactivity, and the effects of medications cause constipation to be a problem for most dying patients—a problem that can add to the discomfort these patients already are experiencing. Knowing that the risk for this problem is high, nursing staff should take measures to promote regular bowel elimination in terminally ill patients. Laxatives usually are administered regularly, and bowel elimination patterns should be recorded and assessed. It must be remembered that what may appear to be diarrhea may actually be seepage of liquid wastes around a fecal impaction.

Poor Nutritional Intake

Many dying patients experience anorexia, nausea, and vomiting that can prevent the ingestion of even the most basic nutrients. Additionally, fatigue and weakness can make the act of eating a monumental task. Serving small-portioned meals that have appealing appearances and smells can stimulate the appetite, as can providing foods that are patients' favorites. An alcoholic drink before meals can boost the appetite of some persons. Nausea and vomiting can be controlled with the use of antiemetics and antihistamines; ginger has been used successfully by many individuals as a natural antiemetic. Also useful are basic nursing measures, such as assisting with oral hygiene, offering a clean and pleasant environment for dining, providing pleasant company during mealtime, and assisting with feeding as necessary.

KEY CONCEPT
The herb ginger has been effective in controlling nausea for some individuals without the side effects of antiemetic drugs.

SPIRITUAL CARE NEEDS

Americans represent a diversity of religious beliefs. Each religion has its own practices related to death, and nursing staff must respect these practices to promote the fulfillment of patients' spiritual needs. Table 41-1 lists some basic differences among religions in beliefs and practices related to death. Nursing staff must be sensitive to differences and ensure that they do not inadvertently disrespect the religious beliefs of patients and their families.

Because it is likely that the importance of religion in patients' lives as they are dying will be a reflection of the role of religion throughout their lives, assessment should explore not only their religious affiliation but also their individual religious practices. Furthermore, nurses must recognize that religion and spirituality are not synonymous; religion is but one aspect of spirituality. Patients can be highly spiritual without religious affiliation. To determine the significance of spirituality and the spiritual needs of patients, nurses can ask questions such as the following.

TABLE 41-1 ● *Religious Beliefs and Practices Related to Death*

Religion	Beliefs and Practices Related to Death
Baptist	Prayer, communion
Buddhist	Last rites by Buddhist priest
Catholic	Prayer, last rites by priest
Christian Science	Visit from Christian Science reader
Episcopal	Prayer, communion, confession, last rites
Friends (Quakers)	Individual communicates with God directly, no belief in afterlife
Greek Orthodox	Prayer, communion, last rites by priest
Hindu	Visit by priest to perform ritual of tying thread around neck or wrist, water put in mouth, family cleanses body after death, cremation accepted
Judaism	After death, body washed by religious person
Lutheran	Prayer, last rites
Mormon	Baptism and preaching to deceased
Muslim	Confession, family prepares body after death, deceased must face Mecca
Pentecostal	Prayer, communion
Presbyterian	Prayer, last rites
Russian Orthodox	Prayer, communion, last rites by priest
Scientologist	Confession, visit with pastoral counselor
Seventh Day Adventist	Baptism, communion
Unitarian	Prayer, cremation accepted

- What gives you the strength to face life's challenges?
- Do you feel a connection with a higher being or spirit?
- What gives your life meaning?

Clergy and congregation members of the religious group to which the patient belongs should be invited to be actively involved with the patient and family, according to their wishes. If nursing staff feel comfortable with the practice, they can offer to pray with patients or read to them from religious texts; of course, nursing staff should ensure that prayers offered are consistent with a patient's belief system.

SIGNS OF IMMINENT DEATH

When death is near, bodily functions will slow and certain signs and symptoms will occur, including:

- decline in blood pressure
- rapid, weak pulse
- dyspnea and periods of apnea
- slower or no pupil response to light
- profuse perspiration
- cold extremities

- bladder and bowel incontinence
- pallor and mottling of skin
- loss of hearing and vision

Identifying the approach of death means that nursing staff can ensure that family is notified and given the opportunity to share the last minutes of the patient's life. If the family is unavailable, a staff member should remain with the patient. Depending on the wishes of the patient and family, clergy may be called to visit the patient at this time. It is important that the patient not be alone during this period; even if it appears that the patient is unresponsive, he or she should be spoken to and touched.

ADVANCE DIRECTIVES

The expression of a patient's desires regarding terminal care and life-sustaining measures can be made through the legal document of an advance directive. All health care facilities and agencies that receive Medicare and Medicaid funding must provide information to patients about the Patient Self-Determination Act, which gives individuals the right to express their choice regarding medical and surgical care and to have those preferences honored if they are unable to communicate at a later time. Nurses should review this issue with patients as they are admitted to a hospital or nursing home setting and discuss the importance of the patient expressing his or her desires in a legally sound manner. For many elders and their families, the discussion of issues pertaining to dying is not a comfortable one; by introducing and guiding the discussion with sensitivity, nurses can assist elders in confronting these important issues and assuring their wishes are known. If an advance directive exists, the nurse should review it with the patient to assure it continues to reflect the patient's preference and a copy should be placed in the medical record for the knowledge of all members of the interdisciplinary team. (Chapter 8 provides more discussion on legal issues pertaining to death and dying.)

> **KEY CONCEPT**
> An advance directive protects the patient's right to make decisions about terminal care and eases some of the burden of family members during this difficult time.

Supporting Family and Friends

Thomas Mann's comment that "a man's dying is more the survivors' affair than his own" is a reminder that the family and friends of the dying person should be considered in the nursing care of that person. They too may have needs requiring therapeutic intervention during the dying process of their loved one. Offering the appropriate support throughout this process may prevent unnecessary stress and provide immense comfort to those involved with the dying person. Just as dying persons experience different reactions as they cope with the reality of their impending death, so may family and friends pass through the stages of denial, anger, bargaining, and depression before they are ready to accept the fact that a special person in their lives is going to die.

Denial. In this stage, family and friends may discourage patients from talking or thinking about death; visit patients less frequently; state that pa-

tients will be better as soon as they return home, start eating, have their intravenous tube removed, and so forth; and shop for a doctor or hospital to find a special cure for the terminal illness.

Anger. Reactions may include criticizing staff for the care they are giving, reproaching a family member for not paying attention to the patient's problem earlier, and questioning why someone who has led such a good life should have this happen.

Bargaining. Family and friends may tell the staff that if they could take the patient home they know they could improve his or her condition. Through prayers or open expression they may agree to take better care of the patient if given another chance. They may consent to some particular action (eg, going to church regularly, volunteering for good causes, giving up drinking) if only the patient could live to a particular time.

Depression. Family and friends may become more dependent on the staff. They may begin crying and limiting contact with the patient.

Acceptance. In this stage, people may react by wanting to spend a great deal of time with the dying person and telling the staff of the good experiences they have had with the patient and how they are going to miss the person. They may request the staff to do special things for the patient (eg, arrange for favorite foods, eliminate certain procedures, provide additional comfort measures). They may frequently remind the staff to be sure to contact them "when the time comes." They may begin making specific arrangements for their own lives without the patient (eg, change of housing, plans for property, strengthening other relationships for support).

Obviously, the type of nursing support will vary depending on the stage at which a family member or friend is assessed to be. Although the nursing actions described for the dying individual during each stage may be applicable for family and friends, the stages experienced by those involved with the dying person may not coincide with the patient's own timetable for these stages. For instance, patients may already have worked through the different stages, come to accept the reality of death, and be ready to openly discuss the impact of their death and make plans for their survivors. However, family members and friends may be at different stages and not be able to deal with the patient's acceptance. The nurse must be aware of these discrepancies in states and provide individualized therapeutic interventions. While providing appropriate support to family and friends as they pass through the stages, the nurse can offer opportunities for dying people to discuss their death openly with a receptive party.

HELPING FAMILY AND FRIENDS AFTER A DEATH

When patients die, the nurse should be available to provide any needed support to family and friends. Some people wish to have several minutes in private with deceased patients to view and touch them. Others want the nurse to accompany them as they visit the deceased. Still others may not want to enter the room at all. The personal desires of the family and friends must be respected; nurses should be careful not to make value judgments of the family's reaction based on their own attitudes and beliefs. It is beneficial to encourage the family and friends to express their grief openly. Crying and shouting may help people cope with and work through their feelings about the death more than suppressing their feelings to achieve a calm composure. Unfortunately, some public figures who have reacted to death in a composed and stoic manner have often been presented as role models for the "proper way" of grieving, thereby conveying the message that an open expression of grief is incorrect.

Funeral and burial arrangements may require guidance by a professional. The survivors of the deceased may be experiencing grief, guilt, or other reactions that place them in a vulnerable position. At this time, they are especially susceptible to sales pitches equating their love for the deceased to the cost of the funeral. Funerals may be arranged costing thousands of dollars more than survivors can actually afford, either depleting any existing savings or leaving a debt that will take years to repay. The family may need to have the extravagant plans presented by a funeral director counterbalanced by realistic questions concerning the financial impact of such a funeral. Someone must take the role of reminding the family that

life does go on and that their future welfare must be considered. Whether it is the nurse, a member of the clergy, or a neighbor, it is valuable to identify some person who can be an advocate for the family at this difficult time and prevent them from being taken advantage of. Rather than waiting for a death to occur before thinking through reasonable funeral plans, people should be encouraged to learn about the funeral industry and plan in advance for funeral arrangements. In addition to books on the topic, a number of memorial societies can assist individuals in their planning.

In addition to assisting the family through the funeral, someone should be available to check on family members several weeks after the death. After the agitation of the funeral has diminished and fewer visitors are calling to pay their respects, the full impact of the death may first be realized. At the time that the most intense grief occurs, fewer resources may be available to provide support. Several studies have revealed higher mortality rates in widowers, especially during the first year following the death. Because there are potential threats to the mourning individual's well-being, planned interventions may prove valuable. The gerontological nurse can arrange for a visiting nurse, a church member, a social worker, or someone else to contact the family members several weeks after the death to make sure they are not experiencing any crisis. Widow-to-widow and similar groups can support individuals through the grieving process. It may also be beneficial to provide the telephone number of a person whom the family can contact if assistance is required.

Nearly three decades ago Edwin Schneidman, who did considerable "postventive" work with survivors, offered the following concise guidance in working with the family and friends of the deceased. His guidance remains relevant today (Schneidman, 1976):

- Total care of a dying person needs to include contact and rapport with the survivors-to-be.
- In working with survivor-victims of dire deaths, it is best to begin as soon as possible after the tragedy, within the first 72 hours if possible.
- Remarkably little resistance is met from survivor-victims; most are willing to talk to a professional person, especially one who has no ax to grind and no pitch to make.

- The role of negative emotions toward the deceased—irritation, anger, envy, guilt—needs to be explored, but not at the beginning.
- The professional plays the important role of reality tester—not so much the echo of conscience as the quiet voice of reason.
- Medical evaluation of the survivors is crucial. One should be alert for possible decline in physical health and in overall mental well-being.

Supporting Nursing Staff

The staff members working with the dying individual have their own set of feelings regarding this significant experience. It may be extremely difficult for staff not only to accept a particular patient's death but also to come to terms with the whole issue of death. Some nursing staff share the difficulty that many persons have in realizing their own mortality. Their experiences with death may be limited, as may their exposure to the subject through formal education. In a health profession in which the emphasis is primarily on "curing," death may be viewed as a dissatisfying failure. Nursing staff may feel powerless as they realize that their best efforts can do little to overcome the reality of impending death. It is not unusual for a nursing caregiver who is involved with a dying patient to also experience the stages of the dying process described by Elisabeth Kübler-Ross. Staff members are commonly observed to avoid contact with dying patients, tell a patient to "cheer up" and not think about death, continue to practice "heroic" measures although a patient is nearing death, and grieve at the death of a patient. Nursing staff may be limited in their ability to support patients and their families if they are at a different stage from them. For example, the nurse may be unable to accept that the patient is dying; avoidance of the topic and unrealistic plans for the patient's future reflect this denial. The patient, however, may be at the point of accepting the reality of the dying process and may want to discuss personal feelings. Recognizing that the nurse is still in denial, the patient may avoid an open discussion of death and be deprived of an important therapeutic activity.

The staff working with a dying patient requires a great deal of support. Colleagues should help coworkers explore their own reactions to dying patients and recognize when those reactions interfere with a therapeutic nurse–patient relationship. The attitude of colleagues and the environment should be such that nursing staff can retreat from a situation that is not therapeutic either for them or the patient. To encourage the nurse to cry or show emotions in other forms may be extremely beneficial. The use of thanatologists, hospice staff, and other resource people may also be valuable in providing support to nurses as they assist an individual through the dying process.

> **KEY CONCEPT**
> Nursing staff should be encouraged to express their own feelings about patients' deaths.

Critical Thinking Exercises
1. Discuss factors that cause Americans to have difficulty discussing and planning for death.
2. Describe the differences between spirituality and religion.
3. In addressing a group of older adults at a senior citizen center, what examples could you offer to support the benefits of developing an advance directive?
4. State some examples of behaviors that could demonstrate reactions of nursing staff to the death of a long-term patient.

Web Connect

Read the American Geriatrics Society Position Statement on the Care of dying Patients at http://americangeriatrics.org/products/positionpapers/careofd.shtml.

● R e f e r e n c e s

Kübler-Ross, E. (1969). *On death and dying.* New York: Macmillan.

Schneidman, E. S. (1976). Postvention and the survivor-victim. In E. S. Schneidman (Ed.), *Death: Current perspectives.* New York: Aronson Jason.

● R e c o m m e n d e d   R e a d i n g s

Ali, N. S. (1999). Promotion of advance care planning in the nonhospitalized elderly. *Geriatric Nursing, 20*(5), 260–265.

Barnum, B. S. (1996). *Spirituality in nursing: From traditional to new age.* New York: Springer.

Blazer, D. (1998). *Emotional problems in later life* (2nd ed.). New York: Springer.

Briggs, L., & Colvin, E. (2002). The nurse's role in end-of-life decision-making for patients and families. *Geriatric Nursing, 23*(5), 302–310.

Davidson, K. M., Tang, J. H., & Titler, M. G. (2003). Evidence-based protocol: Family bereavement support before and after the death of a nursing home resident. *Journal of Gerontological Nursing, 29*(1), 10–19.

Emanuel, L. E. (Ed.). (1998). *Regulating how we die: The ethical, medical, and legal issues surrounding physician-assisted suicide.* Cambridge, MA: Harvard University Press.

Filene, P. G. (1998). *In the arms of others: A cultural history of the right to die in America.* Chicago: I. R. Dee.

Inman, L. (2002). Advance directives: Why community-based older adults do not discuss their wishes. *Journal of Gerontological Nursing, 28*(9), 40–46.

Leder, D. (1997). *Spiritual passages: Embracing life's sacred journey.* New York: Jeremy R. Tarcher/Putnam.

Leming, M. R. (1998). *Understanding dying, death, and bereavement* (4th ed.). Fort Worth, TX: Harcourt Brace College.

Harrold, J. K., & Lynn, J. (1998). *A good dying: Sharing health care for the last months of life.* New York: Haworth Press.

Hegge, M., & Fischer, C. (2000). Grief responses of senior and elderly widows: Practice implications. *Journal of Gerontological Nursing, 26*(2), 35–43.

Isaia, D., Parker, V., & Murrow, E. (1999). Spiritual well-being among older adults. *Journal of Gerontological Nursing, 25*(8), 15–21.

Jacobsen, F. W., & Kindlen, M. (1997). *Living through loss: A training guide for those supporting people facing loss.* Bristol, PA: Jessica Kingsley Publishers.

Jowell, B. T., & Schwisow, D. (1997). *After he's gone: A guide for widowed and divorced women.* Secaucus, NJ: Carol Publishing Group.

Marrone, R. L. (1997). *Death, mourning, and caring.* Pacific Grove, CA: Brooks/Cole.

McKhann, C. F. (1999). *A time to die: The place for physician assistance.* New Haven, CT: Yale University Press.

Morgan, J. D. (1997). *Readings in thanatology.* Amityville, NY: Baywood.

Panke, J. T. (2002). Difficulties in managing pain at the end of life. *American Journal of Nursing, 102*(7), 26–34.

Raudonis, B. M., Kyba, F. C. N., & Kinsey, T. A. (2002). Long-term care nurses' knowledge of end-of-life care. *Geriatric Nursing, 23*(5), 296–299.

Saunders, D. C., & Kastenbaum, R. C. (1997). *Hospice care on the international scene.* New York: Springer.

Steinberg, M., & Younger, S. J. (1998). *End of life decisions: A psychosocial perspective.* Washington, DC: American Psychiatric Press.

Wilson, S. A., & Daley, B. J. (1999). Family perspectives on dying in long-term care settings. *Journal of Gerontological Nursing, 25*(11), 19–25.

Wurzbach, M. E. (2002). End of life treatment decisions in long-term care. *Journal of Gerontological Nursing, 28*(6), 14–21.

Young, D. M., Mentes, J. C., & Titler, M. G. (1999). Acute pain management protocol. *Journal of Gerontological Nursing, 25*(6), 10–21.

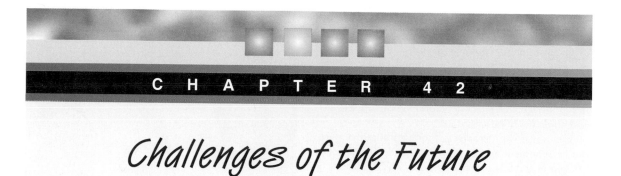

Challenges of the Future

■ Learning Objectives

After reading this chapter, you should be
able to:

• describe efforts that advance
  gerontological nursing research

• list measures to educate caregivers

• identify potential new roles for
  gerontological nurses

• discuss measures to provide quality
  services while controlling health care
  costs

The Past, Present, and Future Status of Gerontological Nursing

Historically, nursing has always carried a significant responsibility for gerontological care. Long before it was popular or profitable for other disciplines to become involved in this specialty, nursing personnel were the major caregivers to the elderly. However, on close examination, one notices that the power and leadership of the nursing profession in the gerontological care arena did not equal the responsibility and workload assumed. Not only did health professionals other than nurses influence the course of this specialty, but also persons with no health background whatsoever influenced services to the aging. The tales are many: entrepreneurs who became millionaires by operating substandard nursing homes, bureaucrats who developed policies with no understanding of their clinical impact, and reimbursement programs that favored highly technical acute services over the chronic and rehabilitative ones that were most needed.

Additional problems lay within the nursing community itself. Rather than aggressively lobbying to effect changes that could have made long-term care settings more attractive to nurses, the nursing community harbored sentiments that nurses who were employed in institutional settings were inferior to the rest. Schools of nursing not only omitted gerontological nursing courses in their programs but also did little to bridge the severe gap between the significant educational and research needs of gerontological care settings and academic resources.

One must wonder why gerontological nurses were not entrepreneurial enough to own and control nursing homes and other service agencies, why they allowed others to mandate practices that diluted quality nursing care, and why they were not assertive enough to demand that their colleagues be constructive problem-solvers rather than critics of the status of gerontological care. Whatever the reasons, one thing is certain: gerontological nurses must now strive to protect both the care of elders and the specialty of gerontological nursing.

Since gerontological nurses have started advocating for advancement of the specialty, tremendous strides have been made. Dynamic professionals are selecting gerontological nursing as a specialty that offers a multitude of opportunities to use a wide range of knowledge and skills and one that presents many challenges that can be independently addressed within the realm of nursing practice. Excellent research for and by nurses is growing to provide a strong scientific foundation for practice. Increasing numbers of nursing schools are adding specialization in gerontological nursing. New opportunities for gerontological nurses to develop practice models are emerging in acute hospitals, assisted living, health maintenance organizations, life-care communities, adult day treatment centers, and other settings (Fig. 42-1). The future of gerontological nursing appears dynamic and exciting. Nevertheless, more challenges exist.

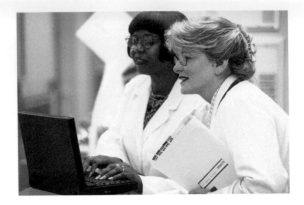

FIGURE 42-1

Opportunities for gerontological nurses to develop new practice models are emerging in a variety of settings.

> **KEY CONCEPT**
> Increasing numbers of nurses are finding gerontological nursing to be a dynamic specialty that affords significant opportunities for independence and creativity.

Challenges

ADVANCE RESEARCH

The growing complexity of and demand for gerontological nursing services is exciting and challenging but is accompanied by the need for a strong knowledge base on which these services can be built. There is no room for the trial and error that flavored nursing actions in the past: the elderly's delicately balanced health status, increased consumer expectations, ever-present risk of litigation, and the requisites of being a professional demand scientific foundations for nursing practice. Fine nursing research is being conducted on a variety of issues, and gerontological nurses must encourage and support these efforts through various actions.

Network with nurse researchers. Local academic institutions, teaching hospitals, and nursing homes may be conducting research that can be relevant to various gerontological settings or in which a service agency can participate. Researchers can be important resources by meshing their research skills with the abilities of those in a service setting to solve clinical problems.

Support research efforts. The support of research comes in many forms. As funding is sought for research projects, letters of support and testimony can help funding agencies understand the full benefit of the effort. Regular contact with leaders who influence the allocation of funds can provide opportunities to educate these persons on the value of supporting research. No less significant to the support of research efforts is the assurance that protocols be followed, for the efforts of researchers can be facilitated or thwarted by colleagues in clinical settings.

Keep abreast of new findings. Gerontological nursing knowledge is continuously expanding, disproving past beliefs and offering new insights. Nurses can engage in independent study, formal courses, and continuing education programs to keep current. Equally important to acquiring knowledge is implementing it to improve the care of older adults.

> **KEY CONCEPT**
> The elderly's delicately balanced health status and high risk for complications, along with rising consumer expectations and a highly litigious society, reinforce the importance of basing practice on a strong scientific foundation.

PROMOTE INTEGRATIVE CARE

In the United States, conventional medicine, with an emphasis on the diagnosis and treatment of diseases, has set the tone for health care practice. Current managed care and reimbursement priorities reinforce the medical model and disease-focused care. Unfortunately, the care of medical conditions is just one aspect of the services elders need to be healthy and experience a high quality of life. In fact, elders' wellness practices, adjustments to life changes, sense of purpose, hopefulness, joy, connections to others, and ability to manage stress can be equally if not more significant to their health and quality of life than medical care.

Nurses must ensure that gerontological care is holistic, meaning that the physical, emotional, social, and spiritual facets of individuals are considered. This implies that nurses not only practice in a holistic manner themselves but also advocate for other disciplines to do so.

Alternative and complementary therapies play a role in holistic care. These therapies tend to be more comforting and safe and less invasive than conventional treatments and empower elders and their caregivers in self-care. Many people who use these therapies report positive experiences with their alternative therapists, who tend to spend more time getting to under-

stand and address the needs of the total person. *However, the use of alternative therapies does not equate with holistic care.* An alternative therapist who has tunnel vision in believing that every malady can be corrected with the one modality he or she practices and excludes effective conventional treatments is no different from the physician who prescribes an analgesic but does not consider imagery, massage, therapeutic touch, and other nonconventional forms of pain relief. Integrating the best of conventional and alternative/complementary therapy supports holistic care.

Part of a holistic approach to care includes care of the caregivers as well. Professional and family caregivers who are in poor health, struggling with psychosocial issues, feeling spiritually empty and disconnected, or managing stress poorly need to heal themselves before they can be effective caregivers. Nurses need to assist these caregivers in identifying their needs and finding the help needed for their healing.

> ✔ **Point to Ponder**
> *Many nurses are in poor physical condition, smoke, regularly eat junk foods, take little time for themselves, and demonstrate other unhealthy habits. What do you think are some of the reasons for this? What can be done to improve nurses' health habits?*

EDUCATE CAREGIVERS

Be it the nursing director, a family member who cares for an older relative, a health aide who has more frequent contact with the patient than the professional nurse, or the physician who only occasionally has an older person in the caseload, caregivers at every level require competency in providing services to the elderly. Gerontological nurses can influence the education of caregivers by:

- helping nursing schools identify relevant issues for inclusion in the curricula
- participating in the classroom and field experiences of students
- evaluating educational deficits of personnel and plan education experiences to eliminate deficits
- promoting interdisciplinary team conferences
- attending and participating in continuing education programs

- reading current nursing literature and sharing information with colleagues
- serving as a role model by demonstrating current practices

With increasing numbers of family members providing more complex care in the home setting than ever before, it is essential that the education of this group not be overlooked. It should not be assumed that because the family has had contact with other providers or has been providing care that they are knowledgeable in correct care techniques. Their knowledge and skills must be evaluated and reinforced periodically.

DEVELOP NEW ROLES

As gerontological subspecialties and settings for care grow, so will the opportunities for nurses to carve new roles for themselves. Nurses can demonstrate creativity and leadership as they break from traditional roles and settings and develop new models of practice, which may include the following:

- geropsychiatric nurse specialist in the assisted living setting
- independent case manager for community-based chronically ill patients
- columnist for local newspaper on issues pertaining to health and aging
- owner or director of elder women's health care center, geriatric day-care program, respite agency, or caregiver training center
- preretirement counselor and educator for private industry
- parish nurse
- consultant, educator, and case manager for geriatric surgical patients

---

KEY CONCEPT
Opportunities exist for nurses to develop new practice models in gerontological care.

This list only begins to describe opportunities awaiting gerontological nurses. It will be important for gerontological nurses to identify nontraditional roles, approach them creatively, test innovative practice models, and share their successes and failures

with colleagues to aid them in their development of new roles. Nurses must recognize that their biopsychosocial sciences knowledge, clinical competencies, and human relations skills give them a strong competitive edge over other disciplines in affecting a wide range of services.

✔ **Point to Ponder**
Based on changes in the health care system and society at large, what unique services could gerontological nurses offer in the future within your community?

BALANCE QUALITY CARE AND HEALTH CARE COSTS

The increasing number of older adults is placing demands for more and more diverse health care services than ever before. At the same time, third-party reimbursers are trying to control the constantly escalating cost of services. Earlier hospital discharges, limited home health visits, more complex nursing home patients, and greater out-of-pocket payment for services by patients demonstrate some of the effects of changes in reimbursement policy. Some health care professionals suspect that as a result of these changes patients are discharged from hospitals prematurely and suffer greater adverse consequences, nursing homes are confronting patients with complex problems for whom they are not adequately prepared or staffed, families are being strained by considerable caregiving burdens, and patients are being deprived of needed but unaffordable services.

Such changes are disconcerting and may cause nurses to feel overwhelmed, frustrated, or dissatisfied. Unfortunately, more cost cutting is likely to occur. Rather than experience burnout or consider a change of occupation, nurses should become involved in cost-containment efforts so that a balance between quality services and budgetary concerns can be achieved. Efforts toward this goal can include the following:

Test creative staffing patterns. Perhaps 6 nurses can be more productive than 3 nurses and 3 nonprofessionals. On the other hand, perhaps some of the high nonproductive time costs associated with nonprofessionals is related to poor hiring and supervision practices; improved management techniques may increase the cost effectiveness of these workers.

Use lay caregivers. Neighbors assisting each other, a family member rooming-in during hospitalizations, and other methods to increase the resources available for service provision can be explored.

Abolish unnecessary practices. Why must nurses spend time administering medications to patients who have successfully administered them before admission and who will continue to administer them after discharge, take vital signs every 4 hours on patients who have shown no abnormalities, bathe all patients on the same schedule regardless of skin condition or state of cleanliness, or rewrite assessments and care plans at specified intervals regardless of a patient's changes or stability? Often regulations and policies are developed under the assumption that, without them, vital signs would never be taken, baths would not be given, and other facets of care would not be completed. Perhaps the time has come for nurses to aggressively convince others that they have the professional judgment to determine the need for and frequency of assessment, care planning, and care delivery.

Ensure safe care. The implementation of cost-containment efforts should be accompanied by concurrent studies of the efforts' impact on rates of complications, readmissions, incidents, consumer satisfaction, and staff turnover, absenteeism, and morale. Specific numbers and documented cases carry more weight than broad criticisms or complaints that care is suffering.

Advocate for older adults. The priorities of society and professions change. History shows us that at different times the spotlight has focused on various underserved groups, such as children, pregnant women, the mentally ill, the handicapped, substance abusers, and, most recently, the aged. As interests and priorities shift to new groups, gerontological nurses must make certain that the needs of the elderly are not forgotten or shortchanged.

As gerontological nursing continues to shed its image of a less-than-*bona-fide* specialty for less-than-competent nurses and fully emerges as the dynamic, multifaceted, and opportunity-filled form of nursing that it is, it will be seen that this is a specialty for the finest talent the profession has to offer. Gerontological nursing has just begun to show its true potential.

KEY CONCEPT

Creativity is needed to deliver high-quality services to the elderly while controlling rising health care costs.

Critical Thinking Exercises

1. What opportunities exist for gerontological nurses to network in your community?
2. Describe several issues that could warrant gerontological nursing research activities.
3. Describe how the increased use of holistic practices could have a positive effect on cost and consumer satisfaction.
4. Outline functions that could be performed by a gerontological nurse in the role of:
   hospital preadmission health screener
   health counselor in a retirement community
   caregiver trainer
   industrial preretirement health educator
   parish or congregational health nurse

Web Connect

Search the Internet using words such as "aging," "geriatrics," "gerontology," and "longevity." Based on some of the information you discover, consider topics that would be intriguing to research.

● Resources

Hartford Institute for Geriatric Nursing
New York University, Steinhardt School of Education
Division of Nursing
246 Green Street
New York, NY 10003

(212) 998-9018
www.hardfordign.org
Disseminates information pertaining to research and education to advance geriatric nursing; provides links to resources of interest to geriatric nursing practice, education, and research.

Index

Note: Page numbers followed by *f* indicate figures; *t* indicates tables; and *d* indicates display text.